Familiar
Medical Quotations

Familiar
Medical Quotations

Edited by
Maurice B. Strauss

Associate Dean and Professor of Medicine
Tufts University School of Medicine

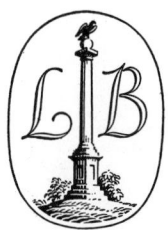

Little, Brown and Company
BOSTON

Library of Congress catalog card No. 68-21620

ISBN 0-316-81915-8

First Edition
Third Printing

PRINTED IN THE UNITED STATES OF AMERICA

MV

Editorial Board

v

Advisory Board

Preface

MEDICINE is concerned with man — his origin and evolution; his social and political organization; his birth, life, and death; his sufferings and happiness; and his relation to the inanimate, the microscopic, the macroscopic, and the universe. In short, medicine is concerned with the biology and ecology of man.

Throughout history, the men of medicine — the physicians of the ages from Huang Ti of nearly five millennia ago to those of today — have sought to delimit the field of medicine, to bring order out of chaos, by adopting a unifying concept based on a popular theory of the time. This is best illustrated by their changing interpretations of the cause of disease: as spirits or supernatural agencies; as an imbalance of the four elements (earth, air, fire, water) or the four humors (blood, phlegm, yellow bile, black bile); as the action of a living microscopic organism (one germ, one disease); or as the action of a chemical determinant (one gene, one enzyme). The history of medicine can be, and usually is, written in terms of the ascendancy of one or another of these theories.

In *Familiar Medical Quotations* the history of medicine can be read from various points of view in the words that physicians, patients, scientists, laymen, philosophers, clergymen, politicians, novelists, playwrights, and poets have said about medicine and its practitioners, their accomplishments and failures, and their virtues, vices, and foibles.

Just when I began collecting quotations remains a mystery. The yellowed scraps of paper suggest a minimum of twenty-five years ago. Although the first intimation of my concern with sources is the correspondence with Sir Hans A. Krebs in 1955, noted below, the actual task of amassing material for publication rather than for private pleasure began in early 1964.

One question that has arisen repeatedly is whether to deny entry to an otherwise qualified quotation because the search for author, source, or both has been fruitless. On one side of the argument is Martin J. Routh: "You will find it a very good practice *always to verify your references,* sir!" [1] Opposing him is Anatole France (whose quotation I considered excluding because I was unable to locate the source): "When a thing has been said and well said, have no scruple: take it and copy it. Give references? Why should you? Either your readers know where you have taken the passage and the precaution is needless, or they do not know and you humiliate them." [2]

To have followed Routh's advice would have eliminated a famous and often-quoted remark ascribed to the great physiologist Ernst Wilhelm von Brücke: "Teleology is a lady without whom no biologist can live. Yet he is ashamed to show himself with her in public." [3]

After years of frustrating search for the source, I wrote to Sir Hans A. Krebs, who had quoted the phrase in his Herter Lecture of 1954. His answer on

[1] See p. 668b.   [2] See p. 670a.   [3] See p. 606b.

January 28, 1955, illustrates the difficulties involved in tracing the sources of "familiar medical quotations":

> I have spent considerable effort in tracing the origin of von Brücke's epigram. A descendant . . . of the same name, told me that it has never appeared in print, but he thought it was authentic. Dr. O. Loewi . . . heard the epigram from E. T. von Brücke, who was a grandson of E. W. von Brücke. . . . Dr. Loewi confirms that the epigram has not appeared in print.

We have undertaken to verify all of the quotations and sources in *Familiar Medical Quotations*. Original or scholarly editions have been used wherever possible, except in the case of medical texts with constantly revised editions. This explains certain peculiarities of spelling and punctuation in quotations from earlier centuries, which we have given in the original provided they are intelligible to the modern reader. We have chosen as most suited to our purpose the King James Version of the Bible and George Lyman Kittredge's 1936 edition of *The Complete Works of Shakespeare*.

When the original source for a quotation could not be located, we have in some cases given a secondary source. For quotations ascribed to several individuals, one source is given with a footnote reference to other versions. Citations from medical journals list the first page of the article in which the quotation appears.

John Bartlett, whose *Familiar Quotations* first appeared in 1855, selected his quotations on the basis of their being "familiar or worthy of being familiar." By the time the fourth edition was ready for press, Bartlett was aware of a difficulty: "It is not easy to determine in all cases the degree of familiarity that may belong to phrases and sentences which present themselves for admission; for what is familiar to one class of readers may be quite new to another." We have followed Bartlett's criterion in selecting material for this book, but have not adhered to his chronological order of presentation by author, since arrangement by categories is more useful for our purposes. Within each category, however, the quotes are given chronologically, permitting the reader a view of the progress of medicine through successive eras. After specific authors these general sources appear in the following sequence: The Bible, The Bible: Apocrypha, The Koran, The Talmud, Anonymous, Proverbs.

More recently Lewis Galantière, in *The New York Times Book Review*, January 19, 1964, enunciated a standard which we have worked to make *Familiar Medical Quotations* reflect:

> A truly serviceable book of quotations is not an expression of its compiler's preferences. . . . It has no preconceptions, takes no stand, is fair to all doctrines and all peoples. The true, the false, the debatable; the tragic and the comic; the wise and the witless come within its compass. A book of quotations is an orderly assembling of those lines . . . which mankind has found itself unable to forget — better yet, to do without. It is a *summum* of human experience.

For the collection of the more than 7000 quotations in this volume I am indebted to, first and foremost, Ruth F. Strauss, who contributed almost half the quotations and performed the duties of co-editor; to the Editorial Board; to the Advisory Board; and to the hundreds who sent in individual contributions. Space does not permit naming them all, but my gratitude is extended to each of them.

I must also express my very considerable indebtedness to Mrs. Roberta W. Francis, who not only supervised the very extensive search for sources, but copy-edited and indexed the entire volume.

Many quotations worthy of entry have, no doubt, been omitted because we did not know them. Some sources for quotations (not too many, we hope) are lacking. Won't you please send them in for the second edition?

M. B. S.

Boston

Contents

CONTENTS

Familiar
Medical Quotations

ABILITY

Propertius [50?–15? B.C.]

Let each man pass his days in that wherein his skill is greatest.
>   *Elegies,* II.i.46 (tr. by H. E. Butler)

Paracelsus [1493?–1541]

Let no one who can be his own belong to another.[1]
>   Motto on various woodcuts of Paracelsus and on title pages of several of his books (tr. by Norbert Guterman in *Selected Writings*)

Oliver Wendell Holmes [1809–1894]

A man of very moderate ability may be a good physician, if he devotes himself faithfully to the work.
>   *Medical Essays,* "Scholastic and Bedside Teaching"

ABORTION

The Zend-Avesta [ca. 550 B.C.]

If a man come near unto a damsel, . . . and she conceives by him, and she says, "I have conceived by thee;" and he replies, "Go then to the old woman and apply to her that she may procure thee miscarriage;"

And the damsel goes to the old woman and applies to her that she may procure her miscarriage; and the old woman brings her some Banga or Shaêta, or Ghnâna or Fraspâta,[2] or some other of the drugs that produce miscarriage and [the man says], "Cause thy fruit to perish!" and she causes her fruit to perish; the sin is on the head of all three, the man, the damsel, and the old woman.
>   *The Vendidad,* XV.ii.13 (tr. by J. Darmesteter)

Tertullian [160?–230?]

To hinder a birth is merely speedier man-killing; nor does it matter whether you take away a life that is born, or destroy one that is coming to the birth. That is a man which is going to be one; you have the fruit already in its seed.
>   *Apoligeticus,* IX (tr. by S. Thelwall)

W. E. H. Lecky [1838–1903]

Abortion . . . was probably regarded by the average Romans of the later days of Paganism much as Englishmen in the last century regarded convivial excesses, as certainly wrong, but so venial as scarcely to deserve censure.
>   *History of European Morals,* Vol. II, Ch. IV

ABSTINENCE

See also ALCOHOL

Robert Herrick [1591–1674]

Against diseases here the strongest fence
Is the defensive vertue, abstinence.
>   *Hesperides,* "Abstinence"

Ambrose Bierce [1842–1914?]

ABSTAINER, n. A weak person who yields to the temptation of denying

---

[1] Alterius non sit qui suus esse potest.
[2] Banga = a narcotic made from hempseed; Shaêta = some yellow plant or liquor; Ghnâna = that which kills; Fraspâta = that which expels.

himself a pleasure. A total abstainer is one who abstains from everything but abstention, and especially from inactivity in the affairs of others.
> *The Devil's Dictionary*

ACCIDENT

John Wilkes [1727–1797]

The chapter of accidents is the longest chapter in the book.
> Quoted by Robert Southey in *The Doctor*, Ch. 118

Ambrose Bierce [1842–1914?]

ACCIDENT, n. An inevitable occurrence due to the action of immutable natural laws.
> *The Devil's Dictionary*

Sir Winston Churchill [1874–1965]

There was a moment . . . of a world aglare, of a man aghast. . . . I do not understand why I was not broken like an eggshell or squashed like a gooseberry. [On being run down by a taxi in New York in 1932.]
> Quoted in *Atlantic Monthly*, January 1949

Evarts A. Graham [1883–1957]

Until homo sapiens becomes more sapient I can see no prospect of his ever avoiding the foolishness of war or of his learning that two automobiles cannot occupy the same spot at the same time, especially when they come from opposite directions. Broken bones and lacerated wounds are therefore likely to require surgical attention for as long as this would-be clairvoyant can see into the future.
> *Postgraduate Medicine* 7:154, 1950

Dorothy L. Sayers [1893–1957]

If accidents happen and you are to blame, take steps to avoid repetition of same.
> *In the Teeth of the Evidence*, "Bitter Almonds"

ADAPTATION

See also EVOLUTION

Helen Keller [1880–   ]

I know that I can feel the heart-throbs of the ancient Greeks in their marble gods and goddesses.
> *The Story of My Life*, Ch. XXII

René J. Dubos [1901–   ]

It can be said that each civilization has a pattern of disease peculiar to it. The pattern of disease is an expression of the response of man to his total environment (physical, biological, and social); this response is, therefore, determined by anything that affects man himself or his environment.
> *Industrial Medicine and Surgery* 30:369, 1961

The study on silkworm diseases constituted for Pasteur an initiation into the problem of infectious diseases. Instead of the accuracy of laboratory procedures he encountered the variability and unpredictability of behavior in animal life, for silkworms differ in their response to disease as do other animals.
> *Louis Pasteur, Free Lance of Science*, Ch. VIII

ADOLESCENCE

See also YOUTH

William Shakespeare [1564–1616]
> My salad days,

When I was green in judgment, cold in blood.
>*Antony and Cleopatra*, I, v, 73

Not yet old enough for a man nor young enough for a boy; as a squash is before 'tis a peascod, or a codling when 'tis almost an apple.
>*Twelfth Night*, I, v, 165

I would there were no age between ten and three-and-twenty, or that youth would sleep out the rest; for there is nothing in the between but getting wenches with child, wronging the ancientry, stealing, fighting.
>*The Winter's Tale*, III, iii, 59

Alexander Pope [1688–1744]

When the brisk Minor pants for twenty-one.
>*Satires and Epistles Imitated,* "First Epistle of the First Book of Horace"

John Armstrong [1709–1779]

Ye Youths and Virgins, when your generous blood
Has drunk the warmth of fifteen Summers, now
The Loves invite; now to new rapture wakes
The finish'd Sense: While stung with keen Desire
The madd'ning Boy his bashful Fetters bursts;
And, urg'd with secret Flames, the riper Maid,
Conscious and shy, betrays her smarting Breast.
>*The Economy of Love*

W. Somerset Maugham [1874–1965]

The feeling of apartness from others comes to most with puberty, but it is not always developed to such a degree as to make the difference between the individual and his fellows noticeable to the individual.
>*Of Human Bondage*, Ch. XIII

Anonymous

A stage between infancy and adultery.

ADULT

See AGE, MATURITY, MIDDLE AGE

ADULTERY

George Gordon, Lord Byron [1788–1824]

What men call gallantry, and gods adultery,
Is much more common where the climate's sultry.
>*Don Juan*, Canto I, Stanza 63

Oliver Wendell Holmes [1809–1894]

I do not think that the breach of the seventh commandment can be shown to have been of advantage to the legitimate owner of his affections.
>*Medical Essays*, "Scholastic and Bedside Teaching"

The Bible

Thou shalt not commit adultery.
>*Exodus* 20:14

Hebrew Proverb

Adultery brings on early old age.

AGE

See also CHILDREN, YOUTH, MATURITY, MIDDLE AGE, OLD AGE, LONGEVITY

Plato [427?–347 B.C.]

What is the prime of life? May it not

be defined as a period of about twenty years in a woman's life, and thirty in a man's?

> *Republic,* V.460.E (tr. by Benjamin Jowett)

Sir Thomas Browne [1605–1682]

Confound not the distinctions of thy Life which Nature hath divided, that is, Youth, Adolescence, Manhood, and old Age; nor in these divided Periods, wherein thou art in a manner Four, conceive thyself but One. Let every division be happy in its proper Virtues, nor one Vice run through all. Let each distinction have its salutary transition, and critically deliver thee from the imperfections of the former, so ordering the whole, that Prudence and Virtue may have the largest Section.

> *Christian Morals,* Pt. III, Sect. 8

Jonathan Swift [1667–1745]

No wise man ever wished to be younger.

> *Thoughts on Various Subjects, Moral and Diverting*

Benjamin Disraeli, Lord Beaconsfield [1804–1881]

Youth is a blunder; manhood a struggle; old age a regret.

> *Coningsby,* Bk. III, Ch. 1

John Shaw Billings [1838–1913]

Ages over 90 are largely overstated, and the ages of women between 25 and 50 are largely understated.

> *Medical Record* 36:589, 1889

Anonymous

An adult is one who has ceased to grow vertically but not horizontally.

Scottish Proverb

A man need not look in your mouth to know how old you are.

AIR POLLUTION

Lucretius [96?–55 B.C.]

Thus when an atmosphere,
Alien by chance to us, begins to heave,
And noxious airs begin to crawl along,
They creep and wind like unto mist
　　and cloud,
Slowly, and everything upon their way
They disarrange and force to change
　　its state.
It happens, too, that when they've
　　come at last
Into this atmosphere of ours, they
　　taint
And make it like themselves and
　　alien.[1]

> *On the Nature of Things,* VI. 1118 (tr. by W. E. Leonard)

Aetios [ca. 535]

Irritations of the eyes, which are caused by smoke, over-heating, dust, or similar injury, are easy to heal; the patient being advised first of all to avoid the irritating causes; . . . next, to bathe the eyes, in the beginning with lukewarm water, later with cold, also to avoid bright light. For the disease ceases without the use of any kind of medicine, if only a proper way of living be adopted.

> *Tetrabiblon,* Sermo II, III.3

William Shakespeare [1564–1616]

Is Brutus sick, and is it physical
To walk unbraced and suck up the
　　humours
Of the dank morning? What, is Brutus
　　sick,
And will he steal out of his whole-
　　some bed
To dare the vile contagion of the
　　night,
And tempt the rheumy and unpurged
　　air
To add unto his sickness?

> *Julius Caesar,* II, i, 261

[1] An explanation of the spread of the plague.

Be as a planetary plague when Jove
Will o'er some high-vic'd city hang
  his poison
In the sick air.
    Timon of Athens, IV, iii, 108

John Arbuthnot [1667–1735]

The first Care in building of Cities, is
to make them airy and well perflated;
infectious Distempers must necessarily
be propagated amongst Mankind living close together.
    An Essay Concerning the Ef-
    fects of Air on Human Bodies,
    Ch. 9, No. 20

Sir William Osler [1849–1919]

Huge blocks of coal that would grace
the doorstep of any multimillionaire
coal dealer as a sign are carried into
the lungs from our coal-polluted air,
and tubercle bacilli ride in on coal-
black chargers three abreast. Coal
barges equal to those on the Susque-
hanna are constantly passing through
unbroken mucosa and along lymph
ducts to the bronchial lymph nodes.
    Quoted by William B. Bean in
    Sir William Osler: Aphorisms,
    Ch. 5

ALCOHOL

See also INTEMPERANCE,
TEMPERANCE

Homer [ca. 850 B.C.]

Inflaming wine, pernicious to mankind,
Unnerves the limbs, and dulls the
  noble mind.
    Iliad, VI.261 (330 as tr. by
    Alexander Pope)

More wine, less wits, you know; wine
makes a man sing even if he is a rare
scholar, makes him titter and chuckle,
aye, makes him dance a jig, and makes

him blurt out what were better kept
to himself.
    Odyssey, XIV.464 (tr. by W. H.
    D. Rouse)

Hippocrates [460?–377? B.C.]

Drinking strong wine cures hunger.
    Aphorisms, II.21 (tr. by Fran-
    cis Adams)

I hold that it is better to give children
only the most diluted wine.
    On Airs, Waters and Places,
    IX (tr. by Francis Adams)

Who could have foretold, from the
structure of the brain, that wine could
derange its functions?

Seneca [4? B.C.–A.D. 65]

Drunkenness is simply voluntary insanity.
    Moral Epistles to Lucilius,
    LXXXIII

Basil the Great [330?–379?]

Drunkenness, the ruin of reason, the
destruction of strength, premature old
age, momentary death.
    Homilies, No. XIV, Ch. 7

St. John Chrysostom [345?–407]

The immoderate drinking of wine produces not fewer diseases of body and
of soul, than much drinking of water,
but far more, and severer; bringing in
as it does upon the mind the war of
the passions, and a tempest of perverse thoughts, besides reducing the
firmness of the body, to a relaxed and
flaccid state.
    Homilies on the Statutes, Hom-
    ily I (tr. by John H. Parker)

Moses ben Maimon (Maimonides) [1135–1204]

Honey and wine are bad for children
but salutary for the elderly.
    Mishneh Torah, "Hilchoth
    De'oth," Ch. 4, No. 12 (tr. by
    Fred Rosner in *Annals of Inter-*
    nal Medicine 62:372, 1965)

William Langland [1332?–1400?]

Dread the delight of drink and thou
  shalt do the better.
Though thou long for more, Measure
  is Medicine.
What the belly asketh is not all good
  for the ghost,
What the soul loveth is not all food
  for the body.
  Piers Plowman, Passus II

John Lyly [1554?–1606]

Long quaffing maketh a short lyfe.
  Euphues

William Shakespeare [1564–1616]

              I have bought
The oil, the balsamum, and aqua-vitae.
  The Comedy of Errors, IV, i,
  88

The second property of your excellent
sherris is the warming of the blood;
which before (cold and settled) left
the liver white and pale, . . . but the
sherris warms it and makes it course
from the inwards to the parts extremes.
  Henry IV, Part II, IV, iii, 111

MACDUFF: What three things does
drink especially provoke?
PORTER: Marry, sir, nose-painting,
sleep, and urine.
  Macbeth, II, iii, 29

              Where should they
Find this grand liquor that hath gilded
  'em?
How cam'st thou in this pickle?
  The Tempest, V, i, 279

Thomas Dekker [1572?–1632?]

To drinke healths, is to drinke sick-
nesse.[1]
  The Honest Whore, Pt. II, Act
  IV, Sc. iii

Tobias Venner [1577–1660]

Stale beer is chiefly to be desired in

[1] Cf. Jerome K. Jerome, p. 9b.

the summer, and it is a drinke (be-
leeve me) for all constitutions, but
especially for the cholericke and mel-
ancholicke most wholsome.
  Via recta ad vitam longam,
  Sect. II

Wine . . . is a great encreaser of the
vitall spirits, and a wonderfull greatly
restorer of all powers and actions of
the bodie: it verie helpeth concoction,
distribution and nutrition, mightily
strengtheneth the natural heat, open-
eth obstruction, discusseth windiness,
taketh away sadness, and other hurt
of melancholy.
  Idem

John Taylor ("The Water Poet")
[1580–1653]

The Saylers in this ship [the *Ca-
rowse*], have taken a use to drinke
other mens healths, to the amplifying
of their owne diseases.[1]
  A Navy of Land Ships, Ch. 6

Francis Beaumont [1584–1616]
and John Fletcher [1579–1625]

Wine works the heart up, wakes the
  wit,
There is no cure 'gainst age but it.
It helps the head-ach, cough and tis-
  sick,
And is for all diseases Physick.[2]
  The Bloody Brother, Act II,
  Sc. ii

George Herbert [1593–1633]

Drink not the third glasse, — which
  thou canst not tame
When once it is within thee.
  The Temple, "The Church
  Porch"

George Wilkins [17th Cent.]

Drinke makes men hungry, or it makes
  them lie.
  *The Miseries of Inforsed Mar-
  riage*, Act II

[1] Cf. Jerome K. Jerome, p. 9b.
[2] Cf. Anonymous, p. 11b.

6

John Milton [1608–1674]

> One sip of this
> Will bathe the drooping spirits in delight
> Beyond the bliss of dreams.
> *Comus*

Samuel Pepys [1633–1703]

Thanks be to God, since my leaving drinking of wine, I do find myself much better and do mind my business better, and do spend less money, and less time lost in idle company.
> *Diary*, January 26, 1662

William Penn [1644–1718]

The smaller the drink, the clearer the head, and the cooler the blood.
> *Fruits of Solitude*, Maxim 66

Drunkenness . . . spoils health, dismounts the mind, and unmans men.
> *Ibid.*, Maxim 72

Henry Aldrich [1647–1710]

> There are five reasons why men drink —
> Good wine, a friend, or being dry,
> Or lest you should by-and-by,
> Or any other reason why.
>> Translation of 16th-century Latin epigram

Matthew Prior [1664–1721]

> I drank; I lik'd it not: 'twas rage, 'twas noise;
> An airy scene of transitory joys.
> In vain I trusted that the flowing bowl
> Would banish sorrow and enlarge the soul.
> To the late revel and protracted feast,
> Wild dreams succeeded and disorder'd rest.
>> *Solomon*, Bk. II

Alexander Pope [1688–1744]

The more you drink, the more you crave.
> *Satires and Epistles Imitated*, "Second Epistle of the Second Book of Horace"

Montesquieu [1] [1689–1755]

In cold countries the aqueous part of the blood is very little evacuated by perspiration. They may, therefore, make use of spiritous liquors, without which the blood would congeal. They are full of humors; consequently strong liquors, which give a motion to the blood, are proper for those countries.
> *The Spirit of Laws*, XIV (tr. by Thomas Nugent)

Philip Stanhope, Lord Chesterfield [1694–1773]

I always naturally hated drinking; and yet I have often drunk, with disgust at the time, attended by great sickness the next day, only because I then considered drinking as a necessary qualification for a fine gentleman and a Man of Pleasure.
> Letter to his son, March 27, 1747

Tobias Smollett [1721–1771]

The fumes of the liquor, mounting into the parson's brain, conspired with his former agitation of spirits, to make him quite delirious.
> *The Adventures of Roderick Random*, Ch. 32

Even here, when the peasants quarrel in their cups (which very seldom happens) they draw their knives, and the one infallibly stabs the other. To such extremities, however, they never proceed, except when there is a woman in the case; and mutual jealousy coop-

[1] Charles de Secondat, baron de la Brède et de Montesquieu.

7

erates with the liquor they have drank, to inflame their passions.
> *Travels through France and Italy,* Letter from Nice, October 22, 1764

Fermented liquors are pernicious to the human constitution.

William Cowper [1731–1800]

He that sips often, at last drinks it up.
> *Progress of Error*

Thomas Jefferson [1743–1826]

I wish to see this beverage [beer] become common instead of the whiskey which kills one-third of our citizens and ruins their families.
> Letter to Col. Charles Yancey, January 6, 1816

Benjamin Waterhouse [1754–1846]

Instances of young gentlemen sinking deep into the scandalous habit of drinking ardent spirits are very rare indeed; yet it would not be difficult to prove, that there is, and has been for several years, six times as much ardent spirit expended annually, as in the days of your grandfathers. Unruly wine and ardent spirits have supplanted sober cider. . . . Many, warmed by the generosity of youth, may think it consonant with prudence to drink so as to produce that exhilaration of spirits, which takes place just on this side of intoxication; but I hesitate not to pronounce, that the repetition of such practices is pernicious to health, and dangerous to morals. Cannot wisdom devise a plan of social intercourse, independent of the stimulus of the bottle?
> *Cautions to Young Persons Concerning Health*

George Gordon, Lord Byron [1788–1824]

'Tis pity wine should be so deleterious,

For tea and coffee leave us much more serious.
> *Don Juan,* Canto IV, Stanza 52

Robert E. Lee [1807–1870]

My experience through life has convinced me that, while moderation and temperance in all things are commendable and beneficial, abstinence from spirituous liquors is the best safeguard of morals and health.
> Letter to S. G. M. Miller and others, December 9, 1869

Oliver Wendell Holmes [1809–1894]

Wine . . . is a food.
> *Medical Essays,* "Currents and Counter-Currents in Medical Science"

Sir Richard Burton [1821–1890]

Who drinks one bowl hath scant delight;
to poorest passion he was born;
Who drains the score must e'er expect to rue the headache of the morn.
> *Kasidah,* Pt. VIII, Stanza 11

Louis Pasteur [1822–1895]

Wine is the most healthful and most hygienic of beverages.
> *Études sur le vin,* Pt. I, Ch. 2, Sect. B

Thomas (Stonewall) Jackson [1824–1863]

I like liquor — its taste and its effects — and that is just the reason why I never drink it. [On being ordered by his physician to take brandy.]
> Quoted by William Jones in *The Life and Letters of Robert Edward Lee, Soldier and Man,* p. 443

Sir Benjamin Ward Richardson [1828–1896]

The devil in solution.
> *Ten Lectures on Alcohol,* "The Liberty of the Abject"

Charles Farrar Browne ("Artemus Ward") [1834–1867]

The Indians on the Overland Route . . . are an intemperate people. They drink with impunity, or anybody who invites them.
> *Works*, Pt. VI, Programme of the Dodworth Hall Lecture

Mark Twain (Samuel L. Clemens) [1835–1910]

Give an Irishman lager for a month, and he's a dead man. An Irishman is lined with copper, and the beer corrodes it. But whiskey polishes the copper and is the saving of him.
> *Life on the Mississippi*, Ch. 23

Henry S. Leigh [1837–1883]

The rapturous, wild, and ineffable pleasure,
Of drinking at somebody else's expense.
> *Carols of Cockayne*, "Stanzas to an Intoxicated Fly"

William James [1842–1910]

The sway of alcohol over mankind is unquestionably due to its power to stimulate the mystical faculties of human nature.
> *The Varieties of Religious Experience*, "Mysticism"

Friedrich Nietzsche [1844–1900]

Two great European narcotics, alcohol and Christianity.
> *The Twilight of the Idols*, "Things the Germans Lack" (tr. by Anthony M. Ludovici)

Sir William Osler [1849–1919]

Throw all the beer and spirits into the Irish Channel, the English Channel and the North Sea for a year, and people in England would be infinitely better. It would certainly solve all the problems with which the philanthropists, the physicians, and the politicians have to deal.
> Lecture to Working Men's College, Camden Town, England, November 17, 1906

Total abstinence varies in different communities. South of the Mason and Dixon line a mint julep, a toddy, or a cocktail before meals or between, is total abstinence; and a profusion of egg-noggs at Christmas a necessity.
> Quoted by William B. Bean in *Sir William Osler: Aphorisms*, Ch. 5

Robert Louis Stevenson [1850–1894]

Fifteen men on the dead man's Chest —
Yo-ho-ho and a bottle of rum!
Drink and the devil had done for the rest —
Yo-ho-ho and a bottle of rum!
> *Treasure Island*, Ch. 1

Philip A. Bruce [1856–1933]

Drinking was much more general than card playing, since it required no previous scientific training for its indulgence.
> *History of the University of Virginia*, Vol. II, Ch. 28

A. E. Housman [1859–1936]

And malt does more than Milton can
To justify God's ways to man.
> *A Shropshire Lad*, No. 62

Jerome K. Jerome [1859–1927]

We drink one another's health and spoil our own.[1]
> *Idle Thoughts of an Idle Fellow*, "On Eating and Drinking"

Anton Chekhov [1860–1904]

I am dying. . . . I haven't drunk champagne for a long time.

---

[1] Cf. Thomas Dekker, p. 6a; John Taylor, p. 6b.

Henri Toulouse-Lautrec
[1864–1901]

I can drink without danger, I am so near to the ground.
> Comment to Charles Bourget

Warren G. Harding [1865–1923]

Constitutional prohibition has been adopted by the Nation. . . . It is the most demoralizing factor in our public life.
> Message to Congress, December 8, 1922

George Ade [1866–1944]

The water-wagon is the place for me. . . .
Last night at twelve I felt immense,
Today I feel like thirty cents. . . .
It is no time for mirth and laughter,
The cold, gray dawn of the morning after.
> *The Sultan of Sulu,* Act II, "Remorse"

Edwin Arlington Robinson [1869–1935]

Miniver Cheevy, born too late,
  Scratched his head and kept on thinking;
Miniver coughed, and called it fate,
And kept on drinking.
> *Miniver Cheevy*

G. K. Chesterton [1874–1936]

Drink because you are happy, but never because you are miserable.

Sir Winston Churchill [1874–1965]

Always remember . . . that I have taken more out of alcohol than alcohol has taken out of me.
> Quoted by Quentin Reynolds in *By Quentin Reynolds*

Herbert Hoover [1874–1964]

Prohibition cast a cloud over all our problems of law enforcement and was generally a constant worry. I should have been glad to have humanity forget all about strong alcoholic drinks. They are moral, physical, and economic curses to the race. But in the present stage of human progress, this vehicle of joy could not be generally suppressed by Federal law.
> *Memoirs,* Ch. 38

Thomas Mann [1875–1955]

Everything depended upon *who* was drunk — a drunken personality was far from being the same as a drunken tinker.
> *The Magic Mountain,* Ch. VI, "Vingt et Un" (tr. by H. T. Lowe-Porter)

Shane Leslie [1885–   ]

Cocktails have all the disagreeability without the utility of a disinfectant.
> *The Observer*

Alvan L. Barach [1895–   ]

An alcoholic has been lightly defined as a man who drinks more than his own doctor.
> *Journal of the American Medical Association* 181:393, 1962

F. Scott Fitzgerald [1896–1940]

The hangover became a part of the day as well allowed-for as the Spanish siesta.[1]
> *The Crack-up* (ed. by Edmund Wilson), "My Lost City"

Alec Waugh [1898–   ]

I am prepared to believe that a dry Martini slightly impairs the palate, but think what it does to the soul.
> *In Praise of Wine,* Ch. 16

Ogden Nash [1902–   ]

Candy
Is dandy

---

[1] Speaking of New York life around 1927.

But liquor
Is quicker.
> *Hard Lines,* "Reflection on Ice-
> Breaking"

T. H. Williams [1909–   ]

Dr. Benjamin Rush . . . was convinced that American commanders drank too much. He proposed that the Congress ration intoxicants to the generals and that any officer who consumed more than one quart of whiskey or got drunk more than once in twenty-four hours be reprimanded at the head of his unit. Moreover, he wanted the Congress to require that generals sleep in their boots and that in battle they remain no more than five hundred yards in the rear of their troops.
> *Americans at War,* Ch. I

Nathan Masor [1913–   ]

The tranquilizer of greatest value since the early history of man, and which may never become outdated, is alcohol, when administered in moderation. It possesses the distinct advantage of being especially pleasant to the taste buds.
> *The New Psychiatry,* Ch. 7

The Bible

Wine that maketh glad the heart of man.
> *Psalms* 104:15

Wine is a mocker, strong drink is raging: and whosoever is deceived thereby is not wise.
> *Proverbs* 20:1

Who hath woe? who hath sorrow? who hath contentions? who hath babbling? who hath wounds without cause? who hath redness of eyes?
They that tarry long at the wine; they that go to seek mixed wine.
Look not thou upon the wine when it is red . . .

At the last it biteth like a serpent, and stingeth like an adder.
> *Proverbs* 23:29

Woe unto them that rise up early in the morning, that they may follow strong drink; that continue until night, till wine inflame them!
> *Isaiah* 5:11

But they also have erred through wine, and through strong drink are out of the way; . . . they err in vision, they stumble in judgment.
> *Isaiah* 28:7

Drink no longer water, but use a little wine for thy stomach's sake and thine often infirmities.
> *I Timothy* 5:23

Anonymous

He that is drunk is as great as a king.[1]
> Old song

He that drinks well, does sleep well;
  he that sleeps well, doth think well;
He that thinks well, doth do well; he that does well, must drink well.
> *The Loyal Garland,* Song 65

Punch cures the gout, the colic, and the 'tisick
And is by all agreed the very best of physic.[2]
> English rhyme (18th Cent.)

Here sleeps in peace a Hampshire Grenadier,
Who caught his death by drinking cold small beer;
Soldiers, take heed from his untimely fall,
And when you're hot, drink strong, or not at all.
> Epitaph of Thomas Thetcher
> at Winchester, England, 1764

[1] Reputedly quoted by Charles II of England.
[2] Cf. Beaumont and Fletcher, p. 6b.

Its [rum's] utility in preserving the planters [of South Carolina] from the effects of the damp and unwholesome air of the morning, has given it the medical name of an *Antifogmatick.* The quantity taken every morning is in exact proportion to the thickness of the fog, and the dampness of the atmosphere. . . . the time we hope is not very distant when these fogs will be measured with much more accuracy, by an instrument called a *Foggrometer,* and which is to be graduated by gills, half pints and quarts.

> *An Oration in Praise of Rum,* University of Pennsylvania Commencement, July 30, 1789 (in *Massachusetts Spy,* November 12, 1789)

An effective and widely available solvent of the super-ego is alcohol.

Proverbs

A hair of the dog that bit me.

A morning sun and a wine-bred child and a Latin-bred woman seldom end well.

Bacchus hath drowned more men than Neptune.[1]

Drunkenness turns a man out of himself, and leaves a beast in his room.

When the wine is in, the wit is out.

French Proverb

Every month, one should get drunk at least once.

French and German Proverb

There are more old drunkards than old doctors.

German Proverb

The brewery is the best drugstore.

[1] German Proverb: More are drowned in the goblet than in the sea.

Irish Proverb

What butter or whiskey will not cure, there is no cure for.

Japanese Proverb

First the man takes a drink, then the drink takes a drink, then the drink takes the man.

Latin Proverbs

In wine there is truth.[1]
> Quoted by Pliny the Elder in *Natural History,* XIV.141

Nothing is more unhealthful than too much wine.

Russian Proverb

Drink a glass of wine after your soup, and you steal a ruble from the doctor.

Welsh Proverb

He who would be healthy let him drink mead.

ALLERGY

Increase Mather [1639–1723]

Some men also have strange antipathies in their natures against that sort of food which others love and live upon. I have read of one that could not endure to eat either bread or flesh; of another that fell into a swoonding fit at the smell of a rose. . . . There are some who, if a cat accidentally come into the room, though they neither see it, nor are told of it, will presently be in a sweat, and ready to die away.
> *Remarkable Providence,* Ch. 4

Sydney Smith [1771–1845]

I am suffering from my old complaint, the hay-fever (as it is called). My fear is, perishing by deliquescence; I melt away in nasal and lachrymal

[1] In vino veritas.

profluvia. My remedies are warm pediluvium, cathartics, topical application of a watery solution of opium to eyes, ears, and the interior of the nostrils. The membrane is so irritable, that light, dust, contradiction, an absurd remark, the sight of a Dissenter, — anything, sets me sneezing; and if I begin sneezing at twelve, I don't leave off till two o'clock, and am heard distinctly in Taunton, when the wind sets that way — a distance of six miles. Turn your mind to this little curse. If consumption is too powerful for physicians, at least they should not suffer themselves to be outwitted by such little upstart disorders as the hay-fever.

> Letter to Dr. Holland, June 1835

Chevalier Jackson [1865–1958]

All that wheezes is not asthma.
> *Boston Medical Quarterly* 16: 86, 1965

AMBITION

Alan Gregg [1890–1957]

Go after *exactly* what you want — not what you want. For you never get anything but the things you exactly wanted.
> Aphorism (Quoted by Wilder Penfield in *The Difficult Art of Giving*, Appendix A)

True inner conflict is between desire and desire, not desire and pain or desire and impossibility.
> *Idem*

ANATOMY

See also BODY

Aristotle [384–322 B.C.]

Those animals that have hairs on their body have lashes on their eyelids: the others (birds and the creatures with horny scales) have none. Of hairy animals, man alone has lashes on both lids.
> *Parts of Animals,* II.xiv (tr. by A. L. Peck)

Pliny the Elder [23–79]

It has been observed, that the height of a man from the crown of the head to the sole of the foot, is equal to the distance between the tips of the middle fingers of the two hands when extended in a straight line.
> *Natural History,* VII.xvii.17 (tr. by J. Bostock and H. T. Riley)

Leonardo da Vinci [1452–1519]

If nature had only one fixed standard for the proportions of the various parts, then the faces of all men would resemble each other to such a degree that it would be impossible to distinguish one from another; but she has varied the five parts of the face in such a way that although she has made an almost universal standard as to their size, she has not observed it in the various conditions to such a degree as to prevent one from being clearly distinguished from another.
> *Codice Atlantico,* 119 (tr. by Edward MacCurdy in *The Notebooks of Leonardo da Vinci,* Vol. II, Ch. XXIX)

And you who think to reveal the figure of man in words, with his limbs arranged in all their different attitudes, banish the idea from you, for the more minute your description the more you will confuse the mind of the reader and the more you will lead him away from the knowledge of the thing described. It is necessary therefore for you to represent and describe.
> *Dell' Anatomia,* Fogli A (*ibid.,* Vol. I, Ch. III)

Begin your anatomy with a man fully grown: then show him elderly and less muscular: then go on to strip him

stage by stage right down to the bones.
And you should afterward make
the child so as to show the womb.
Idem

Then describe the man fully grown
and the woman, and their measurements, and the nature of their com-
plexions, colour and physiognomy.
Ibid., Fogli B (*idem*)

This plan of mine of the human body
will be unfolded to you just as though
you had the natural man before you.
Quaderni d'Anatomia, Vol. I
(*idem*)

But though possessed of an interest
in the subject you may perhaps be
deterred by natural repugnance, or,
if this does not restrain you, then perhaps by the fear of passing the night
hours in the company of these corpses,
quartered and flayed and horrible to
behold.
Idem

With what words O writer can you
with a like perfection describe the
whole arrangement of that of which
the design is here?
For lack of due knowledge you describe it so confusedly as to convey
but little perception of the true shapes
of things, and deceiving yourself as
to these you persuade yourself that
you can completely satisfy the hearer
when you speak of the representation
of anything that possesses substance
and is surrounded by surface.
I counsel you not to cumber yourself with words unless you are speaking to the blind. If however notwithstanding you wish to demonstrate in
words to the ears rather than to the
eyes of men, let your speech be of
things of substance or natural things,
and do not busy yourself in making
enter by the ears things which have to
do with the eyes, for in this you will
be far surpassed by the work of the
painter.

How in words can you describe this
heart without filling a whole book?
Yet the more detail you write concerning it the more you will confuse
the mind of the hearer.
Ibid., Vol. II (*idem*)

You should show first the spine of the
neck with its tendons like the mast of
a ship with its shrouds without the
head; then make the head with its
tendons which give it its motion upon
its axis.
Idem

Jean Fernel [1497–1558]

Anatomy is to physiology as geogra-
phy to history; it describes the theatre
of events.
*On the Natural Part of Medi-
cine*, Ch. 1

Andreas Vesalius [1514–1564]

How much has been attributed to
Galen, easily leader of the professors
of dissection, by those physicians and
anatomists who have followed him,
and often against reason! . . . there
is that blessed and wonderful *plexus
reticularis* which that man everywhere
inculcates in his books. There is nothing of which physicians speak more
often. They have never seen it (for it
is almost non-existent in the human
body), yet they describe it from
Galen's teaching. Indeed, I myself cannot wonder enough at my own stupid-
ity and too great trust in the writings
of Galen and other anatomists.
De Humani Corporis Fabrica,
Bk. VII, Ch. XII (tr. by
Charles Singer as *Vesalius on
the Human Brain*)

No, Domine, even if that is not Galen's
opinion, we shall however demonstrate
here, that in fact it is so.[1]
Quoted by Baldesar Heseler in

[1] While demonstrating the muscles of the
abdomen, Vesalius replied thus to Matthaeus
Curtius, who had remarked, "This, however,
was not Galen's opinion."

Andreas Vesalius' First Public Anatomy at Bologne, 1540, an Eyewitness Report (tr. by Ruben Eriksson)

John Halle [1529–1568]

But chieflye the anatomye
Ye oughte to understande;
If ye will cure well anye thinge,
That ye doe take in hande. . . .

Withoute the knowledge of whyche
   arte,
Thou canste not chose but erre;
In all that thou shalte goe aboute
Thy knowledge to preferre: . . .

He is no true chirurgien
That cannot shewe by arte,
The nature of evrye member,
Eche from other aparte.

For in that noble handye worke,
There dothe nothinge excell,
The knowledge of anatomye,
If it be learned well.
   An Historicall Expostulation

William Shakespeare [1564–1616]

The kingly crowned head, the vigilant
   eye,
The counsellor heart, the arm our
   soldier,
Our steed the leg, the tongue our
   trumpeter.
   Coriolanus, I, i, 119

René Descartes [1596–1650]

And, indeed, there are several great men whom the study of human anatomy has not only lifted to the recognition of a God, but who are impelled to sing his praise observing with what admirable wisdom and singular providence he has perfected the arrangement of every part.
   Discours de la Méthode

Molière [1622–1673]

GERONTE: It was very clearly explained, but there was just one thing which surprised me — that was the positions of the liver and the heart. It seemed to me that you got them the wrong way about, that the heart should be on the left side, and the liver on the right.
SGANARELLE: Yes, it used to be so but we have changed all that. Everything's quite different in medicine nowadays.
   Le Médecin Malgré Lui, Act II, Sc. iv (tr. by John Wood)

Bernard Le Bovier de Fontenelle [1657–1757]

We anatomists are like the porters in Paris, who are acquainted with the narrowest and most distant streets, but who know nothing of what takes place in the houses!

Giovanni Battista Morgagni [1682–1771]

For those who have dissected or inspected many, have at least learn'd to doubt when the others, who are ignorant of anatomy, and do not take the trouble to attend to it, are in no doubt at all.
   De Sedibus et Causis Morborium, Vol. I, Bk. 2, Letter 16 (tr. by B. Alexander)

Alexander Pope [1688–1744]

Like following life through creatures
   you dissect,
You lose it in the moment you detect.
   Moral Essays, Epistle I

William Hunter [1718–1783]

Were I to place a man of proper talents, in the most direct road for becoming truly great in his profession, I would choose a good practical Anatomist and put him into a large hospital to attend the sick and dissect the dead.
   Two Introductory Lectures . . . to his Last Course of Anatomical Lectures, Lect. 2

Oliver Wendell Holmes
[1809–1894]

Gentlemen, damn the sphenoid bone!
> Opening of anatomy lectures
> at Harvard Medical School

These, gentlemen, . . . are the tuberosities of the ischia, on which man was designed to sit and survey the works of Creation.
> Quoted by Dr. Cheever in J. T. Morse, Jr.'s *Life and Letters of Oliver Wendell Holmes*, Vol. I, Ch. VII

Rudolf Virchow [1821–1902]

A cell state in which every cell is a citizen.
> *Die Cellularpathologie*

Mark Twain (Samuel L. Clemens) [1835–1910]

Surgeons and anatomists see no beautiful women in all their lives, but only a ghastly stack of bones with Latin names to them, and a network of nerves and muscles and tissues inflamed by disease.
> Letter to the *Alta Californian*, San Francisco, May 28, 1867

Percy Hammond [1873–1936]

The human knee is a joint and not an entertainment.
> Review of a play, ca. 1912 (Quoted by Mark Sullivan in *Our Times*, Vol. III)

W. Somerset Maugham [1874–1965]

You will have to learn many tedious things, . . . which you will forget the moment you have passed your final examination, but in anatomy it is better to have learned and lost than never to have learned at all.[1]
> *Of Human Bondage*, Ch. LIV

[1] Advice to first-year medical students.

ANEMIA

See also BLOOD

William Shakespeare [1564–1616]

> Lepidus . . . is troubled
With the green sickness.
> *Antony and Cleopatra*, III, ii, 4

There's never none of these demure boys come to any proof; for thin drink doth so over-cool their blood, and making many fish-meals, that they fall into a kind of male green-sickness.
> *Henry IV, Part II*, IV, iii, 96

PANDER: Now the pox upon her green-sickness for me!
BAWD: Faith, there's no way to be rid on't but by the way to the pox.
> *Pericles*, IV, vi, 14

Out, you green-sickness carrion! out,
> you baggage!
You tallow-face!
> *Romeo and Juliet*, III, v, 157

Austin Flint [1812–1886]

Fatal anaemia must follow degenerative disease reducing the amount of gastric juice so far that the assimilation of food is rendered wholly inadequate to the wants of the body.
> *American Medical Times* 1:181, 1860

Anthony Trollope [1815–1882]

American lads and lasses are all pale. Men at thirty and women at twenty-five have had all semblance of youth baked out of them. Infants even are not rosy, and the only shades known on the cheeks of children are those composed of brown, yellow, and white. All this comes of those damnable hot-air pipes with which every tenement in America is infested.
> *North America*, Ch. 12

Samuel Fenwick [1821–1902]

The progressive atrophy of the stomach had prevented the digestion of the albuminous materials of the food, at the same time that the healthy condition of the liver, pancreas, and intestines admitted of a free supply of the other constituents of the body.[1]
> *Lancet* 2:78, 1870

W. Somerset Maugham [1874–1965]

She was very anaemic. Her thin lips were pale, and her skin was delicate, of a faint green colour, without a touch of red even in the cheeks.
> *Of Human Bondage,* Ch. LV

She was dreadfully anaemic and suffered from the dyspepsia which accompanies that ailing.
> *Ibid.,* Ch. LIX

Her anaemia made her rather short of breath, and she held her mouth slightly open.
> *Ibid.,* Ch. LX

William D. Snively, Jr. [1911–   ]

There is a vast army of pale and peaked children abroad in the land, an army of children in the "pastel tints."[2]

ANESTHESIA

Thomas Middleton [1570?–1627]

I'll imitate the pities of old surgeons
To cast this lost limb, who, ere they show their art,
Cast one asleep, then cut the diseas'd part.
> *Women Beware Women,* Act IV, Sc. i

[1] Report of an autopsy on a pernicious anemia victim.
[2] Preston A. McLendon of Georgetown University has referred to malnourished preschoolers as "pastel children."

John C. Warren [1778–1856]

Gentlemen, this is no humbug.[1]

Oliver Wendell Holmes [1809–1894]

Three natural anaesthetics . . . — sleep, fainting, death.
> *Medical Essays,* "The Medical Profession in Massachusetts"

J. Marion Sims [1813–1883]

My hands are then henceforth, washed of chloroform and devoted to ether.
> Letter to his wife, November 21, 1861 (in *The Story of My Life,* Appendix A)

Victoria of England [1819–1901]

Dr. Snow gave that blessed Chloroform & the effect was soothing, quieting & delightful beyond measure.[2]
> *Journal*

S. Weir Mitchell [1829–1914]

Nature had not waited for man to supply her anaesthetics, and the disturbed chemistries of failing life were flooding nerve and brain with potent sedatives.
> *In War Time,* Ch. IV

William Ernest Henley [1849–1903]

BEFORE . . .
Behold me waiting — waiting for the knife.
A little while, and at a leap I storm
The thick, sweet mystery of chloroform,
The drunken dark, the little death-in-life.

[1] Comment after his first operation on a patient under the influence of ether, which was administered by Dr. William T. G. Morton at the Massachusetts General Hospital on October 16, 1846.
[2] Dr. John Snow, of Edinburgh, gave Queen Victoria chloroform at the birth of Prince Leopold, April 7, 1853.

OPERATION . . .
And you gasp and reel, and shudder
In a rushing, swaying rapture,
While the voices at your elbow
Fade — receding — fainter —
farther. . . .

Then the lights grow fast and furious,
And you hear a noise of waters,
And you wrestle, blind and dizzy,
In an agony of effort,

Till a sudden lull accepts you,
And you sound an utter dark-
ness . . .
And awaken . . . with a strug-
gle . . .
On a hushed, attentive audience.

AFTER
Like as a flamelet blanketed in smoke,
So through the anaesthetic shows my
life; . . .
Faces look strange from space — and
disappear.
Far voices, sudden loud, offend my
ear —
And hush as sudden. . . .
Time and the place glimpse on to me
again;
And, unsurprised, out of uncertainty,
I wake — relapsing — somewhat faint
and fain,
To an immense, complacent dreamery.
In Hospital, Sects. iv–vi

Sir William Osler [1849–1919]

The extraordinary controversy which
has raged, and re-raged every few
years, on the question to whom the
world is indebted for the introduction
of anaesthesia, illustrates the absence
of true historical perspective, and a
failure to realize just what priority
means in the case of a great discovery.
> Remarks on presenting William
> Morton's original papers to the
> Royal Society of Medicine,
> May 15, 1918

August Bier [1861–1949]

In America there exist professional
anesthetists. This specialty is also being praised in Germany. I cannot
think of anything more dull.

Wilfred Trotter [1872–1939]

Mr. Anaesthetist, if the patient can
keep awake, surely you can.
> Quoted in *Lancet* 2:1340, 1965

Elizabeth Longford [1906–   ]

Dr. Simpson's [1] first patient, a doctor's wife in 1847, had been so carried
away with enthusiasm that she chris-
tened her child, a girl, "Anaesthesia."
> *Queen Victoria,* Ch. 17

The Bible

And the Lord God caused a deep sleep
to fall upon Adam, and he slept: and
he took one of his ribs, and closed up
the flesh instead thereof.
> *Genesis* 2:21

ANGINA

William Heberden [1710–1801]

There is a disorder of the breast
marked with strong and peculiar
symptoms, considerable for the kind
of danger belonging to it, and not
extremely rare, which deserves to be
mentioned more at length. The seat
of it, and sense of strangling, and
anxiety with which it is attended, may
make it not improperly be called
angina pectoris.

They who are afflicted with it, are
seized while they are walking, (more
especially if it be up hill, and soon
after eating) with a painful and most
disagreeable sensation in the breast,
which seems as if it would extinguish
life, if it were to increase or to continue; but the moment they stand
still, all this uneasiness vanishes. [2]
> *Commentaries on the History
> and Cure of Diseases,* Ch. 70

[1] Sir James Young Simpson [1811–1870]
of Edinburgh, the pioneer of chloroform.
[2] On the syndrome he named without
knowledge of the coronary mechanism.

John Hunter [1728–1793]

My life is in the hands of any rascal who chooses to annoy and tease me.[1]
> Quoted by Arturo Castiglioni in *A History of Medicine*, Ch. 18

ANTIBIOTICS

Hilary Koprowski [1916–   ]

If a universal antibiotic is found, immediately organize societies to prevent its use. It should be dealt with as we should have treated, and did not treat, the atomic bomb. Use any feasible national and international deterrents to prevent it falling into the hands of stupid people who probably will still be in the majority in your time as they were in mine.
> *Man and His Future* (ed. by Gordon Wolstenholme), "Future of Infectious and Malignant Diseases"

ANTISEPSIS

See also INFECTION

Joseph, Lord Lister [1827–1912]

Since the antiseptic treatment has been brought into full operation, and wounds and abscesses no longer poison the atmosphere with putrid exhalations, my wards, though in other respects under precisely the same circumstances as before, have completely changed their character; so that during the last nine months not a single instance of pyaemia, hospital gangrene or erysipelas has occurred in them.

[1] Hunter suffered from angina pectoris. Opposition at a board meeting to the appointment of his successor at St. George's Hospital so roused his ire that an attack caused his death at the meeting.

As there appears to be no doubt regarding the cause of this change, the importance of the fact can hardly be exaggerated.
> *British Medical Journal* 2:246, 1867

In order, Gentlemen, that you may get satisfactory results with this sort of treatment, you must be able to see with your mental eye the septic ferments as distinctly as we see flies or other insects with the corporeal eye. If you can really see them in this distinct way with your intellectual eye, you can be properly on your guard against them; if you do not so see them, you will be constantly liable to relax in your precautions.
> *Edinburgh Medical Journal* 21:193, 1875

The irritation of the wound by antiseptic irrigation and washing may therefore now be avoided, and nature left quite undisturbed to carry out her best methods of repair.
> *Report of the British Association for the Advancement of Science*, 1896

Robert Bridges [1844–1930]

Who dream'd that living air poison'd
  our SURGERY, coating
All our sheeny weapons with germs of
  an invisible death,
Till he saw the sterile steel work with
  immunity, and save
Quickly as its warring scimitars of
  victory had slain?
> *Now in Wintry Delights*

Sir William Osler [1849–1919]

Neatness is the asepsis of clothes.
> *Johns Hopkins Hospital Nurses Alumnae Magazine* 12:72, 1913

Soap and water and common sense are the best disinfectants.
> Quoted by William B. Bean in *Sir William Osler: Aphorisms*, Ch. 5

Sir William Watson Cheyne [1852–1932]

Surgeons noted that Lister was constantly changing his technique and dressings and came to the conclusion that this was because his results were not good. They apparently did not listen to his statements, as he altered his methods with the object of reducing or removing the irritation of the antiseptic and at the same time simplifying his technique.

Antiseptic Treatment of Wounds

Martin H. Fischer [1879–1962]

When in doubt as to which disinfectant to use, try soap and water.

Quoted by Howard Fabing and Ray Marr in *Fischerisms*

ANTIVIVISECTION

John Caius [1510–1573]

That plausible proverbe verified upon a Tyraunt, namely that he loved his sowe better then his Sonne, may well be applyed to these kinde of people who delight more in dogges that are deprived of all possibility of reason, than they doe in children that be capeable of wisedome and judgement.

Works, "A Treatise of English Dogs" (tr. by A. Fleming)

Samuel Johnson [1709–1784]

I know not, that by living dissections any discovery has been made by which a single malady is more easily cured.

The Idler, No. 17 (August 5, 1758)

Charles Darwin [1809–1882]

Vivisection . . . is justifiable for real investigations on physiology; but not for mere damnable and detestable curiosity.

Letter to E. Ray Lankester, March 22, 1871

Joseph, Lord Lister [1827–1912]

There are people who do not object to eating a mutton chop — people who do not even object to shooting a pheasant with the considerable chance that it may be only wounded and may have to die after lingering in pain, unable to obtain its proper nutriment — and yet who consider it something monstrous to introduce under the skin of a guinea pig a little inoculation of some microbe to ascertain its action. These seem to me to be most inconsistent views.

British Medical Journal 1:317, 1897

William H. Welch [1850–1934]

The main cause of this unparalleled progress in physiology, pathology, medicine and surgery has been the fruitful application of the experimental method of research, just the same method which has been the great lever of all scientific advance in modern times.

Argument against Antivivisection Bill (Senate #34), February 21, 1900

Sir Charles Sherrington [1861–1952]

[My portrait by Augustus John] should be used by the Anti-Vivisection Society to show how cruel and callous these physiologists are!

Quoted by Lord Cohen of Birkenhead in *The Sherrington Lectures*, Vol. IV, Lect. I

Rudyard Kipling [1865–1936]

[Doctors] have been exposed — you will always be exposed — to the attacks of those persons who consider their own undisciplined emotions more important than the world's most bitter agonies — those people who would limit, and cripple, and hamper research because they fear research may be accompanied by a little pain and suffering.

A Doctor's Work, address to students at London's Middlesex Hospital, October 1, 1908

Irvin S. Cobb [1876–1944]

I would rather that any white rabbit on earth should have the Asiatic cholera twice than that I should have it just once.

J. B. S. Haldane [1892–1964]

There are a few honest antivivisectionists. . . . I have not met any of them, but I am quite prepared to believe that they exist.

Possible Worlds, "Some Enemies of Science"

ANXIETY

See also WORRY

Ali ibn-Hazm [994–1064]

No one is moved to act, or resolves to speak a single word, who does not hope by means of this action or word to release anxiety from his spirit.

Epistle on the Medicine to Apply to Souls, Sect. I

Joseph Addison [1672–1719]

A continual Anxiety for Life vitiates all the Relishes of it, and casts a Gloom over the whole Face of Nature; as it is impossible we should take Delight in any thing that we are every Moment afraid of losing.

The Spectator, Vol. 1, No. 25 (March 29, 1711)

Karl Jaspers [1883–　]

As the order of existence becomes increasingly rational and is applied to everyone, its extraordinary success carries with it a feeling of impending doom and of an anxiety which develops because it is no longer apparent what makes life worthwhile.

The terrifying spectre of the future is responsible for the anxiety of the individual: removed from his background, he is left without a function which he can recognize. Consequently, an overwhelming anxiety, unlike any that has been known before, is the uncanny companion of modern man. The anxiety refers not only to his threatened existence as an individual within his society, a threat of which he has become increasingly aware, but also to the threatened loss of his own identity, which he cannot maintain. . . .

The anxiety affects the body. In spite of increasing longevity, the growing feeling of insecurity is unmistakable. Demands for medical care go far beyond the limit which is justified by medical science. If the mind cannot cope with existence, if man can no longer tolerate the lack of meaning, he escapes into illness which affords him protection because he does understand it.

Die geistige Situation der Zeit, Pt. I, Ch. 3 (tr. by Max Samter)

Japanese (Shinto) Proverb

Every little yielding to anxiety is a step away from the natural heart of man.

APHORISMS

Howard Fabing [1907–　]

Since the days of Hippocrates, our father, the aphorism has been the literary vehicle of the doctor. . . . Laymen have stolen the trick from time to time, but the aphorism remains the undisputed contribution of the doctor to literature.

Fischerisms, "To Martin H. Fischer"

APPENDICITIS

Richard Clarke Cabot [1868–1939]

There are two kinds of appendicitis — acute appendicitis and appendicitis for revenue only.
> Clinicopathological conference discussion, ca. 1925

Delbert H. Nickson [1890–1951]

The patient suffered from chronic remunerative appendicitis.

APPETITE

See also FASTING, HUNGER

Hippocrates [460?–377? B.C.]

When a person who is recovering from a disease has a good appetite, but his body does not improve in condition, it is a bad symptom.
> *Aphorisms,* II.31 (tr. by Francis Adams)

Cicero [106–43 B.C.]

The appetites of the belly and the palate, far from diminishing as men grow older, go on increasing.
> *Pro Caelio,* 191

Epictetus [60?–120?]

Let the first satisfaction of appetite be always the measure to you of eating and drinking; and appetite itself the sauce and the pleasure.
> *Fragments,* XXV (tr. by E. Carter)

François Rabelais [1494?–1553]

'Appetite comes as you eat,' said Bishop Hangest of Le Mans; but thirst vanishes as you drink!
> *Gargantua,* Bk. I, Ch. 5 (tr. by Jacques Le Clercq)

Michel de Montaigne [1533–1592]

My appetite comes to me as I eat.
> *Essays,* Bk. III, Ch. 9, "Of Vanity" (tr. by Donald M. Frame)

Leonard Lessius [1554–1623]

The most ordinary meats, yea and drie bread itself, do better taste and relish a sober man, and yeeld him greater pleasure, then the greatest dainties that can be do to those who are given to Gluttonie. For the evil juices that did infect the stomack and the Organ of Taste, and which bred a loathing and offence, being removed and cleared, the Appetite returneth of it self, and the pure relish and naturall delight in meats is felt.
> *Hygiasticon,* Ch. VIII (tr. by Timothy Smith)

William Shakespeare [1564–1616]

But, like a sickness, did I loathe this food;
But, as in health, come to my natural taste,
Now I do wish it, love it, long for it.
> *A Midsummer Night's Dream,* IV, i, 176

Doth not the appetite alter? A man loves the meat in his youth that he cannot endure in his age.
> *Much Ado About Nothing,* II, iii, 247

To make our appetites more keen,
With eager compounds we our palate urge.
> *Sonnet CXVIII*

Sir John Suckling [1609–1642]

'Tis not the meat, but 'tis the appetite
Makes eating a delight.
> *Fragmenta Aurea,* "Of Thee, Kind Boy"

William Penn [1644–1718]

If thou rise with an appetite, thou art sure never to sit down without one.
    Fruits of Solitude, Maxim 64

Jonathan Swift [1667–1745]

Does it make your mouth water?
    Polite Conversation, Dialogue III

Joseph Addison [1672–1719]

The most violent Appetites in all Creatures are LUST and HUNGER: The first, is a perpetual Call upon them to propagate their Kind; the latter, to preserve themselves.
    The Spectator, Vol. II, No. 120 (July 18, 1711)

Ivan Turgenev [1818–1883]

Illness isn't the only thing that spoils the appetite.
    A Month in the Country, Act IV (tr. by Constance Garnett)

The Bible

All the labour of man is for his mouth, and yet the appetite is not filled.
    Ecclesiastes 6:7

Anonymous

A boy is an appetite with a skin pulled over it.

English Proverb

New meat begets a new appetite.

French Proverbs

No sauce like appetite.[1]

Eating and drinking takes away one's stomach.

German Proverb

When the boy is growing he has a wolf in his belly.

[1] French, Danish, Dutch, Italian Proverb: Hunger is the best sauce.

ARTERIES

William Shakespeare [1564–1616]

These pipes and these conveyances of our blood.
    Coriolanus, V, i, 54

Why, universal plodding prisons up The nimble spirits in the arteries.
    Love's Labour's Lost, IV, iii, 305

                Stuff'd within With bloody veins.
    Pericles, I, iv, 93

Thomas Sydenham [1624–1689]

A man is as old as his arteries.
    Quoted by F. H. Garrison in *Bulletin of the New York Academy of Medicine* 4:993, 1928

ARTERIOSCLEROSIS

Leonardo da Vinci [1452–1519]

[Cause of death in the old]
Veins which by the thickening of their tunicles in the old restrict the passage of the blood, and by this lack of nourishment destroy their life without any fever, the old coming to fail little by little in slow death.
    Dell' Anatomia, Fogli B (tr. by Edward MacCurdy in *The Notebooks of Leonardo da Vinci,* Vol. I, Ch. III)

ASTHMA

See ALLERGY

AUTOPSY

Leonardo da Vinci [1452–1519]

And this old man, a few hours before his death, told me that he had lived a hundred years, and that he did not feel any bodily ailment other than weakness, and thus while sitting upon a bed in the hospital of Santa Maria Nuova at Florence, without any movement or sign of anything amiss, he passed away from this life.

And I made an autopsy in order to ascertain the cause of so peaceful a death, and found that it proceeded from weakness through the failure of blood and of the artery that feeds the heart and the other lower members, which I found to be very parched and shrunk and withered. . . . The other autopsy was on a child of two years, and here I found everything the contrary to what it was in the case of the old man.

> *Dell' Anatomia*, Fogli B (tr. by Edward MacCurdy in *The Notebooks of Leonardo da Vinci*, Vol. I, Ch. III)

O speculator concerning this machine of ours let it not distress you that you impart knowledge of it through another's death, but rejoice that our Creator has ordained the intellect to such excellence of perception.

> *Quaderni d'Anatomia*, Vol. II (*idem*)

Hermann Boerhaave [1668–1738]

A disease which is new and obscure to you, Doctor, will be known only after death; and even then not without an autopsy will you examine it with exacting pains. But rare are those among the extremely busy Clinicians who are willing or capable of doing this correctly.

> *Atrocis, nec Descripti Prius, Morbi Historia* (tr. in *Bulletin of the Medical Library Association* 43:217, 1955)

Richard Bright [1789–1858]

To connect accurate and faithful observations after death with symptoms displayed during life must be in some degree to forward the objects of our noble art.

> *Reports of Medical Cases,* Vol. I

Hughlings Jackson [1835–1911]

We have long heard that old maids' husbands are always well behaved, and on the same principle the pathology of those who do not make post-mortem examinations is often confident and definite.

> *British Medical Journal* 2:305, 1882

Hobart Amory Hare [1862–1931]

[Osler] went into the post-mortem room with the joyous demeanor of the youthful Sophocles leading the chorus of victory after the Battle of Salamis. He cared little, and admitted he knew less, as to how the victory could perhaps have been reached by proper treatment before death took place.

> *Therapeutic Gazette* 36: 160, 1920

H. L. Mencken [1880–1956]

When I die my kidneys go to the Municipal Museum of Altoona, Pa., and my liver to Oberlin College, but it would take much eloquence to make me leave even my thyroid gland to Milwaukee.

> Letter to Theodore Dreiser, October 30, 1922

W. Russell, Lord Brain [1895–1966]

In the post-mortem room we witness the final result of disease, the failure of the body to solve its problems, and there is an obvious limit to what one can learn about normal business transactions from even a daily visit to the bankruptcy court.

> *Canadian Medical Association Journal* 83:349, 1960

Anonymous

My friend was ill: I attended him. He died: I dissected him.

> French saying ascribed to various celebrated physicians

BACTERIA

See INFECTION, MICROBES

BALDNESS

Hippocrates [460?–377? B.C.]

The wasting of the brain which leads to baldness.

> *Epidemics,* VI.iii.1

Ovid [43 B.C.–A.D. 17?]

Ugly are hornless bulls, a field without grass is an eyesore,
So is a tree without leaves, so is a head without hair.

> *The Art of Love,* III.249 (tr. by R. Humphries)

Martial [fl. 1st Cent.]

You manufacture, with the aid of unguents, a false head of hair, and your bald and dirty scalp is covered with dyed locks. There is no need to have a hairdresser for your head. A sponge, Phoebus, would do the business better.

> *Epigrams,* VI.57 (tr. by Henry G. Bohn)

You collect your straggling hairs on either side, Marinus, endeavoring to conceal the vast expanse of your shining bald pate by the locks which still grow on your temples. . . . Why not confess yourself an old man? Be content to seem what you really are, and let the barber shave off the rest of your hair. There is nothing more contemptible than a bald man who pretends to have hair.

> *Ibid.,* X.83

Apuleius [fl. 2nd Cent.]

But I, poor wretch, have first married a husband older than my father, more bald than a coot, more weak than a child.

> *The Golden Ass,* V.9 (tr. by W. Adlington, rev. by S. Gaselee)

School of Salerno [1095–1224]

For ointment juice of Onyons is assign'd
To heads whose haire falls faster than it growes.

> *Regimen Sanitatis Salernitanum* (tr. by Sir John Harington as *The Englishman's Doctor*)

John Lydgate [1370?–1451?]

He was ballid as a cote.

> *Troy-Book,* Bk. II

William Shakespeare [1564–1616]

There's no time for a man to recover his hair that grows bald by nature.

> *The Comedy of Errors,* II, ii, 73

Mark Twain (Samuel L. Clemens) [1835–1910]

Trouble has brung these grey hairs and this premature balditude.

> *The Adventures of Huckleberry Finn,* Ch. 19

Oliver Herford [1863–1935]

A hair in the head is worth two in the brush.

Samuel Hoffenstein [1890–1947]

Babies haven't any hair:
Old men's heads are just as bare; —
From the cradle to the grave
Lies a haircut and a shave.

> *Poems in Praise of Practically Nothing,* "Songs of Faith in the Year after Next"

English Proverb

A bald head is soon shaven.

BASIC SCIENCE

Thomas Sydenham [1624–1689]

This is all very fine, but it won't do — Anatomy — Botany — Nonsense! Sir, I know an old woman in Covent Garden who understands botany better, and as for anatomy, my butcher can dissect a joint full and well; no, young man, all that is stuff; you must go to the bedside, it is there alone you can learn disease.[1]

> Quoted by John Comrie in *Selected Works of Thomas Sydenham, M.D.*, "Life of Thomas Sydenham"

Oliver Goldsmith [1728–1774]

The circle of science which I have run through, before I undertook the study of physic, is not only useful but absolutely necessary to the making a skilful physician. Such sciences enlarge our understanding, and sharpen our sagacity; and what is a practitioner without both but an empiric, for never yet was a disorder found entirely the same in two patients?

> Letter to T. Contarine, 1753

Thomas Jefferson [1743–1826]

Harvey's discovery of the circulation of the blood was a beautiful addition to our knowledge of the animal economy, but on a review of the practice of medicine before and since that epoch, I do not see any great amelioration which has been derived from that discovery.

> Letter to Edward Jenner, May 14, 1806 (Quoted by John Baron in *Life of Edward Jenner*, Vol. II, Ch. 3)[2]

[1] Comment to Hans Sloane on Robert Boyle's letter to him (1684) describing Sloane as a "ripe scholar, a good botanist, and a skilled anatomist."

[2] This version, identified as a letter to the Reverend Doctor G. C. Jenner, is found in the 1903 edition of Jefferson's *Writings* by the Thomas Jefferson Memorial Association.

Abraham Colles [1773–1843]

Be assured, that no man can know his own profession perfectly, who knows nothing else; and that he who aspires to eminence in any particular science, must first acquire the habit of philosophizing on matters of science in general.

> *A Treatise on Surgical Anatomy*, Pt. I, Sect. I

Peter Mere Latham [1789–1875]

It is all very fine to insist that the eye cannot be understood without a knowledge of optics, nor the circulation without hydraulics, nor the bones and the muscles without mechanics: that metaphysics may have their use in leading us through the intricate functions of the nervous system, and the mysterious connection of mind and matter. It is a truth; and it is a truth also that the whole circle of the sciences is required to comprehend a single particle of matter: but the most solemn truth of all is, *that the life of man is three-score years and ten.*

> *Lectures on Clinical Medicine*, Lect. I

BATHING

See HYGIENE

BEDSIDE MANNER

See also PATIENT–PHYSICIAN RELATIONSHIP

George du Maurier [1834–1896]

"What sort of doctor is he?"
"Oh, well, I don't know much about his ability; but he's got a very good bedside manner!"

> Caption to drawing in *Punch*, March 15, 1884

George W. E. Russell [1853–1919]

Such, exactly, were the Family Physicians of my youth. They always dressed in shiny black,—trousers, neckcloth and all; they were invariably bald, and had shaved upper lips and chins, and carefully-trimmed whiskers. They said "Hah!" and "Hum!" in tones of omniscience which would have converted a Christian Scientist; and, when feeling one's pulse, they produced the largest and most audibly-ticking gold watches conceivable by the horologist's art. They had what are called "the courtly manners of the old school"; were diffuse in style, and abounded in periphrasis. Thus they spoke of "the gastric organ" where their successors talk of the stomach, and referred to brandy as "the domestic stimulant." When attending families where religion was held in honour, they were apt to say to the lady of the house, "We are fearfully and wonderfully made."
One Look Back, Ch. I

BELLY

See also STOMACH

Homer [ca. 850 B.C.]

It's this damned belly that gives a man his worst troubles.
Odyssey, XV.344 (tr. by W. H. D. Rouse)

Saadi (Muslih-ud-Din)
[1184?–1291]

When belly with bad pains doth swell,
It matters nought what else goes well.
Gulistān, III.9 (tr. by E. Arnold)

William Shakespeare [1564–1616]
                     He was a man
Of an unbounded stomach.
Henry VIII, IV, ii, 33

My belly's as cold as if I had swallow'd snowballs for pills.
The Merry Wives of Windsor, III, v, 23

The Bible

Behold, my belly is as wine which hath no vent; it is ready to burst like new bottles.
Job 32:19

Proverb

The belly robs the back.

BIOCHEMISTRY

Otto Tachenius [d. 1670]

In all things you shall find everywhere the *Acid* and the *Alcaly*.
Hyppocrates Chymacus, Ch. 21

Robert Boyle [1627–1691]

He that thoroughly understands the nature of Ferments, and Fermentations, shall probably be much better able then he that ignores them, to give a fair account of divers *Phenomena* of several diseases (as well Fevers as others) which will perhaps be never thoroughly understood, without an insight into the doctrine of Fermentation.
The Usefulness of Natural Philosophy, Pt. II, Essay II

Elisha Bartlett [1804–1855]

Let chemistry push her researches into the remotest accessible recesses of the living economy, and let her claim, for her own, every process, every act, every transformation, over which she can establish a legitimate jurisdiction.
Philosophy of Medical Science, Pt. II, Ch. 15

Louis Pasteur [1822–1895]

If the mysterious influence to which the dissymmetry of natural products is due should come to change in sense or direction, the constituting elements of all living beings would take an inverse dissymmetry. Perhaps a new world would be presented to us. Who could foresee the organization of living beings, if the cellulose, which is right, should become left, if the left albumen of the blood should become right? There are here mysteries which prepare immense labors for the future, and from this hour invite the most serious meditations of science.

> Lecture, Chemical Society of Paris, February 3, 1860

Barry Commoner [1917–   ]

The theory of the DNA code is sometimes epitomized by the statement "DNA is the secret of life," an aphorism which appears increasingly to guide the course of current biological investigations. The viewpoint developed here suggests that biology might be more wisely guided by the aphorism, "Life is the secret of DNA."

> *American Scientist* 52:365, 1964

BIOLOGY

Leonardo da Vinci [1452–1519]

Man and the animals are merely a passage and channel for food, a tomb for other animals, a haven for the dead, giving life by the death of others, a coffer full of corruption.

> *Codice Atlantico*, 76 (tr. by Edward MacCurdy in *The Notebooks of Leonardo da Vinci*, Vol. I, Ch. I)

Elisha Bartlett [1804–1855]

With certain limited exceptions, the laws of physical science are positive and absolute, both in their aggregate and in their elements, — in their sum, and in their details; but the ascertainable laws of the science of life are approximative only, and not absolute.

> *Philosophy of Medical Science*, Pt. II, Ch. 11

Ernst Haeckel [1834–1919]

The cell never acts; it reacts.

> *Generelle Morphologie*

Donald Culross Peattie [1898–1964]

I say that it touches a man that his blood is sea water and his tears are salt, that the seed of his loins is scarcely different from the same cells in a seaweed, and that of stuff like his bones are coral made. I say that a physical and biologic law lies down with him, and wakes when a child stirs in the womb, and that the sap in a tree, uprushing in the spring, and the smell of the loam, where the bacteria bestir themselves in darkness, and the path of the sun in the heaven, these are facts of first importance to his mental conclusions, and that a man who goes in no consciousness of them is a drifter and a dreamer, without a home or any contact with reality.

> *An Almanac for Moderns*, "April First"

George Orwell [1903–1950]

ALL ANIMALS ARE EQUAL BUT SOME ANIMALS ARE MORE EQUAL THAN OTHERS.

> *Animal Farm*, Ch. X

BIRTH

See also BIRTH AND DEATH, CHILDBIRTH

Pliny the Elder [23–79]

Man alone, at the very moment of his birth cast naked upon the naked earth.

> *Natural History*, VII.i (tr. by J. Bostock and H. T. Riley)

William Wordsworth [1770–1850]

Our birth is but a sleep and a forgetting.
>*Ode. Intimations of Immortality*

Elisha Bartlett [1804–1855]

Certainly, nothing can be more doubtful or contingent, in any single instance, than the birth of a male or a female child. One event is almost as likely to happen as the other.
>*Philosophy of Medical Science,* Pt. II, Ch. 11

Harriet Beecher Stowe
[1811–1896]

"Do you know who made you?"

"Nobody as I knows on," said the child, with a short laugh.

The idea appeared to amuse her considerably; for her eyes twinkled, and she added, "I spect I grow'd. Don't think nobody never made me."
>*Uncle Tom's Cabin,* Ch. XX

George Macdonald [1824–1905]

Where did you come from, baby dear?
Out of the everywhere into here.
>*At the Back of the North Wind,* Ch. 33

BIRTH AND DEATH

See also BIRTH, DEATH

Marcus Manilius [1st Cent. B.C.?]

We begin to die at birth; the end flows from the beginning.
>*Astronomica,* IV

St. John Chrysostom [345?–407]

If thou grievest for the dead, mourn also for those who are born into the world; for as the one thing is of nature, so is the other too of nature.
>*Homilies on the Statutes,* Homily VI (tr. by John H. Parker)

Sir Francis Bacon [1561–1626]

It is as natural to die as to be born; and to a little infant, perhaps, the one is as painful as the other.
>*Essays,* "Of Death"

What then remaines, but that we still
>should cry,
Not to be borne, or being borne, to die.
>*The World*

Joseph Hall [1574–1656]

Death borders upon our birth; and our cradle stands in our grave.
>*Epistles,* Decade III, Epistle 2

Sir Thomas Browne [1605–1682]

With what shift and pains we come into the World we remember not; but 'tis commonly found no easy matter to get out of it.
>*Christian Morals,* Pt. II, Sect. 13

They carried them out of the world with their feet forward, not inconsonant with reason: As contrary unto the native posture of man, and his production first into it.
>*Urne-Buriall,* Ch. IV

Jean de La Bruyère [1645–1696]

There are but three events which concern man: birth, life, and death. They are unconscious of their birth, they suffer when they die, and they neglect to live.
>*Characters,* "Of Mankind" (tr. by Henri van Laun)

Benjamin Franklin [1706–1790]

A man is not completely born until he be dead.
>Letter to Elizabeth Hubbart, February 22, 1756

Thomas Lovell Beddoes
[1803–1849]

>While men are here,
They should keep close and warm and
>thick together,

Many abreast. Our middle life is
broad;
But birth and death, the turnstiles that
admit us
On earth and off it, send us, one by
one,
A solitary walk.
>*Death's Jest-Book,* Act IV,
>Sc. iv

Alfred, Lord Tennyson
[1809–1892]

Every moment dies a man,
Every moment one is born.
>*The Vision of Sin,* Pt. IV

Mark Twain (Samuel L. Clemens)
[1835–1910]

Why is it that we rejoice at a birth
and grieve at a funeral: It is because
we are not the person involved.
>*The Tragedy of Pudd'nhead
Wilson,* Ch. 9, "Pudd'nhead
Wilson's Calendar"

Anatole France [1844–1924]

They were born, they suffered, they
died.[1]
>*The Opinions of Jérôme Coign-
ard,* Ch. 16 (tr. by Mrs. Wilfred Jackson)

George Santayana [1863–1952]

There is no cure for birth and death
save to enjoy the interval.
>*Soliloquies in England,* 24,
>"War Shrines"

Dying is something ghastly, as being
born is something ridiculous.
>*Three Philosophical Poets,* Ch.
>II

T. S. Eliot [1888–1965]

I believe the moment of birth
Is when we have knowledge of death.
>*The Family Reunion,* Pt. I,
>Sc. ii

[1] A one-sentence "history of man."

Anonymous

The childe was borne: and cryed, became man, after fell sicke, and dyed.
>*The London Prodigall,* I (1605)

Proverbs

The first breath is the beginning of
death.

We are born crying, live complaining,
and die disappointed.

Serbian Proverb

There is only one way to be born and
a thousand ways to die.

BIRTH CONTROL

Hugh Downman [1740–1809]

She who refuses to her young one's lip
Her swelling bosom, each returning
year
Conceives, and each returning year
sustains
The pangs of child-birth. Harrass'd by
fatigue
The strongest constitution fails, but
soon
The weaker system, like a blighted
flower,
Falls under the shock. The nursing
time
Was meant by wisest nature, as a stay,
A vacant interspace, in which the
nerves,
And threads of life unstrung, might
re-assume
Their native tone, endued again with
strength,
And corresponding vigour, to support
The day of toil.
>*Infancy,* "On Infant Nursing"

Ralph Waldo Emerson
[1803–1882]

If government knew how, I should like
to see it check, not multiply the population. When it reaches its true law of

action, every man that is born will be hailed as essential.
The Conduct of Life, Ch. VII

Charles Dickens [1812–1870]

Accidents will occur in the best-regulated families.
David Copperfield, Ch. 28

Rudolf Virchow [1821–1902]

Marriages are not normally made to avoid having children.
Quoted by F. H. Garrison in *Bulletin of the New York Academy of Medicine* 4:995, 1928

George Bernard Shaw [1856–1950]

The most revolutionary invention of the XIX century was the artificial sterilization of marriage.
Man and Superman, "Maxims for Revolutionists"

Laurence Housman [1865–1959]

If Nature had arranged that husbands and wives should have children alternatively, there would never be more than *three* in a family.

Dora Russell [1894–   ]

We want far better reasons for having children than not knowing how to prevent them.
Hypatia, Ch. IV

BLADDER

See also KIDNEY, URINE

Dr. Dunlop [fl. 20th Cent.]

You notice that the tabetic has the power of holding water for an indefinite period. He is also impotent — in fact two excellent properties to possess for a quiet day on the river.
Teaching at Charing Cross Hospital, London

Anonymous

As men draw near the common goal
Can anything be sadder
Than he who, master of his soul,
Is servant to his bladder?
The Speculum, Melbourne, No. 140 (1938)

BLINDNESS

See also EYE, SIGHT

John Skelton [1460?–1529]

But have ye not heard this, —
How an one-eyed man is
Well-sighted when
He is among blind men? [1]
Why Come Ye Not to Courte?

William Shakespeare [1564–1616]

O heavens, this is my true-begotten father! who, being more than sand-blind, high-gravel-blind, knows me not.
The Merchant of Venice, II, ii, 36

He that is strucken blind cannot forget
The precious treasure of his eyesight lost.
Romeo and Juliet, I, i, 239

John Milton [1608–1674]

Why, in truth, should I not bear gently the deprivation of sight, when I may hope that it is not so much lost as revoked and retracted inwards, for the sharpening rather than the blunting of my mental edge?
The Familiar Letters, No. 21, to Emeric Bigot, March 24, 1656 (tr. from Latin by David Masson)

O loss of sight, of thee I most complain!

[1] Cf. Proverb, p. 33a.

Blind among enemies, O worse then
    chains.
Dungeons, or beggery, or decrepit age!
    Samson Agonistes

O dark, dark, dark, amid the blaze of
    noon,
Irrecoverably dark, total Eclipse
Without all hope of day!
    Idem

Doth God exact day-labour, light
    deny'd,
I fondly ask.
    Sonnet XIX, "When I consider
    how my light is spent"

           These eyes, though clear
To outward view, of blemish or of
    spot,
Bereft of light their seeing have forgot;
Nor to their idle orbs doth sight appear
Of sun or moon or star throughout the
    year,
Or man or woman. Yet I argue not
Against Heaven's hand or will, nor
    bate a jot
Of heart or hope, but still bear up
    and steer
Right onward.
    Sonnet XXII, "To Cyriack
    Skinner"

Samuel Pepys [1633–1703]

And so I betake myself to that course,
which is almost as much as to see myself go into my grave: for which, and
all the discomforts that will accompany my being blind, the good God
prepare me!
    Diary, May 31, 1669 (final
    entry)

Colley Cibber [1671–1757]

O say what is that Thing call'd Light,
    Which I must ne'er enjoy;
What is the Blessing of the Sight,
    O tell your poor blind boy?
    The Blind Boy

Alexander Pope [1688–1744]

He from thick films shall purge the
    visual ray,
And on the sightless eyeball pour the
    day.
    Messiah

Tobias Smollett [1721–1771]

A Frenchman wi'l sooner part with
his religion than ·with his hair, which,
indeed, no consideration will induce
him to forego. I know a gentleman
afflicted with a continual head-ach,
and a defluxion on his eyes, who was
told by his physician that the best
chance he had for being cured, would
be to have his head close shaved,
and bathed every day in cold water.
"How (cried he) cut my hair? Mr.
Doctor, your most humble servant!"
He dismissed his physician, lost his
eye-sight, and almost his senses, and
is now led about with his hair in a bag,
and a piece of green silk hanging like
a screen before his eyes.
    *Travels through France and
    Italy*, "Letter from Paris, Oc-
    tober 12, 1763"

Horatio, Lord Nelson
[1758–1805]

I have only one eye — I have a right
to be blind sometimes.[1]
    Quoted by Robert Southey in
    Life of Nelson, Ch. 7

Alfred, Lord Tennyson
[1809–1892]

Thrice as blind as any noon-tide
    owl . . .
Being too blind to have desire to see.
    The Holy Grail

Alice Cary [1820–1871]

My soul is full of whispered song;
    My blindness is my sight;

[1] Putting a telescope to his blind eye,
Nelson used this excuse to ignore a signal
flag that ordered his squadron to retreat
from the Battle of Copenhagen.

The shadows that I feared so long
Are all alive with light.
Dying Hymn

David Seegal [1899–   ]

Why does man have compassion for the
blind
And for the deaf an irritable bind?
*The Pharos of Alpha Omega
Alpha* 28:128, 1965, "Anachronism"

The Bible

Isaac was old, and his eyes were dim,
so that he could not see.
Genesis 27:1

Thou shalt not curse the deaf, nor
put a stumblingblock before the blind.
Leviticus 19:14

But Ahijah could not see; for his eyes
were set by reason of his age.
I Kings 14:4

I was eyes to the blind, and feet was
I to the lame.
Job 29:15

O foolish people, and without understanding; which have eyes, and see
not; which have ears, and hear not.
Jeremiah 5:21

And if the blind lead the blind, both
shall fall into the ditch.
Matthew 15:14

The halt, and the blind.
Luke 14:21

Proverbs

Among the blind, the one-eyed man
is king.[1]

As blind as a bat at noon.

[1] Scottish, African Proverb: In the country [land] of the blind, the one-eyed man
is king.
Cf. John Skelton, p. 31b.

Who so blind as they that will not
see?

German and Spanish Proverb

Better one-eyed than stone blind.

Greek Proverb

A blind man leaned against a wall;
— "This is the boundary of the
world," he said.

BLOOD

See also ANEMIA, ARTERIES,
CIRCULATION

William Shakespeare [1564–1616]

The veins unfill'd, our blood is cold,
and then
We pout upon the morning, are unapt
To give or to forgive; but when we
have stuff'd
These pipes and these conveyances of
our blood
With wine and feeding, we have suppler souls
Than in our priest-like fasts.
Coriolanus, V, i, 51

My heart drops blood.
Cymbeline, V, v, 148

I'll empty all these veins,
And shed my dear blood drop by drop.
Henry IV, Part I, I, iii, 133

The blood weeps from my heart.
Henry IV, Part II, IV, iv, 58

The tide of blood in me
Hath proudly flow'd in vanity till
now.
Now doth it turn and ebb back to the
sea,
Where it shall mingle with the state
of floods
And flow henceforth in formal majesty.
Ibid., V, ii, 129

There is . . .
Scarce blood enough in all their sickly
    veins
To give each naked curtleaxe a stain.
        Henry V, IV, ii, 19

These words of yours draw lifeblood
    from my heart.
        Henry VI, Part I, IV, vi, 43

                            I cannot rest
Until the white rose that I wear be
    dy'd
Even in the lukewarm blood of
    Henry's heart.
        Henry VI, Part III, I, ii, 32

            That surly spirit, melancholy,
Had bak'd thy blood and made it
    heavy, thick,
Which else runs tickling up and down
    the veins.
        King John, III, iii, 42

Yet who would have thought the old
man to have had so much blood in
him?
        Macbeth, V, i, 43

Only my blood speaks to you in my
    veins.
        The Merchant of Venice, III,
        ii, 176

And from the purple fountain Brutus
    drew
    The murd'rous knife, and, as it left
        the place,
    Her blood, in poor revenge, held it
        in chase;

And bubbling from her breast, it doth
    divide
In two slow rivers, that the crimson
    blood
Circles her body in on every side. . . .
    Some of her blood still pure and red
        remain'd,
    And some look'd black, and that
        false Tarquin stain'd.
        The Rape of Lucrece, line 1734

Corrupted blood some watery token
    shows,
And blood untainted still doth red
    abide,
Blushing at that which is so putre-
    fied.
        Ibid., line 1748

With purple fountains issuing from
    your veins!
        Romeo and Juliet, I, i, 92

I am sure my heart wept blood.
        The Winter's Tale, V, ii, 97

Would you not deem it breath'd? and
    that those veins
Did verily bear blood?
        Ibid., V, iii, 63

John Mayow [1640–1679]

The animal spirit is "spiritus nitro-
aeriens" [the oxygen of Lavoisier].
. . . the blood returning from the
brain to the heart is in great part deprived of the nitro-aeric particles which
it has left in the cerebrum and cerebellum for the production of the animal spirits.
        Tractus Quinque, Pt. IV, Ch. 4

Johann Wolfgang von Goethe [1749–1832]

Blood is a very special juice.
        Faust, Part I, Act I, Sc. iv

The Bible

The blood is the life.
        Deuteronomy 12:23

The Talmud

Blood is the originating cause of all
men's diseases.
        Baba Bathra, III.58a

Proverbs

Blood is thicker than water.

Human blood is all of one color.

There's no getting blood out of a turnip.

BLOODLETTING

Moses ben Maimon (Maimonides) [1135–1204]

A person should not accustom himself to constant bloodletting. He should not phlebotomize [himself] except if there is extraordinary need. One should not let blood either in the sunny [summer] months nor in the rainy [winter] season. . . . After 50 years of age, he should not phlebotomize [himself] at all. A person should not be bled and take a bath the same day nor be bled and then undertake a journey nor [be bled] on the day he returns from a journey. On the day of phlebotomy, he should eat and drink less than he is accustomed to, and he should rest on the day of phlebotomy.

> *Mishneh Torah,* "Hilchoth De'oth," Ch. IV, No. 18 (tr. by Fred Rosner in *Annals of Internal Medicine* 62:372, 1965)

Council of Tours [1163]

The church abhors bloodletting.

Jean Fernel [1497–1558]

The physician today seems athirst for blood. Blood-letting, like wine-drinking, is right enough in moderation, but in excess it leads to disaster.

> *Treatise,* 1545 (Quoted by Sir Charles Sherrington in *The Endeavour of Jean Fernel,* Pt. 3)

William Shakespeare [1564–1616]

Let's purge this choler without letting blood.
This we prescribe, though no physician; . . .
Our doctors say this is no month to bleed.

> *Richard II,* I, i, 153

John Donne [1573–1631]

Sometimes, as soon as the *Phisicians* foote is in the *chamber,* his *knife* is in the patients *arme.*

> *Devotions Upon Emergent Occasions,* IX

Robert Burton [1577–1640]

In letting of blood three main circumstances are to be considered, "who, how much, when."

> *The Anatomy of Melancholy,* Pt. 2, Sect. 4, Memb. 3

Samuel Pepys [1633–1703]

Mr. Holliard come to me, and let me blood, about sixteen ounces, I being exceedingly full of blood and very good. I begun to be sick; but lying upon my back I was presently well again, and did give him 5 s. for his pains. . . . after dinner, my arm tied up with a black ribbon, I walked with my wife to my brother Tom's.

> *Diary,* May 4, 1662

Voltaire [1694–1778]

When it [smallpox] is accompanied by malignant fever, when the vessels are so overfilled with blood as to be at the point of bursting, when the blood is about to fly to the brain, and the body is filled with bile and foreign substances which, fermenting, adversely affect the whole organism, then mere commonsense tells us that bleeding is indispensable.

> Letter to Louis de Breteuil, baron de Preuilly, ca. December 5, 1723 (tr. by S. G. Tallentyre)

Oliver Wendell Holmes [1809–1894]

The lancet was the magician's wand of the dark ages of medicine.

> *Medical Essays,* "Some of My Early Teachers"

Hester W. Chapman [1899–   ]

Charles developed a high fever and became so ill that he was let blood five times in as many days. His magnificent constitution survived both the illness and the remedy.

> *The Tragedy of Charles II,*
> Pt. III, Ch. 7

BODY

See also ANATOMY, BODY AND MIND, BODY SNATCHER

Sushruta [5th Cent.? B. C.]

Excessively corpulent and excessively lean persons are alike condemnable. A body which is neither too stout nor too lean, but strikes the mean as regards plumpness, is the best. A lean frame should have the preference to a stout one.

> *Sushruta-Samhitá,* "Sutrasthánam," Ch. 15 (tr. by K. K. L. Bhishagratna)

Plato [427?–347 B.C.]

We are imprisoned in the body, as in an oyster-shell.

> *Phaedrus,* 250.C (tr. by Benjamin Jowett)

Seneca [4? B.C.–A.D. 65]

The body is not a permanent dwelling, but a sort of inn (with a brief sojourn at that) which is to be left behind when one perceives that one is a burden to the host.

> *Moral Epistles to Lucilius,* CXX (tr. by Richard M. Gummere)

Galen [fl. 2nd Cent.]

[Hippocrates] enjoins a thorough study of the nature of the body which we are endeavoring to heal, as well as the properties of all those factors from daily exposure to which the body be-

comes of itself more healthy or more sickly.

> *De Sectis ad eos, qui introducuntur,* III

St. John Chrysostom [345?–407]

This body of ours, so low and small, consists of four elements; viz. of what is warm, that is, of blood; of what is dry, that is, of yellow bile; of what is moist, that is, of phlegm; of what is cold, that is, of black bile.

> *Homilies on the Statutes,* Homily X (tr. by John H. Parker)

Elizabeth I of England [1533–1603]

I know I have the body of a weak and feeble woman, but I have the heart and stomach of a king, — and of a king of England too.

> Speech to the troops at Tilbury on the approach of the Spanish Armada, 1588

Sir Francis Bacon [1561–1626]

Of all substances which nature hath produced, man's body is the most extremely compounded. . . . This variable composition of man's body hath made it as an instrument easy to distemper.

> *The Advancement of Learning,* Bk. II

Sir Thomas Browne [1605–1682]

Now for the wals of flesh, wherein the soule doth seem to be immured before the Resurrection, it is nothing but an elementall composition, and a fabricke that must fall to ashes; *All flesh is grasse,* is not onely metaphorically, but literally true, for all those creatures which we behold, are but the hearbs of the field, digested into flesh in them, or more remotely carnified in our selves. Nay further, we are what we all abhorre, *Antropophagi* and Cannibals, devourers not onely of men, but of our selves; and that not in an allegory, but a positive truth; for all this masse of flesh which wee behold, came in at our mouths: this frame wee looke upon, hath beene upon our trenchers; In briefe, we have devoured our selves and yet do live and remaine our selves.

Religio Medici, Pt. I, Sect. 37

Robert Boyle [1627–1691]

It seems to me . . . highly dishonourable for a Reasonable Soul to live in so Divinely built a Mansion, as the Body she resides in, altogether unacquainted with the exquisite Structure of it.

The Usefulness of Natural Philosophy, Pt. I, Essay V

Baruch Spinoza [1632–1677]

The human body is composed of a number of individual parts, of diverse nature, each one of which is in itself extremely complex.

Ethics, Pt. II, Prop. XIII

John Arbuthnot [1667–1735]

Am I but what I seem, mere flesh and
  blood;
A branching channel, with a mazy
  flood?
The purple stream that through my
  vessels glides,
Dull and unconscious flows like common tides:
The pipes through which the circling
  juices stray,
Are not that thinking I, no more than
  they:
This frame, compacted with tran-
  scendent skill,
Of moving joints, obedient to my will:
Nurs'd from the fruitful glebe, like
  yonder tree,
Waxes and wastes; I call it mine, not
  me.

Know Yourself

Joseph Addison [1672–1719]

I consider the Body as a System of Tubes and Glands, or to use a more Rustick phrase, a Bundle of Pipes and Strainers, fitted to one another after so wonderful a manner as to make a proper Engine for the Soul to work with.

The Spectator, Vol. II, No. 115
(July 12, 1711)

Julien Offroy de La Mettrie [1709–1751]

The human body is a machine which winds its own springs: the living image of perpetual movement.

L'Homme Machine

Thomas Jefferson [1743–1826]

No knowledge can be more satisfactory to a man than that of his own frame, its parts, their functions and actions.

Letter to Dr. Thomas Cooper,
October 7, 1814

Friedrich von Schiller [1759–1805]

Providence, it seems to me, has organized our bodies so miserly that despite constant renewal there is always an excess of consumption.

Prosäische Schriften (Erste Periode), "Ueber den Zusammenhang der thierischen Natur des Menschen mit seiner geistigen," Sect. 27 (tr. by Hans Waine)

Ralph Waldo Emerson [1803–1882]

The human body is the magazine of inventions, the patent office, where are the models from which every hint is taken. All the tools and engines on earth are only extensions of its limbs and senses.

Society and Solitude, "Works and Days"

Oliver Wendell Holmes [1809–1894]

This body in which we journey across

the isthmus between the two oceans is not a private carriage, but an omnibus.
The Guardian Angel, Ch. 3

Herman Melville [1819–1891]

The human body . . . indeed is like a ship; its bones being the stiff standing-rigging, and the sinews the small running ropes, that manage all the motions.
Redburn, Ch. XIII

Walt Whitman [1819–1892]

If any thing is sacred the human body is sacred,
And the glory and sweet of a man is the token of manhood untainted,
And in man or woman a clean, strong, firm-fibred body, is more beautiful than the most beautiful face.
Leaves of Grass, "I Sing the Body Electric"

Samuel Butler [1835–1902]

The body is but a pair of pincers set over a bellows and a stewpan and the whole fixed upon stilts.
Note-Books, Ch. 1

Friedrich Nietzsche [1844–1900]

There is more wisdom in your body than in your deepest philosophy.
Human, All Too Human, Pt. II (tr. by Hans Waine)

Hermann M. Biggs [1859–1923]

The human body is the only machine for which there are no spare parts.
Radio talk (Quoted by Laurence Farmer in *Doctors' Legacy*)

Marcel Proust [1871–1922]

It is in moments of illness that we are compelled to recognise that we live not alone but chained to a creature of a different kingdom, whole worlds apart, who has no knowledge of us and by whom it is impossible to make ourselves understood: our body.
The Guermantes Way, Pt. II, "My Grandmother's Illness" (tr. by C. K. Scott-Moncrieff)

Béla Schick [1877–1967]

The human body is like a bakery with a thousand windows. We are looking into only one window of the bakery when we are investigating one particular aspect of a disease.
Quoted by I. J. Wolf in *Aphorisms and Facetiae of Béla Schick,* "Early Years"

Edna St. Vincent Millay [1892–1950]

For the body at best
Is a bundle of aches,
Longing for rest.
The Buck in the Snow, "Moriturus"

The Bible

All flesh is grass.
Isaiah 40:6

BODY AND MIND

See also BODY, MIND

Huang Ti (The Yellow Emperor) [2697–2597 B.C.]

People . . . should not weary during daytime and they should not allow their minds to become angry.
Nei Ching Su Wên, Bk. 1, Sect. 2 (tr. by Ilza Veith in *The Yellow Emperor's Classic of Internal Medicine*)

Evil customs affect the body as much as wind and rain affect the body.
Ibid., Bk. 2, Sect. 5

When the minds of the people are closed and wisdom is locked out they

remain tied to disease. Yet their feelings and desires should be investigated and made known, their wishes and ideas should be followed; and then it becomes apparent that those who have attained spirit and energy are flourishing and prosperous, while those perish who lose their spirit and energy.
> *Ibid.*, Bk. 4, Sect. 13

Homer [ca. 850 B.C.]

A faultless body and a blameless mind.
> *Odyssey*, III.111 (138 as tr. by Alexander Pope)

Euripides [484–406 B.C.]

Bodies devoid of mind are as statues in the market place.
> *Electra*, 386

Plato [427?–347 B.C.]

The cure of many diseases is unknown to the physicians of Hellas, because they are ignorant of the whole, which ought to be studied also; for the part can never be well unless the whole is well. . . . This . . . is the great error of our day in the treatment of the human body, that the physicians separate the soul from the body.
> *Charmides*, 156.E (tr. by Benjamin Jowett)

Aristotle [384–322 B.C.]

The body is most fully developed from thirty to thirty-five years of age, the mind at about forty-nine.
> *Rhetoric*, II.xiv (tr. by J. H. Freese)

Plautus [254?–184 B.C.]

>   Well in body,
> But sick in mind.
> *Epidicus*, Act I, Sc. ii

Cicero [106–43 B.C.]

In proportion as the strength of the mind is greater than that of the body, so those ills are more severe that are contracted in the mind than those contracted in the body.
> *Philippic Orations*, XI.iv.9 (tr. by W. C. A. Ker)

Lucretius [96?–55 B.C.]

The mind is begotten along with the body, and grows up with it, and with it grows old.
> *On the Nature of Things*, III. 455 (tr. by W. H. D. Rouse)

Ovid [43 B.C.–A.D. 17?]

I am no better in mind than in body; both alike are sick and I suffer double hurt.
> *Tristia*, III.viii.33 (tr. by A. L. Wheeler)

My body is sick but my mind is worse, engrossed in gazing endlessly upon its suffering.
> *Ibid.*, IV.vi.43

Juvenal [60?–140?]

Pray first for a sound mind in a sound body.
> *Satires*, X.356 (tr. by J. Mazzaro)

Pliny the Younger [62–113]

The body must be repaired and supported, if we would preserve the mind in all its vigour.
> *Epistles*, I.9 (tr. by W. Melmoth)

Martin Luther [1483–1546]

Heavy thoughts bring on physical maladies; when the soul is oppressed so is the body.
> *Table-Talk*, Sect. DCXLV, "Of Temptation and Tribulation" (tr. by William Hazlitt)

Sir Francis Bacon [1561–1626]

We see all wise physicians in the prescriptions of their regiments to their patients do ever consider *accidentia animi* [the nature of the

mind], as of great force to further or hinder remedies or recoveries.
> *The Advancement of Learning,* Bk. II

A healthy body is the guest-chamber of the soul; a sick one, its prison.[1]

René Descartes [1596–1650]

The mind is so intimately dependent upon the condition and relation of the organs of the body, that if any means can ever be found to render men wiser and more ingenious than hitherto, I believe that it is in Medicine they must be sought for.
> *Discours de la Méthode,* Pt. VI (tr. by John Veitch)

Duc François de La Rochefoucauld [1613–1680]

Intellectual strength and intellectual weakness are ill-named; they are, in fact, only the manifestation of good or poor functioning on the part of our physical organs.
> *Maxims,* No. 44 (tr. by Constantine FitzGibbon)

John Locke [1632–1704]

As the Strength of the Body lies chiefly in being able to endure Hardships, so also does that of the Mind.
> *Some Thoughts Concerning Education,* Sect. 33

David Hartley [1705–1757]

Thus it may appear, that there ought to be a great reciprocal Influence between the mind and alimentary Duct.
> *Observations on Man,* Vol. 1, Ch. II, Sect. 2

Samuel Johnson [1709–1784]

Are you sick, or are you sullen?
> Letter to James Boswell, November 5, 1784

[1] Attributed to Sir Francis Bacon.

David Hume [1711–1776]

All our perceptions are dependent on our organs and the disposition of our nerves and animal spirits.
> *A Treatise of Human Nature,* I

Georg Christoph Lichtenberg [1742–1799]

When it comes to the body, there are as many imaginary invalids as invalids in fact. When it comes to the mind, there are as many who are only supposed to have sound ones as there are persons who have them in fact.
> *Aphorismen* (1789–1793)

Thomas Jefferson [1743–1826]

A strong body makes the mind strong.
> Letter to Peter Carr, August 19, 1785

Knowledge indeed is a desirable, a lovely possession, but I do not scruple to say that health is more so. It is of little consequence to store the mind with science if the body be permitted to become debilitated. If the body be feeble, the mind will not be strong.
> Letter to Thomas M. Randolph, Jr., August 27, 1786

The most uninformed mind with a healthy body, is happier than the wisest valetudinarian.
> *Ibid.,* July 6, 1787

Friedrich von Schiller [1759–1805]

All significant diseases, especially those issuing from a malignancy of the abdomen, are heralded by a greater or lesser upheaval of personality.
> *Prosäische Schriften* (Erste Periode), "Ueber den Zusammenhang der thierischen Natur des Menschen mit seiner geistigen," Sect. 19 (tr. by Hans Waine)

Charles C. Colton [1780?–1832]

Body and mind, like man and wife, do not always agree to die together.
Lacon, Vol. I, Ch. 324

Leigh Hunt [1784–1859]

The mind may undoubtedly affect the body; but the body also affects the mind. There is a re-action between them; and by lessening it on either side, you diminish the pain on both.
The Indicator, VII, "Advice to the Melancholy"

George Gordon, Lord Byron [1788–1824]

'Tis very certain the desire of life
  Prolongs it: this is obvious to physicians,
When patients, neither plagued with friends nor wife,
  Survive through very desperate conditions,
Because they still can hope. . . .
Despair of all recovery spoils longevity,
And makes men's miseries of alarming brevity.
Don Juan, Canto II, Stanza 64

Peter Mere Latham [1789–1875]

Now the will, I fear, is far less master of the mind than of the body. A man may resolve never to move from his chair, but he cannot resolve never to be angry.
Diseases of the Heart, Lect. XXXVIII

Charles Dickens [1812–1870]

Minds, like bodies, will often fall into a pimpled, ill-conditioned state from mere excess of comfort.
Barnaby Rudge, Ch. 7

Mary Baker Eddy [1821–1910]

Health is not a condition of matter, but of Mind; nor can the material senses bear reliable testimony on the subject of health.
Science and Health, Ch. VI

Mortal mind and body are one. Neither exists without the other, and both must be destroyed by immortal Mind.
Ibid., Ch. VII

Thomas Huxley [1825–1895]

Our mental conditions are simply the symbols in consciousness of the changes which take place automatically in the organism.
Method and Results, "On the Hypothesis that Animals Are Automata, and its History"

Edward L. Trudeau [1848–1915]

I have seen souls grow while bodies shrivel and the really great things of life unfold to a man when all that the world prizes most has been denied.
Letter to James J. Waring, December 23, 1907

George Bernard Shaw [1856–1950]

Mens sana in corpore sano is a foolish saying. The sound body is a product of the sound mind.
Man and Superman, "Maxims for Revolutionists"

A. E. Housman [1859–1936]

Experience has taught me, when I am shaving of a morning, to keep watch over my thoughts, because, if a line of poetry strays into my memory, my skin bristles so that the razor ceases to act. . . . The seat of this sensation is the pit of the stomach.
The Name and Nature of Poetry

Nikolai Lenin [1870–1924]

Sensation is nothing but a direct connection of the mind with the external world; it is the transformation of

energy of external excitation into a mental state.
Materialism and Empirio-Criticism

The most important thing in illness is never to lose heart.
Quoted by Hewlett Johnson in *The Secret of Soviet Strength*, Bk. II, Ch. 3, Sect. 2

Sir Winston Churchill [1874–1965]

When I have had to stand up on parade, or even, I regret to say, in church, for half an hour at a time, I have always felt that the erect position is not natural to man, has only been painfully acquired, and is only with fatigue and difficulty maintained. But no one who is fond of painting finds the slightest inconvenience, as long as the interest holds, in standing to paint for three or four hours at a stretch.
Painting as a Pastime

C. Jeff Miller [1874–1936]

Body and soul cannot be separated for purposes of treatment, for they are one and indivisible. Sick minds must be healed as well as sick bodies.
Surgery, Gynecology & Obstetrics 52:488, 1931

Francis Weld Peabody [1881–1927]

Sickness produces an abnormally sensitive emotional state in almost everyone, and in many cases the emotional state repercusses, as it were, on the organic disease.
The Care of the Patient

J. B. S. Haldane [1892–1964]

I have never yet met a healthy person who worried very much about his health, or a really good person who worried much about his own soul.
The Inequality of Man

Sir Robert Platt [1900–   ]

Future generations, paying tribute to the medical advances of our time, will say: "Strange that they never seemed to realize that the real causes of ill-health were to be found largely in the mind, and that even in 1965 there was hardly a teacher who could talk about sex except in biological terms" (which I must say takes most of the interest out of it).
British Medical Journal 2:551, 1965

Chinese Proverb

The body may be healed, but not the mind.

German Proverb

Sickly body, sickly mind.

BODY SNATCHER

Ambrose Bierce [1842–1914?]

BODY-SNATCHER, n. A robber of grave-worms. One who supplies the young physicians with that with which the old physicians have supplied the undertaker.
The Devil's Dictionary

GRAVE, n. A place in which the dead are laid to await the coming of the medical student.
Ibid.

Anonymous

If anyone shall dig up and plunder a buried corpse and it be proved of him, he shall be outlawed until he comes to an agreement with the relatives of the dead man, and they ask that he be allowed to come among men again.
The Salic Law, LV.2 (ca. 490)

Her body dissected by fiendish men,
Her bones anatomized,

Her soul, we trust, has risen to God,
Where few physicians rise.
          Epitaph of Ruth Sprague [1]

BONES

John Lyly [1554?–1606]

The broken bone, once set together, is
stronger than ever.
          Euphues

William Shakespeare [1564–1616]

Charles in a moment threw him and
broke three of his ribs, that there is
little hope of life in him.
          As You Like It, I, ii, 135

Thy bones are marrowless.
          Macbeth, III, iv, 94

Thy bones are hollow.
          Measure for Measure, I, ii, 56

Is this the poultice for my aching
     bones?
          Romeo and Juliet, II, v, 65

               I love and honour him,
But must not break my back to heal
     his finger.
          Timon of Athens, II, i, 23

Ben Jonson [1573?–1637]

The bones of her fingers ran out at
length, when you prest 'hem, they are
so gently delicate!
          Cynthia's Revels, Act V, Sc. iv

John Webster [1580?–1625?]

Like bones which, broke in sunder,
     and well set,

Knit the more strongly.
          The White Devil, Act II, Sc. i

Anonymous

Old bones are brittle.

BOWELS

See also CONSTIPATION, DYS-
ENTERY, GASTROINTESTIN-
AL TRACT, STOMACH

Moses ben Maimon (Maimonides)
[1135–1204]

Man should always strive to have his
intestines relaxed all the days [of his
life] and that [bowel function] should
approximate diarrhea. This is a fundamental principle in medicine,
[namely] whenever the stool is withheld or is extruded with difficulty,
grave illnesses result.
          Mishneh Torah, "Hilchoth
          De'oth," Ch. IV, No. 13 (tr.
          by Fred Rosner in *Annals of
          Internal Medicine* 62:372,
          1965)

One should examine oneself prior to
entering the bath and after leaving it,
lest excretion of wastes be necessary.
A person should always similarly examine himself before meals and after
meals, before sexual intercourse and
after sexual intercourse, before and
after he exercises and exerts himself,
and before and after he goes to sleep.
The total number of circumstances is
thus ten.
          Ibid., No. 16

Samuel Johnson [1709–1784]

Dear Doctor (said he one day to a
common acquaintance, who lamented
the tender state of his *inside*), do not
be like the spider, man; and spin con-

---

[1] The inscription explains: "Ruth Sprague,
Daughter of Gibson and Elizabeth Sprague.
Died June 11, 1846, aged 9 years, 4 mos.,
and 3 days. She was stolen from the grave
by Roderick R. Clow, dissected at Dr. P. M.
Armstrong's office, in Hoosick, N. Y., from
which place her mutilated remains were obtained and deposited here."

versation thus incessantly out of thy own bowels.

> Quoted by G. B. Hill in *Johnsonian Miscellanies*, Vol. I, "Recollections of Dr. Johnson by Miss Reynolds"

John Abernethy [1764–1831]

One day, for example, a lady took her daughter, evidently most tightly laced, a practice which we believe mothers now are aware is mischievous, but scarcely to the extent known to medical men. She complained of Abernethy's rudeness to her, as well she might; still he gave her, in a few words, a useful lesson. "Why, Madam," said he, "do you know there are upward of thirty yards of bowels squeezed underneath that girdle of your daughter's? Go home and cut it; let Nature have fair play, and you will have no need of my advice."

> Quoted by George Macilwain in *Memoirs of John Abernethy*, Ch. 33

Sir Astley Paston Cooper [1768–1841]

An old Scotch physician, for whom I had a great respect, and whom I frequently met professionally in the city, used to say, as we were entering the patient's room together, "Weel, Mister Cooper, we ha' only twa things to keep in meend, and they'll searve us for here and herea'ter; one is always to have the fear of the Laird before our ees; that'll do for herea'ter; and the t'other is to keep your booels open, and that will do for here.

> *Lectures on Surgery*, Lect. 3

Sir William Withey Gull [1816–1890]

The jejunum is more exempt from morbid conditions than any other portion of the alimentary canal.

> *St. Bartholomew's Hospital Reports* 52:45, 1916

Henry Wheeler Shaw ("Josh Billings") [1818–1885]

I hav finally kum to the konklusion, that a good reliable sett ov bowels iz wurth more tu a man, than enny quantity ov brains.

> *Josh Billings: His Sayings*, Ch. 29

Chinese Proverb

For colic, get the bowels open.

BRAIN

See also MIND, STROKES

Hippocrates [460?–377? B.C.]

From the brain, and from the brain only, arise our pleasures, joys, laughter and jests, as well as our sorrows, pains, griefs and tears. . . . It is the same thing which makes us mad or delirious, inspires us with dread or fear, whether by night or by day, brings sleeplessness, inopportune mistakes, aimless anxieties, absent-mindedness, and acts that are contrary to habit. These things that we suffer all come from the brain, when it is not healthy, but becomes abnormally hot, cold, moist, or dry.

> *The Sacred Disease*, Sect. XVII (tr. by W. H. S. Jones)

Pliny the Elder [23–79]

The brain is the highest of the organs in position, and it is protected by the vault of the head; it has no flesh or blood or refuse. It is the citadel of sense-perception.

> *Natural History*, XI.49 (tr. by H. Rackham)

David Hartley [1705–1757]

The white medullary substance of the brain is the immediate instrument by which ideas are presented to the mind;

or in other words, whatever changes are made in this substance, corresponding changes are made in our ideas, and vice versa.

Observations on Man, I

Julien Offroy de La Mettrie [1709–1751]

The brain has muscles for thinking as the legs have muscles for walking.

L'Homme Machine

William Cullen [1710–1790]

Sensation and volition, so far as they are connected with corporeal motions, are functions of the brain alone. . . . the will operating in the brain only, by a motion begun there, and propagated along the nerves, produces the contraction of the muscles.

Institutions of Medicine, Pt. I, Sect. ii

Alexander Monro II [1733–1817]

For, as the substance of the brain, like that of the other solids of our body, is nearly incompressible, the quantity of blood within the head must be the same, or very nearly the same, at all times, whether in health or disease, in life or after death.

Observations of the Structure and Functions of the Nervous System, Ch. 1, Sect. 4

Pierre Cabanis [1757–1808]

Impressions arriving at the brain make it enter into activity, just as food falling into the stomach excites it to more abundant secretion of gastric juice.

Traité du physique et du moral de l'homme, Second Mémoir

Sir William Lawrence [1783–1867]

Sensation, perception, memory, judgment, reasoning, thought, in a word all the manifestations called mental or intellectual are the animal functions of their appropriate organic apparatus,

the central organ of the nervous system. . . . In opposition to these views it has been contended that thought is not an act of the brain, but of an immaterial substance residing in or connected with it.

Lectures on Comparative Anatomy, Physiology and Zoology

Karl Vogt [1817–1895]

The brain secretes thought as the stomach secretes gastric juice, the liver bile, and the kidneys urine.

Köhlerglaube und Wissenschaft

Johann Wagner [1800?–1833]

The auditory nerves were atrophied. . . . The convolutions of the brain, which was rather soft and edematous, seemed to be twice as deep and twice as numerous as normal.

Report of his autopsy on Ludwig van Beethoven (Quoted by Theodor von Frimmel in *Beethoven Handbuch,* Vol. I, "Leichenöffnung," tr. by Hans Waine)

Emily Dickinson [1830–1886]

The Brain — is wider than the Sky —
For — put them side by side —
The one the other will contain
With ease — and You — beside —

Poems, "The Brain Is Wider Than the Sky"

Auguste Forel [1848–1931]

Every act of thinking is identical with the molecular activity of the brain-cortex that coincides with it.

Die psychischen Fühigkeiten der Ameisen

Santiago Ramón y Cajal [1852–1934]

As long as our brain is a mystery, the universe, the reflection of the structure of the brain, will also be a mystery.

Charlas de Café

The human brain is a world consisting of a number of explored continents and great stretches of unknown territory.
Idem

Sir Charles Sherrington [1861–1952]

Suppose we choose the hour of deep sleep. Then only in some sparse and out of the way places are nodes flashing and trains of light-points running. Such places indicate local activity still in progress. At one such place we can watch the behaviour of a group of lights perhaps a myriad strong. They are pursuing a mystic and recurrent manoeuver as if of some incantational dance. They are superintending the beating of the heart and the state of the arteries so that while we sleep the circulation of the blood is what it should be. The great knotted headpiece of the whole sleeping system lies for the most part dark, and quite especially so the roof-brain. Occasionally at places in it lighted points flash or move but soon subside. Such lighted points and moving trains of light are mainly far in the outskirts, and wink slowly and travel slowly. At intervals even a gush of sparks wells up and sends a train down the spinal cord, only to fail to arouse it. Where however the stalk joins the headpiece, there goes forward in a limited field a remarkable display. A dense constellation of some thousands of nodal points bursts out every few seconds into a short phase of rhythmical flashing. At first a few lights, then more, increasing in rate and number with a deliberate crescendo to a climax, then to decline and die away. After due pause the efflorescence is repeated. With each such rhythmic outburst goes a discharge of trains of travelling lights along the stalk and out of it altogether into a number of nerve branches. What is this doing? It manages the taking of our breath the while we sleep.
Man on His Nature, Ch. 7

Martin H. Fischer [1879–1962]

The brain is our pacemaker.
Quoted by Howard Fabing and Ray Marr in *Fischerisms*

Aleksandr Blok [1880–1921]

The brain is not an organ to be relied upon. It is developing monstrously. It is swelling like a goitre.

BREATHING

Huang Ti (The Yellow Emperor) [2697–2597 B.C.]

When man grows old . . . there is much gas within his thorax, resulting in panting and troubled breathing.
Nei Ching Su Wên, Bk. 6, Sect. 19 (tr. by Ilza Veith in *The Yellow Emperor's Classic of Internal Medicine*)

Leonardo da Vinci [1452–1519]

These muscles have a voluntary and an involuntary movement seeing that they are those which open and shut the lung. When they open they suspend their function which is to contract, for the ribs which at first were drawn up and compressed by the contracting of these muscles then remain at liberty and resume their natural distance as the breast expands. And since there is no vacuum in nature the lung which touches the ribs from within must necessarily follow their expansion; and the lung therefore opening like a pair of bellows draws in the air in order to fill the space so formed.
Dell' Anatomia, Fogli A (tr. by Edward MacCurdy in *The Notebooks of Leonardo da Vinci,* Vol. I, Ch. III)

Philip Thicknesse [1719–1792]

If diseases are conveyed from man, to man, by the breath (a fact which cannot be disputed) why may we not conclude that youthful breath conveys Health and Long Life to the aged? Every body has experienced the sweetness of the breath of cows, and, for that reason it is esteemed wholesome, and as the fragrancy of young people's breath, who are brought up under a proper regimen, falls little short of that of cows, it is natural to suppose, that it is productive of the same virtue.[1]

> *The Valetudinarian's Bath Guide, or The Means of Obtaining Long Life and Health,* Ch. 5, Sect. 8

William Morris [1834–1896]

Some folk seem glad even to draw their breath.
> *The Earthly Paradise,* "Bellerophon at Argos"

Kenneth T. Bird [1917–   ]

A medical chest specialist is long-winded about the short-winded.

BRUISES

Charles Dickens [1812–1870]

My pa is one mask of brooses both blue and green.
> *Nicholas Nickleby,* Ch. 15

CANCER

Andrew Boorde [1490–1549]

Carcinoma is the greke worde. In englyshe it is named the sickenes of the prison. And some auctours doth say

[1] Thicknesse states that he got his hints on wholesome breathing (taking in great gulps of pure air) from Hermippus Redivius, who he thinks was either a tutor or a director of a college of young virgins.

that it is a Canker, the whiche doth corode and eate the superial partes of the body, but I do take it for the sickenes of the prison.
> *Brevyary,* Fol. XXVI, Ch. 59

William Heberden [1710–1801]

Cancers of the tongue and mouth begin with a small hard lump, and sometimes with a little sore; both of which are attended with pricking pains, and they spread in the same manner with cancerous sores in other parts. This is so great an evil, that the slightest suspicion of it occasions very great uneasiness.
> *Commentaries on the History and Cure of Diseases,* Ch. 56

Elisha Bartlett [1804–1855]

Cancerous disorganization of the stomach, in some instances, gives no indication of its existence, sufficiently distinct to render its detection possible, during life, even by the most competent and careful observers: and the same thing is true in the case of most other diseases.
> *Philosophy of Medical Science,* Pt. II, Ch. 10

Rutherford Morison [1853–1939]

In men nine out of ten abdominal tumours are malignant; in women nine out of ten abdominal swellings are the pregnant uterus.
> Quoted in *The Practitioner,* October 1965

August Bier [1861–1949]

There is a tremendous literature on cancer, but what we know for sure about it can be printed on a calling card.

Charles H. Mayo [1865–1939]

While there are several chronic diseases more destructive to life than cancer none is more feared.
> *Annals of Surgery* 83:357, 1926

Marcel Proust [1871–1922]

After a certain lapse of time the cancer patient dies. It is very rare that at the end of the same amount of time the inconsolable widower is not cured.
> *The Sweet Cheat Gone,* Ch. 3, "Venice" (tr. by Justin O'Brien)

William Boyd [1885–   ]

When we think of cancer in general terms we are apt to conjure up a process characterized by a steady, remorseless and inexorable progress in which the disease is all-conquering, and none of the immunological and other defensive forces which help us to survive the onslaught of bacterial and viral infections can serve to halt the faltering footsteps to the grave.
> *The Spontaneous Regression of Cancer*

Anonymous

A story circulated [at a medical meeting] about a man who had decided gradually to give up everything that scientists have linked to cancer.
The first week, he cut out smoked fish and charcoal steaks.
The second week, he cut out smoking.
The third week, he cut out having relations with women.
The fourth week, he cut out drinking.
The fifth week, he cut out paper dolls.
> Quoted in the *Boston Herald,* September 4, 1965

CASTRATION

Ovid [43 B.C.–A.D. 17?]

He who first robbed boys of their nature should himself have suffered the wounds he made.
> *The Art of Love,* II.iii.3 (tr. by G. Showerman)

William Shakespeare [1564–1616]

Does your worship mean to geld and splay all the youth of the city?
> *Measure for Measure,* II, i, 242

I'll geld 'em all.
> *The Winter's Tale,* II, i, 147

CAUSES

Mo-tze [fl. 5th–4th Cents. B.C.]

The physician who is attending a patient . . . has to know the cause of the ailment before he can cure it.
> *Ethical and Political Works,* Bk. IV, Ch. XIV (tr. by Yi-pao Mei)

Aristotle [384–322 B.C.]

Conscientious and careful physicians allocate causes of disease to natural laws, while the ablest scientists go back to medicine for their first principles.

Cicero [106–43 B.C.]

Physicians consider that, when they have discovered the cause of disease, they have also discovered the method of treating it.
> *Tusculan Disputations,* III.x.23 (tr. by J. E. King)

Celsus [25 B.C.–A.D. 50]

A reckoning up of the cause often solves the malady.
> *De Medicina,* Prooemium (tr. by W. G. Spencer)

I am of the opinion that the Art of Medicine ought to be rational, but to draw instruction from evident causes, all obscure ones being rejected from the practice of the Art, although not from the practitioner's study.
> *Idem*

Marcus Aurelius [121–180]

In the series of things, those which follow are always aptly fitted to those which have gone before: for this series is not like a mere enumeration of disjointed things, which has only a necessary sequence, but it is a rational connection: and all existing things are arranged together harmoniously, so the things which come into existence exhibit no mere succession, but a certain wonderful relationship.

Meditations, IV.45 (tr. by G. Long)

John Hunter [1728–1793]

All the causes of things cannot be seen, because they appear to depend on circumstances which are unknown, or appear to be accidental.

Quoted by S. R. Gloyne in *John Hunter*

Baron Justus von Liebig [1803–1873]

We are too much accustomed to attribute to a single cause that which is the product of several, and the majority of our controversies come from that.

Louis Pasteur [1822–1895]

All things are hidden, obscure and debatable if the cause of the phenomena be unknown, but everything is clear if this cause be known.

The Germ Theory and Its Application to Medicine and Surgery, Ch. 2 (tr. by H. C. Ernst)

Marcel Proust [1871–1922]

In pathology certain conditions similar in appearance are due, some to an excess others to an insufficiency of tension, of secretion and so forth.

Within a Budding Grove, Pt. I (tr. by C. K. Scott-Moncrieff)

Wilfred Trotter [1872–1939]

The fundamental activity of medical science is to determine the ultimate causation of disease.

Collected Papers, "De Minimus," Sect. 5

Henry E. Sigerist [1891–1957]

Disease has social as well as physical, chemical, and biological causes.

CHARACTER

Ralph Waldo Emerson [1803–1882]

A dome of brow denotes one thing, a pot-belly another; a squint, a pug-nose, mats of hair, the pigment of the epidermis, betray character.

The Conduct of Life, Ch. I

Benjamin Disraeli, Lord Beaconsfield [1804–1881]

There is no index of character so sure as the voice.

Tancred, Bk. II, Ch. 1

Alan Gregg [1890–1957]

Probably other psychological approaches should be added to the conditioned reflexes — in order to reveal the slow and cumulative experiences by which an individual becomes unique.

Scientific Monthly 58:365, 1944

Proverb

The choleric drinks, the melancholic eats, the phlegmatic sleeps.

CHARITY

Hippocrates [460?–377? B.C.]

Sometimes give your services for nothing. . . . And if there be an opportunity of serving one who is a stranger in financial straits, give full assistance

to all such. For where there is love of man, there is also love of the art.
> *Precepts,* Sect. VI (tr. by W. H. S. Jones)

St. Jerome [340?–420]

Of gold she would not wear so much as a seal-ring, choosing to store her money in the stomachs of the poor rather than to keep it at her own disposal.
> *Letter CXXVII* (tr. by W. H. Fremantle)

Judah ibn-Tibbon [1120–1190]

If thou receivest payment from the rich, attend gratuitously upon the poor.
> *The Last Will of Rabbi Judah Aben Tibbon* (tr. by Hirsch Edelman in *The Path of Good Men*)

Hermann Boerhaave [1668–1738]

My best patients are the poor because the Lord has taken it upon Himself to pay me for them.
> Quoted by Jean Cruveilhier in a letter

John Morgan [1735–1789]

I shall always esteem it a favourable circumstance, that puts it in my power to administer relief to persons, whose indigence forbids them to expect it upon any other terms.
> *A Discourse Upon the Institution of Medical Schools in America,* Preface

John Abernethy [1764–1831]

Private patients, if they do not like me, can go elsewhere; but the poor devils in the hospital I am bound to take care of.
> Quoted by George Macilwain in *Memoirs of John Abernethy,* Ch. 5

Jesse R. Burden [1798–1875]

If you attend a poor person gratis, you will seldom be called into the family of a rich and aspiring relative, and if the poor person become rich you are the last, probably, that he will employ. If you complain of this treatment, it will show that your charity is like sounding brass or a tinkling cymbal. He who confers a benefit ought never to remember it, if he be wise and good.
> Valedictory address, Philadelphia College of Medicine, July 19, 1850

Think not of the return of gratitude, and never expose yourselves by repeating what you have done, or of complaining of the ingratitude of the recipients.
> *Idem*

Robert Browning [1812–1889]

> Who studious in our art
> Shall court a little labor unrepaid.
> *Strange Medical Experience of Karshish, the Arab Physician*

Abraham Coles [1813–1891]

O it is well that ye have hearts to feel
And ears not deaf to pity's soft appeal,
Putting no difference 'twixt rich and poor,
Plying with equal zeal the means of cure,
Not deeming it becoming to regard
Color or rank or person or reward.
> *The Microcosm,* "Physician's Character and Aims — Science Progressive"

Harvey Cushing [1869–1939]

To the medical profession, if not to the community in general, *The Dispensary* [by Samuel Garth] must always remain of historic import, commemorating as it does the first attempt to establish those out-patient rooms, which since have become such a universal charity.
> Quoted by Mary Lou McDonough in *Poet Physicians*

Alan Gregg [1890–1957]

In medicine, charity offers to the poor the gains in medical skill, not the leavings.
The Bampton Lectures

When society cannot afford to have what it cannot afford to be without, it is the occasion for intelligent giving.

The Bible

Charity suffereth long, and is kind; charity envieth not; charity vaunteth not itself, is not puffed up.
　Doth not behave itself unseemly, seeketh not her own, is not easily provoked, thinketh no evil;
　Rejoiceth not in iniquity, but rejoiceth in the truth;
　Beareth all things, believeth all things, hopeth all things, endureth all things. . . .
　And now abideth faith, hope, charity, these three; but the greatest of these is charity.
I Corinthians 13:4

The Talmud

The house which is not opened for charity will be opened to the physician.

CHEERFULNESS

Pindar [522?–443 B.C.]

The best of healers is good cheer.
Nemean Ode, IV.1 (tr. by J. Sandys)

Nicholas Udall [1505–1556]

For mirth prolongeth life, and causeth health.
Ralph Roister Doister, Prologue

Sir Francis Bacon [1561–1626]

To be free-minded and cheerfully disposed at hours of meat and of sleep and of exercise, is one of the best precepts of long lasting.
Essays, "Of Regiment of Health"

Joseph Addison [1672–1719]

Health and Chearfulness mutually beget each other.
The Spectator, Vol. V, No. 387 (May 24, 1712)

Laurence Sterne [1713–1768]

I live in a constant endeavour to fence against the infirmities of ill health, and other evils of life, by mirth.
Tristram Shandy, Dedication

Arthur Murphy [1727–1805]

Chearfulness, Sir, is the principal Ingredient in the Composition of Health.
The Apprentice (1764), Act II, Sc. iv

John Wolcot ("Peter Pindar") [1738–1819]

Care to our coffin adds a nail, no doubt,
And ev'ry grin, so merry, draws one out.
Expostulatory Odes, Ode XV

William James [1842–1910]

Happiness is no positive feeling, but a negative condition of freedom from a number of restrictive sensations of which our organism usually seems to be the seat.

Santiago Ramón y Cajal [1852–1934]

The joviality of friends is the best antidote for the venom of the world and the fatigues of life. In the words of the old song: "He loves me who makes me laugh."
Charlas de Café

Elbert G. Hubbard [1856–1915]

Optimism: A kind of heart stimulant — the digitalis of failure.
The Roycroft Dictionary

The Bible

Pleasant words are as an honeycomb, sweet to the soul, and health to the bones.

Proverbs 16:24

A merry heart doeth good like a medicine: but a broken spirit drieth the bones.

Proverbs 17:22

CHILBLAINS

Thomas Hood [1799–1845]

Another weepeth over chilblains fell, Always upon the heel, yet never to be well!

The Irish Schoolmaster

CHILD HEALTH

See also CHILDREN

Hippocrates [460?–377? B.C.]

I hold that it is better to give children only the most diluted wine.

On Airs, Waters and Places, IX (tr. by Francis Adams)

Moses ben Maimon (Maimonides) [1135–1204]

Honey and wine are bad for children but salutary for the elderly.

Mishneh Torah, "Hilchoth De'oth," Ch. 4, No. 12 (tr. by Fred Rosner in *Annals of Internal Medicine* 62:372, 1965)

Thomas Phaer [1510?–1560]

Slepe is the nouryshment and food of a sucking child.

The Boke of Chyldren

Felix Würtz [1518–1576]

None will grow more straight in his body than those who are laid free and loose in the limbs in a sheltered, ample-spaced cradle.

Quoted by A. V. Neale in *The Advancement of Child Health*

William Cadogan [1711–1797]

Children, in general, are overclothed and overfed. To these causes, I impute most of their diseases.

Essays upon Nursing and Management of Children

George Armstrong [d. 1781]

If you take away a sick Child from its Parent or Nurse you break its Heart immediately: also, if there must be a Nurse to each Child what kind of an Hospital must there be to contain any Number of them. . . . Add to all this it very seldom happens that a Mother can conveniently leave the Rest of her Family to go into an Hospital to attend her sick infant.

Catherine II of Russia [1729–1796]

Go to any village: The number of children born to most peasant families is ten, twelve, often as many as twenty. Yet only one, two or maybe four of these are living. Reduce the mortality rate, consult doctors, do something about the care of young children. . . . They run about naked in their shifts in the snow and ice. Those who survive are healthy, but nineteen out of twenty die, *and what a loss to the state.*

Quoted by Zoé Oldenbourg in *Catherine the Great,* Ch. 35 (tr. by Anne Carter)

William Black [1771–1811]

Up to this century the management of these tender creatures in sickness was left to ignorant old nurses and rude quackery.

History of Medicine

Sir Winston Churchill
[1874–1965]

There is no finer investment for any community than putting milk into babies.
> Radio broadcast, March 21, 1943

Béla Schick [1877–1967]

After nine months of pregnancy a mother is entitled to have her baby get safe care. To expose her newborn to infection is criminal.
> Quoted by I. J. Wolf in *Aphorisms and Facetiae of Béla Schick,* "Early Years"

Edward Anthony [1895–   ]

Eat no green apples or you'll droop,
Be careful not to get the croup,
Avoid the chicken-pox and such
And don't fall out of windows much.
> *Advice to Small Children*

A. V. Neale [1899–   ]

As the Lord Chancellor has said of good judges, so we may say of good child-health experts — they must have impartiality, the gift of wise silence, wide knowledge of human and natural laws, a quick grasp of fact, and vast experience of human nature.
> *The Advancement of Child Health,* Ch. 5

Meyer A. Perlstein [1902–   ]

Pediatricians eat because children don't.

John F. Kennedy [1917–1963]

The needs of children should not be made to wait.
> *Message to Congress on the Nation's Youth,* February 14, 1963

We can say with some assurance that, although children may be the victims of fate, they will not be the victims of our neglect.
> Remarks on signing the Maternal and Child Health and Mental Retardation Planning Bill, October 24, 1963

Anonymous [ca. 1470]

Till now the babes oft died with ills unknown, for none was there with skill to aid.
> Quoted by A. V. Neale in *The Advancement of Child Health*

Proverb

A naughty child is better sick than whole.

Chinese Proverb

If a child is constantly sick, it is due to overfeeding.

CHILDBIRTH

See also BIRTH, BIRTH CONTROL, MIDWIFE, TWINS

Euripides [484–406 B.C.]

What they say of us is that we have a
    peaceful time
Living at home, while they do the
    fighting in war.
How wrong they are! I would very
    much rather stand
Three times in the front of battle
    than bear one child.
> *Medea,* 248 (tr. by R. Warner)

Pliny the Elder [23–79]

There is nothing encourageth a woman sooner to be barren than hard travail in child bearing.
> *Natural History*

It is contrary to nature for children to come into the world with feet first.
> *Ibid.,* VII.8 (tr. by J. Bostock and H. T. Riley)

Sir Thomas More [1478–1535]

It is for trouth reported, that the Duches his mother had so muche a doe in her travaile, that shee coulde not bee delivered of hym uncutte: and that hee [Richard III] came into the worlde with the feete forwarde, as menne bee borne outwarde, and (as the fame runneth) also not untothed.
The History of King Richard III

William Shakespeare [1564–1616]

Thy mother felt more than a mother's pain,
And yet brought forth less than a mother's hope,
To wit, an indigested and deformed lump,
Not like the fruit of such a goodly tree.
Teeth hadst thou in thy head when thou wast born.
Henry VI, Part III, V, vi, 49

I came into the world with my legs forward.
Ibid., V, vi, 71

The Queen's in labour,
They say in great extremity, and fear'd
She'll with the labour end.
Henry VIII, V, i, 18

Finger of birth-strangled babe
Ditch-deliver'd by a drab.
Macbeth, IV, i, 30

What shall be done, sir, with the groaning Juliet?
She's very near her hour.
Measure for Measure, II, ii, 15

The lady shrieks and, well-a-near,
Does fall in travail with her fear.
Pericles, III, Chorus, 51

Divinest patroness and midwife gentle
To those that cry by night, . . .
make swift the pangs
Of my queen's travails!
Ibid., III, i, 11

A terrible childbed hath thou had.
Ibid., III, i, 57

In childbed died she, but brought forth
A maid child.
Ibid., V, iii, 5

This child was prisoner to the womb, and is
By law and process of great Nature thence
Freed and enfranchis'd.
The Winter's Tale, II, ii, 59

John Hall [1627–1656]

Great births are hard in the labour, and many glorious men have been cut out of the womb.
The Dissolution of the Late Parliament

William Blake [1757–1827]

My mother groan'd! my father wept.
Into the dangerous world I leapt:
Helpless, naked, piping loud:
Like a fiend hid in a cloud.
Songs of Experience, "Infant Sorrow"

John Greenleaf Whittier [1807–1892]

But care and sorrow, and childbirth pain,
Left their traces on heart and brain.
Maud Muller

Ignaz Semmelweis [1818–1865]

When I look back upon the past, I can only dispel the sadness which falls upon me by gazing into that happy future when the infection will be banished. . . . The conviction that such a time must inevitably sooner or later arrive will cheer my dying hour.[1]
Etiology, Foreword

[1] Semmelweis discovered the infectious nature of childbirth fever and how physicians transmitted it, but was not believed at the time.

Clarence Darrow [1857–1938] **and William Jennings Bryan** [1860–1925]

MR. DARROW: Do you believe that after Eve ate the apple, or gave it to Adam — whichever way it was — God cursed Eve, and at that time decreed that all womankind thenceforth and forever should suffer the pains of childbirth in the reproduction of the earth?
MR. BRYAN: I believe what it says, and I believe the fact as fully.
> Cross-examination of Bryan by Darrow at the Scopes trial, July 21, 1925 (Quoted by Leslie H. Allen in *Bryan and Darrow at Dayton*)

W. W. Chipman [1866–1950]

Parturition is a physiological process — the same in the countess and in the cow.

Boris Pasternak [1890–1960]

At the moment of child-birth, every woman has the same aura of isolation, as though she were abandoned, alone. . . . It is the woman, by herself, who brings forth her progeny, and carries it off upstairs, to some top storey of life, a quiet, safe place for a cradle. Alone, in silence and humility, she feeds and rears the child.
> *Doctor Zhivago*, Ch. 9, Sect. 3 (tr. by Max Hayward and Manya Harari)

The Bible

Unto the woman he said, I will greatly multiply thy sorrow and thy conception; in sorrow thou shalt bring forth children.
> *Genesis* 3:16

Give me children, or else I die.
> *Genesis* 30:1

The Hebrew women are not as the Egyptian women; for they are lively, and are delivered ere the midwives come in unto them.
> *Exodus* 1:19

A woman when she is in travail hath sorrow, because her hour is come: but as soon as she is delivered of the child, she remembereth no more the anguish, for joy that a man is born into the world.
> *John* 16:21

CHILDREN

See also CHILD HEALTH, CHILDBIRTH, MATERNITY, PARENTS

Plato [427?–347 B.C.]

But at three, four, five, and even six years the childish nature will require sports; now is the time to get rid of self-will in him, punishing him, but not so as to disgrace him.
> *Laws*, VII.794 (tr. by Benjamin Jowett)

Ferrarius [16th Cent.]

Infants do not cry without some legitimate cause.
> Quoted by A. V. Neale in *The Advancement of Child Health*

Infants savour of the nature of the person by whom they are suckled.
> *Idem*

William Shakespeare [1564–1616]

How sharper than a serpent's tooth it is
To have a thankless child!
> *King Lear*, I, iv, 297

A grievous burthen was thy birth to me;
Tetchy and wayward was thy infancy.
> *Richard III*, IV, iv, 168

George Herbert [1593–1633]

The growth of flesh is but a blister;
Childhood is health.
> *The Temple*, "Holy Baptism"

John Milton [1608–1674]

The childhood shews the man,
As morning shews the day.
Paradise Regained, Bk. IV

William Wordsworth [1770–1850]

Him whom you love, your Idiot Boy.
The Idiot Boy

The child is father of the man.
My Heart Leaps Up

Sydney Smith [1771–1845]

What is childhood but a series of happy delusions?
Quoted by Lady Holland in *A Memoir of the Rev. Sydney Smith*, Ch. 11

Robert Southey [1774–1843]

The days of childhood are but days of woe.
The Retrospect

Charles Brown [1786–1842]

Between you & me, I think an infant is disagreeable, — it is all gut and squall.
Letter to John Keats, December 21, 1820

Oliver Wendell Holmes [1809–1894]

Children betray their tendencies in their way of dealing with the breasts that nourish them.
Medical Essays, "Border Lines of Knowledge in Some Provinces of Medical Science"

Prince Otto von Bismarck [1815–1898]

You can do anything with children if you only play with them.

Sir John Lubbock, Baron Avebury [1834–1913]

It is customary, but I think it is a mistake, to speak of happy childhood. Children, however, are often over-anxious and acutely sensitive. Man ought to be man and master of his fate; but children are at the mercy of those around them.
The Pleasures of Life, Pt. I, Ch. I

William G. Sumner [1840-1910]

It used to be believed that the parent had unlimited claims on the child and rights over him. In a truer view of the matter, we are coming to see that the rights are on the side of the child and the duties on the side of the parent.
The Forgotten Man's Almanac, October 14

Ambrose Bierce [1842–1914?]

CHILDHOOD, n. The period of human life intermediate between the idiocy of infancy and the folly of youth — two removes from the sin of manhood and three from the remorse of age.
The Devil's Dictionary

Luther Burbank [1849–1926]

If we had paid no more attention to plants than we have to our children, we would now be living in a jungle of weeds.

Eugene Field [1850–1895]

Here we have a baby. It is composed of a Bald Head and a Pair of Lungs.
The Tribune Primer, "The Baby"

Albert Schweitzer [1875–1965]

I was a very sickly child when we moved to Günsbach. On the occasion of my father's induction my mother had decked me out as finely as she could in a white frock with coloured ribbons, but not one of the pastors' wives that had come to the ceremony

56

ventured to compliment her on her thin and yellow-faced baby, and none of them went beyond embarrassed commonplaces. So at last my mother — she has often told me about it — could restrain herself no longer: she fled with me in her arms to the bedroom, and there wept hot tears over me.

> *Memoirs of Childhood and Youth,* Ch. 1 (tr. by C. T. Campion)

There was another incident of my earliest childhood which I remember as the first occasion on which I consciously, and on account of my own conduct, felt ashamed of myself. I was still in petticoats, and was sitting on a stool in the yard while my father was busy about the beehives. Suddenly a pretty little creature settled on my hand, and I watched it with delight as it crawled about. Then all at once I began to shriek. The pretty little creature was a bee, which had a good right to be angry when the pastor was robbing him of the honey-filled combs in his hive, and to sting the robber's little son in revenge! My cries brought the whole household round me, and everyone pitied me. The servant-girl took me in her arms and tried to comfort me with kisses, while my mother reproached my father for beginning to work at the hives without first putting me in a place of safety. My misfortune having made me so interesting an object, I went on crying with much satisfaction, till I suddenly noticed that, although the tears were still pouring down, the pain had disappeared. My conscience told me to stop, but in order to be interesting a bit longer I went on with my lamentations, so getting a lot more comforting than I really needed. However, this made me feel such a little rogue that I was miserable over it all the rest of the day. How often in after life, when assailed by tempta-

tion, has this experience warned me against exaggerating, or making too much of, whatever has happened to me!

> *Idem*

Béla Schick [1877–1967]

Children are not simply micro-adults, but have their own specific problems.

> Quoted by I. J. Wolf in *Aphorisms and Facetiae of Béla Schick,* "Early Years"

Will Durant [1885–   ]

The tired mothers found that spanking took less time than reasoning, and penetrated sooner to the seat of memory. My mother spared the rod, because she preferred to use her hand.

> *Transition,* Ch. 1

André Maurois [1885–1967]

A child's feelings are none the less acute for being in part unwarranted. There are bastards of the imagination, born in wedlock, who nevertheless feel themselves to be rejected by their parents, without knowing why. These more than others long for worldly triumphs, to compensate for their deep-rooted sense of loss.

> *Prometheus: The Life of Balzac,* Pt. I, Ch. 1 (tr. by Norman Denny)

Alan Gregg [1890–1957]

Our national inclination to suffer children gladly, prolong adolescence patiently, and deliberately defer maturity.

> *Scientific Monthly* 58:365, 1944

Theodor S. Geisel ("Dr. Seuss") [1904–   ]

A child . . . is the last container of a sense of humor, which disappears as he gets older and he laughs only according to the way the boss, society,

politics or the race want him to. Then he becomes an adult. And an adult is an obsolete child.
> *New York Mirror,* May 18, 1958

John Ciardi [1916–]

Among the hopes of this world, none shines more promisingly than the external resilience with which some children manage to escape into humanity from even the dreariest of parents.
> *Saturday Review,* August 10, 1963

Anonymous

Not so much attention is paid to our children's minds as is paid to their feet.
> Quoted by A. V. Neale in *The Advancement of Child Health*

The pediatric psychiatrist vehemently defended his viewpoint that he liked children in the abstract but not in the concrete as he watched them track through his newly poured cement walk.

Proverb

Late children, early orphans.

English Proverb

Children suck the mother when they are young, and the father when they are old.

Estonian Proverb

A child [remains a child] until there is another child.

Italian Proverb

When children are little they make our heads ache; when grown, our hearts.[1]

[1] Czech Proverb: Small children stamp on your lap, big ones on your heart.
Romany Proverb: When they are young they are arm-achy, and when they are old they are heart-achy.

CIRCULATION

See also ARTERIES, BLOOD, HEART

Leonardo da Vinci [1452–1519]

All the veins and arteries proceed from the heart; and the reason is that the maximum thickness that is found in these veins and arteries is at the junction that they make with the heart; and the farther away they are from the heart the thinner they become and they are divided into more minute ramifications.
> *Dell' Anatomia,* Fogli B (tr. by Edward MacCurdy in *The Notebooks of Leonardo da Vinci,* Vol. I, Ch. III)

William Shakespeare [1564–1616]

I send it through the rivers of your blood
Even to the court, the heart, to th' seat o' th' brain,
And, through the cranks and offices of man,
The strongest nerves and small inferior veins
From me receive that natural competency
Whereby they live.
> *Coriolanus,* I, i, 139

As dear to me as are the ruddy drops
That visit my sad heart.
> *Julius Caesar,* II, i, 288

William Harvey [1578–1657]

What remains to be said upon the quantity and source of the blood which thus passes, is of so novel and unheard-of a character that I not only fear injury to myself from the envy of a few, but I tremble lest I have mankind at large for my enemies, so much doth wont and custom, that become as a second nature, and doctrine once sown and that hath struck deeproot, and respect for antiquity influence all men: Still the die is cast, and my trust is in my love of truth, and the candour that inheres in cultivated minds.

> *On the Motion of the Heart and Blood in Animals,* Ch. 8 (tr. by Robert Willis)

Sir William Osler [1849–1919]

The physics of a man's circulation are the physics of the waterworks of the town in which he lives, but once out of gear, you cannot apply the same rules for the repair of the one as of the other.

> *Aequanimitas, with Other Addresses,* "On the Educational Value of the Medical Society"

Anonymous [ca. 1550 B.C.]

Everywhere he feels his Heart because its vessels run to all his limbs.

> *The Ebers Papyrus,* Ch. XX, "The Beginning of the Secret Book of the Physician" (tr. by Cyril P. Bryan) [1]

CIRCUMCISION

Ralph Waldo Emerson [1803–1882]

The circumcision is an example of the power of poetry to raise the low and offensive.

> *Essays* (Second Series), "The Poet"

The Bible

Ye shall circumcise the flesh of your foreskin; and it shall be a token of the covenant betwixt me and you.

> *Genesis* 17:11

[1] This manuscript is a collection of extracts and jottings from about forty written and oral sources, some of which may predate it by two millennia; because it survives intact, Bryan calls it "the most ancient book in the world."

Circumcised the eighth day, of the stock of Israel, of the tribe of Benjamin, an Hebrew of the Hebrews.[1]

> *Philippians* 3:5

CLIMATE

Lucretius [96?–55 B.C.]

As we see these four climates to be diverse under the four winds and quarters of heaven, so the colour and aspect of men are seen to be widely different and diseases to possess the nations after their kind.

> *On the Nature of Things,* VI. 1110 (tr. by W. H. D. Rouse)

Sir Thomas Browne [1605–1682]

He is happily seated who lives in Places whose Air, Earth, and Water, promote not the Infirmities of his weaker Parts, or is early removed into Regions that correct them. He that is tabidly inclined, were unwise to pass his days in *Portugal:* Cholical Persons will find little Comfort in *Austria* or *Vienna:* He that is Weak-legg'd must not be in Love with *Rome,* nor an infirm Head with *Venice* or *Paris.* Death hath not only particular Stars in Heaven, but malevolent Places on Earth, which single out our Infirmities, and strike at our weaker Parts.

> *A Letter to a Friend*

John Arbuthnot [1667–1735]

The Air has an Influence in forming the Languages of Mankind: The serrated close way of Speaking of Northern Nations, may be owing to their Reluctance to open their Mouth wide in cold Air, which must make their Language abound in Consonants; whereas from a contrary Cause, the inhabitants of warmer Climates open-

[1] Paul's description of himself.

ing their Mouths, must form a softer Language, abounding in Vowels.
> *An Essay Concerning The Effects of Air on Human Bodies,* Ch. 6, Sect. 20

Ogden Nash [1902–   ]

Winter comes but once a year,
And when it comes it brings the doctor good cheer.
> *I'm a Stranger Here Myself,* "Summergreen for President"

Richard Armour [1906–   ]

Some hoist the windows, gasp for air,
While others find it chilly.
Some turn up thermostats a hair,
While others think them silly.

Some like it cold, some like it hot,
Some freeze, while others smother.
And by some fiendish, fatal plot
They marry one another.
> *Light Armour,* "Room Temperature"

American Proverb

The California climate makes the sick well and the well sick, the old young and the young old.

Danish Proverb

Fresh air impoverishes the doctor.

Flemish Proverb

Where there is sunshine no doctors are wanted.[1]

CLINICIAN

See also PHYSICIANS

Thomas Addis [1881–1949]

A clinician is complex. He is part craftsman, part practical scientist, and

part historian; so his several classifications involve, in varying degree, all these elements. It is only if we look at him when he is working with his patients that we find him single-minded. Then he is wholly pragmatic and utilitarian. His only design is to bring relief, and he is not at all scrupulous about how he does it.
> *Glomerular Nephritis, Diagnosis and Treatment,* Ch. 5

Young clinicians, dazzled by new experimental methods, are in danger of becoming poor doctors, and they should remember that they are doctors, first, last and all the time.
> Quoted in *Journal of the Mount Sinai Hospital* 10:41, 1943

Anonymous

CLINICIAN: learns less and less about more and more until he knows nothing about everything.
RESEARCHER: learns more and more about less and less until he knows everything about nothing.

COFFEE

Sydney Smith [1771–1845]

If you want to improve your understanding, drink coffee.
> Quoted by Lady Holland in *A Memoir of the Rev. Sydney Smith,* Ch. 11

Jesse Torrey [1787–1834]

Coffee, though a useful medicine, if drank constantly, will at length induce a decay of health, and hectic fever.
> *The Moral Instructor,* Pt. IV, Sect. II, Ch. 10

Hungarian Proverb

Good coffee should be black like the devil, hot like hell, and sweet like a kiss.

[1] Italian (Sardinian) Proverb: When the sun enters, the doctor remains outside.

COLDS

William Shakespeare [1564–1616]

Let him walk from whence he came, lest he catch cold on 's feet.
The Comedy of Errors, III, i, 37

'Tis dangerous to take a cold.
Henry IV, Part I, II, iii, 9

A whoreson cold, sir, a cough, sir, which I caught with ringing in the King's affairs upon his coronation day, sir.
Henry IV, Part II, III, ii, 193

You will catch cold, and curse me.
Troilus and Cressida, IV, ii, 15

John Webster [1580?–1625?]

I have caught
An everlasting cold; I have lost my voice
Most irrecoverably.
The White Devil, Act V, Sc. vi

Thomas Jefferson [1743–1826]

A person not sick will not be injured by getting wet. It is but taking a cold bath which never gives a cold to any one.
Letter to Thomas M. Randolph, Jr., August 27, 1786

Jane Austen [1775–1817]

My sore-throats, you know, are always worse than anybody's.
Persuasion, Ch. 18

Charles Lamb [1775–1834]

Do you know what it is to succumb under an insurmountable day mare — a whoreson lethargy, Falstaff calls it — an indisposition to do any thing — a total deadness and distaste — a suspension of vitality — an indifference to locality — a numb soporifical good-fornothingness — an ossification all over — an oyster-like insensibility to the passing events — a mind-stuper — a brawny defiance to the needles of a thrusting-in conscience — did you ever have a very bad cold with a total irresolution to submit to water gruel processes? . . . Who shall deliver me from the body of this death?
Letter to Bernard Barton, January 9, 1824

Henry David Thoreau [1817–1862]

There are sure to be two prescriptions diametrically opposite. Stuff a cold and starve a cold are but two ways.
A Week on the Concord and Merrimack Rivers, "Wednesday"

William Ralph Inge [1860–1954]

I am thinking not only of their [doctors'] great skill — though I think I should think even more of them if they had discovered how to prevent and how to cure a common cold.
Address to students of the London Hospital, 1933

Frank (Kin) Hubbard [1868–1930]

A bad cold wouldn' be so annoyin' if it wuzn' fur th' advice of our friends.
Brown County Primer

Bernarr MacFadden [1868–1955]

If you feed a cold, as is often done, you frequently have to starve a fever.
Physical Culture, February 1934

Sir Alexander Fleming [1881–1955]

A good gulp of hot whisky at bedtime — it's not very scientific, but it helps.
News summary, March 22, 1954

Robert Benchley [1889–1945]

If you think that you have caught a cold, call in a good doctor. Call in three good doctors and play bridge.
From Bed to Worse, "How to Avoid Colds"

Woods Hutchinson [20th Cent.]

A person's age is not dependent upon the number of years that have passed over his head, but upon the number of colds that have passed through it.
Quoted by Dr. Shirley W. Wynne

English Proverbs

A May cold is a thirty-day cold.

Stuff a cold and starve a fever.

German Proverb

Sauerkraut is good for a cold.

Indian (Telugu) Proverb

One cold in the head is as bad as ten diseases.

COMMITTEE MEETINGS

Sir Robert Christison [1797–1882]

We shall have long sittings, much fighting is anticipated.
Quoted by W. K. Pyke-Lees in *Medical Ethics,* Ch. II

Sir James Paget [1814–1899]

We sat for eight days, and on six of them decided to do nothing.
Idem

Irvine H. Page [1901–   ]

I came, I saw, I concurred! [1]
Journal of the American Medical Association 194:1355, 1965

[1] A medical committeeman's complaint.

COMMUNICATION

See also TERMINOLOGY, WRITING

Voltaire [1694–1778]

Why then, asked the Sirian, do you quote this Aristotle in Greek? It is, the learned man replied, because it is wiser to quote that which one does not understand at all, in the language that one comprehends least.[1]

René Laënnec [1781–1826]

Do not fear to repeat what has already been said. Men need [the truth] dinned into their ears many times and from all sides. The first rumor makes them prick up their ears, the second registers, and the third enters.

Peter Mere Latham [1789–1875]

Beware of language, for it is often a great cheat.
Diseases of the Heart, Lect. XI

Almost all language is figurative, and so far may obscure as well as illustrate the subject which it is used to denote.
General Remarks on the Practice of Medicine, Ch. XVI

Men are apt to talk largely and at random about what they are agreed to praise.
Ibid., Ch. XVII

Karl F. H. Marx [1796–1877]

More than the hand is the tongue the organ which can do most good and evil.
Quoted by F. H. Garrison in *Bulletin of the New York Academy of Medicine* 4:1001, 1928

[1] Cf. Richard Asher, p. 612b.

Edward Bulwer-Lytton
[1803–1873]

In science, address the few, in literature, the many. In science, the few must dictate opinion to the many; in literature, the many, sooner or later, force their judgment on the few.
> *Caxtoniana,* "Readers and Writers"

Sir William Osler [1849–1919]

In the life of every successful physician there comes the temptation to toy with the Delilah of the press—daily and otherwise. There are times when she may be courted with satisfaction, but beware! Sooner or later she is sure to play the harlot, and has left many a man shorn of his strength, viz., the confidence of his professional brethren.
> *Aequanimitas, with Other Addresses,* "Internal Medicine as a Vocation"

You may learn to consume your own smoke. The atmosphere is darkened by the murmurings and whimperings of men and women over the non-essentials, the trifles that are inevitably incident to the hurly-burly of the day's routine. Things cannot always go your way. Learn to accept in silence the minor aggravations, cultivate the gift of taciturnity and consume your own smoke with an extra draught of hard work, so that those about you may not be annoyed with the dust and soot of your complaints.
> *Ibid.,* "The Master-Word in Medicine"

Never hide the work of others under your own name.
> Quoted by William B. Bean in *Sir William Osler: Aphorisms,* Ch. 2

William J. Mayo [1861–1939]

Begin with an arresting sentence; close with a strong summary; in between speak simply, clearly, and always to the point; and above all be brief.
> Quoted by Helen Clapesattle in *The Doctors Mayo*

Edward H. Goodman [1879–   ]

It is a distinct art to talk medicine in the language of the non-medical man.

Alphonse Raymond Dochez
[1882–1964]

The performance of an experiment in basic science or clinical medicine is not enough; it is the investigator's moral as well as scientific obligation to make the new fact known to the profession.
> Quoted in *P & S Quarterly* 11:18, June 1966

Lawrence K. Frank [1890–   ]

Our language is a "verbal tissue slice" which abstracts the living process from time and space and immobilizes it for discussion.
> *Annals of the New York Academy of Sciences* 50:189, 1948

Don't quote me, that's what you heard, not what I said.

Arthur M. Walker [1896–1955]

The resounding brass of ill-considered claims in the public press.
> Quoted by Julius L. Wilson in *Walkerisms*

CONCEPTION

See also PREGNANCY, SEX

Ashurbanipal [669–626 B.C.]

Does a woman conceive when a virgin, or grow fat without eating?

Pliny the Elder [23–79]

If ten dayes after a woman hath had the company of a man shee feele an

extraordinary ache in the head, and perceive giddinesse in the brain as if all things went round; find a dazling and mistinesse, in the eies, abhorring and loathing meat, and withall a turning and wambling in the stomacke; it is a signe that she is conceived, and beginneth to breed.[1]
> *Natural History,* VII.vi (tr. by Philemon Holland)

Plutarch [46?–120?]

It is said that no woman ever produced a child without the cooperation of a man.
> *Moralia,* "Advice to Bride and Groom" (tr. by F. C. Babbitt)

Marcus Aurelius [121–180]

A man passes seed into a womb and goes his way, and anon another cause takes it in hand and works upon it and perfects a babe — what a consummation from what a beginning!
> *Meditations,* X.26 (tr. by C. R. Haines)

Charles Darwin [1809–1882]

Man is developed from an ovule, about the 125th of an inch in diameter, which differs in no respect from the ovules of other animals.
> *The Descent of Man,* Ch. 1

Rutherford Morison [1853–1939]

Never neglect the history of a missed menstrual period.
> Quoted in *The Practitioner,* October 1965

The Bible: Apocrypha

And in my mother's womb was fashioned to be flesh in the time of ten months, being compacted in blood, of the seed of man, and the pleasure that came with sleep.
> *The Wisdom of Solomon* 7:2

CONSCIENCE

Michel de Montaigne [1533–1592]

The laws of conscience, which we say are born of nature, are born of custom.
> *Essays,* Bk. I, Ch. 23, "Of Custom, and Not Easily Changing an Accepted Law" (tr. by Donald M. Frame)

William E. Gladstone [1809–1898]

The disease of an evil conscience is beyond the practice of all the physicians of all the countries in the world.
> Speech at Plumstead, 1878

T. S. Eliot [1888–1965]

What people call their conscience . . . is just the cancer
That eats away the self.
> *The Family Reunion,* Pt. I, Sc. i

It is not my conscience,
Not my mind, that is diseased, but the world I have to live in.
> *Idem*

CONSERVATISM

Lucius Cary, Viscount Falkland [1610?–1643]

When it is not necessary to change, it is necessary not to change.
> *A Discourse of Infallibility*

Samuel Johnson [1709–1784]

How many men in a year die through the timidity of those they consult for health!

---

[1] Holland's elaboration is considerably more graphic than a literal translation (by H. Rackham) of the Latin:
> On the tenth day from conception pains in the head, giddiness and dim sight, distaste for food, and vomiting are symptoms of the formation of the embryo.

Emil Du Bois-Reymond
[1818–1896]

Where we do not know, let us be cautious.[1]

Camille Flammarion [1842–1925]

There are men who would even be afraid to commit themselves to the doctrine that castor oil is a laxative.

CONSTIPATION

See also BOWELS

Moses ben Maimon (Maimonides)
[1135–1204]

How can a person heal his intestines if they are slightly constipated? If he is a young boy, he should eat salty foods, cooked and spiced with olive oil, fish brine and salt, without bread, every morning; or he should drink the liquid of boiled spinach or cabbage in olive oil and fish brine and salt. If he is an old man, he should drink honey mixed with warm water in the morning and wait approximately four hours, and then he should eat his meal. He should do this for one day or three or four days if it is necessary, until his intestines soften [and move freely].
> *Mishneh Torah*, "Hilchoth De'oth," Ch. IV, No. 13 (tr. by Fred Rosner in *Annals of Internal Medicine* 62:372, 1965)

Anyone who lives a sedentary [life] and does not exercise or he who postpones his excretions or he whose intestines are constipated, even if he eats good foods and takes care of himself according to [proper] medical principles — all his days will be painful ones and his strength will wane.
> *Ibid.*, No. 15

[1] Ignorabimus, dubitemus.

Tobias Smollett [1721–1771]

Doctor, the pills are good for nothing — I might as well swallow snow-balls to cool my reins — I have told you over and over, how hard I am to move; and at this time of day, I ought to know something of my own constitution.
> *The Expedition of Humphry Clinker*, Letter 1

CONSULTATION

See also SPECIALIST

Hippocrates [460?–377? B.C.]

Physicians who meet in consultation must never quarrel, or jeer at one another.
> *Precepts*, VIII (tr. by W. H. S. Jones)

John Halle [1529–1568]

When thou arte callde at anye time,
A patient to see:
And dost perceave the cure too grate,
And ponderous for thee:

See that thou laye disdeyne aside,
And pride of thyne owne skyll:
And thinke no shame counsell to take,
But rather wyth good wyll.

Gette one or two of experte men,
To helpe thee in that nede;
And make them partakers wyth thee
In that work to procede. . . .

But one thinge note, when two or moe
Together joygned be;
Aboute the paynfull patient,
See that ye doe agree.

See that no discorde doe arise,
Nor be at no debate;
For that shall sore discomforte hym,
That is in sycke estate. . . .

For noughte can more discomforte him,
That lies in griefe and peyne,
Then heare that one of you dothe beare
To other suche disdeine.
> *An Historiall Expostulation . . . with a goodlye Doctrine and Instruction*

John Donne [1573–1631]

But where there is room for *consultation,* things are not desperate. They *consult;* so there is nothing *rashly, inconsideratly* done; and then they *prescribe,* they *write,* so there is nothing *covertly, disguisedly, unavowedly* done.
> *Devotions Upon Emergent Occasions,* IX

Sir Samuel Garth [1] [1661–1719]

See, one physician, like a sculler plies,
The patient lingers and by inches dies,
But two physicians, like a pair of oars
Waft him more swiftly to the Stygian shores.

Thomas Jefferson [1743–1826]

Whenever he saw three physicians together, he looked up to discover whether there was not a turkey buzzard in the neighborhood.
> Quoted by Dr. Everett, private secretary to President James Monroe

Oliver Wendell Holmes [1809–1894)

Now when a doctor's patients are perplexed,
A *consultation* comes in order next —
You know what that is? In a certain place
Meet certain doctors to discuss a case
And other matters, such as weather, crops,
Potatoes, pumpkins, lager-beer, and hops.

[1] Attributed to Sir Samuel Garth.

For what's the use? — there's little to be said,
Nine times in ten your man's as good as dead;
At best a talk (the secret to disclose)
Where three men guess and *sometimes* one man knows.
> *Rip Van Winkle, M.D.,* Canto II

William Green Brownson [1830–1899]

In manner brusk, pompous in air and style,
He greets his brother with the blandest smile,
With new found friends shakes hands with relish keen,
Happy to see them, happier to be seen.
His conversation he directs to these,
With studied effort to attract and please; . . .
His fine impression made, he condescends
To interview the doctor and the friends;
And, ere he sees the case, states his belief
That he can soon suggest a prompt relief.
He quickly scans the case, and feigns to see
At once the lesion and the remedy;
Tells of a dozen cases he has had
Within a year, with symptoms quite as bad.
And thus the farce of consultation ends;
What further he discloses to the friends
We ne'er shall know; but sometimes it transpires,
He gets the case — his brother soon retires.
> *The Country Doctor,* "The Consultation"

Louis A. Duhring [1845–1913]

Remember that the sufferer is entitled to every aid and suggestion that can be obtained, and that in the event of a fatal issue the blame of not seeking consultations with more experienced heads may rest upon you. Keep in mind that some one else may possess experience, skill, or knowledge that you do not happen to have.

> Valedictory address, University of Pennsylvania Medical School, June 7, 1894

Sir William Osler [1849–1919]

Can anything be more doleful than a procession of four or five doctors into the sick man's room?

> *Montreal Medical Journal* 24: 518, 1896

Proverb

While doctors consult, the patient dies.[1]

Chinese Proverb

In a dangerous illness call in three doctors.

German Proverb

No doctor is better than three.

CONTAGION

See INFECTION, MICROBES

CONTROVERSY

William Clowes [1544–1604]

I have heretofore said there is no book so profitable for matter or so pleasant for penning which has not had from time to time some that have misliked it in both parts, not only backbiters and whisperers, but also such as will seem to say somewhat, lest they should be suspected to know little or nothing, who have not sticked to set themselves as it were in a despiteful

and mortall hatred against many profitable works.

> *A Profitable and Necessarie Booke of Observations* (ed. by F. N. L. Poynter in *Selected Writings*, Ch. 21)

William Harvey [1578–1657]

It cannot be helped that dogs bark and vomit their foul stomachs, or that cynics should be numbered among philosophers; but care can be taken that they do not bite or inoculate their mad humours, or with their dogs' teeth gnaw the bones and foundations of truth.

> *On the Circulation of the Blood*, "Second Essay to Jean Riolan" (tr. by Robert Willis)

Alexander Pope [1688–1744]

Like Doctors thus, when much dispute has past,
We find our tenets just the same at last.

> *Moral Essays*, Epistle III

John Jones [1729–1791]

Thus men of more enlighten'd genius and more intrepid spirit must compose themselves to the risque of public censure, and the contempt of their jealous contemporaries, in order to lead ignorant and prejudic'd minds into more happy and successful methods.

> Introductory lecture to his course in surgery

William Hazlitt [1778–1830]

When a thing ceases to be a subject of controversy, it ceases to be a subject of interest.

> *The Atlas*, January 31, 1830, "The Spirit of Controversy"

Hermann von Helmholtz [1821–1894]

Metaphysicians, like all those who cannot give any decisive reasons to their

---

[1] Cf. Italian Proverb, p. 371b.

opponents, are usually not very polite in their controversy; one's own success may approximately be estimated from the increasing want of politeness in the replies.

> *Das Denken in der Medizin*
> (tr. by E. Atkinson in *Popular Lectures on Scientific Subjects,* Vol. II)

Rudolf Virchow [1821–1902]

Has not science the noble privilege of carrying on its controversies without personal quarrels?

> Quoted by F. H. Garrison in *Bulletin of the New York Academy of Medicine* 4:995, 1928

Louis Pasteur [1822–1895]

I do not forget that Medicine and Veterinary practice are foreign to me. I desire judgment and criticism upon all my contributions. Little tolerant of frivolous or prejudiced contradiction, contemptuous of that ignorant criticism which doubts on principle, I welcome with open arms the militant attack which has a method in doubting and whose rule of conduct has the motto "More light."

> *The Germ Theory and Its Applications to Medicine and Surgery,* Ch. 12, Sect. III (tr. by H. C. Ernst)

Thomas Huxley [1825–1895]

Gladstone's first article [an attack on science] caused such a flow of bile that I have been the better for it ever since.

> Letter to Sir John Skelton, January 21, 1886

A polemic is as little abhorrent to me as gin to a reclaimed drunkard.

Mark Twain (Samuel L. Clemens) [1835–1910]

It were not best that we should all think alike; it is difference of opinion that makes horse-races.

> *The Tragedy of Pudd'nhead Wilson,* Ch. 19, "Pudd'nhead Wilson's Calendar"

Santiago Ramón y Cajal [1852–1934]

It is best to attenuate the virulence of our adversaries with the chloroform of courtesy and flattery, much as bacteriologists disarm a pathogen by converting it into a vaccine.

> *Charlas de Café*

The most effective and economical of all reactions to injury is silence.

> *Idem*

Sir F. M. R. Walshe [1888–   ]

Criticism is dead only in fields of knowledge that are not advancing. In periods of high intellectual ferment in any branch of knowledge, creation and criticism are equal and equally active partners. Destroy one, you destroy the other.

> *Perspectives in Biology and Medicine* 2:197, 1959

William E. Tanner [1889–   ]

The surgeon's ideas, even if abstract, must be put into practice before they can be judged. The man who puts his thoughts into action will always excite opposition, for the mind is more conscious of the effect of deeds than of words.

> *Sir W. Arbuthnot Lane,* Epilogue

Work which is useful may receive approbation and become a standard for others. Work which excites opposition and criticism is also valuable if it leads to ideas of permanent value. Even if wrong in conception or execution it may be valuable if it directs thought and action into new and previously unexplored paths.

> *Idem*

Alan Gregg [1890–1957]

Be sparing of criticism, since the habit of trivial comment weakens the force of real protest.
> Aphorism (Quoted by Wilder Penfield in *The Difficult Art of Giving*, Appendix A)

CONVALESCENCE

George Bernard Shaw [1856–1950]

I enjoy convalescence. It is the part that makes the illness worth while.
> *Back to Methuselah*, Pt. II, "Gospel of the Brothers Barnabas"

CORNS

William Shakespeare [1564–1616]
> Ladies that have their toes
> Unplagu'd with corns will have a bout with you.
> *Romeo and Juliet*, I, v, 18

Jonathan Swift [1667–1745]

A coming shower your shooting corns presage,
Old a-ches throb, your hollow tooth will rage.
> *A Description of a City Shower*

John Gay [1685–1732]

And when too short the modish shoes are worn,
You'll judge the seasons by your shooting corn.
> *Trivia*, Bk. I

James Gibbons Huneker [1860–1921]

My corns ache, I get gouty, and my prejudices swell like varicose veins.
> *Old Fogy*, Ch. I

COSMETICS

Samuel Butler [1835–1902]

In their eagerness to stamp out disease, these people overshot their mark; for people had become so clever at dissembling — they painted their faces with such consummate skill — they repaired the decay of time and the effects of mischance with such profound dissimulation — that it was really impossible to say whether any one was well or ill till after an intimate acquaintance of months or years. Even then the shrewdest were constantly mistaken in their judgements, and marriages were often contracted with most deplorable results, owing to the art with which infirmity had been concealed.
> *Erewhon*, Ch. XIV

COUGH

Sir Thomas Browne [1605–1682]

The ancient Inhabitants of this Island were less troubled with Coughs when they went naked, and slept in Caves and Woods, than Men now in Chambers and Feather-beds.
> *A Letter to a Friend*

Samuel Johnson [1709–1784]

Cough: A convulsion of the lungs, vellicated by some sharp serosity.
> *Dictionary*

Charles Lamb [1775–1834]

My bedfellows are Cough and cramp, we sleep 3 in a bed.
> Letter to Edward Moxon, April 27, 1833

English Proverb

A dry cough is the trumpeter of death.

Latin Proverb

Love and a cough cannot be hidden.[1]

CRAMPS

William Shakespeare [1564–1616]

He would have liv'd many a fair year
. . . if it had not been for a hot midsummer night; for (good youth) he
went but forth to wash him in the
Hellespont, and being taken with the
cramp, was drown'd.
> *As You Like It,* IV, i, 100

To-night thou shalt have cramps,
Side-stitches that shall pen thy breath
up.
> *The Tempest,* I, ii, 325

I'll rack thee with old cramps,
Fill all thy bones with achës.
> *Ibid.,* I, ii, 369

Go, charge my goblins that they grind
their joints
With dry convulsions, shorten up their
sinews
With aged cramps.
> *Ibid.,* IV, i, 259

O, touch me not! I am not Stephano,
but a cramp.
> *Ibid.,* V, i, 286

Charles Lamb [1775–1834]

My bedfellows are Cough and cramp,
we sleep 3 in a bed.
> Letter to Edward Moxon, April
> 27, 1833

Charles Dickens [1812–1870]

In came a fiddler . . . and tuned like
fifty stomach-aches.
> *A Christmas Carol,* Stave II

---

[1] French Proverb: Love, a cough, smoke,
and money cannot long be hid.
　German Proverb: Love, fire, the itch, a
cough, and gout are not to be concealed.
　Indian (Hindi) Proverb: Lust, fire, cough,
these three are not concealed.
　Venetian Proverb: Love, a cough, the itch,
and the stomach cannot be hid.

CRIPPLES

Sir Francis Bacon [1561–1626]

Deformed persons commonly take revenge on nature.
> *The Advancement of Learning,*
> Bk. VI, Ch. 3

William Shakespeare [1564–1616]

Would ye not think his cunning to be
great that could restore this cripple to
his legs again?
> *Henry VI, Part II,* II, i, 133

Where's that valiant crookback prodigy?
> *Henry VI, Part III,* I, iv, 75

She did corrupt frail nature with some
bribe
To shrink mine arm up like a wither'd
shrub;
To make an envious mountain on my
back,
Where sits deformity to mock my
body;
To shape my legs of an unequal size;
To disproportion me in every part.
> *Ibid.,* III, iii, 155

If thou . . . wert grim,
Ugly, and sland'rous to thy mother's
womb,
Full of unpleasing blots and sightless
stains,
Lame, foolish, crooked, swart, prodi-
gious,
Patch'd with foul moles and eye-
offending marks,
I would not care.
> *King John,* III, i, 43

I, that am curtail'd of this fair pro-
portion,
Cheated of feature by dissembling
Nature,
Deform'd, unfinish'd, sent before my
time
Into this breathing world, scarce half
made up,

And that so lamely and unfashionable
That dogs bark at me as I halt by
them.
>　*Richard III*, I, i, 18

That bottled spider, that foul bunch-
back'd toad.
>　*Ibid.*, IV, iv, 81

William Hay [1695–1755]

Another great Advantage of Deformity
is, that it tends to the Improvement
of the Mind. A man, that cannot shine
in his Person, will have recourse to his
Understanding: and attempt to adorn
that Part of him, which alone is capable of ornament.
>　*Essay on Deformity*

Walter B. Pitkin [1878–1953]

Many people are better off with grave
handicaps than with trifling ones. The
grave handicaps release copious energies.
>　*Life Begins at Forty*

The Bible

I was eyes to the blind, and feet was
I to the lame.
>　*Job* 29:15

The halt, and the blind.
>　*Luke* 14:21

Latin Proverb

If you dwell with a lame man, you will
learn to limp.

CULTS

Samuel Hahnemann [1755–1843]

Like cures like.[1]
>　Motto for homeopathy

Ralph Waldo Emerson
[1803–1882]

Homeopathy is insignificant as an act

[1] Cf. Hippocrates, p. 492a.

of healing, but of great value as criticism on the hygeia or medical practice
of the time.
>　*Essays* (Second Series), "Nom-
>　inalist and Realist"

Oliver Wendell Holmes
[1809–1894]

A disease for Hahnemann consists essentially in a group of symptoms. The
proper medicine for any disease is the
one which is capable of producing a
similar group of symptoms when given
to a healthy person.
>　*Medical Essays*, "Homoeopathy
>　and Its Kindred Delusions"

As one humble member of a profession
which for more than two thousand
years has devoted itself to the pursuit
of the best earthly interests of mankind, always assailed and insulted
from without by such as are ignorant
of its infinite perplexities and labors,
always striving in unequal contest
with the hundred-armed giant who
walks in the noonday, and sleeps not
in the midnight, yet still toiling, not
merely for itself and the present moment, but for the race and the future, I
have lifted my voice against this lifeless delusion, rolling its shapeless bulk
into the path of a noble science it is
too weak to strike, or to injure.
>　*Idem*

Homoeopathy [is] . . . a mingled mass
of perverse ingenuity, of tinsel erudition, of imbecile credulity, and of
artful misrepresentation, too often
mingled in practice . . . with heartless and shameless imposition.
>　*Idem*

The vulgar quackeries drop off, atrophied, one after another. Homoeopathy has long been encysted, and is
carried on the body medical as quietly
as an old wen.
>　*Ibid.*, "Scholastic and Bedside
>　Teaching"

Mary Baker Eddy [1821–1910]

Christian Science explains all cause and effect as mental, not physical.
Science and Health, Ch. VI

Frank Kittredge Paddock
[1841–1901]

It is interesting how infrequently one hears ill spoken of those who are carried along on the coattails of medicine: the osteopaths, chiropractors, naturopaths and such. It may be that those who consult them are ashamed to spread about the horrid result brought about by reputation being greater than result.
Aphorism

Ambrose Bierce [1842–1914?]

HOMEOPATHY, n. A school of medicine midway between Allopathy and Christian Science. To the last both the others are distinctly inferior, for Christian Science will cure imaginary diseases, and they can not.
The Devil's Dictionary

Finley Peter Dunne ("Mr. Dooley") [1867–1936]

"I think," said Mr. Dooley, "that if th' Christyan Scientists had some science an' th' doctors more Christianity, it wudden't make anny diff'rence which ye called in — if ye had a good nurse."
Mr. Dooley's Opinions, "Christian Science"

H. L. Mencken [1880–1956]

Any plumber of today, when he loses hope of setting up a studio of his own, is free to become an osteopath, a bootlegger or a labor leader. It is hard for a man with that possibility always before him to become class conscious.
Baltimore Evening Sun, August 11, 1924

Noah D. Fabricant [1904–   ]

Most medical fads are like some women's fashions — frail, fickle and costly.
Amusing Quotations for Doctors and Patients, "Fads"

Once a medical fad is dead, its evils are soon forgotten — but so are its victims.
Idem

South Carolina Legislature

Osteopathy shall be defined as a complete system of therapeutics embracing all scientific subjects pertaining to the healing art except materia medica. Instead it places emphasis on structural integrity as a major essential to health and that any derangement of structural integrity is a fundamental cause of disease, by interfering with the natural function of immunity and nutrition. Practice consists principally in the correction of all structural derangement by manipulative measures including physio and electro therapy, minor surgery, diet, hygiene and obstetrics.
Acts of the Legislature, 1938

CURES

See also REMEDIES, TREATMENT

Hippocrates [460?–377? B.C.]

For extreme diseases, extreme methods of cure, as to restriction, are most suitable.
Aphorisms, I.6 (tr. by Francis Adams)

Marius [155?–86 B.C.]

The cure is not worth the pain.[1]
Quoted by Plutarch in *Lives,* VI.3 (tr. by John Dryden)

[1] Said after having had a varicose vein cut from his leg.

Seneca [4? B.C.–A.D. 65]

It is part of the cure to wish to be cured.
> *Hippolytus,* 249

Nothing hinders a cure so much as frequent change of medicine; no wound will heal when one salve is tried after another.
> *Moral Epistles to Lucilius,* II.iii (tr. by Richard M. Gummere)

Tacitus [55?–after 117]

From the nature of human frailty, cure operates more slowly than disease, and . . . the body itself is slow to grow and quick to decay.
> *Agricola,* 3 (tr. by M. Hutton)

William Roper [1496–1578]

There in his [Sir Thomas More's] Chappell, . . . incontynentt [1] came into his mynd that a glister [2] should be thonly way to helpe her. [3] Which, when he told the phisitions, they by and by confessed that, if there were any hope of health, that was the very best helpe indeed, much marvailinge of themselfes that they had not before remembred it.

Then was it ymmediately ministred unto her sleapinge, which she could by no meanes have bine brought unto wakinge. And albeit after that she was therby throughly awaked, gods markes, an evident undoubted token of death, plainely appeared upon her, yeat she, contrary to all their expectacions, was, as it was thought, by her fathers fervent prayer myraculously recoverid, and at length againe to perfect health restored. Whom, if it had pleased god at that tyme to have taken to his mercye, her father said he wold never have medled with worldly matters after.
> *The Life of Sir Thomas More, Knight*

Michael Servetus (Villanovanus) [1511–1553]

The king [Francis I of France] himself by his touch cures those suffering from struma or scrofula. I myself have seen the king touch many attacked by this ailment but I have never seen any cured.
> Observations added to his 1535 edition of Ptolemy's *Geography* (tr. by Charles D. O'Malley in *Michael Servetus,* Ch. 1)

Michel de Montaigne [1533–1592]

The sick man is not to be pitied who has a cure up his sleeve.
> *Essays,* Bk. III, Ch. 3, "Of Three Kinds of Association" (tr. by Donald M. Frame)

William Clowes [1544–1604]

> *Hippocrates* in his aphorisme, as *Galen* writeth sure,
> Saith, foure things are needfull to every kinde of cure.
> The first, saith he, to God belongeth the chiefest part,
> The second to the Surgeon, who doth apply the art.
> The third unto the medicine, that is dame Natures friend,
> The fourth unto the patient, with whom I heere will end.
> How then may a Surgeon appoint a time, a day or houre,
> When three parts of the cure are quite without his power.
> *Profitable and Necessarie Book of Observations*

---

[1] incontynent(ly) = immediately.
[2] glister = clyster, enema.
[3] Margaret More Roper, daughter of Sir Thomas More and wife of the author, was suffering from the sweating sickness.

Sir Francis Bacon [1561–1626]

As for the just cure, it must answer to the particular disease; and so be left to counsel rather than rule.

> *Essays,* "Of Seditions and Troubles"

William Shakespeare [1564–1616]

We thank you, maiden;
But may not be so credulous of cure,
When our most learned doctors leave us.

> *All's Well That Ends Well,* II, i, 118

DOCTOR: There are a crew of wretched souls
That stay his cure. Their malady convinces
The great assay of art; but at his touch,
Such sanctity hath heaven given his hand,
They presently amend.
MALCOLM: I thank you, doctor.
MACDUFF: What's the disease he means?
MALCOLM: 'Tis call'd the evil:
A most miraculous work in this good king,
Which often since my here-remain in England
I have seen him do. How he solicits heaven
Himself best knows; but strangely-visited people,
All swol'n and ulcerous, pitiful to the eye,
The mere despair of surgery, he cures,
Hanging a golden stamp about their necks,
Put on with holy prayers.

> *Macbeth,* V, iii, 141

Death may usurp on nature many hours,
And yet the fire of life kindle again
The o'erpress'd spirits. I heard of an Egyptian
That had nine hours lien dead,
Who was by good appliance recovered.

> *Pericles,* III, ii, 82

I pray you give her air.
Gentlemen,
This queen will live; nature awakes; a warmth
Breathes out of her. She hath not been entranc'd
Above five hours. See how she gins to blow
Into life's flower again! . . .
Lend me your hands; to the next chamber bear her.
Get linen. Now this matter must be look'd to,
For her relapse is mortal. Come, come!
And Aesculapius guide us!

> *Ibid.,* III, ii, 91

Sir Thomas Browne [1605–1682]

I can cure vices by Physicke, when they remaine incurable by Divinity, and shall obey my pils, when they contemne their precepts.

> *Religio Medici,* Pt. II, Sect. 9

John Bunyan [1628–1688]

Physicians get neither name nor fame by pricking of wheals, or picking out of thistles, or by laying of plaisters to the scratch of a pin: every old woman can do this. But if they would have a name and fame — if they will have it quickly, they must, as I said, do some great and desperate cures. Let them fetch one to life that was dead; let them recover one to his wits that was mad; let them make one that was born blind to see; or let them give ripe wits to a fool; these are notable cures; and he that can do thus, and if he doth thus first, he shall have the name and fame he desires; he may lie abed till noon.

> *The Jerusalem Sinner Saved; or Good News for the Vilest of Men*

Thomas Latta [d. 1833]

She had apparently reached the last moments of her earthly existence and now nothing could injure her — indeed, so entirely was she reduced, that

I feared that I should be unable to get my apparatus ready ere she expired. Having inserted a tube into the basilic vein, cautiously — anxiously, I watched the effects: ounce after ounce was injected, but no visible change was produced. Still persevering, I thought she began to breathe less laboriously, soon the sharpened features, and sunken eye and fallen jaw, pale and cold, bearing the manifest impress of death's signet, began to glow with returning animation; the pulse, which had long ceased, returned to the wrist; at first small and quick, by degrees it became more distinct, fuller, slower, and firmer, and in the short space of half an hour, when six pints had been injected she expressed in a firm voice that she was free from all uneasiness, actually became jocular, and fancied all she needed was a little sleep; her extremities were warm, and every feature bore the aspect of comfort and health.[1]

> *Lancet* 2:274, 1831

Thomas Hardy [1840–1928]

> And ill it therefore suits
> The mood of one of my high temperature
> To pause inactive while await me means
> Of desperate cure for these so desperate ills!
>> *The Dynasts*, Pt. I, Act IV, Sc. iii

Henry Cuyler Bunner [1855–1896]

The Doctor fared even better. The fame of his new case spread far and wide. People seemed to think that if he could cure an elephant he could cure anything.
> *Short Sixes*, "The Infidelity of Zenobia"

[1] The first known use of replacement therapy in medicine; the patient had been depleted of extracellular fluid volume by the diarrhea of cholera.

Anonymous

> A fire with water we defeat,
> With parasols the midday heat,
> Mad elephants with goads that prick,
> Oxen and asses with a stick. . . .
> Science has cures for every ill
> Except the fool; he prospers still.
>> Sanskrit poem (tr. by A. W. Ryder)

Chinese Proverb

Medicine cures the man who is fated not to die.

Irish Proverb

A good laugh and a long sleep are the best cures in the doctor's book.

Polish Proverb

The poor are cured by work, the rich by the doctor.

CURIOSITIES

Johannes de Gorter [1689–1762]

It is surprising that the basic sciences single out, for observation and intensive study, phenomena which are most uncommon and hardly of intrinsic significance.

Similarly, medicine discusses diseases which are so rare that one does not encounter them more than once or twice during a lifetime with extraordinary thoroughness as if the salvation of the art would depend on it.
> *De motu vitali* (tr. by Max Samter)

DEAFNESS

See also EAR, HEARING

Thomas Churchyard [1520?–1604]

Dumme and deaffe as a post.
> *Chippes*

Nicholas Breton [1545?–1626?]

Hee is as deafe as a doore.
The Wil of Wit, "The Miseries of Mauillia"

William Shakespeare [1564–1616]

FALSTAFF: It is a kind of deafness.
JUSTICE: I think you are fall'n into the disease, for you hear not what I say to you.
FALSTAFF: Very well, my lord, very well. Rather, an't please you, it is the disease of not list'ning, the malady of not marking, that I am troubled withal.
Henry IV, Part II, I, ii, 133

Ears more deaf than adders.
Troilus and Cressida, II, ii, 172

Jonathan Swift [1667–1745]

Deaf, giddy, helpless, left alone,
To all my Friends a Burden grown.[1]
Written by the Reverend Dr. Swift on His Own Deafness

Oliver Goldsmith [1728–1774]

When they talk'd of their Raphaels, Correggios, and stuff,
He [2] shifted his trumpet and only took snuff.
Retaliation

Ludwig van Beethoven [1770–1827]

Yet it was not possible for me to say to men: speak louder, shout, for I am deaf. Alas! how could I declare the weakness of a *sense* which in me *ought to be* more acute than in others — a sense which *formerly* I possessed in highest perfection, a perfection such

---

[1] Vertiginosus, inops, surdis, male gratus amicis.
Swift wrote this poem in Latin; the English translation is from Faulkner's edition of 1747.
[2] Sir Joshua Reynolds, who was very deaf.

as few in my profession enjoy, or ever have enjoyed.
Letter to his brothers Carl and Johann, October 6, 1802 (tr. by J. S. Shedlock)

Sir William Wilde [1815–1876]

There are two kinds of deafness. One is due to wax and is curable; the other is not due to wax and is not curable.

David Seegal [1899–   ]

Why does man have compassion for the blind
And for the deaf an irritable bind?
The Pharos of Alpha Omega Alpha 28:128, 1965, "Anachronism"

Merrill Moore [1903–1957]

Deaf men live in a world divorced from sound;
By consequence their own thoughts are increased,
Louder, longer are the noises leased
That they can think, like voices in a swound;

But there is no sweet wedding in this sound
With words accompanying from such outside source
As you and I possess —
                          theirs is far worse,
Yet none falls in a fit upon the ground
Complaining of deafness; there are advantages
That are the deaf man's and are only his —

Much he does not have to listen to
Of true, or trivial, and the untrue,

And some (some do not) learn an inner poise
That does not hang from soundlessness or noise.
M: One Thousand Autobiographical Sonnets, Ch. II, "Deaf Men"

The Bible

O foolish people, and without understanding; which have eyes, and see not; which have ears, and hear not.
Jeremiah 5:21

Proverbs

Deaf men are quick-ey'd and distrustful.

Who so deaf as they that will not hear?

American Proverb

Deaf people always hear better than they say they do (or, than you think they do).

DEATH

See also BIRTH AND DEATH, LIFE AND DEATH, MURDER, SLEEP AND DEATH, SUICIDE

I. GENERAL

Ibycus [ca. 550 B.C.]

You cannot find a medicine for life when once a man is dead.
Chrysippus (tr. by J. M. Edmonds in *Lyra Graeca*, Vol. II)

Sophocles [496?–406 B.C.]

Death is not the greatest of ills; it is worse to want to die, and not be able to.
Electra, 1007

Seneca [4? B.C.–A.D. 65]

Death is a punishment to some, to some a gift, and to many a favor.
Hercules Oetaeus

Juvenal [60?–140?]

Death alone proclaims how small are our poor human bodies!
Satires, X.172 (tr. by G. G. Ramsay)

Marcus Aurelius [121–180]

Think continually how many physicians are dead after often contracting their eyebrows over the sick; and how many astrologers after predicting with great pretensions the deaths of others; and how many philosophers after endless discourses on death or immortality.
Meditations, IV.48 (tr. by G. Long)

Avicenna [980–1037]

From Earth's dark Centre unto Saturn's Gate
I've solved all Problems of this World's Estate,
From every Snare of Plot and Guile set free,
Each bond resolved — saving alone Death's Fate.
The Canon

William Langland [1330?–1400?]

Ded as a dore-nayle.
Piers Plowman, Passus II

Ambroise Paré [1517?–1590]

When youth is wakeful and old age drowsy, death is nigh.
Quoted by F. H. Garrison in *Bulletin of the New York Academy of Medicine* 4:992, 1928

Sir Walter Raleigh [1552?–1618]

O eloquent, just, and mighty Death! whom none could advise, thou hast perswaded; what none hath dared thou hast done; and whom all the world hath flattered, thou only hast cast out of the world and despised: thou hast drawn together all the far stretched greatness, all the pride, cruelty, and ambition of man, and covered it all over with these two narrow words, *Hic jacet.*
History of the World, Bk. V, Ch. vi, Sect. 12

William Shakespeare [1564–1616]

Death —

The undiscover'd country, from whose bourn
No traveller returns.
Hamlet, III, i, 78

The jaws of death.
Twelfth Night, III, iv, 394

John Donne [1573–1631]

Any man's *death* diminishes *me,* because I am involved in *Mankinde;*
And therefore never send to know for whom the *bell* tolls; It tolls for *thee.*
Devotions Upon Emergent Occasions, XVII

Death be not proud, though some have called thee
Mighty and dreadfull, for, thou art not soe,
For, those, whom thou think'st, thou dost overthrow,
Die not, poore death, nor yet canst thou kill mee.
Holy Sonnets, X

One short sleepe past, wee wake eternally,
And death shall be no more; death, thou shalt die.
Idem

Duc François de La Rochefoucauld [1613–1680]

No man may gaze fixedly at the sun, nor at death.
Maxims, No. 26 (tr. by Constantine FitzGibbon)

Henry Vaughan [1622–1695]

They are all gone into the world of light!
And I alone sit ling'ring here;
Their very memory is fair and bright,
And my sad thoughts doth clear.
Friends Departed

My Soul, there is a Countrie
Afar beyond the stars,

Where stands a wingèd Sentrie
All skilful in the wars.
Silex Scintillans, Pt. I, "Peace"

John Wilmot, Earl of Rochester [1647–1680]

Dead, we become the lumber of the world.
After Death

Joseph Addison [1672–1719]

The Fear of Death often proves Mortal, and sets People on Methods to save their Lives, which infallibly destroy them.
The Spectator, Vol. I, No. 25 (March 29, 1711)

Edward Young [1683–1765]

All men think all men mortal, but Themselves.
Night Thoughts, Night I

Jonathan Edwards [1703–1758]

The bodies of those that made such a noise and tumult when alive, when dead, lie as quietly among the graves of their neighbours as any others.
Practical Sermons, Sermon XV, Sect. V

Tobias Smollett [1721–1771]

I'll warrant him as dead as a herring.
The Adventures of Roderick Random, Ch. 4

Walter Savage Landor [1775–1864]

Absence and death are the same — only that in death there is no suffering.
Letter to Robert Browning, 1862

Thomas Lovell Beddoes [1803–1849]

That will be all eternal heaven distilled
Down to one thick rich minute.
Death's Jest-Book, Act II, Sc. iii

Oliver Wendell Holmes
[1809–1894]

Why can't a fellow hear the fine things
   said
About a fellow when a fellow's dead?
    Rip Van Winkle, M.D., Canto
    I

John Bright [1811–1889]

The Angel of Death has been abroad
throughout the land; you may almost
hear the beating of his wings.
    Speech, House of Commons,
    February 23, 1855

Robert Browning [1812–1889]

How he lies in his rights of a man!
Death has done all death can.
    After

Fear death? — to feel the fog in my
   throat,
   The mist in my face.
    Prospice

Charles Dickens [1812–1870]

Marley was dead, to begin with. . . .
Old Marley was as dead as a door-nail.
    A Christmas Carol, Stave I

Emily Dickinson [1830–1886]

The Bustle in a House
The Morning after Death
Is solemnest of industries
Enacted upon Earth, —

The Sweeping up the Heart,
And putting Love away
We shall not want to use again
Until Eternity.
    Poems, "The Bustle in a
    House"

Sir William S. Gilbert
[1836–1911]

For twenty years I have been dead
and buried. Don't dig me up now.
    Ruddigore, Act I

Robert Bridges [1844–1930]

When Death to either shall come, —
   I pray it be first to me, —
Be happy as ever at home,
   If so, as I wish, it be.

Possess thy heart, my own;
   And sing to the child on thy knee,
Or read to thyself alone
   The songs that I made for thee.
    *When Death to Either Shall
    Come*

Elie Metchnikoff [1845–1916]

It must surprise my readers to find
how little science really knows about
death.
    *The Prolongation of Life: Op-
    timistic Studies,* Pt. III, Ch. I

Thomas Mann [1875–1955]

The ancients . . . knew how to pay
homage to death. For death is worthy
of homage, as the cradle of life, as
the womb of palingenesis. Severed
from life, it becomes a spectre, a distortion, and worse. For death, as an
independent power, is a lustful power,
whose vicious attraction is strong indeed; to feel drawn to it, to feel sympathy with it, is without any doubt
at all the most ghastly aberration to
which the spirit of man is prone.
    The Magic Mountain, Ch. V,
    "Soup-Everlasting" (tr. by
    H. T. Lowe-Porter)

Otto Weininger [1880–1903]

It is often a cause for astonishment
that men with quite ordinary, even
vulgar, natures experience no fear of
death. But it is quite explicable: it
is not the fear of death which creates
the desire for immortality, but the desire for immortality which causes fear
of death.
    Sex and Character, Pt. II, Ch.
    5

Women are as much afraid of death as are men, but they have not the longing for immortality.
Idem

Francis Weld Peabody
[1881–1927]

Death is not the worst thing in the world, and to help a man to a happy and useful career may be more of a service than the saving of life.
The Care of the Patient

Alan Gregg [1890–1957]

A thousand goodbyes come after death — the first six months of bereavement.
Aphorism (Quoted by Wilder Penfield in *The Difficult Art of Giving*, Appendix A)

Sidney Hook [1902–   ]

The fear of death, the desire to survive at any cost or price in human degradation, has been the greatest ally of tyranny, past or present.

The Bible

The land of darkness and the shadow of death.
Job 10:21

Yea, though I walk through the valley of the shadow of death, I will fear no evil.
Psalms 23:4

We have made a covenant with death.
Isaiah 28:15

O death, where is thy sting? O grave, where is thy victory?
I Corinthians 15:55

And I looked, and behold a pale horse: and his name that sat on him was Death.
Revelation 6:8

Anonymous

Feare of death is worse than death it selfe.
The True Chronicle History of King Leir, Sc. xix

French Proverbs

After death the doctor.

When one is dead, it is for a long time.

Latin Proverbs

Death defies the doctor.

The fear of death is crueler than death itself.

II. DYING

Epicharmus [6th–5th Cents. B.C.]

I dread to die, but dread not being dead.
Quoted by Cicero in *Tusculan Disputations*, I.viii.15 (tr. by A. P. Peabody)

Aristotle [384–322 B.C.]

It is best to quit life, just as we leave a banquet, neither thirsty or drunken.

Menander [343?–291? B.C.]

Whom the Gods love die young.
Fragments, 125

Poseidippus [fl. 289 B.C.]

Of all the boons that man asks of the gods, he prays most fervently for an easy death.
Fragment from *Myrmex*

Plautus [254?–184 B.C.]

He whom the gods love dies young, while he has his strength and senses and wits.
Bacchides, IV.vii.816

Lucretius [96?–55 B.C.]

We often see a man pass away by degrees, and limb by limb lose the sensation of life: first the toes of the feet grow livid, and the nails, next die feet and legs, afterwards over the other limbs go creeping the cold footsteps of death.
> *On the Nature of Things,* III.526 (tr. by W. H. D. Rouse)

Martial [fl. 1st Cent.]

The mode of death is sadder than death itself.
> *Epigrams,* XI.91

Petrarch [1304–1374]

A good death does honor to a whole life.
> *Canzoniere,* XVI

Ambroise Paré [1517?–1590]

I prefer to die by the hand of God.
> Comment to colleague who proposed amputation of his toes

Michel de Montaigne [1533–1592]

All days travel toward death, the last one reaches it.
> *Essays,* Bk. I, Ch. 20, "That to Philosophize Is to Learn to Die" (tr. by Donald M. Frame)

The most voluntary death is the fairest.
> *Ibid.,* Bk. II, Ch. 3, "A Custom of the Island of Cea"

If you don't know how to die, don't worry; Nature will tell you what to do on the spot, fully and adequately. She will do this job perfectly for you; don't bother your head about it.
> *Ibid.,* Bk. III, Ch. 12, "Of Physiognomy"

William Shakespeare [1564–1616]

The King himself hath a heavy reck-oning to make when all those legs and arms and heads, chopp'd off in a battle, shall join together at the latter day and cry all 'We died at such a place!' some swearing, some crying for a surgeon.
> *Henry V,* IV, i, 140

Her blue blood, chang'd to black in in every vein,
Wanting the spring that those shrunk pipes had fed,
Show'd life imprison'd in a body dead.
> *The Rape of Lucrece,* line 1454

She's cold,
Her blood is settled, and her joints are stiff;
Life and these lips have long been separated.
Death lies on her like an untimely frost
Upon the sweetest flower of all the field.
> *Romeo and Juliet,* IV, v, 25

Thomas Campion [1567–1620]

Leave prolonging thy distresse!
All delayes afflict the dying.
Many lost sighes long I spent, to her for mercy crying;
But now, vain mourning, cease!
I'll dye, and mine owne griefes release.

Thus departing from this light
To those shades that end in sorrow,
Yet a small time of complaint, a little breath Ile borrow,
To tell my once delight
I dye alone through her despight.
> *The Fourth Booke of Ayres,* "Leave Prolonging"

John Webster [1580?–1625?]

Death hath ten thousand several doors For men to take their exits.
> *The Duchess of Malfi,* Act IV, Sc. ii

Francis Beaumont [1584–1616]
and John Fletcher [1579–1625]

Death hath so many doors to let out
life.
> *The Custom of the Country,*
> Act II, Sc. ii

Sir Thomas Browne [1605–1682]

Many have studied to exasperate the
ways of Death, but fewer hours have
been spent to soften that necessity.
. . . To learn to dye is better than to
study the ways of dying. Death will
find some way to unty or cut the most
Gordian Knots of Life, and make
men's miseries as mortal as themselves.
> *Christian Morals,* Pt. II, Sect.
> 13

Pierre Corneille [1606–1684]

Pierced to the depth of my heart by
a blow unforeseen — and mortal.
> *Le Cid,* Act I, Sc. vii

Sir William Davenant [1606–1668]

I shall ask leave to desist, when I am
interrupted by so great an experiment
as dying.
> *Gondibert,* "Postscript to the
> Reader"

Jeremy Taylor [1613–1667]

*The Soul by the help of sickness
knocks off the fetters of Pride and
vainer complacencies.* Then she draws
the curtains, and stops the light from
coming in, and takes the pictures
down, those fantastic images of self-
love, and gay remembrances of vain
opinion, and popular noises. Then the
spirit stoops into the sobrieties of
humble thoughts, and feels corruption chiding the forwardness of fancy,
and allaying the vapours of conceit
and factious opinions. For humility
is the Soul's grave, into which she
enters, not to die, but to meditate and
inter some of its troublesome appen-
dages. There she sees the dust, and
feels the dishonours of the body, and

reads the register of all its sad ad-
herences; and then she lays by all her
vain reflections, beating upon her
Crystal and pure mirror from the
fancies of strength and beauty, and
little decayed prettinesses of the body.
> *The Rule and Exercises of Holy
> Dying,* Ch. 3, Sect. 6

Jean de La Fontaine [1621–1695]

Death never takes the wise man by
surprise;
He is always ready to go.
> *Fables,* "La Mort et le
> Mourant"

John Dryden [1631–1700]

And, dying, bless the hand that gave
the blow.
> *The Spanish Friar,* Act II,
> Sc. i

Book of Common Prayer [1662]

From lightning and tempest; from
plague, pestilence and famine; from
battle and murder, and from sudden
death, *Good Lord, deliver us.*
> *The Litany*

Voltaire [1694–1778]

He who has plenty of witnesses of his
death, dies always with courage.
> *Age of Louis XIV,* Ch. XXVIII

Nathaniel Cotton [1705–1788]

Would you extend your narrow span,
And make the most of life you can;
Would you, when medicines cannot
save,
Descend with ease into the grave;
Calmly retire, like evening light,
And cheerful bid the world goodnight?
> *Visions in Verse,* III, "Health"

Henry Fielding [1707–1754]

It hath been often said that it is not
death, but dying, which is terrible.
> *Amelia,* Bk. III, Ch. 4

Samuel Johnson [1709–1784]

The truth is that every death is violent which is the effect of accident; every death, which is not gradually brought on by the miseries of age, or when life is extinguished for any other reason than that it is burnt out. He that dies before sixty, of a cold or consumption, dies, in reality, by a violent death.

> Letter to Bennet Langton, September 21, 1758

Then with no throbbing fiery pain,
No cold gradation of decay,
Death broke at once the vital chain
And free'd his soul the nearest way.
> *On the Death of Mr. Robert Levet, a Practiser in Physic*

I will take no more physick, not even my opiates; for I have prayed that I may render up my soul to GOD unclouded.
> Quoted by James Boswell in *Life of Samuel Johnson*, December 1784

Oliver Goldsmith [1728–1774]

The doctors found, when she was dead —
Her last disorder mortal.
> *Elegy on Mrs. Mary Blaize*

I am told he makes a very handsome corpse, and becomes his coffin prodigiously.
> *The Good-Natured Man*, Act I

Thomas Jefferson [1743–1826]

There is a ripeness of time for death . . . when it is reasonable we should drop off, and make room for another growth. When we have lived our generation out, we should not wish to encroach on another.
> Letter to John Adams, August 1, 1816

I enjoy good health; I am happy in what is around me, yet I assure you I am ripe for leaving all, this year, this day, this hour.
> *Idem*

Maria Edgeworth [1767–1849]

I've a great fancy to see my own funeral afore I die.
> *Castle Rackrent*, "Continuation of Memoirs"

Sydney Smith [1771–1845]

Death must be distinguished from dying, with which it is often confounded.
> Quoted by Lady Holland in *A Memoir of the Rev. Sydney Smith*, Ch. 6

Thomas Campbell [1777–1844]

O Death! if there be quiet in thy arms,
  And I must cease — gently, O, gently come
To me! and let my soul learn no alarms,
  But strike me, ere a shriek can echo, dumb,
Senseless, and breathless.
> *Lines Written in Sickness*

Baron Guillaume Dupuytren [1777–1835]

I prefer to die by the decree of God rather than by the hand of man.
> Quoted by Arpad G. Gerster in *Proceedings of the Charaka Club* 4:113, 1916

Jacob Bigelow [1786–1879]

It is in vain that the unhappy inquirer resorts to his statistical tables to inform himself whether there is most danger in a steamboat or on a railroad, — he unfortunately learns that the most dangerous thing a man can do is to go to bed, for more people die in bed than anywhere else.
> *Proceedings and Debates of the Fourth National Quarantine and Sanitary Convention*, 1860, Banquet Address

George Gordon, Lord Byron
[1788–1824]

Yet what is
Death, so it be but glorious? 'Tis a
sunset.
Sardanapalus, Act II, Sc. i

Peter Mere Latham [1789–1875]

The way of death is often smoother
than the path of life; and great bodily
anguish (there is reason to believe)
does not often enter largely into the
process of dissolution.
Lectures on Clinical Medicine,
Lect. VI

Percy Bysshe Shelley
[1792–1822]

First our pleasures die — and then
Our hopes, and then our fears — and
when
These are dead, the debt is due,
Dust claims dust — and we die too.
Death

Mild was the slow necessity of death:
The tranquil spirit failed beneath its
grasp,
Without a groan, almost without a
fear,
Calm as a voyager to some distant
land,
And full of wonder, full of hope as he.
Queen Mab, Sect. IX

William Cullen Bryant
[1794–1878]

So live, that when thy summons comes
to join
The innumerable caravan which moves
To that mysterious realm where each
shall take
His chamber in the silent halls of
death,
Thou go not, like the quarry-slave at
night,
Scourged to his dungeon, but, sustained and soothed
By an unfaltering trust, approach thy
grave,

Like one who wraps the drapery of
his couch
About him, and lies down to pleasant
dreams.
Thanatopsis

John Keats [1795–1821]

There is a great difference between
going off in warm blood like Romeo,
and making one's exit like a frog in
a frost.
Letter to Fanny Brawne,
March 1820

Henry Wadsworth Longfellow
[1807–1882]

'Tis the cessation of our breath.
Silent and motionless we lie;
And no one knoweth more than this.
Christus: A Mystery, Pt. II,
Sect. ii

Abraham Lincoln [1809–1865]

If I am killed, I can die but once; but
to live in constant dread of it, is to
die over and over again.[1]
Quoted by John T. Morse in
Abraham Lincoln, Vol. II, Ch.
13

Henri Amiel [1821–1881]

To die quickly is a privilege; I shall
die by inches.
Journal Intime, September 1,
1874 (tr. by Mrs. Humphrey
Ward)

Matthew Arnold [1822–1888]

I ask but that my death may find
The freedom to my life denied;
Ask but the folly of mankind,
Then, then at last, to quit my side.

Spare me the whispering, crowded
room,
The friends who come, and gape, and
go;
The ceremonious air of gloom —
All, that makes death a hideous show!
A Wish

[1] Cf. William Shakespeare, p. 91b.

Benjamin Harrison [1833–1901]

I'd rather have a bullet inside of me than to be living in constant dread of one.[1]

> Quoted by Henry L. Stoddard in *As I Knew Them*

Samuel Butler [1835–1902]

Death in anything like luxury is one of the most expensive things a man can indulge himself in. It costs a lot of money to die comfortably, unless one goes off pretty quickly.

> *Note-Books*, Ch. II, "A Luxurious Death"

Mark Twain (Samuel L. Clemens) [1835–1910]

The reports of my death are greatly exaggerated.[2]

> Cable from London to the Associated Press, June 2, 1897

W. Winwood Reade [1838–1875]

As the atoms are to the human unit, so the human units are to the human whole. There is only One Man upon the earth; what we call men are not individuals, but components; what we call death is merely the bursting of a cell.

> *The Martyrdom of Man*, Ch. IV

William G. Sumner [1840–1910]

I think of it about as I think of going upstairs to bed.

> *The Forgotten Man's Almanac*, April 12

Sir William Osler [1849–1919]

I have careful records of about five hundred death-beds, studied particu-

larly with reference to the modes of death and the sensations of the dying. . . . Ninety suffered bodily pain or distress of one sort or another, eleven showed mental apprehension, two positive terror, one expressed spiritual exaltation, one bitter remorse. The great majority gave no signs one way or the other; like birth, their death was a sleep and a forgetting.

> *Science and Immortality*

Patients rarely die of the disease from which they suffer. (Secondary or terminal infections are the real cause of death.)

> Quoted in *St. Bartholomew's Hospital Reports* 52:39, 1916

William M. Beaumont [1851–1928]

The one object of most doctors seems to be to make a competence and then retire, after which they patiently wait on the platform for the train to bear them into eternity. When my time comes, may I rush into the station without time to think of the ticket or where I am going and jump into the Express as it is on the move.[1]

> Passage from his will

Rudolph Matas [1860–1957]

The transition between life and death should be gentle in the winter of life. Death, under these conditions, is invested with a certain grandeur and poetry, if it comes to a man when he has completed his mission. . . . There is nothing to fear, nothing to dread.

> *The Soul of a Surgeon*

Marcel Proust [1871–1922]

We may, indeed, say that the hour of death is uncertain, but when we say so we represent that hour to ourselves as situated in a vague and remote expanse of time, it never occurs to us that it can have any connexion with the day that has already dawned, or

---

[1] Upon dismissing the White House detectives, 1889.

[2] According to *Mark Twain, Wit and Wisdom,* edited by Cyril Clemens, Twain instructed a reporter to cable: "The report of Mark Twain's death is greatly exaggerated."

[1] Dr. Beaumont died suddenly as he was showing a patient out of his office.

may signify that death — or its first assault and partial possession of us, after which it will never leave hold of us again — may occur this very afternoon, so far from uncertain, this afternoon every hour of which has already been allotted to some occupation. . . . you have no suspicion that death, which has been making its way towards you along another plane, shrouded in an impenetrable darkness, has chosen precisely this day of all days to make its appearance.

> *The Guermantes Way,* Pt. II, "My Grandmother's Illness" (tr. by C. K. Scott-Moncrieff)

Charles Péguy [1873–1914]

When a man lies dying, he does not die from the disease alone. He dies from his whole life.

> *Basic Verities,* "The Search for Truth" (tr. by A. and J. Green)

W. Somerset Maugham [1874–1965]

Dying is the most hellishly boresome experience in the world! Particularly when it entails dying of "natural causes."

> Quoted by Wilmon Menard in *The Two Worlds of Somerset Maugham,* Ch. 22

Thomas Mann [1875–1955]

A man's dying is more the survivors' affair than his own.

> *The Magic Mountain,* Ch. VI, "A Soldier, and Brave" (tr. by H. T. Lowe-Porter)

Sir Charles Singer [1876–   ]

Medicine cannot give immortality, but it should enable us all to live out our full lives. Death, coming in due and not undue time, is shorn of all his terrors, when every man and every woman
> Shall come to his grave in a full age,

Like as a shock of corn cometh in, in his season.
> (*Job* 5:26)
> *A Short History of Medicine,* Epilogue

Martin H. Fischer [1879–1962]

We die of the things we know nothing about.

> Quoted by Howard Fabing and Ray Marr in *Fischerisms*

André Maurois [1885–1967]

I knew a man who had been virtually drowned and then revived. He said that his death had not been painful.

Aline (Mrs. Joyce) Kilmer [1888–1941]

Things have a terrible permanence
> When people die.
> *Things*

Alden Hatch [1898–   ]

Finally God had granted him [1] the ultimate boon that neither forethought, science, nor character can command — a quick and easy death.

> *The Mountbattens,* Pt. I, Ch. 17

Meyer A. Perlstein [1902–   ]

If your time hasn't come, not even a doctor can kill you.

John W. Thompson [1906–   ]

That I shall die before the winter snow
Awakes to join the singing gush of streams,
Is better far than death when violets grow,

[1] Louis, Prince of Battenberg [1854–1921], father of the present Lord Mountbatten and grandfather of Prince Philip, Duke of Edinburgh.

And lilacs lace the fringe of summer
  dreams.

For in the dancing springtime of the
    year
With myriad sounds of whispering
    trees is born
The symphony of life; then mine's
    too dear,
Too great the pain from these forever
    torn.

But now a tomb-like coldness stills
    the air
Alike on earth and there between the
    stars;
With it I merge my soul without de-
    spair,

No sound of thrush this final union
    mars
As endless restful death bids me share
    soon
The silence of the drifting timeless
    moon.
          That I Shall Die

The Bible

Then Abraham gave up the ghost . . .
and was gathered to his people.
          Genesis 25:8

Anonymous

Don't know. Died without the aid of
    a physician.
Had never been fatally ill before.
Went to bed feeling fine, woke up dead.
Died suddenly. Nothing serious.
          Death notices (19th Cent.)

There is a dignity in dying that doctors should not dare to deny.

You have two chances — one of get-
ing the germ and one of not. And if
you get the germ you have two
chances — one of getting the disease
and one of not. And if you get the
disease you have two chances — one
of dying and one of not. And if you
die — well, you still have two chances!

III. DEATH AS FRIEND

Aeschylus [525–456 B.C.]

O Death the Healer, scorn thou not,
    I pray,
To come to me: of cureless ills thou art
The one physician. Pain lays not its
    touch
Upon a corpse.
          Fragment 229 (tr. by E. H.
          Plumptre)

Herodotus [484–424 B.C.]

Death is a delightful hiding-place for
weary men.
          Histories, VII.xlvi

Marcus Aurelius [121–180]

Death is a release from the impressions of sense, and from impulses that
make us their puppets, from the va-
garies of the mind, and the hard service of the flesh.
          Meditations, VI.28 (tr. by C.
          R. Haines)

Despise not death, but welcome it,
for Nature wills it like all else.
          Ibid., IX.3

Tertullian [160?–230?]

There is nothing dreadful in that
which delivers from all that is to be
dreaded.
          The Soul's Testimony, IV (tr.
          by S. Thelwall)

Agathias Scholasticus [536–582]

Why fear death, the mother of rest,
death that puts an end to sickness and
the pains of poverty? It happens but
once to mortals, and no man ever saw
it come twice.
          Greek Anthology, X.69 (tr. by
          W. R. Paton)

Anne Boleyn [1507–1536]

Oh, Death! rock me asleep,
    Bring on my quiet rest,

Let pass my very guiltless ghost
Out of my careful breast.
Ring out the doleful knell,
Let its sound my death tell —
For I must die,
There is no remedy,
For now I die.
> Written after her death sentence (Quoted by N. Brysson Morrison in *The Private Life of Henry VIII*, Ch. 14)

Sir Francis Bacon [1561–1626]

I have often thought upon death, and find it the least of all evils.
> *An Essay on Death*, Sect. I [1]

Sir Thomas Browne [1605–1682]

I boast nothing, but plainely say, we all labour against our owne cure, for death is the cure of all diseases. There is no Catholicon, or universall remedy I know but this, which thogh nauseous to queasier stomachs, yet to prepared appetites is Nectar and a pleasant potion of immortality.
> *Religio Medici*, Pt. II, Sect. 9

Jeremy Taylor [1613–1667]

Of all the evils of the world which are reproached with an evil character, death is the most innocent of its accusation.
> *The Rule and Exercises of Holy Dying*, Ch. II, Sect. VII

Jean de La Bruyère [1645–1696]

A long illness seems to be placed between life and death, in order to make death a comfort both to those who die and to those who remain.
> *Caractères*, Ch. XI

Johann Gottlieb Fichte [1762–1814]

The sure end of all pain, and of all sensibility to pain, is death; and of all things which the mere natural man is wont to regard as evils, this is to me the least.
> *The Vocation of Man*, Bk. III, Ch. 4 (tr. by W. Smith)

Sydney Smith [1771–1845]

Every one must go to his grave with his heart scarred like a soldier's body, — sometimes a parent, sometimes a child, a friend, a husband, or a wife. Thus the bands of this life are gradually loosened, and death at last is more welcome than the comfortless solitude of the world.
> Quoted by Lady Holland in *A Memoir of the Rev. Sydney Smith*, Ch. 2

Robert Southey [1774–1843]

My name is DEATH: THE LAST BEST FRIEND AM I.
> *Carmen Nuptiale: The Lay of the Laureate*, "The Dream"

Charles C. Colton [1780?–1832]

Death . . . a friend that alone can bring the peace his treasures cannot purchase, and remove the pain his physicians cannot cure.
> *Lacon*, Vol. II, Ch. CX

John Keats [1795–1821]

I have been half in love with easeful Death.
> *Ode to a Nightingale*

Now more than ever seems it rich to die,
To cease upon the midnight with no pain.
> *Idem*

Henry Wadsworth Longfellow [1807–1882]

Death is better than disease.
> *Christus: A Mystery*, Pt. II, Sect. i

[1] The authorship of this work is questionable; it has also been attributed to Sir Thomas Browne [1605–1682].

Pliny Earle [1809–1892]

What is it, then, to die, that it should
    be
Essential to our happiness? It is
To throw off all things worldly, all
    the dross
That man is heir to, and go forth,
    again,
Clad in the vestment of immortal
    life. . . .
'Tis to depart from this precarious
    scene,
Where life is bounded, and its little
    span
Measured by moments, — where the
    material world
Marks transient days and seasons, and
    to go
Where time has never wandered,
    where long years
Dwindle to moments, and a moment
    grows
Into the length of ages; where the
    past
And future meet, in one eternal
    present.
    What Is It To Die?

John Bruce MacCallum
[1876–1906]

Strong men have trembled at thy
    name, O Death,
And nations lifted up their hands in
    prayer
To crave the senseless boon that thou
    wilt spare
Their little lives, their wasted sup-
    pliant breath.

Great beasts have feared thee, and in
    shrieking herds
Have fled before thee on the burning
    plain.
And their proud masters to escape thy
    pain
Have howled unto their gods, strange
    vows, vain words.

But I here on the borders of thy land
With cold damp winds against my
    aching brow
Am not afraid of thee, for in thy hand

I see no gift but rest, and only thou
Canst comfort me, for thou dost un-
    derstand,
O Death, and I await thee even now.
    Death

Spirit of death, so soft, so sweet,
Be fleet, be fleet,
If I must feel your breath upon mine
    eyes,
If I must reach that vale where twi-
    light flies
Mistladen to the night,
Oh come, be swift, and strike while I
    am free,
When life is sweet and joy has raised
    for me
Its wavering light.

Spirit of death, so dark, so cold,
Must I grow old
In ever fearing that your voice will
    come,
Bidding my soul forever to be dumb,
Mine eyes to lose their light?
Oh come be swift while I am strong
    and free,
Break this thin web that binds the
    mystery,
Before the grey of twilight bids me
    see
The terrors of the night.

Spirit of death, so still, so slow,
Must I too go
To twilight years, the tedious down-
    ward path?
Must I too live this fading aftermath
And feel my heart grow cold?
Oh come be swift and take me while
    I stand,
My work still strong beneath a steady
    hand,
A life that ne'er grew old.
    Epitaph

Oliver St. John Gogarty
[1878–1957]

But for your Terror
Where would be Valour?
What is Love for
    But to stand in your way?
Taker and Giver,

For all your endeavour
You leave us with more
   Than you touch with decay!
    An Offering of Swans, "To
    Death"

The Bible

Which long for death, but it cometh
not; and dig for it more than for hid
treasures.
    Job 3:21

Irish Proverb

Death is the poor man's best physician.[1]

IV. DEATH AS ENEMY

Antiphanes [408?–334? B.C.]

None ever die who wish; 'tis those
   that gloat
On life that Charon hurries to his
   boat;
Seized by the leg, dragged off against
   their will,
E'en while of food and drink they take
   their fill.
    Fragments, 86 (tr. by F. A.
    Paley)

Paracelsus [1493?–1541]

Consider with what vigour nature
strives against death. She resorts to
heaven and earth and all their powers
and virtues to help her. So also the
soul must fight the devil with all her
might. . . . Nature too is full of
anxiety; she has recourse to everything that God has given her in order
to repel death; she tries to drive out
harsh, bitter death, who fights against
her; dreadful death, whom our eyes
cannot see, nor our hands clutch. But
nature sees, touches and knows him.
Therefore she summons all the powers

[1] Swedish Proverb: Death is the last
doctor.

of heaven and earth to resist the terrible one.
    Opus Paramirum, Pt. I, Bk. II,
    Ch. ii (tr. by Norbert Guter-
    man in *Selected Writings*)

Sir Francis Bacon [1561–1626]

Men fear Death, as children fear to
go in the dark; and as that natural
fear in children is increased with tales,
so is the other.
    Essays, "Of Death"

Philip Massinger [1583–1640]

Grim Death.
    The Roman Actor, Act IV, Sc. ii

Sir Thomas Browne [1605–1682]

I am not so much afraid of death, as
ashamed thereof; tis the very disgrace
and ignominy of our natures, that in
a moment can so disfigure us that our
nearest friends, wives and Children
stand afraid and start at us.
    Religio Medici, Pt. I, Sect. 40

John Milton [1608–1674]

      With one stroke of this Dart
Strange horror seise thee, and pangs
   unfelt before.
So spake the grieslie terrour.
    Paradise Lost, Bk. II

Duc François de La Rochefoucauld [1613–1680]

Everything has been written which
could by possibility persuade us that
death is not an evil. . . . Nevertheless, I doubt whether any man of good
sense ever believed it.
    Maxims, No. 504

Alexander Smith [1830–1867]

To have to die is a distinction of
which no man is proud.
    Dreamthorp, Ch. II

Death is the ugly fact which nature
has to hide, and she hides it well.
    Ibid., Ch. III

The Bible

The last enemy that shall be destroyed is death.
> *I Corinthians* 15:26

V. DEATH AS INEVITABLE

Euripides [484–406 B.C.]

Death is a debt we all must pay.
> *Alcestis,* 419

Socrates [470?–399 B.C.]

Must not all things at last be swallowed up in death?
> Quoted by Plato in *Phaedo,* 72.D (tr. by Benjamin Jowett)

Cicero [106–43 B.C.]

The elements of which . . . all things are composed are liable to change; therefore every body is liable to change. But if any body were not liable to death, then not every body would be liable to change. Hence it follows that every body is liable to death.
> *On the Nature of the Gods,* III.xii.30 (tr. by H. Rackham)

Horace [65–8 B.C.]

Pale Death with foot impartial knocks at the poor man's cottage and at princes' palaces.
> *Odes,* I.iv.13 (tr. by C. E. Bennett)

Epictetus [60?–120?]

What is death? A bugbear.[1] Turn it about and learn what it is; see, it does not bite. The paltry body must be separated from the bit of spirit, either now or later, just as it existed apart from it before.
> *Discourses,* II.i.17 (tr. by W. Oldfather)

[1] bugbear = a terrifying mask.

Tertullian [160?–230?]

It is a poor thing for anyone to fear what is inevitable.
> *The Soul's Testimony,* IV (tr. by S. Thelwall)

John Lydgate [1370?–1451?]

Against Death is worth no medicine.
> *The Daunce of Machabree*

William Shakespeare [1564–1616]

CORNELIUS: The Queen is dead.
CYMBELINE: Who worse than a physician
Would this report become? But I consider
By med'cine life may be prolong'd, yet death
Will seize the doctor too.
> *Cymbeline,* V, v, 27

A man can die but once; we owe God a death. I'll ne'er bear a base mind. An't be my destiny, so; an't be not, so. No man's too good to serve's prince; and let it go which way it will, he that dies this year is quit for the next.
> *Henry IV, Part II,* III, ii, 250

Cowards die many times before their deaths;
The valiant never taste of death but once.[1]
Of all the wonders that I yet have heard,
It seems to me most strange that men should fear,
Seeing that death, a necessary end,
Will come when it will come.
> *Julius Caesar,* II, ii, 32

John Donne [1573–1631]

Death . . . comes equally to us all, and makes us all equall when it comes.
> Sermon preached at Whitehall, March 8, 1622

[1] Cf. Abraham Lincoln, p. 84b.

John Webster [1580?-1625?] and Thomas Dekker [1572?-1632?]

I saw him now going the way of all flesh.
> *Westward Hoe,* Act II, Sc. ii

Bishop Joseph Henshawe [1603-1679]

How time runs away, and we meet with Death alway, e're wee have time to thinke ourselves alive: One doth but *breake-fast* here, another *dine,* he that lives longest doth but *suppe:* We must all *goe to bed* in another World.
> *Horae Succisivae,* Pt. I

Sir Thomas Browne [1605-1682]

This reasonable moderator, and equal piece of justice, Death.
> *Religio Medici,* Pt. I, Sect. 38

Bernard Le Bovier de Fontenelle [1657-1757]

In vain we shall penetrate more and more deeply the secrets of the structure of the human body, we shall not dupe nature; we shall die as usual.
> *Dialogues des Morts,* Dialogue V (tr. by Harvey and Erasistratos)

Book of Common Prayer [1662]

Man, that is born of a woman, hath but a short time to live.
> *Burial of the Dead*

In the midst of life we are in death.
> *Idem*

John Gay [1685-1732]

The rich, the poor, the great, the small
Are levell'd. Death confounds 'em all.
> *Fables,* Series II, Fable 16

Laurence Sterne [1713-1768]

To die, is the great debt and tribute due unto nature.
> *Tristram Shandy,* Bk. V, Ch. 3

Richard Brinsley Sheridan [1751-1816]

Death's a debt; his mandamus binds all alike — no bail, no demurrer.
> *St. Patrick's Day,* Act II, Sc. iv

Thomas Lovell Beddoes [1803-1849]

Death is the one condition of our life:
To murmur were unjust; our buried sires
Yielded their seats to us, and we shall give
Our elbow-room of sunshine to our sons.
From first to last the traffic must go on;
Still birth for death.
> *The Second Brother,* Act III, Sc. ii

Henri Amiel [1828-1881]

The only certainty in this world of vain agitations and infinite anxieties, is the certainty of death, and that which is the foretaste and small change of death — pain.
> *Journal Intime,* April 17, 1860 (tr. by Mrs. Humphrey Ward)

Friedrich Nietzsche [1844-1900]

The certainty of death could add a blithe zest to life, but your drug-store minds spoil it with nauseous poisons.
> *Human, All Too Human,* Pt. II (tr. by Hans Waine)

Oscar Wilde [1854-1900]

The Doctor said that Death was but
A scientific fact.
> *The Ballad of Reading Gaol,* Pt. III

One can survive everything nowadays, except death.
> *A Woman of No Importance,* Act I

W. Somerset Maugham
[1874-1965]

The verdict for him too was death, not the inevitable death that horrified and yet was tolerable because science was helpless before it, but the death which was inevitable because the man was a little wheel in the great machine of a complex civilisation, and had as little power of changing the circumstances as an automaton. Complete rest was his only chance. The physician did not ask impossibilities.

Of Human Bondage, Ch. LXXXI

Merrill Moore [1903-1957]

Doctors must die, too; all their knowledge of
Digitalis, adrenalin, henbane,
Matters little if death raps again —
Once he may be forestalled, but their great love
Or little love of life is merely human:
Doctors must die like other men and women.

Ah, yes, they know the coronary well,
The lenticulo-striate artery, like a bell
In the village church; and when those strike their knell
What may have been well is no longer well.

Knowledge of nature gives exemption to
No one, his father, and to no one's son;
No one is probably the only one
Who lives any longer than other mortals do.

M: One Thousand Autobiographical Sonnets, Ch. IX, "Les Savants Ne Sont Pas Curieux"

The Bible

Dust thou art, and unto dust shalt thou return.

Genesis 3:19

Let us eat and drink; for tomorrow we die.

Isaiah 22:13 and *I Corinthians* 15:32

Proverbs

Against the evil of death there is no remedy in the gardens.

Death devours lambs as well as sheep.

English Proverbs

Old men go to death, and death comes to young men.

Young men may die, old men must.

German Proverb

No herb grows that will cure death.

Scottish Proverb

There's a cure for everything but stark dead.

DELIRIUM

Lucretius [96?-55 B.C.]

In bodily disease a wandering mind
Is often found; devoid of reason then,
The patient raves and roams delirious.

On the Nature of Things, III. 464

William Shakespeare [1564-1616]

O vanity of sickness! Fierce extremes
In their continuances will not feel themselves.
Death, having prey'd upon the outward parts,
Leaves them insensible; and his siege is now
Against the mind, the which he pricks and wounds
With many legions of strange fantasies,
Which, in their throng and press to that last hold,
Confound themselves.

King John, V, vii, 13

George Gordon, Lord Byron
[1788–1824]

Delirium is our best deceiver.
The Spell Is Broke, The Charm Is Flown!

Francis Brett Young [1884–1954]

To-night I lay with fever in my veins,
Consumed, tormented creature of fire
and ice,
And, weaving the enhavock'd brain's
device,
Dreamed that for evermore I must
walk these plains
Where sunlight slayeth life, and where
no rains
Abated the fierce air, nor slaked its
fire:
So that death seemed the end of all
desire,
To ease the distracted body of its
pains.
And so I died, and from my eyes the
glare
Faded, nor had I further need of
breath;
But when I reached my hand to find
you there
Beside me, I found nothing. . . .
Lonely was death,
And with a cry I wakened, but to
hear
Thin wings of fever singing in my ear.
104° Fahrenheit

DEPRESSION

See MELANCHOLY

DERMATOLOGY

See SKIN

DIABETES

Martin H. Fischer [1879–1962]

Many a diabetic has stayed alive by
stealing the bread denied him by his
doctor.
Quoted by Howard Fabing and
Ray Marr in *Fischerisms*

Wilfrid G. Oakley [1905–   ]

Man may be the captain of his fate,
but he is also the victim of his blood
sugar.
*Transactions of the Medical So-
ciety of London* 78:16, 1962

DIAGNOSIS

Huang Ti (The Yellow Emperor)
[2697–2597 B.C.]

By observing myself I know about
others and their diseases are revealed
to me, and by observing the external
symptoms one gathers knowledge
about internal disturbances.
Nei Ching Su Wên, Bk. 2, Sect.
2 (tr. by Ilza Veith in *The
Yellow Emperor's Classic of
Internal Medicine*)

The most important requirement of
the art of healing is that no mistakes
or neglect occur. There should be no
doubt or confusion as to the application of the meaning of complexion and
pulse. These are the maxims of the
art of healing.
Ibid., Bk. 4, Sect. 13

Menander [343?–291? B.C.]

Physicians, you know, by way of
building a towering reputation, are
wont to diagnose insignificant troubles
as greater ones and to exaggerate real
dangers.
Fragments, 497 (tr. by F. G.
Allinson)

St. Justin [100?–165?]

By examining the tongue of the patient, physicians find out the diseases

of the body, and philosophers the diseases of the mind.

Chang Chung-ching [fl. 170–196]

The skilful doctor knows by observation, the mediocre doctor by interrogation, the ordinary doctor by palpation.

> Quoted by K. C. Wong and Wu Lien-teh in *History of Chinese Medicine*

John of Mirfield [1362–1407]

If there is any doubt as to whether a person is or is not dead, apply lightly roasted onion to his nostrils, and if he is alive, he will immediately scratch his nose.

> *Breviarum Bartholomei,* "De Signis Malis" (tr. by H. R. Aldridge)

Paracelsus [1493?–1541]

Now they say when I come to a patient, I know not immediately what ails him, but I need time to find out. It is true. That they judge immediately is the fault of foolishness; for in the end the first judgment is false and from day to day they know the longer, the less, what it is, and make liars of themselves. Whereas I desire to approach from day to day, the longer, the closer to the truth. For with hidden diseases it is not as with the recognising of colours: in colours one sees well what is black, green, blue, etc. But if there were a curtain before it, thou also wouldst not know. To see through a curtain requires effort where there has been none before. What the eyes see can well be judged hurriedly, but what is hidden from the eyes it is in vain to conceive as though it were visible.

> *Seven Defensiones,* "The Seventh Defence" (tr. by Lilian Temkin)

J. J. F. Vicarius [1664– ?]

Oh, how fallacious sometimes are diagnostics!

> Quoted by Giovanni Battista Morgagni in *The Seats and Causes of Diseases,* Vol. I, Bk. 2, Letter 16 (tr. by B. Alexander)

Immanuel Kant [1724–1804]

Physicians think they do a lot for a patient when they give his disease a name.

Nicholas de Belleville [1753–1831]

When you are called to a sick man, be sure you know what the matter is — if you do not know, nature can do a great deal better than you can guess.

> Quoted by Fred B. Rogers in *Help-Bringers,* "Belleville"

Jacob Bigelow [1786–1879]

He is a great physician who, above other men, understands diagnosis.

> *Nature in Disease,* Ch. 2

Peter Mere Latham [1789–1875]

The diagnosis of disease is often easy, often difficult, and often impossible.

> *Diseases of the Heart,* Lect. XIV

The physiognomy of disease . . . can never be adequately described, and I urge you always to remark it and to dwell much on it; for some acute observers have drawn such secrets from the expression of the countenance, that it has been to them in the place of almost all other symptoms.

> *Lectures on Clinical Medicine,* Lect. III

Alfred Stillé [1813–1900]

I . . . have devoted whatever knowledge and skill I possessed to the simple, if difficult, task of knowing and curing diseases. . . . Medicine is, first of all, an art, but an art that can only be successfully practised when the physician is able to recognize the individual diseases he must meet with in practice, and distinguish from one another those which are similar in appearance, but unlike in nature.

> *Medical News* 44:433, 1884

Sir James Paget [1814-1899]

As no two persons are exactly alike in health so neither are any two in disease; and no diagnosis is complete or exact which does not include an estimate of the personal character, or the constitution of the patient.

There used to be a French saying that "French physicians treat the disease, English the patient." So far as this is true it is to the honour of the English, for to treat a sick man rightly requires the diagnosis not only of the disease but of all the manner and degrees in which its supposed essential characters are modified by his personal qualities, by the mingled inheritances that converge in him, by the changes wrought in him by the conditions of his past life, and by many things besides.

> Address to Abernethian Society, 1885 (Quoted by Sir James Patterson Ross in *St. Bartholomew's Hospital Journal* 54:50, 1950)

Henri Amiel [1821-1881]

Why do doctors so often make mistakes? Because they are not sufficiently individual in their diagnoses or their treatment. They class a sick man under some given department of their nosology, whereas every invalid is really a special case, a unique example. How is it possible that so coarse a method of sifting should produce judicious therapeutics?

> *Journal Intime*, August 22, 1873 (tr. by Mrs. Humphrey Ward)

Jean Martin Charcot [1825-1893]

Clinical medicine is made up of anomalies, while nosography is the description of phenomena that occur regularly. What we look for in the clinics is almost always exceptional; what we study in nosography is the rule. It is well to know that, in the practice of medicine, a nosographer is not always a clinician.

To learn how to treat disease, one must learn how to recognize it. The diagnosis is the best trump in the scheme of treatment.

Joseph Bell [1] [1837-1911]

The precise and intelligent recognition and appreciation of minor differences is the real essential factor in all successful medical diagnosis. . . . Eyes and ears which can see and hear, memory to record at once and to recall at pleasure the impressions of the senses, and an imagination capable of weaving a theory or piecing together a broken chain or unravelling a tangled clue, such are the implements of his trade to a successful diagnostician.

> Lecture to students in the Faculty of Medicine, University of Edinburgh

Ambrose Bierce [1842-1914?]

DIAGNOSIS, n. A physician's forecast of disease by the patient's pulse and purse.

> *The Devil's Dictionary*

Sir William Osler [1849-1919]

Adhesions are the refuge of the diagnostically destitute.

> Quoted by William B. Bean in *Sir William Osler: Aphorisms*, Ch. 5

---

[1] Dr. Bell was Sir Arthur Conan Doyle's professor and gave him the idea of Sherlock Holmes and his adventures.

Samuel J. Meltzer [1851–1921]

The fact that your patient gets well does not prove that your diagnosis was correct.

Rutherford Morison [1853–1939]

Beware of the diagnosis of hysteria, neurosis or neuralgia, unless organic disease can be excluded with certainty.
> Quoted in *The Practitioner*, October 1965

Remember that exploratory incisions should not be made a cloak for diagnostic incompetence.
> *Idem*

Robert Tuttle Morris [1857–1945]

There is no royal road to diagnosis.
> *Doctors Versus Folks*, Ch. 4

Sir Arthur Conan Doyle [1859–1930]

It is an old maxim of mine that when you have excluded the impossible, whatever remains, however improbable, must be the truth.
> *The Adventures of Sherlock Holmes*, "The Adventure of the Beryl Coronet"

August Bier [1861–1949]

A smart mother makes often a better diagnosis than a poor doctor.

It is more important to cure people than to make diagnoses.

James B. Herrick [1861–1954]

The doctor may also learn more about the illness from the way the patient tells the story than from the story itself.
> *Memories of Eighty Years*, Ch. VIII

J. Chalmers Da Costa [1863–1933]

Diagnosis by intuition is a rapid method of reaching a wrong conclusion.
> *The Trials and Triumphs of the Surgeon*, Ch. I

Charles Norris [1867–1935]

If you have to choose between a brilliant and a common sense diagnosis, your percentage of correct ones will be much higher with the latter.

Sir Robert Hutchison [1871–1960]

If you once get into the habit of guessing you are diagnostically damned.
> *The Principles of Diagnosis, Prognosis and Treatment*

Wilfred Trotter [1872–1939]

Disease often tells its secrets in a casual parenthesis.
> *Collected Papers*, "Art and Science in Medicine," Sect. 6

Karl Kraus [1874–1936]

Diagnosis is one of the commonest diseases.

Russell John Howard [1875–1942]

Diagnosis precedes treatment.
> Quoted by F. G. St. Clair Strange in *The Hip*, Ch. 7

Martin H. Fischer [1879–1962]

Diagnosis is not the end, but the beginning of practice.
> Quoted by Howard Fabing and Ray Marr in *Fischerisms*

Do you ever ponder the advisability of *not* making a diagnosis and thereby avoiding a death sentence?
> *Idem*

If your diagnosis is wrong, you're ruined — because the patient never forgets; but if your diagnosis is right, you're also ruined — unless you forget.
> *Idem*

In diagnosis, think of the easy first.
> *Idem*

Make a diagnosis and get hanged for it. You can't sail a boat on your *impressions* of where the north lies.
Idem

When you no longer know what headache, heartache, or stomach-ache means without cistern punctures, electrocardiograms, and six x-ray plates, you are slipping.
Idem

Thomas Addis [1881–1949]

[The physician] will use scientific methods, he will for a time dismember his patient — isolate, for instance, his kidneys or his heart and observe their action under very specialized conditions — but in the end he has to put these parts together again in his "diagnosis." This "diagnosis" is his total conception of the relationships between the patient as a person, the disease as a part of the patient, and the patient as a part of the world in which he lives.
Glomerular Nephritis, Diagnosis and Treatment, Ch. 5

Sir Thomas Lewis [1881–1945]

Diagnosis is a system of more or less accurate guessing, in which the endpoint achieved is a name. These names applied to disease come to assume the importance of specific entities, whereas they are for the most part no more than insecure and therefore temporary conceptions.
Lancet 1:619, 1944

James Howard Means
[1885–1967]

So much of the diagnostic process is now done through technological procedures that the doctor has lost some of his apparent omniscience, prestige and mystique.
Daedalus 92:701, 1963

Sir Heneage Ogilvie [1887–　　]

A misleading symptom is misleading only to one able to be misled.
Surgery, Orthodox and Heterodox, Ch. 11

Sir F. M. R. Walshe [1888–　　]

For the clinician judgment depends upon the primary clinical assessment. How often do we see the clinician shooting off all he has before he has really seen his target or put his hands upon his patient and, in the process, what discomforts, hazards and pains he may inflict upon him.
Canadian Medical Association Journal 67:395, 1952

J. Burns Amberson [1890–　　]

If you make the right diagnosis, the treatment is easy.

J. B. S. Haldane [1892–1964]

Early diagnosis of disease is the business of the general public even more than of the medical profession.
Possible Worlds, "The Time Factor in Medicine"

Robert Graves [1895–　　]

His case is not uncommon,
The doctors pronounce;
But prescribe no cure.
The Halls of Bedlam

Francis Scott Smyth [1895–　　]

To know what kind of a person has a disease is as essential as to know what kind of a disease a person has.
Journal of Medical Education 37:495, 1962

Paul Reznikoff [1896–　　]

When laboratory reports conflict with clinical judgment, don't discard the latter before repeating the laboratory tests.

William Dock [1898–   ]

DR. DOCK: Why don't you follow Sutton's Law?
STUDENT: What is that?
DR. DOCK: Willy Sutton, the notorious bank-robber, was asked by reporters why he always robbed banks rather than hotel clerks, filling stations, or other easy marks. He replied, "Because that's where the money is." [1]

David Seegal [1899–   ]

Balanced compulsiveness is a "must" for the effective clinician because the management of today's patient is often divided among many hands. The family physician must assess divergent opinions and lead his patient through a series of examinations which may be hazardous, time-consuming, and expensive. Here his abilities are tested exactly; this is not to say that he must be a Toscanini, a tyrant, or a nit-picker, but he cannot afford to be lax in his responsibilities. Casualness may lead to disaster; other factors being equal, controlled compulsiveness is the best antidote for this failing.
Journal of Chronic Diseases
17:105, 1964

The sound clinician attacks the core of the problem and avoids being mousetrapped by tangential data.
The Pharos of Alpha Omega Alpha 26:7, 1963

John L. McClenahan [1915–   ]

A sick man may wear a wrong diagnosis around his neck like a millstone, and the doctor's task may be first to *un*diagnose him so recovery can begin.
Medical Affairs 3:8, 1962

[1] Comment during ward rounds at the Yale–New Haven Hospital when he discovered that every test except the critical one had been done.

Anonymous

For most diagnoses all that is needed is an ounce of knowledge, an ounce of intelligence, and a pound of thoroughness!

In diagnosis, the young are positive and the middle-aged tentative; only the old have flair.
Lancet 1:795, 1951

There's a lot of it going around.

Chinese Proverb

To be uncertain is to be uncomfortable, but to be certain is to be ridiculous.

DIAPHRAGM

Leonardo da Vinci [1452–1519]

[The diaphragm] is shaped like a deeply hollowed spoon. If it were not arched so that it could receive the stomach and other viscera into its concavity it could not afterward contract . . . and exert pressure on the intestines, and drive the food from the stomach into the intestines, nor could it help the abdominal muscles to expel the feces, nor could it by contracting enlarge the thoracic cavity and compel the lung to expand, so that they may inspire air to refresh the veins coming from the heart.
Quaderni d'Anatomia, Vol. I

Ambrose Bierce [1842–1914?]

DIAPHRAGM, n. A muscular partition separating disorders of the chest from disorders of the bowels.
The Devil's Dictionary

DIARRHEA

See BOWELS, DYSENTERY, INFECTION

DIET

See also EATING, FASTING,
HUNGER, NUTRITION, SALT,
VEGETARIANISM, VITAMINS

Hippocrates [460?–377? B.C.]

Those bodies which have been slowly
emaciated should be slowly recruited;
and those which have been quickly
emaciated should be quickly recruited.
> *Aphorisms*, II.7 (tr. by Francis
> Adams)

It is easier to fill up with drink than
with food.
> *Ibid.*, II.11

An article of food or drink which is
slightly worse, but more palatable, is
to be preferred to such as are better
but less palatable.
> *Ibid.*, II.38

Plato [427?–347 B.C.]

Cookery simulates the disguise of
medicine, and pretends to know what
food is the best for the body; and if
the physician and the cook had to
enter into a competition in which children were the judges, or men who had
no more sense than children, as to
which of them best understands the
goodness or badness of food, the
physician would be starved to death.
> *Gorgias*, 465.B (tr. by Ben-
> jamin Jowett)

Demosthenes [385?–322 B.C.]

Like the diet prescribed by doctors,
which neither restores the strength of
the patient nor allows him to succumb.
> *Third Olynthiac*, 33 (tr. by
> J. H. Vince)

Horace [65–8 B.C.]

Hear what blessings the simple life
  confers
And how great they are. First and
  foremost, good health.

You'll realize how harmful a many-
  course dinner is
If you think of old-fashioned food,
  which sat so well
On your stomach. Mixing boiled and
  roast meat, or shellfish
And fricaseed thrush, sours your liver
  and makes the phlegm
Act up in your stomach.
> *Satires*, II.ii.70 (tr. by S. P.
> Bovie)

A man will pass his summers in health,
who will finish his luncheon with black
mulberries which he has picked from
the tree before the sun is trying.
> *Ibid.*, II.iv.21 (tr. by H. R.
> Fairclough)

Ovid [43 B.C.–A.D. 17?]

Now to perform a true physician's
  part,
And show I am a perfect master of my
  art,
I will prescribe what diet you should
  use,
What food you ought to take, and
  what refuse.
> *The Remedies of Love*, 796

Galen [fl. 2nd Cent.]

Hunger is not a fitting reason to fill
one's belly greedily and to excess, nor
does thirst justify draining the whole
cup in a single gulp. . . . be on our
guard in order that we may take less
to eat than those who are dining with
us and that we may keep away from
the dainty foods while we eat the
healthful foods in moderation.
> *De Cognoscendis Curandisque
> Animi Morbis*, Ch. 6 (tr. by
> P. W. Harkins as *On the Pas-
> sions and Errors of the Soul*)

Moses ben Maimon (Maimonides)
[1135–1204]

A person should not eat until his stomach is replete but should diminish [his
alimentary intake] by approximately
one fourth of satiation. One should

not drink water during meals save a little and mixed with wine. When the food commences to be digested in the intestines, one may drink as much water as one finds necessary. However, even after the food has been digested, he should not imbibe water excessively.
Mishneh Torah, "Hilchoth De'oth," Ch. IV, No. 2 (tr. by Fred Rosner in *Annals of Internal Medicine* 62:372, 1965)

In the warm [summer] months, one should eat cooling foods, not use seasoning to excess, and consume vinegar. In the rainy [winter] months, one should eat warming foods, abundantly spice [the food]. . . . In this manner should one prepare [food] in cold climates and warm climates, [that is] in each and every place that which is best suited thereto.
Ibid., No. 8

There are some foods which are extremely detrimental and it is proper for man never to eat them, such as large salted old fish, old salted cheese, truffles, mushrooms, old salted meat, wine must, and a cooked dish which has been kept until it acquired a foul odor. Likewise, any food whose odor is bad or excessively bitter is like a fatal poison unto the body. There are other foods which are also detrimental but are not as injurious as the aforementioned ones. Therefore, of these, one should eat only a little and only after [intervals of] many days. . . . Examples [of this type of food] are large fish, cheese, and milk that is kept for 24 hours after milking. The meat of large oxen and large he-goats, beans, lentils, peas, barley bread, unleavened bread, cabbage, leeks, onions, garlic, mustard, and radishes — all of these are detrimental foods.
Ibid., No. 9

There are other foods which are [also] detrimental but not as much as the [aforementioned ones]. They are water fowl, small young pigeons, dates, bread toasted in oil or bread that was kneaded with oil, fine meal that was completely sifted so that not a trace of bran remains, gravy, and brine [of salted fish]. One should not consume these foods excessively. A person that is wise and can control his inclinations and does not yield to his appetite, and does not eat any of the aforementioned [detrimental foods] unless he needs them as a medicine, is indeed a strong man.
Ibid., No. 10

A person should always abstain from fruits of trees and not consume them excessively even when they are dried, and needless to say when they are fresh. . . . Figs, grapes, and almonds, however, are always good whether fresh or dried, and a person may eat therefrom as much as he requires. One should not eat them constantly even though they are better than all the [other] fruits of trees.
Ibid., No. 11

Honey and wine are bad for children but salutary for the elderly especially in the rainy [winter] season. A person should eat in the warm [summer] months two thirds of what he eats in the rainy [winter] months.
Ibid., No. 12

Another major principle of bodily health, [physicians] state, is that as long as a person labors and becomes greatly fatigued and does not satiate [himself by overeating] and keeps his bowels soft, no illness will befall him and [on the contrary] his strength becomes fortified even if he eats detrimental foods.
Ibid., No. 14

Andrew Boorde [1490–1549]
The chefe physycke (the counceyll of

a physycyon excepte) dothe come from the Kytchyn.
A Dyetary of Helthe, Ch. XVIII

The physycyon and the coke for sycke men must consult togyther for the preparacion of meate for sycke men.
Idem

Edward Hall [d. 1547]

Their [the English soldiers'] victaile was muche part Garlike, and the Englieshmen did eate of the Garlike with all meates, and drank hote wynes in the hote wether, and did eate all the hote frutes that thei could gette, which caused their bloudde so to boyle in their belies, that there fell sicke three thousande of the flixe.
The Triumphant Reigne of Kyng Henry the VIII

William Bullein [d. 1576]

A good Kitchen, is a good Apothicaries shop.
The Bulwark Against All Sickness

Eate good broth made of chickens, leane Mutton, roste a little Partriche, eate light leavened breade; beware of grosse meates, Beefe, Porke, &c, and salletes, strong wine, Spice, sweete meates, and rawe fruites. I praie you remember this, and drink your Diacodion at night to reconcile slepe again, and be somewhat laxative.
A Dialogue

Michel de Montaigne [1533–1592]

Our doctors . . . eat the melon and drink the new wine while they keep their patient tied down to syrups and slops.
Essays, Bk. III, Ch. 9, "Of Vanity" (tr. by Donald M. Frame)

Sir Francis Bacon [1561–1626]

Examine thy customs of diet, sleep, exercise, apparel, and the like. . . .

I commend rather some diet for certain seasons, than frequent use of physic.
Essays, "Of Regiment of Health"

William Shakespeare [1564–1616]

But I am a great eater of beef, and I believe that does harm to my wit.
Twelfth Night, I, iii, 90

Tobias Venner [1577–1660]

[Milk] causeth the bodie to waxe grosse, and for amending of a dry constitution, and for them that are extenuated by long sicknes, or are in a consumption, it is by reason of the excellent moistning, cooling and nourishing facultie of it, of singular efficacie.
Via recta ad vitam longam, Sect. V

It [lettuce] is of all hearbes, the best and wholesomest for hot seasons, for young men, and them that abound with choler, and also for the Sanguine, and such as have hot stomachs.
Ibid., Sect. VII

I . . . advertise all such as have plethoricke and full bodies, especially living at rest, and which are of a phlegmaticke temperature, that they not onely eschew the use of breakefasts, but also oftentimes content themselves with one meale in a day.
Ibid., Sect. VIII

William Lithgow [1582?–1645?]

He that eateth well, drinketh well, he that drinketh well, sleepeth well, he that sleepeth well, sinneth not, and he that sinneth not, goeth straight through Purgatory to Paradize.[1]
The Totall Discourse of the Rare Adventures, Pt. II

[1] This is a phrase which Lithgow, a Protestant who thought all Catholics were sinners, claimed he heard "lascivious Friars" uttering to each other in Italy.

Randle Cotgrave [d. 1634?]

Eat bread at pleasure, drinke wine by measure.[1]
> *A Dictionarie of the French and English Tongues,* "Vin"

Sir Thomas Browne [1605–1682]

I have no antipathy, or rather Idiosyncrasie, in dyet, humour, ayre, any thing; I wonder not at the *French,* for their dishes of frogges, snailes, and toadstooles, nor at the Jewes for Locusts and Grasse-hoppers, but being amongst them, make them my common viands; and I finde they agree with my stomach as well as theirs; I could digest a Sallad gathered in a Church-yard, as well as in a Garden.
> *Religio Medici,* Pt. II, Sect. 1

Jonathan Swift [1667–1745]

Kitchen Physic is the best Physic.
> *Polite Conversation,* Dialogue II

Montesquieu [1689–1755]

That kind of health which can be preserved only by a careful and constant regulation of diet is but a tedious disease.

Voltaire [1694–1778]

I observe, walking about the country, that the children of the soil eat much less than they require: it is difficult to conceive this immoderate passion for abstinence.
> Letter to M. de Bastide, 1760 (tr. by S. G. Tallentyre)

Matthew Green [1696–1737]

I always choose the plainest food
To mend viscidity of blood.
Hail! water-gruel, healing power,
Of easy access to the poor. . . .
To thee I fly, by thee dilute —
Through veins my blood doth quicker shoot.
> *The Spleen*

[1] Pain tant qu'il dure, vin à mesure.

Samuel Johnson [1709–1784]

Some people . . . have a foolish way of not minding, or pretending not to mind, what they eat. For my part, I mind my belly very studiously, and very carefully; for I look upon it, that he who does not mind his belly will hardly mind anything else.[1]
> Quoted by James Boswell in *Life of Samuel Johnson,* August 5, 1763

Thomas Jefferson [1743–1826]

I fancy it must be the quantity of animal food eaten by the English which renders their character insusceptible of civilisation. I suspect it is in their kitchens & not in their churches that their reformation must be worked, & that Missionaries of that description from hence would avail more than those who should endeavor to tame them by precepts of religion.
> Letter to Mrs. John (Abigail) Adams, September 25, 1785

Anthelme Brillat-Savarin [1755–1826]

Tell me what you eat, and I will tell you what you are.
> *La Physiologie du Goût,* "Fundamental Truths" (tr. by R. E. Anderson as *Gastronomy as a Fine Art*)

Sydney Smith [1771–1845]

              Oh, herbacious treat!
'Twould tempt the dying anchorite to eat.[2]
> Quoted by Lady Holland in *A Memoir of the Rev. Sydney Smith,* Ch. 11

Richard Bright [1789–1858]

The great rule is, to avoid everything which obviously deranges the stomach.
> *Guy's Hospital Reports* 1:338, 1836

[1] Cf. Charles W. Eliot, p. 131b.
[2] In reference to his recipe for salad.

Chauncey Depew [1834–1928]

[Butter:] That delightful substance which comes out of the wonderful chemistry which God has given the cow for the delight of the world and the sustenance of children.

> Speech in the Senate, April 2, 1902

Henry S. Leigh [1837–1883]

If you wish to grow thinner, diminish your dinner,
And take to light claret instead of pale ale;
Look down with an utter contempt upon butter,
And never touch bread till it's toasted — or stale.

> *Carols of Cockayne,* "On Corpulence"

Ambrose Bierce [1842–1914?]

OYSTER, n. A slimy, gobby shellfish which civilization gives men the hardihood to eat without removing its entrails! The shells are sometimes given to the poor.

> *The Devil's Dictionary*

August Bier [1861–1949]

What is worse than keeping a diet! It can make your whole life miserable.

Sir Robert Hutchison [1871–1960]

One swears by wholemeal bread, one by sour milk; vegetarianism is the only road to salvation of some, others insist not only on vegetables alone, but on eating those raw. At one time the only thing that matters is calories; at another time they are crazy about vitamins or about roughage.

The scientific truth may be put quite briefly; eat moderately, having an ordinary mixed diet, and don't worry.

> *Newcastle Medical Journal,* Vol. 12, 1932

Martin H. Fischer [1879–1962]

Diets were invented of the church, the workhouse and the hospital. They were started for the punishment of the spirit and have ended in the punishment of the body.

> Quoted by Howard Fabing and Ray Marr in *Fischerisms*

Doctors confuse color with chemistry. The white meat of chicken is therefore the essence of a light diet and dark meat is poison.

> *Idem*

First need in the reform of hospital management? That's easy! The death of all dietitians, and the resurrection of a French chef.

> *Idem*

The first rule to proper diet? Ask them what they want and then give it to them. There are few exceptions.

> *Idem*

The proper concept of a strengthening diet is a chicken wrung out in hot water.

> *Idem*

Lin Yutang [1895–   ]

The Chinese do not draw any distinction between food and medicine.

> *The Importance of Living,* Ch. IX, Sect. vii

René J. Dubos [1901–   ]

Whenever shortages of bread or brandy develop, jealousies and conflicts arise, emotional tensions mount, regulations become necessary, and liberties are lost.

> *The Dreams of Reason,* Ch. III

The Bible

Thou shalt not seethe a kid in his mother's milk.

> *Exodus* 23:19

Thou mayest eat flesh, whatsoever thy soul lusteth after.
Deuteronomy 12:20

A feast of fat things.
Isaiah 25:6

Man shall not live by bread alone.
Matthew 4:4 and *Luke* 4:4

Strong meat belongeth to them that are of full age.
Hebrews 5:14

The Talmud

In eating, a third of the stomach should be filled with food, a third with drink, and the rest left empty.
Gittin

Until the age of forty food is more beneficial; thenceforth drink is more beneficial.
Shabbath XXIII.152a (tr. by H. Freedman)

Anonymous

A scientist says: Roast beef made England what she is today. Moral: Eat more vegetables.

Milk before wine
I would 'twere mine;
Milk taken after,
Is poison's daughter.
Old English rhyme

There was an old man of Tobago
Who lived on rice, gruel and sago;
Till, much to his bliss
His physician said this —
To a leg, sir, of mutton you may go.
The Oxford Book of Nursery Rhymes, No. 507

Proverbs

A little with quiet is the only diet.

Jack Sprat he loved no fat, and his wife she loved no lean:
And yet betwixt them both they lick'd the platters clean.

To lengthen thy life, lessen thy meals.

What one relishes, nourishes.

Whatsoever was the father of a disease, an ill diet was the mother.

Chinese Proverb

He that takes medicine and neglects to diet himself, wastes the skill of the physician.

Czech Proverb

Eat a little, inquire a little, but don't be curious, and you'll live long.

Dutch Proverb

Herring in the land, the doctor at a stand.

English Proverb

Feed sparingly and defy the physician.

French Proverb

Bread and cheese is medicine for the well.

German Proverb

A man is what he eats.[1]

Japanese Proverb

When the oranges are golden, physicians' faces grow pale.

Latin Proverb

From a great supper comes a great pain; that you may sleep lightly sup lightly.

Scottish Proverb

Light supper makes long life.

Scottish and Italian Proverb

He that eats but one dish seldom needs the doctor.

Spanish Proverb

Diet cures more than the lancet.

[1] Der Mensch ist, was er isst.

DIGESTION

See also EATING, INDIGESTION

Lucretius [96?–55 B.C.]

Nor does it matter a whit with what food the body is nourished, so long as you can digest what you take, and distribute it abroad through the limbs, and preserve the moisture of the stomach uninterrupted.
> *On the Nature of Things,* IV.630 (tr. by W. H. D. Rouse)

Paracelsus [1493?–1541]

If the physician is to understand the correct meaning of health, he must know that there are more than a hundred, indeed more than a thousand, kinds of stomach; consequently, if you gather a thousand persons, each of them will have a different kind of digestion, each unlike the others.
> *Three Books on Surgery,* Bk. III, Foreword (tr. by Norbert Guterman)

William Stevenson [1] [1530?–1575]

I can not eate, but lytle meate,
    my stomacke is not good:
But sure I thinke, that I can drynke
    with him that wears a hood.
> *Gammer Gurton's Needle,* Act II

Michel de Montaigne [1533–1592]

What good does it do us to have our belly full of meat if it is not digested?
> *Essays,* Bk. I, Ch. 25, "Of Pedantry" (tr. by Donald M. Frame)

William Shakespeare [1564–1616]

Will Fortune never come with both hands full,
But write her fair words still in foulest letters?

[1] Attributed to William Stevenson.

She either gives a stomach, and no food
(Such are the poor, in health), or else a feast,
And takes away the stomach.
> *Henry IV, Part II,* IV, iv, 103

Now good digestion wait on appetite,
And health on both!
> *Macbeth,* III, iv, 38

Things sweet to taste prove in digestion sour.
> *Richard II,* I, iii, 236

For your health and your digestion sake,
An after-dinner's breath.
> *Troilus and Cressida,* II, iii, 120

George Herbert [1593–1633]

A good digestion turneth all to health.
> *The Temple,* "The Church Porch"

William Penn [1644–1718]

The receipts of cookery are swelled to a volume, but a good stomach excels them all: to which nothing contributes more than industry and temperance.
> *Fruits of Solitude,* Maxim 61

John Fothergill [1712–1780]

The stomach is in general the best director; what ever it takes with pleasure, I mean with regard to quality, is always preferable to any other; but to regulate the quantity is not always easy; yet to leave off rather short is sometimes necessary, even though the appetite seems yet lively. . . . This abstemious method has likewise another good effect; it allows a glass of wine to be drunk without injury; nay it renders it necessary and beneficial.
> Letter to a young patient, 1749

Sydney Smith [1771–1845]

I am convinced digestion is the great secret of life; and that character,

talents, virtues, and qualities are powerfully affected by beef, mutton, pie-crust, and rich soups.
> Letter to Arthur Kinglake, September 30, 1837

Benjamin Disraeli, Lord Beaconsfield [1804–1881]

A good eater must be a good man; for a good eater must have a good digestion, and a good digestion depends upon a good conscience.
> *The Young Duke*

Samuel Butler [1835–1902]

The healthy stomach is nothing if not conservative. Few radicals have good digestions.
> *Note-Books,* Ch. VI, "Indigestion"

Joseph Conrad [1857–1924]

You can't ignore the importance of a good digestion. The joy of life . . . depends on a sound stomach, whereas a bad digestion inclines one to skepticism, incredulity, breeds black fancies and thoughts of death.
> *Under Western Eyes,* Pt. III, Ch. 3

Charles T. Copeland [1860–1952]

To eat is human, to digest divine.

Don Marquis [1878–1937]

it is a cheering thought to think that god is on the side of the best digestion
> *archy does his part,* "the big bad wolf"

how beautiful is the universe
when something digestible meets
with an eager digestion
> *the lives and times of archy and mehitabel,* "robin and the worm"

Lin Yutang [1895–]

Happiness for me is largely a matter of digestion.

Proverbs

A man has often more trouble to digest meat than to get it.

The guts uphold the heart, and not the heart the guts.

DIGITALIS

See FOXGLOVE

DISCOVERY

See also RESEARCH

Michel de Montaigne [1533–1592]

Whenever a new discovery is reported to the scientific world, they say first, "It is probably not true." Thereafter, when the truth of the new proposition has been demonstrated beyond question, they say, "Yes, it may be true, but it is not important." Finally, when sufficient time has elapsed to fully evidence its importance, they say, "Yes, surely it is important, but it is no longer new."

Sir Francis Bacon [1561–1626]

Brutes by their natural instinct have produced many discoveries, whereas men by discussion and the conclusions of reason have given birth to few or none.
> *Novum Organum,* "Aphorisms," LXXIII

Sir Humphry Davy [1778–1829]

I thank God I was not made a dextrous manipulator; the most important of my discoveries have been suggested to me by my failures.

Claude Bernard [1813–1878]

A great discovery is a fact whose appearance in science gives rise to shining ideas, whose light dispels many obscurities and shows us new paths.

An Introduction to the Study of Experimental Medicine, Pt. I, Ch. 2, Sect. ii (tr. by H. C. Greene)

A discovery is generally an unforeseen relation not included in theory, for otherwise it would be foreseen.

Ibid., Sect. iii

Ardent desire for knowledge, in fact, is the one motive attracting and supporting investigators in their efforts; and just this knowledge, really grasped and yet always flying before them, becomes at once their sole torment and sole happiness. Those who do not know the torment of the unknown cannot have the joy of discovery, which is certainly the liveliest that any man can feel.

Ibid., Pt. III, Ch. 4, Sect. iv

Louis Pasteur [1822-1895]

Oersted [1] . . . suddenly saw, by chance you will say, but chance only favours the prepared mind, the needle move and take up a position quite different from the one assigned to it by terrestrial magnetism.

Address, December 7, 1854

To be astonished at anything is the first movement of the mind towards discovery.

S. Weir Mitchell [1829-1914]

The success of a discovery depends upon the time of its appearance.

Quoted by F. H. Garrison in *Bulletin of the New York Academy of Medicine* 4:1002, 1928

William H. Welch [1850-1934]

Of the half dozen great discoveries which in their day have revolutionized

[1] Hans Christian Oersted [1777-1851], founder of the science of electromagnetism.

the science and the art of medicine, only that of the circulation of the blood belongs to a past century, while surgical anaesthesia, cellular pathology, the demonstration of the germ doctrine of infectious diseases, antiseptic surgery, and the prophylactic and therapeutic applications of the principles underlying artificial immunity have all been introduced during the nineteenth century.

Papers and Addresses, Vol. III, "The Material Needs of Medical Education"

Theobald Smith [1859-1934]

Great discoveries which give a new direction to currents of thought and research are not, as a rule, gained by the accumulation of vast quantities of figures and statistics. These are apt to stifle and asphyxiate and they usually follow rather than precede discovery. The great discoveries are due to the eruption of genius into a closely related field, and the transfer of the precious knowledge there found to his own domain.

Boston Medical and Surgical Journal 172:121, 1915

J. Chalmers Da Costa [1863-1933]

Many a man who is brooding over alleged mighty discoveries reminds me of a hen sitting on billiard balls.

The Trials and Triumphs of the Surgeon, Ch. 1

Sir Berkeley Moynihan [1865-1936]

A discovery is rarely, if ever, a sudden achievement, nor is it the work of one man; a long series of observations, each in turn received in doubt and discussed in hostility, are familiarized by time, and lead at last to the gradual disclosure of truth.

Surgery, Gynecology & Obstetrics 31:549, 1920

Martin H. Fischer [1879–1962]

Every discovery in science is a tacit criticism of things as they are. That is why the wise man is invariably called the fool.

> Quoted by Howard Fabing and Ray Marr in *Fischerisms*

None of the great discoveries was made by a "specialist" or a "researcher."
> *Idem*

The greatest discoveries of surgery are anesthesia, asepsis, and roentgenology — and none was made by a surgeon.
> *Idem*

Wilder Penfield [1891–   ]

One evening in the late eighteenth century an Italian woman stood in her kitchen watching the frogs' legs which she was preparing for the evening meal. "Look at those muscles moving. . . . They always seem to come alive when I hang them on the copper wire."

Her husband [Luigi Galvani] looked. . . . The cut end of the frog's nerve was in contact with the copper wire, and electric current produced by the contact was passing along the nerve to the muscle. As a result, the muscle was twitching and contracting. . . .

He had discovered the key to electricity, and to nerve conduction, and to muscle action. Here was the basis of all animal movement, reflex and voluntary, in frog and man.
> *The Second Career,* "The Physiological Basis of the Mind"

Henry E. Sigerist [1891–1957]

We must also keep in mind that discoveries are usually not made by one man alone, but that many brains and many hands are needed before a discovery is made for which one man receives the credit.
> *A History of Medicine,* Vol. I, Introduction

Albert Szent-Györgyi [1893–   ]

As far as I can remember, it was very rarely that I found the answer to any of my problems by conscious thinking. This conscious thinking only acted as a primer for my brain, which seemed to work much better without my muddling when I was asleep or fishing. I think that without such concentration and devotion nothing can be achieved, be it in art or in science. When Newton was asked how he made his discoveries, he replied: "By always thinking into them."
> *Perspectives in Biology and Medicine* 5:173, 1962

David and Beatrice C. Seegal [1899–   ] [1898–   ]

Scientific discovery is not a monopoly of the fully matured investigator. It is not unusual for a student to present interesting and promising ideas. Best was a medical student when he was associated with Banting in the experiment which led to the discovery of insulin. Cannon was a medical student when he suggested the use of bismuth for visualization of hollow organs by X ray. It is never too soon to be alert and to question all rules as well as all exceptions.
> *The Diplomate* 22:125, 1950

Maurice B. Strauss [1904–1974]

Discoveries do not arise *de novo,* like Athene from the brow of Zeus, but are more akin to the living layers of a coral reef built on the past labors of countless predecessors.
> *Medicine* 43:619, 1964

W. I. B. Beveridge [1908–   ]

Probably the majority of discoveries in biology and medicine have been come upon unexpectedly, or at least had an element of chance in them, especially the most important and revolutionary ones.
> *The Art of Scientific Investigation,* Ch. III

One of the best illustrations of such a discovery [originating from hypotheses] is provided by the story of Christopher Columbus' voyage; it has many of the features of a classic discovery in science. (a) He was obsessed with an idea. . . . (b) the idea was by no means original. . . . (c) he met great difficulties in getting someone to provide the money to enable him to test his idea as well as in the actual carrying out of the experimental voyage, (d) when finally he succeeded he did not find the expected new route, but instead found a whole new world, (e) despite all evidence to the contrary he clung to the bitter end to his hypothesis. . . . (f) he got little credit or reward during his lifetime and neither he nor others realised the full implications of his discovery, (g) since his time evidence has been brought forward showing that he was by no means the first European to reach America.
> *Ibid.*, Ch. IV

DISEASE

See also INFECTION, OBSERVATION, SICKNESS, TREATMENT

Hesiod [fl. 8th Cent. B.C.]

Of themselves diseases come upon men continually by day and by night, bringing mischief to mortals silently.
> *Works and Days* (tr. by H. G. Evelyn-White)

Aeschylus [525–456 B.C.]

Of a truth lusty health resteth not content within its due bounds; for disease ever presseth close against it, its neighbour with a common wall.
> *Agamemnon*, 1001 (tr. by H. W. Smyth)

Hippocrates [460?–377? B.C.]

Those diseases that medicines do not cure are cured by the knife. Those that the knife does not cure are cured by fire. Those that fire does not cure must be considered incurable.
> *Aphorisms*, VII.87 (tr. by W. H. S. Jones)

Plato [427?–347 B.C.]

To require the help of medicine, not when a wound has to be cured, or on occasion of an epidemic, but just because, by indolence and a habit of life such as we have been describing, men fill themselves with waters and winds, as if their bodies were a marsh, compelling the ingenious sons of Asclepius to find more names for diseases, such as flatulence and catarrh; is not this, too, a disgrace? . . . I do not believe that there were any such diseases in the days of Asclepius. . . . the guild of Asclepius did not practice our present system of medicine, which may be said to educate diseases.
> *Republic*, III.405 (tr. by Benjamin Jowett)

Pien Ch'iao [fl. 255 B.C.]

Men worry over the great number of diseases, while doctors worry over the scarcity of effective remedies.
> Quoted by K. C. Wong and Wu Lien-teh in *History of Chinese Medicine*, Bk. I, Ch. 5

Ovid [43 B.C.–A.D. 17?]

'Tis not the same story to feel and to cure a disease; all men can feel, skill must remove the trouble.
> *Pontic Epistles*, III.ix.16 (tr. by A. L. Wheeler)

Seneca [4? B.C.–A.D. 65]

A disease also is farther on the road to being cured when it breaks forth from concealment and manifests its power.
> *Moral Epistles to Lucilius*, LVI (tr. by Richard M. Gummere)

You need not wonder that diseases are beyond counting: count the cooks!
Ibid., XCV.xxiii

St. Augustine [354–430]

All diseases of Christians are to be ascribed to demons.

Rhazes [850–923]

When the disease is stronger than the patient, the physician will not be able to help him at all, and if the strength of the patient is greater than the strength of the disease, he does not need a physician at all. But when both are equal, then one needs a physician who will support the patient's strength and help him against the disease.
Quoted by Moses ben Maimon in *The Preservation of Youth* (tr. by Fi Tadbir as-Sihha)

Paracelsus [1493?–1541]

Once a disease has entered the body, all parts which are healthy must fight it: not one alone, but all. Because a disease might mean their common death. Nature knows this; and Nature attacks the disease with whatever help she can muster. Therefore, the medicines that you prescribe must encompass the entire expanse of the firmament, the close and distant celestial spheres.
Opus Paramirum, Pt. I, Bk. II, Ch. ii (tr. by Max Samter)

Barnabe Rich [1540?–1617]

The diseases of Ireland are many, and the sickness is grown to that contagion that it is almost past cure.
The Anothomy of Ireland

George Pettie [1548–1589]

When hope and hap, when health and wealth, are highest, then woe and wrack, disease and death, are nighest.
A Petite Pallace of Pettie His Pleasure, "Alexius"

Thomas Moffett [1553–1604]

Every disease will have his course.
Health's Improvement, Ch. 1

William Shakespeare [1564–1616]

We would not understand what was most fit
But, like the owner of a foul disease,
To keep it from divulging, let it feed
Even on the pith of life.
Hamlet, IV, i, 20

Before the curing of a strong disease,
Even in the instant of repair and health,
The fit is strongest.
King John, III, iv, 112

For thine own bowels which do call thee sire,
The mere effusion of thy proper loins,
Do curse the gout, serpigo, and the rheum
For ending thee no sooner.
Measure for Measure, III, i, 29

His dissolute disease will scarce obey this medicine.
The Merry Wives of Windsor, III, iii, 203

Now the rotten diseases of the South, the guts-griping, ruptures, catarrhs, loads o' gravel i' th' back, lethargies, cold palsies, raw eyes, dirt-rotten livers, whissing lungs, bladders full of imposthume, sciaticas, limekilns i' th' palm, incurable boneache, and the rivelled fee simple of the tetter, take and take again such preposterous discoveries!
Troilus and Cressida, V, i, 20

Till then I'll sweat and seek about for eases,
And at that time bequeath you my diseases.
Ibid., V, x, 56

As burning fevers, agues pale and faint,

Life-poisoning pestilence, and frenzies
wood,
The marrow-eating sickness, whose at-
taint
Disorder breeds by heating of the
blood,
Surfeits, imposthumes, grief, and
damn'd despair
Swear Nature's death for framing
thee so fair.
Venus and Adonis, line 739

Robert Burton [1577–1640]

Diseases . . . crucify the soul of man,
attenuate our bodies, dry them, wither
them, rivel them up like old apples,
make them as so many Anatomies.
The Anatomy of Melancholy,
Pt. I, Sect. 2, Memb. 3, Subsect. 10

James Howell [1594?–1666]

Ther is a common saying that says,
He hath as many diseases as a horse,
but 'tis false, for *man* hath many
more.
The Parley of Beasts, Sect. 5

Sir Thomas Browne [1605–1682]

Some will allow no Diseases to be new,
others think that many old ones are
ceased; and that such which are esteemed new, will have but their time:
However, the Mercy of God hath scattered the great heap of Diseases, and
not loaded any one Country with all:
some may be new in one Country
which have been old in another. New
Discoveries of the Earth discover new
Diseases.
A Letter to a Friend

Samuel Butler [1612–1680]

Diseases of their own Accord,
But *Cures* come difficult and hard.
*Satyr upon the Weakness and
Misery of Man*

Thomas Sydenham [1624–1689]

The generality have considered that

disease is but a confused and disordered effort of Nature, thrown down
from her proper state, and defending
herself in vain.
Medical Observations (3rd ed.),
Preface (tr. by R. G. Latham
in *Works,* Vol. I)

A disease, however much its cause
may be adverse to the human body, is
nothing more than an effort of Nature,
who strives with might and main to
restore the health of the patient by
the elimination of the morbific humor.
Ibid., Sect. 1, Ch. 1

John Ward [1629–1681]

Friend, thou hast two diseases, and
whilst I kill one, the other will kill
thee!
Diary

Michael Wigglesworth
[1631–1705]

New-England, where for many yeers
You scarcely heard a cough,
And where Physicians had no work,
Now finds them work enough.

One wave another followeth
And one disease begins
Before another cease, because
We turn not from our sins.
*God's Controversy with New-
England*

John Locke [1632–1704]

All doctors up to the present century
seem to me to have failed, because in
the cure of diseases they have given
little thought, or none at all, to the
specific nature of each disease, and
considered only the external symptoms, which are no more concerned
with their specific nature than the
type and richness of the soil are with
species of plants which may grow in
it.
*An Essay Concerning Human
Understanding*

Hermann Boerhaave [1668–1738]

What Doctor is there, who while he treats a disease unknown to him, might be at ease, until he had clearly perceived the nature of this disease and its hidden causes?

> *Atrocis, nec Descripti Prius, Morbi Historia* (tr. in *Bulletin of the Medical Library Association* 43:217, 1955)

Edward Young [1683–1765]

Old-age *will* come; disease *may* come before;
Fifteen is full as mortal as *threescore.*
> *Love of Fame,* Satire VI

Alexander Pope [1688–1744]

The young disease, that must subdue at length,
Grows with his growth, and strengthens with his strength.
> *An Essay on Man,* Epistle II

Henry Fielding [1707–1754]

Every physician, almost, hath his favourite disease, to which he ascribes all the victories obtained over human nature. The gout, the rheumatism, the stone, the gravel, and the consumption have all their several patrons in the faculty; and none more than the nervous fever, or the fever on the spirits. And here we may account for those disagreements in opinion concerning the cause of a patient's death which sometimes occur between the most learned of the college.
> *Tom Jones,* Bk. II, Ch. 9

Samuel Johnson [1709–1784]

Disease generally begins that equality which death completes.
> *The Rambler,* No. 48 (September 1, 1750)

Thomas Jefferson [1743–1826]

The disorders of the animal body, & the symptoms indicating them, are as various as the elements of which the body is composed.
> Letter to Dr. Caspar Wistar, June 21, 1807

Johann Wolfgang von Goethe [1749–1832]

I have learned much from disease which life could have never taught me anywhere else.
> Quoted by Johann Peter Eckermann in *Conversations with Goethe*

Edward Jenner [1749–1823]

The deviation of man from the state in which he was originally placed by nature seems to have proved to him a prolific source of diseases.
> *An Inquiry into the Causes and Effects of the Variolae Vaccinae, or Cow-Pox*

Sydney Smith [1771–1845]

I hope that Lord Grey and you are well — no easy thing seeing that there are above 1500 diseases to which Man is subjected.
> Letter to Lady Grey, February 1, 1836

Jacob Bigelow [1786–1879]

Most men form an exaggerated estimate of the powers of medicine, founded on the common acceptance of the name, that medicine is the art of curing diseases. That this is a false definition is evident from the fact that many diseases are incurable, and that one such disease must at last happen to every living man. A far more just definition would be that medicine is the art of understanding diseases, and of curing or relieving them when possible. Under this acceptation our science would, at least, be exonerated from reproach, and would stand on a basis capable of supporting a reason-

able and durable system for the amelioration of human maladies.
Nature in Disease, Ch. 2

Peter Mere Latham [1789–1875]

We should always presume the disease to be curable until its own nature prove it otherwise.
Diseases of the Heart, Lect. XIV

Perfect health, like perfect beauty, is a rare thing; and so, it seems, is perfect disease.
General Remarks on the Practice of Medicine, Ch. X, Pt. 2

Thomas Carlyle [1795–1881]

Self-contemplation ... is infallibly the symptom of disease.
Characteristics

Heinrich Heine [1797–1856]

So it appears: disease was then
The cause for that creative urge,
Creating was a fiery purge,
Creating I grew well again.
Songs of Creation, No. 7 (tr. by Ernst Feise)

Armand Trousseau [1801–1867]

A knowledge of the specific element in disease is the key of medicine.
Clinical Medicine, Vol. I, Introduction

Elisha Bartlett [1804–1855]

There are certain pathological processes and conditions, one characteristic element of which consists in a distinct and well marked periodicity in their recurrence. These processes and conditions differ very widely from each other in many important particulars; but they agree in this.
Philosophy of Medical Science, Pt. II, Ch. 8

It is not easy to show, that any disease is absolutely local, on the one hand, or absolutely general, on the other.
Ibid., Ch. 10

Any definition is inadequate and defective, unless it does really define, or describe, the disease.
Ibid., Ch. 14

Alonzo Clark [1807–1887]

Every man's disease is his personal property.
Quoted by F. H. Garrison in *Bulletin of the New York Academy of Medicine* 5:154, 1929

Henry Wadsworth Longfellow [1807–1882]

Death is better than disease.
Christus: A Mystery, Pt. II, Sect. i

Alfred, Lord Tennyson [1809–1892]

Ring out old shapes of foul disease.
In Memoriam, Sect. CVI

Sir William Withey Gull [1816–1890]

You will soon learn that diseases, like other natural facts, require no peculiar mode of study. . . . Man is naturally unwilling to feel himself but a part, though the highest part as yet, of the course of nature, however deeply he may be convinced that all is ruled by the wisest providence. He desires to feel himself an exception from the common laws of nature. . . . The sense of mystery is so indigenous, . . . that, although I do not for a moment suppose any well-educated medical man could think that disease ever comes but through discoverable natural courses, we assume almost as much when we are satisfied not to have traced them to their beginnings. . . .

Diseases are but parts of a course of natural history.
>　*British Medical Journal* 2:425, 1874

Rudolf Virchow [1821–1902]

Ever since we recognized that diseases are neither self-subsistent, circumscribed, autonomous organisms, nor entities which have forced their way into the body, nor parasites rooted on it, but . . . the course of physiological phenomena under altered conditions . . . the goal of therapy has had to be the maintenance or the reestablishment of normal physiological conditions.
>　*Disease, Life, and Man,* "Standpoints in Scientific Medicine" (tr. by L. J. Rather)

Jean Martin Charcot [1825–1893]

Disease is very old, and nothing about it has changed. It is we who change, as we learn to recognize what was formerly imperceptible.
>　*De l'expectation en médecine*

Samuel Butler [1835–1902]

They regard bodily ailments as the more venial in proportion as they have been produced by causes independent of the constitution. Thus if a person ruin his health by excessive indulgence at the table or by drinking, they count it to be almost a part of the mental disease which brought it about, and so it goes for little, but they have no mercy on such illnesses as fevers or catarrhs or lung diseases, which to us appear to be beyond the control of the individual.
>　*Erewhon,* Ch. X

Henry Maudsley [1835–1918]

To despise the little things of functional disorder is to fall by little and little into organic disease.

Sir Clifford Allbutt [1836–1925]

I have often said figuratively, that, by the stepping-stones of borderland cases, one may walk from any one disease round the whole continent of morbid principalities and return dryshod to the starting-point.
>　*Diseases of the Arteries, including Angina Pectoris*

The name of a disease is not, as it is continually regarded, a thing.
>　Quoted by F. H. Garrison in *Bulletin of the New York Academy of Medicine* 4:1000, 1928

We are led to think of diseases as isolated disturbances in a healthy body, not as the phases of certain periods of bodily development.
>　*Idem*

Sir William Osler [1849–1919]

To talk of diseases is a sort of Arabian Nights' entertainment.
>　*Aequanimitas, with Other Addresses,* "Nurse and Patient"

Variability is the law of life, and as no two faces are the same, so no two bodies are alike, and no two individuals react alike and behave alike under the abnormal conditions which we know as disease.
>　*Ibid.,* "On the Educational Value of the Medical Society"

Credulity in matters relating to disease remains a permanent fact in our history, uninfluenced by education.
>　*British Medical Journal* 2:185, 1909

Sir Frederick Treves [1853–1923]

The symptoms of disease are marked by purpose, and the purpose is beneficent. The processes of disease aim not at the destruction of life, but at the saving of it.
>　Address to the Edinburgh Philosophical Institution, October 31, 1905

Sir Arthur Conan Doyle
[1859–1930]

Men die of the diseases which they have studied most. . . . It's as if the morbid condition was an evil creature which, when it found itself closely hunted, flew at the throat of its pursuer.

> *Round the Red Lamp,* "The Surgeon Talks"

August Bier [1861–1949]

When a disease is named after some author, it is very likely that we don't know much about it.

Charles H. Mayo [1865–1939]

Disease at times creates experiments that physiology completely fails to duplicate, and the wise physiologist can obtain clues to the resolution of many problems by studying the sick.

Claude Bragdon [1866–1946]

Health and disease, thought and emotion, are communicable, contagious.

Wilfred Trotter [1872–1939]

Disease often tells its secrets in a casual parenthesis.

> *Collected Papers,* "Art and Science in Medicine," Sect. 6

Thomas Mann [1875–1955]

But the disease makes him ailing within and fevered without; disease makes men more physical, it leaves them nothing but body.

> *The Magic Mountain,* Ch. IV, "The Thermometer" (tr. by H. T. Lowe-Porter)

Disease has nothing refined about it, nothing dignified. Such a conception is in itself pathological, or at least tends in that direction. Perhaps I may best arouse your mistrust of it if I tell you how ancient and ugly this conception is. It comes down to us from a past seething with superstition, in which the idea of humanity had degenerated and deteriorated into sheer caricature; a past full of fears, in which well-being and harmony were regarded as suspect and emanating from the devil, whereas infirmity was equivalent to a free pass to heaven. Reason and enlightenment have banished the darkest of these shadows that tenanted the soul of man — not entirely, for even yet the conflict is in progress.

> *Ibid.,* "Necessary Purchases"

Thomas Addis [1881–1949]

We are accustomed to speak of "disease entities" as though they had an independent, individual existence and could be recognized as friends — or better, perhaps, as enemies. This is obviously one of those abstractions that do violence to the reality of the concrete situation, for there is no disease apart from the patient. The disease is the change produced in the patient by a pathological process. Diagnosis involves the observation of the patient as he is, and also a reconstruction in imagination of the patient as he was, before he was afflicted. The disease is the difference between these two pictures. But this, also, is an abstraction.

> *Glomerular Nephritis, Diagnosis and Treatment,* Ch. 1

Francis Weld Peabody
[1881–1927]

Disease in man is never exactly the same as disease in an experimental animal, for in man the disease at once affects and is affected by what we call the emotional life. Thus, the physician who attempts to take care of a patient while he neglects this factor is as unscientific as the investigator who neglects to control all the conditions that may affect his experiment.

> *The Care of the Patient*

Ralph H. Major [1884–　]

Disease and destiny — as we survey the sweep of history and the panorama of life through the centuries, we are compelled to admit the role, often decisive, that disease plays.
>*Disease and Destiny,* Logan Clendening Lectures, 8th Series

Dame Rebecca West [1892–　]

To those who fall and hurt themselves, one runs with comfort; by those who lie dangerously stricken by a disease, one sits and waits.

Lin Yutang [1895–　]

Eventually we have to come to a conception of health and disease by which the two merge into each other.
>*The Importance of Living,* Ch. IX, Sect. vii

David Seegal [1899–　]

We all are plagued by diseases and disorders; we all shall become sick and die; but in the often long latent period between the diseases and/or disorders of early life and the illnesses of later years, medical science offers opportunity after opportunity for amelioration of the human condition.
>*Journal of Chronic Diseases* 16:196, 1963

René J. Dubos [1901–　]

Complete freedom from disease . . . is almost incompatible with the process of living.
>*Mirage of Health,* Ch. I

Proverb

A disease known is half cured.

Chinese Proverb

Before thirty, men seek disease; after thirty, diseases seek men.

English Proverb

Diseases are the tax on ill pleasures.

Irish Proverbs

A long disease does not always tell a lie; it will kill at last.

Every disease is a physician.

Scottish (Gaelic) Proverb

Wealth breeds a pleurisy, ambition a fever, liberty a vertigo, and poverty is a dead palsy.

Spanish Proverb

The disease a man dreads, that he dies of.

Welsh Proverb

Disease and sleep keep far apart.

DREAMS

Herodotus [484–424 B.C.]

Dreams in general originate from those incidents which have most occupied the thoughts during the day.
>*Histories,* VII.16 (tr. by William Beloe)

Plato [427?–347 B.C.]

In sleep, when the rest of the soul, the rational, gentle and dominant part, slumbers, . . . the beastly and savage part, replete with food and wine, gambols and, repelling sleep, endeavors to sally forth and satisfy its own instincts. . . . there is nothing it will not venture to undertake as being released from all sense of shame and all reason. It does not shrink from attempting to lie with a mother in fancy or with anyone else, man, god, or brute. It is ready for any foul deed of blood. . . . there exists in every one of us, even in some reputed most respectable, a terrible, fierce and lawless brood of desires, which it seems are revealed in our sleep.
>*Republic,* IX.571 (tr. by P. Shorey)

Menander [343?–291? B.C.]

For what one has dwelt on by day,
these things he sees in visions of the
night.
> *Fragments,* 734 (tr. by F. G.
> Allinson)

Cato [1] [234–149 B.C.]

Reck not of dreams; in things which
men pursue,
Sleep sees the hopes of waking hours
come true.
> *The Sayings of Cato* (tr. by
> J. W. Duff)

Leonardo da Vinci [1452–1519]

Why does the eye see a thing more
clearly in dreams than the imagination
when awake?
> Arundel MSS., British Mu-
> seum (tr. by Edward Mac-
> Curdy in *The Notebooks of
> Leonardo da Vinci,* Vol. I,
> Ch. I)

Michel de Montaigne [1533–1592]

Dreams are faithful interpreters of our
inclinations; but there is art to sort-
ing and understanding them.
> *Essays,* Bk. III, Ch. 13, "Of
> Experience" (tr. by Donald
> M. Frame)

Sir Thomas Browne [1605–1682]

Hippocrates wisely considered Dreams
as they presaged Alterations in the
Body, and so afforded hints toward
the preservation of Health, and prevention of Diseases; and therein was
so serious as to advise Alteration of
Diet, Exercise, Sweating, Bathing and
Vomiting.
> *A Letter to a Friend*

John Dryden [1631–1700]

All Dreams, as in old *Gallen* I have
read,
Are from Repletion and Complexion
bred:

[1] Attributed to Cato.

From rising Fumes of indigested Food,
And noxious Humors that infect the
Blood.
> *Fables Ancient and Modern,*
> "The Cock and the Fox"

Alexander Pope [1688–1744]

Yet ate, in dreams, the custard of the
day.
> *The Dunciad,* Bk. I

Tobias Smollett [1721–1771]

Had it been simply waking, he would
have been obliged to them for the
noise that disturbed him; for, in that
case, he would have been relieved from
the tortures of hell-fire, to which, in
his dream, he fancied himself exposed.
But this dreadful vision had been the
result of that impression, which was
made upon his brain by the intolerable anguish of his joints; so that,
when he awaked, the pain instead of
being allayed, was rather aggravated
by a great acuteness of sensation.
> *The Adventures of Peregrine
> Pickle,* Ch. 70

Christopher Anstey [1724–1805]

If ever I ate a good supper at night,
I dream'd of the devil, and wak'd in a
fright.
> *The New Bath Guide,* Letter
> IV

Charles Churchill [1731–1764]

>   Dreams,
Children of night, of indigestion bred,
Which, Reason clouded, seize and turn
the head.
> *The Candidate*

Thomas Lovell Beddoes
[1803–1849]

If there were dreams to sell,
  What would you buy?
Some cost a passing bell;
  Some a light sigh,
That shakes from Life's fresh crown
Only a rose-leaf down.

If there were dreams to sell,
Merry and sad to tell,
And the crier rang the bell,
    What would you buy?
        Dream-Pedlary

Edgar Allan Poe [1809–1849]

All that we see or seem
Is but a dream within a dream.
        A Dream within a Dream

Alfred, Lord Tennyson
[1809–1892]

                Maybe wildest dreams
Are but the needful preludes of the
    truth.
        The Princess, "Conclusion"

Henry David Thoreau [1817–1862]

Dreams are the touchstones of our
characters.
        *A Week on the Concord and
        Merrimack Rivers,* "Wednes-
        day"

Henri Amiel [1821–1881]

Dreams are excursions into the limbo
of things, a semi-deliverance from the
human prison.
        Journal Intime, December 3,
        1872 (tr. by Mrs. Humphrey
        Ward)

Sigmund Freud [1856–1939]

Obviously one must hold oneself responsible for the evil impulses of one's
dreams. In what other way can one
deal with them? Unless the content of
the dream rightly understood is inspired by alien spirits, it is part of
my own being.
        Collected Papers, Vol. V,
        "Some Additional Notes Upon
        Dream Interpretation as a
        Whole," Pt. B

It seems to be my fate to discover
only the obvious; that children have
sexual feelings, which every nursemaid knows; and that night dreams
are just as much wish-fulfillment as
daydreams.

Franklin P. Adams (F.P.A.)
[1881–1960]

Don't tell me what you dreamt last
    night, for I've been reading Freud.
        *Don't Tell Me What You
        Dreamt Last Night*

T. S. Eliot [1888–1965]

When you're alone in the middle of the
    night and you wake in a sweat
    and a hell of a fright
When you're alone in the middle of the
    bed and you wake like someone
    hit you in the head
You've had a cream of a nightmare
    dream and you've got the hoo-
    ha's coming to you.
        Fragment of an Agon

The Bible: Apocrypha

Your old men shall dream dreams,
your young men shall see visions.
        Joel 2:28

The Talmud

A dream which is not interpreted is
like a letter which is not read.
        Berakoth, IX.55b (tr. by M.
        Simon)

Hebrew Proverb

Dreams are a sixtieth part of prophecy.

DROPSY

Plautus [254?–184 B.C.]

I walk as I were girdled with my
    spleen;
And look as if my belly carried
    twins —
Wretch that I am! I fear me I shall
    burst.
        Curculio, Act II, Sc. 1

Horace [65–8 B.C.]

The dropsy by indulgence nursed
Pursues us with increasing thirst,
Till art expels the cause and drains
The watery languor from our veins.
> *Odes*, II.ii.13 (tr. by P. Francis)

Ovid [43 B.C.–A.D. 17?]

So he whose belly swells with dropsy,
the more he drinks, the thirstier he
grows.
> *Fasti*, I.215 (tr. by G. J. Frazer)

Celsus [25 B.C.–A.D. 50]

Hydrops . . . is relieved more easily
in slaves than in freemen, for since it
demands hunger, thirst, and a thousand other troublesome treatments and
prolonged endurance, it is easier to
help those who are easily constrained
than those who have an unserviceable
freedom.
> *De Medicina*, III.21 (tr. by
> W. G. Spencer)

Dante Alighieri [1265–1321]

[I] saw one there whose shape was
　like a lute,
　Had but his legs, between the groin
　　and haunch,
　Where the fork comes, been lopt off
　　at the root.

The heavy dropsy, whose indigested
　bunch
　Of humours bloats the swollen frame
　　within,
　Till the face bears no proportion to
　　the paunch,

Puffed his parched lips apart, with
　stiffened skin
　Drawn tight, as the hectic gapes,
　　one dry lip curled
　Upward by thirst, the other toward
　　the chin.
> *The Divine Comedy*, "Hell,"
> Canto XXX (tr. by Dorothy L.
> Sayers)

William Shakespeare [1564–1616]

It is a dropsied honour.
> *All's Well That Ends Well*, II,
> iii, 135

There is a devil haunts thee in the
likeness of an old fat man. . . . that
swoll'n parcel of dropsies.
> *Henry IV, Part I*, II, iv, 493

The dropsy drown this fool!
> *The Tempest*, IV, i, 230

William Heberden [1710–1801]

Swellings of the ancles or legs towards
evening, which vanish, or are greatly
lessened in the morning, are very common in women while they are breeding, and in hot weather.
> *Commentaries on the History
> and Cure of Diseases*, Ch. 48

Where persons after having laboured
for some time under complaints of the
lungs, or of the bowels, begin to find a
swelling in the legs, it is a sign of some
deep mischief in the breast or abdomen, the swelling will most probably
increase to a just dropsy, and the case
end fatally.
> *Idem*

Erasmus Darwin [1731–1802]

Bolster'd with down, amid a thousand
　wants,
Pale Dropsy reared his bloated form,
　and pants;
"Quench me, ye cool pellucid rills!"
　he cries,
Wets his parch'd tongue, and rolls his
　hollow eyes.
So bends tormented TANTALUS to
　drink,
While from his lips the refluent waters
　shrink; . . .
Divine HYGEIA, from the bending
　sky
Descending, listens to his piercing cry;
Assumes bright DIGITALIS' dress
　and air; . . .

O'er Him She waves her serpent-
wreathed wand,
Cheers with her voice, and raises with
her hand,
Warms with rekindling bloom his visage wan,
And charms the shapeless monster
into man.
> *The Botanic Garden,* Pt. II,
> Canto II

DRUGGIST

Alexander Pope [1688–1744]

So modern 'Pothecaries, taught the art
By Doctor's bills to play the Doctor's
part,
Bold in the practice of mistaken rules,
Prescribe, apply, and call their masters
fools.
> *An Essay on Criticism,* Pt. I

David Hume [1711–1776]

It appears to me that apothecaries
bear the same relation to physicians,
that priests do to philosophers; the
ignorance of the former makes them
positive, and dogmatical, and assuming, and enterprising, and pretending,
and consequently much more taking
with the people.
> Letter to John Clephane, Feb-
> ruary 18, 1751

Ambrose Bierce [1842–1914?]

APOTHECARY, n. The physician's
accomplice, undertaker's benefactor
and grave worm's provider.
> *The Devil's Dictionary*

DRUGS

See also OPIUM, REMEDIES,
TREATMENT

Virgil [70–19 B.C.]

He preferred to know the power of
herbs and their value for curing purposes, and, heedless of glory, to exercise that quiet art.
> *Aeneid,* XII.396

William Harrison [1534–1593]

Great thanks therefore be given unto
the physicians of our age and countrie,
who not onelie indeavour to search out
the use of such simples as our soile
doth yeeld and bring foorth, but also
to procure such as grow elsewhere,
upon purpose so to acquaint them with
our clime, that they in time through
some alteration received from the nature of the earth, maie likewise turne
to our benefit and commoditie, and be
used as our owne.
> *Holinshed's Chronicles,* Vol. I,
> Bk. II, Ch. 20

The greater number of simples that go
unto anie compound medicine, the
greater confusion is found therein, because the qualities and operations of
verie few of the particulars are thor-
oughlie knowne.
> *Idem*

John Lyly [1554?–1606]

The camomile the more it is trodden
and pressed down the more it spread-
eth.
> *Euphues*

Sir Francis Bacon [1561–1626]

If you fly physic in health altogether,
it will be too strange for your body
when you shall need it. If you
make it too familiar, it will work no
extraordinary effect when sickness
cometh.
> *Essays,* "Of Regiment of
> Health"

William Shakespeare [1564–1616]

Give me to drink mandragora . . .
That I might sleep.
> *Antony and Cleopatra,* I, v, 4

[You wish]
To jump a body with a dangerous
physic
That's sure of death without it.
Coriolanus, III, i, 154

The drug he gave me, which he said
was precious
And cordial to me, have I not found it
Murd'rous to th' senses?
Cymbeline, IV, ii, 326

The sovereignest thing on earth
Was parmacity for an inward bruise.
Henry IV, Part I, I, iii, 57

That gentle physic, given in time, had
cur'd me;
But now I am past all comforts here
but prayers.
Henry VIII, IV, ii, 122

What rhubarb, senna, or what purga-
tive drug,
Would scour these English hence?
Macbeth, V, iii, 55

Not poppy nor mandragora,
Nor all the drowsy syrups of the
world,
Shall ever medicine thee to that sweet
sleep
Which thou ow'dst yesterday.
Othello, III, iii, 330

Take thou this vial, being then in bed,
And this distilled liquor drink thou
off;
When presently through all thy veins
shall run
A cold and drowsy humour; for no
pulse
Shall keep his native progress, but
surcease;
No warmth, no breath, shall testify
thou livest;
The roses in thy lips and cheeks shall
fade
To paly ashes, thy eyes' windows fall
Like death when he shuts up the day
of life;

Each part, depriv'd of supple government,
Shall, stiff and stark and cold, appear
like death;
And in this borrowed likeness of
shrunk death
Thou shalt continue two-and-forty
hours,
And then awake as from a pleasant
sleep.
Romeo and Juliet, IV, i, 93

Then recover'd again with aqua-vitae
or some other hot infusion.
The Winter's Tale, IV, iv, 814

John Dryden [1631–1700]

Like him, who, being in good health,
lodged himself in a physician's house,
and was over-persuaded by his land-
lord to take physic (of which he died),
for the benefit of the doctor.
Aeneïs, "Dedication to the
Marquis of Normanby"

Joseph Glanvill [1636–1680]

The Physitian looks with another Eye
on the Medicinal hearb, then the graz-
ing Oxe, which swoops it in with the
common grass.
The Vanity of Dogmatizing,
Ch. XXIV

Joseph Addison [1672–1719]

Physick, for the most part, is nothing
else but the Substitute of Exercise or
Temperance.
The Spectator, Vol. III, No.
195 (October 13, 1711)

John Gay [1685–1732]

Man may escape from Rope and Gun;
Nay, some have out-liv'd the Doctor's
Pill.
The Beggar's Opera, Act II,
Sc. 8, Air 26

Alexander Pope [1688–1744]

Learn from the beasts the physic of
the field.
An Essay on Man, Epistle III

Johannes Gaub [1704–1780]

No scientific discipline is currently as hotly pursued as chemistry; is one not compelled, therefore, to apply its astounding results to man?

. . . Chemists concentrate the fragrance of cinnamon into a few drops; and distill — from treacherous poisons and innocent plants — the most amazing medications. Yet, there is more to come! If chemistry keeps its promises . . . whatever is alive, will be perfect; and, in the end, man will live for centuries, free from pain and suffering, in indestructible health, until he dissolves, serenely, in peace.

. . . How far removed is the harsh reality from such dreams! One can only admire ambition undeterred by distant goals, but we cannot transgress, ever, the limits set for us by nature. As the giants failed when they piled Pelion on Ossa to take the lightning out of Jupiter's hands, so will chemists fail. Swelled by extraordinary, almost supernatural experimental success, they have been tempted by fallacious fantasies to try their hand on medicine, even though their awareness of the elegant precision of the human organism should have kept them away.

> Address, October 18, 1734, "De vana vitae longae, a chemicis promissae spectatione" (tr. by Max Samter)

David Hume [1711–1776]

Nor has Rhubarb prov'd always a Purge, or Opium a Soporific to everyone who has taken these Medicines.
> *An Enquiry Concerning Human Understanding*, Sect. VI

Thomas Jefferson [1743–1826]

Patsy in convent. My health good till lately. James's illness and recovery. Remind of Umbrella, Seneca snake root and ginseng.
> Entry in journal, November 11, 1784, summarizing letter to Nicholas Lewis

Philippe Pinel [1745–1826]

For, in diseases of the mind, as well as in all other ailments, it is an art of no little importance to administer medicines properly: but, it is an art of much greater and more difficult acquisition to know when to suspend or altogether to omit them.
> *A Treatise on Insanity*, Sect. I (tr. by D. D. Davis)

Anthelme Brillat-Savarin [1755–1826]

Look at that patient, who is ordered by the faculty to take a black draught such as our grandfathers drank. That trusty adviser, the sense of smell, warns him against the repulsive flavour of the treacherous fluid; his eyes stare as at the approach of danger; disgust is on his lips; and already his stomach rises. Nevertheless, on being urged, he arms himself with determination, gargles his throat with brandy, holds his nose, and drinks.

While the detestable beverage is in the mouth and in contact with the organ, the sensation is confused and the suspense intolerable; but as soon as the last drop is swallowed, the after-taste is felt, sickening flavours act and the patient's countenance in every feature, expresses a horror and disgust such as no one dare encounter unless under the fear of death.
> *La Physiologie du Goût*, Ch. 2 (tr. by R. E. Anderson as *Gastronomy as a Fine Art*)

George Colman, the Younger [1762–1836]

When taken,
To be well shaken.
> *Broad Grins*, "The Newcastle Apothecary"

Napoleon Bonaparte [1769–1821]

Medicine is a collection of uncertain prescriptions which kill the poor, and succeed sometimes with the rich; and the results of which, collectively taken, are more fatal than useful to mankind. Speak to me no more about these fine things; I am not a man for drugs.

> Quoted by F. Antommarchi in *The Last Days of the Emperor Napoleon*, Vol. I

Thomas Moore [1779–1852]

How the Doctor's brow should smile Crown'd with wreaths of camomile.
> *Wreaths for the Ministers*

Peter Mere Latham [1789–1875]

Poisons and medicine are oftentimes the same substance given with different intents.
> *General Remarks on the Practice of Medicine*, Ch. IV

Thomas Hood [1799–1845]

Home-made physic, that sickens the sick.
> *Miss Kilmansegg and Her Precious Leg*, "Her Misery"

Elisha Bartlett [1804–1855]

Long abused humanity is likely, at no very remote period, to be finally delivered from the abominable atrocities of wholesale and indiscriminate drugging.
> *Philosophy of Medical Science*, Pt. II, Ch. 16

Oliver Wendell Holmes [1809–1894]

No families take so little medicine as those of doctors, except those of apothecaries.
> *Medical Essays*, "Currents and Counter-Currents in Medical Science"

Throw out opium, which the Creator himself seems to prescribe, for we often see the scarlet poppy growing in the cornfields, as if it were foreseen that wherever there is hunger to be fed there must also be pain to be soothed; throw out a few specifics which our art did not discover, and is hardly needed to apply; throw out wine, which is a food, and the vapors which produce the miracle of anaesthesia, and I firmly believe that if the whole materia medica, *as now used*, could be sunk to the bottom of the sea, it would be all the better for mankind, — and all the worse for the fishes.[1]
> *Idem*

The disgrace of medicine has been that colossal system of self-deception, in obedience to which mines have been emptied of their cankering minerals, the vegetable kingdom robbed of all its noxious growths, the entrails of animals taxed for their impurities, the poison-bags of reptiles drained of their venom, and all the inconceivable abominations thus obtained thrust down the throats of human beings suffering from some fault of organization, nourishment, or vital stimulation.
> *Ibid.*, "Border Lines of Knowledge in Some Provinces of Medical Science"

Sir William S. Gilbert [1836–1911]

What time the poet hath hymned
The writhing maid, lithe-limbed,
  Quivering on amaranthine asphodel,
How can he paint her woes,
Knowing, as well he knows,
  That all can be set right with calomel?
> *Patience*, Act I

John Shaw Billings [1838–1913]

We are a bitters-and-pill-taking people.
> *Boston Medical and Surgical Journal* 124:349, 1891

Ambrose Bierce [1842–1914?]

BELLADONNA, n. In Italian a beautiful lady; in English a deadly poison. A striking example of the essential identity of the two tongues.
> *The Devil's Dictionary*

[1] Cf. Martin H. Fischer, p. 125b.

MEDICINE, n. A stone flung down the Bowery to kill a dog in Broadway.
> *Idem*

Sir William Osler [1849–1919]

Imperative drugging — the ordering of medicine in any and every malady — is no longer regarded as the chief function of the doctor.
> *Aequanimitas, with Other Addresses,* "Medicine in the Nineteenth Century"

A desire to take medicine is, perhaps, the great feature which distinguishes man from other animals.
> *Science* 17:170, 1891

Nickel-in-the-slot, press-the-button therapeutics are no good. You cannot have a drug for every malady.
> Quoted by William B. Bean in *Sir William Osler: Aphorisms,* Ch. 3

One of the first duties of the physician is to educate the masses not to take medicine.
> *Idem*

One should treat as many patients as possible with a new drug while it still has the power to heal.

Sir Arthur Conan Doyle [1859–1930]

"For me," said Sherlock Holmes, "there still remains the cocaine bottle."
> *The Sign of Four,* "The Strange Story of Jonathan Small"

Karel Frederik Wenckebach [1864–1940]

I owe my reputation to the fact that I use digitalis in doses the text books say are dangerous and in cases that the text books say are unsuitable.
> Quoted in *Lancet* 2:633, 1937

Richard Clarke Cabot [1869–1939]

I believe that we not only feed the public demand for useless and harmful drugs, but also go far to create that very demand. We educate our patients and their friends to believe that every or almost every symptom and disease can be benefited by a drug.
> *Journal of the American Medical Association* 47:982, 1906

W. Somerset Maugham [1874–1965]

He set his face firmly against all the discoveries of the last thirty years: he had no patience with the drugs which became modish, were thought to work marvellous cures, and in a few years were discarded; he had stock mixtures which he had . . . used all his life; he found them just as efficacious as anything that had come into fashion since.
> *Of Human Bondage,* Ch. CXVI

Martin H. Fischer [1879–1962]

A man who cannot work without his hypodermic needle is a poor doctor. The amount of narcotic you use is inversely proportional to your skill.
> Quoted by Howard Fabing and Ray Marr in *Fischerisms*

Half the modern drugs could well be thrown out the window, except that the birds might eat them.[1]
> *Idem*

There is only one reason why men become addicted to drugs; they are weak men. Only strong men are cured, and they cure themselves.
> *Idem*

Aldous Huxley [1894–1963]

A hundred doses of happiness are not enough: send to the drug-store for another bottle — and, when that is finished, for another. . . . There can be no doubt that, if tranquillizers could be bought as easily and cheaply

---

[1] Cf. Oliver Wendell Holmes, p. 124b.

as aspirin, they would be consumed, not by the billions, as they are at present, but by the scores and hundreds of billions. And a good, cheap stimulant would be almost as popular.
Brave New World Revisited, Ch. 8

Malcolm Muggeridge [1903–　　]

I will lift up mine eyes unto the pills. Almost everyone takes them, from the humble aspirin to the multi-coloured, king-sized three deckers, which put you to sleep, wake you up, stimulate and soothe you all in one. It is an age of pills.
The New Statesman, August 3, 1962, "London Diary"

Ah, the paradise that awaits us in 1984! . . . For every ill a pill. Tranquilizers to overcome angst, pep pills to wake us up, life pills to ensure blissful sterility. I will lift up mine eyes unto the pills whence cometh my help.

John Bowle [1905–　　]

[King Henry VIII] would concoct medicines for his own use; a plaster "designed to heal ulcers without pain," and an unguent "devised by his Majesty at Greenwich to cool inflammation to take away the itch"; in his mature age, he invented "The King's Grace's oyntment made at St James's to coole and dry and comfort the Member."
Henry VIII, Ch. I

Frank M. Berger [1913–　　]

Tranquilizers at times do much more than eliminate agitation; they may facilitate social adjustment, eliminate delusions and hallucinations, or make mute patients communicative. An important characteristic of tranquilizers which is often overlooked is their ability to affect patients suffering from mental disturbances. Tranquilizers, as a rule, do not bring "peace of mind" to normal persons; they may not af-

fect them at all or may make them feel worse.
Drugs and Behavior (ed. by Leonard Uhr and James G. Miller), Ch. 3

Frederick W. Hanley [1917–　　]

Give me a button of wild peyote
To munch in my den at night,
That I may set my id afloat
In the country of queer delight.

So ho! it's off to the land of dreams
With never a stop or stay,
Where psychiatrists meet with fairy queens
To sing a roundelay.

Give me a flagon of mescaline
To wash o'er my mundane mind,
That I may feel like a schizophrene
Of the catatonic kind.

So hey! let in the visions of light
To banish banality,
Then will I surely catch a sight
Of the Real Reality.

Give me a chalice of lysergic
To quaff when day is done,
That I may get a perceptual kick
From my diencephalon.

So ho! let all resistance down
For a transcendental glance
Past the superego's frosty frown
At the cosmic underpants.

Give me a pinch of psilocybin
To sprinkle in my beer,
That my psychopathic next-of-kin
May not seem quite so queer.

So hey! it's off for the visions bizarre,
Past the ego boundary,
For a snort at the psychedelic bar
Of the new psychiatry.
Canadian Medical Association Journal 90:686, 1964, "Psychedelics"

John F. Kennedy [1917–1963]

It has been estimated that consumers

waste $500 million a year on medical quackery and another $500 million dollars annually on some "health foods" which have no beneficial effect. . . . Unnecessary deaths, injuries, and financial loss . . . can be expected to continue until the law requires adequate testing for safety and efficacy of products and devices before they are made available to consumers.

> *Message to Congress on Problems of the Aged,* February 21, 1963

Samuel E. Stumpf [1918–   ]

Some drugs have been appropriately called "wonder-drugs" inasmuch as one wonders what they will do next.

> *Annals of Internal Medicine* 64:460, 1966

Harold A. Kaminetzky
[1923–   ]

There are no really "safe" biologically active drugs. There are only "safe" physicians.

> *Obstetrics and Gynecology* 21: 512, 1963

Louis Lasagna [1923–   ]

[There is] the myth that the merit of a drug can be measured . . . by continued use. As others have pointed out, if survival is the test of fitness, then we should all forthwith pay homage to the oyster, which has endured essentially unchanged for 200,000,000 years.

> Review of Morton Mintz's *The Therapeutic Nightmare* in *The New York Times Book Review,* November 28, 1965

The Bible

Dead flies cause the ointment of the apothecary to send forth a stinking savour.

> *Ecclesiastes* 10:1

The Bible: Apocrypha

The Lord hath created medicines out of the earth; and he that is wise will not abhor them.

> *Ecclesiasticus* 38:4

Anonymous

Physicians of the highest rank
(To pay their fees, we need a bank),
Combine all wisdom, art and skill,
Science and sense, in Calomel.

> *Calomel*

Quinine is made of the sweat of ships' carpenters.

> Sailors' saying

A drug is a substance that, when injected into a rat, produces a scientific paper.

Chinese Proverb

No medicine is medium [quality] medicine.

French and German Proverb

Pills are to be swallowed, not chewed.

German Proverbs

Each physician thinks his pills best.

The garden is the poor man's apothecary.

Japanese Proverb

Good medicine always has a bitter taste.[1]

Latin Proverb

Who lives medically lives miserably.

DYSENTERY

William Heberden [1710–1801]

The Dysentery is common in camps.

> *Commentaries on the History and Cure of Diseases,* Ch. 31

[1] German Proverb: Bitter in the mouth, health in the body.

T. E. Lawrence [1888–1935]

Dysentery of this Arabian coast sort used to fall like a hammer blow, and crush its victims for a few hours, after which the extreme effects passed off; but it left men curiously tired.
Seven Pillars of Wisdom, Ch. 31

The Bible

I am poured out like water, and all my bones are out of joint: my heart is like wax; it is melted in the midst of my bowels.
Psalms 22:14

Chinese Proverb

Diarrhea is a river-fish complaint.

EAR

See also DEAFNESS, HEARING

St. Jean Baptiste de la Salle [1651–1719]

The ears should be kept perfectly clean; but it must never be done in company. It should never be done with a pin, and still less with the fingers, but always with an ear-picker.
The Rules of Christian Manners and Civility, I

The Bible

The hearing ear, and the seeing eye.
Proverbs 20:12

EARLY RISING

Huang Ti (The Yellow Emperor) [2697–2597 B.C.]

After a night of sleep people should get up early (in the morning); they should walk briskly around the yard; they should loosen their hair and slow down their movements (body); by these means they can (fulfill) their wish to live healthfully.
Nei Ching Su Wên, Bk. 1, Sect. 2 (tr. by Ilza Veith in *The Yellow Emperor's Classic of Internal Medicine*)

Aristotle [384–322 B.C.]

Rising before daylight is also to be commended; it is a healthy habit, and gives more time for the management of the household as well as for liberal studies.
Economics, I (tr. by G. Cyril Armstrong)

School of Salerno [1094–1224]

Rise earely in the morne.
Regimen Sanitatis Salernitanum (tr. by Sir John Harington as *The Englishman's Doctor*)

Sir Anthony Fitzherbert [1470–1538]

Erly rysyng maketh a man hole in body, holer in soule, and rycher in goodes.
Book of Husbandry, Ch. 149

Benjamin Franklin [1706–1790]

He that riseth late, must trot all day, and shall scarce overtake his business at night.
Poor Richard's Almanack, 1742

Leigh Hunt [1784–1859]

It is universally acknowledged that lying late in the morning is a great shortener of life. At least, it is never found in company with longevity. It also tends to make people corpulent.
The Indicator, XXI, "A Few Thoughts on Sleep"

George Gordon, Lord Byron [1788–1824]

I have sat up on purpose all the night,
   Which hastens, as physicians say,
   one's fate;

And so all ye, who would be in the
right
  In health and purse, begin your day
  to date
From daybreak, and when coffin'd at
four-score
Engrave upon the plate, you rose at
four.
> *Don Juan,* Canto II, Stanza
> 140

Dorothy Parker [1893–1967]

Early to bed, and you'll wish you were
dead. Bed before eleven, nuts before
seven.
> *The Little Hours*

James Thurber [1894–1961]

Early to rise and early to bed makes
a male healthy and wealthy and dead.
> *Fables for Our Time,* "The
> Shrike and the Chipmunks"

Proverbs

Early to bed, and early to rise, makes
a man healthy, wealthy and wise.

Go to bed with the lamb and rise with
the lark.

Scottish Proverb

Get a name to rise early, and you may
lie all day.

EATING

See also DIET, DIGESTION,
FASTING, HUNGER, INDI-
GESTION

Socrates [470–399 B.C.]

Base men live to eat and drink, and
good men eat and drink to live.
> Quoted by Plutarch in *Moralia,*
> "How the Young Man Should
> Study Poetry" (tr. by F. C.
> Babbitt)

Cicero [106–43 B.C.]

One should eat to live, not live to eat.
> *Rhetoricorum,* LV

Lucretius [96?–55 B.C.]

In those days again, it was lack of
food that drove fainting bodies to
death; now contrariwise it is the abundance that overwhelms them.
> *On the Nature of Things,*
> V.1007 (tr. by W. H. D. Rouse)

Catullus [84?–54 B.C.]

           I shook off
A most abominable cough
My stomach caused me, t'other day —
And right it served me, I must say,
For loving with too keen a zest
Luxurious dinners highly drest.
> *Carmina,* XLIV

Ovid [43 B.C.–A.D. 17?]

Don't just pick at your food, as if you
  had had a big dinner;
  Don't, on the other hand, gobble as
  much as you can.
> *The Art of Love,* III.257 (tr.
> by R. Humphries)

Juvenal [60?–140?]

See, the lone glutton craves whole
  boars, a beast
Designed by Nature for a social feast.
But speedy wrath o'ertakes him;
  gorged with food,
Swollen and fretted by the peacock
  crude,
He seeks the bath his feverish pulse
  to still.
Hence sudden death and age without
  a will.
> *Satires,* I.144 (tr. by J. War-
> rington)

Moses ben Maimon (Maimonides) [1135–1204]

When a person eats, he should always
be sitting in his place or reclining on
the left side. He should not walk nor
ride nor exercise nor agitate his body,

nor should he promenade until the food is digested in his intestines. Any one who promenades [immediately] after his meal or who fatigues himself brings upon himself serious and grave illnesses.

> *Mishneh Torah,* "Hilchoth De'oth," Ch. IV, No. 3 (tr. by Fred Rosner in *Annals of Internal Medicine* 62:372, 1965)

Excessive eating is like a deadly poison to the body of any man and it is the principle [cause] of all illnesses. Most diseases that man is afflicted with are due to bad foods or because he fills his abdomen and eats excessively, even of good [wholesome] foods.

> *Ibid.,* No. 15

François Rabelais [1494?–1553]

My first masters taught me this habit, for breakfast, they said, gave man a good mind. So they started the day by drinking.

> *Gargantua,* Bk. I, Ch. 21 (tr. by Jacques Le Clercq)

Henry IV of France [1553–1610]

Great eaters and great sleepers are incapable of anything else that is great.

William Shakespeare [1564–1616]

Surfeit is the father of much fast.

> *Measure for Measure,* I, ii, 130

They are as sick that surfeit with too much as they that starve with nothing.

> *The Merchant of Venice,* I, ii, 6

SIR TOBY: Does not our life consist of four elements?
SIR ANDREW: Faith, so they say; but I think it rather consists of eating and drinking.

> *Twelfth Night,* II, iii, 9

Tobias Venner [1577–1660]

Great and late suppers are very of-fensive to the whole body, especially to the head and eyes, by reason of the multitude of vapors, that ascend from the meats that have been plentifully received.

> *Via recta ad vitam longam,* Sect. VIII

John Selden [1584–1654]

In Gluttony there must be Eating, in Drunkenness there must be drinking: 'tis not the eating, nor 'tis not the drinking that is to be blamed, but the Excess.

> *Table Talk,* "Humility"

Thomas Fuller [1608–1661]

[King Edward IV] by intemperance in his diet, in some sort digged his grave with his own teeth.

> *Church History,* Bk. IV, Sect. 3

Benjamin Franklin [1706–1790]

If, after exercise, we feed sparingly, the digestion will be easy and good, the body lightsome, the temper cheerful, and all the animal functions performed agreeably.

> *The Art of Procuring Pleasant Dreams*

In general, mankind, since the improvement of cookery, eats twice as much as nature requires.

> *Poor Richard's Almanack*

Henry Taylor [1711–1785]

I have heard it remarked by a statesman of high reputation, that most great men have died of over-eating themselves.

> *Sermons*

Thomas Jefferson [1743–1826]

We never repent of having eaten too little.

> Letter to Thomas Jefferson Smith, February 21, 1825

Thomas Malthus [1766–1834]

I think I may fairly make two postulata.

First, That food is necessary to the existence of man.

Secondly, That the passion between the sexes is necessary, and will remain nearly in its present state.

> *An Essay on the Principle of Population* (1798), Ch. 1

Napoleon Bonaparte [1769–1821]

An army travels on its stomach.[1]

Sydney Smith [1771–1845]

All gentlemen and ladies eat too much. I made a calculation, and found I must have consumed some waggonloads too much in the course of my life. Lock up the mouth, and you have gained the victory.

> Quoted by Lady Holland in *A Memoir of the Rev. Sydney Smith*, Ch. 11

Thomas Brown [1778–1820]

If, morrow's headache knowing,
Stomach sick and overflowing,
Gives to-day, while spoons are going,
Not another inch for stowing, —
Shall we, future fasts foreknowing,
When the soup divine is flowing,
Sigh, and wish to see it going?

What though, morrow's ails inviting,
Doctors come, in ails delighting,
Shall they stop us now? — O never!
How provoking!
While 'tis smoking,
Sure *even they* would eat forever.
> *The Warning*

[1] In *The Mind of Napoleon*, J. C. Herold suggests that the closest Napoleon ever came to this famous aphorism was in a 1795 memorandum: "The basic principle that we must follow in directing the armies of the Republic is this: that they must feed themselves on war at the expense of the enemy territory."

George Gordon, Lord Byron [1788–1824]

But man is a carnivorous production,
    And must have meals, at least one
        meal a day;
He cannot live, like woodcocks, upon
        suction,
    But, like the shark and tiger, must
        have prey;
Although his anatomical construction
    Bears vegetables, in a grumbling
        way,
Your labouring people think beyond
        all question
Beef, veal, and mutton, better for
        digestion.
> *Don Juan*, Canto II, Stanza 67

Ralph Waldo Emerson [1803–1882]

We do not eat for the good of living, but because the meat is savory and the appetite is keen.
> *Essays* (Second Series), "Nature"

Charles W. Eliot [1834–1926]

Taking food and drink is a great enjoyment for healthy people, and those who do not enjoy eating seldom have much capacity for enjoyment or usefulness of any sort.[1]
> *The Happy Life*

Ambrose Bierce [1842–1914?]

EAT, v.i. To perform successively (and successfully) the functions of mastication, humectation, and deglutition.
> *The Devil's Dictionary*

EDIBLE, adj. Good to eat, and wholesome to digest, as a worm to a toad, a toad to a snake, a snake to a pig, a pig to a man, and a man to a worm.
> *Idem*

GLUTTON, n. A person who escapes the evils of moderation by committing dyspepsia.
> *Idem*

[1] Cf. Samuel Johnson, p. 103b.

Sir William Osler [1849–1919]

A greatly distended stomach is an epigastric swill barrel which should be turned up and emptied occasionally.
> Quoted by William B. Bean in *Sir William Osler: Aphorisms,* Ch. 5

George Bernard Shaw [1856–1950]

There is no love sincerer than the love of food.
> *Man and Superman,* Act I

Sir Walter Raleigh [1861–1922]

Eat slowly; only men in rags
And gluttons old in sin
Mistake themselves for carpet bags
And tumble victuals in.
> *Stans Puer ad Mensam*

Mahatma Gandhi [1869–1948]

I eat to live, to serve, and also, if it so happens, to enjoy, but I do not eat for the sake of enjoyment.

Hilaire Belloc [1870–1953]

M was a Millionaire who sat at Table,
And ate like this — as long as he was able;
At half-past twelve the waiters turned him out:
He lived impoverished and died of gout.

MORAL

Disgusting exhibition! Have a care
When, later on you are a Millionaire,
To rise from table feeling you could still
Take something more, and not be really ill.
> *Cautionary Verses,* "A Moral Alphabet"

René J. Dubos [1901–]

Death on the expense account is a characteristic feature of the affluent society.
> *Man Adapting,* Ch. III

The Bible

Meats for the belly, and the belly for meats.
> *I Corinthians* 6:13

The Bible: Apocrypha

And if thou hast been forced to eat, arise, go forth, vomit, and thou shalt have rest.
> *Ecclesiasticus* 31:21

The Talmud

One should not converse at meals lest the windpipe acts before the gullet and his life will thereby be endangered.
> *Ta'anith,* I.5b (tr. by J. Rabbinowitz)

Anonymous

Gluttony is no sin if it doesn't injure health.
> Doctrine condemned by Pope Alexander VII

I eat, therefore I am.
[Edo, ergo sum.]
> Parody of Descartes' "Cogito, ergo sum"

The way to a man's heart is through his stomach.

Proverbs

A little in the morning, nothing at noon,
And a light supper doth make to live long.

Better belly burst than good drink or meat be lost.

By suppers more have been killed than Galen ever cured.

Full bellies make empty skulls.

More die by food than famine.[1]

The eye is bigger than the belly.

[1] Hunger scarce kills any, but gluttony and drunkenness multitudes.
I saw few die of hunger, of eating a hundred thousand.

Chinese Proverb

He who toils with pain will eat with pleasure.

English Proverb

He that eats till he is sick must fast till he is well.

French Proverbs

A glutton digs his grave with his teeth.

Short men eat more than tall ones.

Latin Proverbs

A belly full of gluttony will never study willingly.

Many dishes, many diseases.[1]

ECONOMICS

See also FEES

Peter Mere Latham [1789–1875]

Superfluity of means leads to their useless expenditure.
> *General Remarks on the Practice of Medicine,* Ch. VIII, Pt. 2

Thomas Huxley [1825–1895]

What men of science want is only a fair day's wages for more than a fair day's work.
> *Method and Results,* "Administrative Nihilism"

John Shaw Billings [1838–1913]

The problem is to induce people to pay twenty-five cents for the liver-encouraging, silent-perambulating, family pills, which cost three cents.
> *Boston Medical and Surgical Journal* 124:349, 1891

[1] Much meat, much malady.

J. Chalmers Da Costa [1863–1933]

It won't help a young man much to be 100 years ahead of his time if he is a month behind in his rent.
> *The Trials and Triumphs of the Surgeon,* Ch. 1

Walter B. Cannon [1871–1945]

I *have* all the money I want. My wife gives me ten dollars a month and with that I pay my carfare, buy my lunches, and get my hair cut.
> *The Way of an Investigator,* "Many Happy Returns"

Ernst Ferdinand Sauerbruch [1875–1951]

BANK DIRECTOR: I don't understand why, with such an income, your account is so frequently overdrawn.
SAUERBRUCH: If you as a banker don't know, how can I possibly understand it? [1]
> Quoted by Thorwald in *The Dismissal,* Ch. 4 (tr. by R. and C. Winston)

Franklin D. Roosevelt [1882–1945]

The problem of economic loss due to sickness [is] a very serious matter for many families with and without incomes, and therefore, an unfair burden upon the medical profession.
> *Address on the Problems of Economic and Social Security,* November 14, 1934

J. Glenn Gray [1913–   ]

Affluence, not religion, might be called the opiate of the 'sixties.
> *Harper's Magazine,* May 1965, "Salvation on the Campus"

John F. Kennedy [1917–1963]

No costs have increased more rapidly in the last decade than the cost of

[1] Conversation which took place during the years of Sauerbruch's greatest glory and highest income; often told by Sauerbruch himself, who lived lavishly and was disinterested in business matters.

medical care. And no group of Americans has felt the impact of these skyrocketing costs more than our older citizens.

Address on the 25th Anniversary of the Social Security Act, August 14, 1960

Latin Proverb

Ready money is ready medicine.[1]

EDUCATION

See also LEARNING, MEDICAL SCHOOLS, STUDENTS, TEACHERS, TEACHING

Hippocrates [460?–377? B.C.]

Whoever is to acquire a competent knowledge of medicine, ought to be possessed of the following advantages: a natural disposition; instruction; a favorable position for the study; early tuition; love of labour; leisure. First of all, a natural talent is required; for, when Nature opposes, everything else is vain; but when Nature leads the way to what is most excellent, instruction in the art takes place, which the student must try to appropriate to himself by reflection, becoming an early pupil in a place well adapted for instruction. He must also bring to the task a love of labour and perseverance, so that the instruction taking root may bring forth proper and abundant fruits.

The Law, II (tr. by Francis Adams)

Instruction in medicine is like the culture of the productions of the earth. For our natural disposition is, as it were, the soil; the tenets of our teacher are, as it were, the seed; instruction in youth is like the planting of the seed in the ground at the proper

[1] Bulgarian Proverb: Ready money is the safest medicine.

season; the place where the instruction is communicated is like the food imparted to vegetables by the atmosphere; diligent study is like the cultivation of the fields; and it is time which imparts strength to all things and brings them to maturity.

Ibid., III

Haly Abbas [d. 994]

Those things which are incumbent on the student of the Art are that he should constantly attend the hospitals and sick-houses; pay unremitting attention to the conditions and circumstance of their inmates, in company with the most acute professors of Medicine; and enquire frequently as to the state of the patients and the symptoms apparent in them, bearing in mind what he has read about these variations, and what they indicate of good or evil. If he does this, he will reach a high degree in this Art. . . . his treatment of the sick will be successful; people will have confidence in him and be favorably disposed towards him, and he will win their affection and respect and a good reputation; nor withal will he lack profit and advantage from them.

Paracelsus [1493?–1541]

Knowledge makes the physician, not the name or the school.

John Milton [1608–1674]

Then also in course might be read to them out of some not tedious Writer the Institution of Physick; that they may know the tempers, the humours, the seasons, and how to manage a crudity [indigestion]: which he who can wisely and timely do, is not only a great Physitian to himself, and to his friends, but also may at some time or other, save an Army by this frugal and expenseless means only; and not let the healthy and stout bodies of young men rot away under him for want of this discipline; which is a

great pity, and no less a shame to the Commander.
Of Education

John Armstrong [1709–1779]

Much had he read,
Much more had seen: he studied from
the life,
And in th' original perus'd mankind.
The Art of Preserving Health,
Bk. 4

William Heberden [1710–1801]

There has lately been established in several of the London hospitals, a plan of courses of lectures in all the branches of knowledge useful to a student of physic. Such plans, if rightly executed, as I have no reason to doubt they will be, must make London a school of physic superior to most in Europe. The experience afforded in an hospital will keep down the luxuriance of plausible theories. Many such have been delivered in lectures, by celebrated teachers, with great applause; but the students, though perfectly masters of them, not having corrected them with what nature exhibits in an hospital, have found themselves more at a loss in the cure of a patient than an elder apprentice of an apothecary.
Letter to Dr. Thomas Percival,
October 15, 1794

Edward Augustus Holyoke [1728–1829]

As to your Inquiry whether a collegiate Education be necessary, I answer No, but then, I am fully persuaded that at least a moderate Acquaintance with the Latin, and some even slight knowledge of the Greek Language is necessary; and still more that initiation into the Newtonian Philosophy and Chemistry, and in general into that Circle of Science which is taught by the Professor of Natural Philosophy in the Apparratus Chamber.
Opinion given to the Massachusetts Medical Society

John Hunter [1728–1793]

[Pointing out several cadavers to Philip Syng Physick's father:] These are the books your son will learn under my direction, the others are fit for very little.
Quoted by Stephen Paget in
John Hunter, Ch. 8

John Morgan [1735–1789]

Young men ought to come well prepared for the study of Medicine, by having their minds enriched with all the aids they can receive from the languages, and the liberal arts. Latin and Greek are very necessary to be known by a Physician. The latter contains the rich original treasures of ancient medical science, and of the first parents of the healing arts. The former contains all the wealth of more modern literature. It is the vehicle of knowledge in which the learned men of every nation in Europe choose to convey their sentiments, and communicate their discoveries to the world.
A Discourse Upon the Institution of Medical Schools in America

There is no art yet known which may not contribute somewhat to the improvement of Medicine; nor is there any one which requires more assistance than that of Physic from every other science. Let young men therefore, who would engage in the pursuit of Medicine or Surgery, make use of all their industry, to possess themselves in good time of these acquisitions. They are necessary to facilitate a progress in the healing arts; they embellish the understanding, and give many peculiar advantages, unattainable without them.
Idem

Thomas Jefferson [1743–1826]

He [1] is at present disposed for Physic. We have not absolutely decided in it's favor. But in the mean time Greek and French will be essential for that profession and proper should he adopt any other.

> Letter to the Rev. Matthew Maury, January 8, 1790

His [the medical student's] mind must be strong indeed, if, rising above juvenile credulity, it can maintain a wise infidelity against the authority of his instructors, & the bewitching delusions of their theories.

> Letter to Dr. Caspar Wistar, June 21, 1807

John Abernethy [1764–1831]

There is no short cut, nor "royal road," to the attainment of medical knowledge. The path which we have to pursue is long, difficult, and unsafe. In our progress, we must frequently take up our abode with death and corruption; we must adopt loathsome diseases for our familiar associates, or we shall never be thoroughly acquainted with their nature and dispositions; we must risk, nay even injure, our own health in order to be able to preserve or restore that of others.

> *Hunterian Oration*, 1819

Sir Astley Paston Cooper [1768–1841]

Nothing is known in our profession by guess; and I do not believe, that from the first dawn of medical science to the present moment, a single correct idea has ever emanated from conjecture: it is right therefore, that those who are studying their profession should be aware that there is no short road to knowledge; and that observations on the diseased living, examination of the dead, and experiments upon living animals, are the only sources of true knowledge; and that inductions

[1] Jefferson's nephew, Dabney Carr.

from these are the sole bases of legitimate theory.

> *A Treatise on Dislocations and Fractures of the Joints*

Peter Mere Latham [1789–1875]

In universities, so that the things taught be good in themselves, education may be as miscellaneous and omnifarious and even as redundant as you please. The object is to rouse the mind and let it make acquaintance with its powers and inclinations, so that it may judge of its own natural fitness by what it is able to do the best.

> *Collected Works*, Vol. II, "A Word or Two on Medical Education"

There is not a more difficult problem in the world than the education for a particular profession.

> *Idem*

When you would teach a man to read, you do not begin with the history of letters.

> *Idem*

Here I am not so much striving to teach, as I am encouraging you to learn.

> *Lectures on Clinical Medicine*, Lect. IX

Karl F. H. Marx [1796–1877]

The education of most people ends upon graduation; that of the physician means a lifetime of incessant study.

> Quoted by F. H. Garrison in *Bulletin of the New York Academy of Medicine* 5:156, 1929

James Syme [1799–1870]

It is as difficult to bring a boy up to be a medical man as it is to educate him for a bishop.

> Quoted by W. K. Pyke-Lees in *Medical Ethics*, Ch. II

John Henry, Cardinal Newman [1801–1890]

General culture of mind is the best aid to professional and scientific study, and educated men can do what illiterate men cannot.

Knowledge in Relation to Culture

Oliver Wendell Holmes [1809–1894]

The most essential part of a student's instruction is obtained, as I believe, not in the lecture room, but at the bedside. Nothing seen there is lost; the rhythms of disease are learned by frequent repetition; its unforeseen occurrences stamp themselves indelibly in the memory.[1]

Medical Essays, "Scholastic and Bedside Teaching"

Philip A. Austin [b. 1819?]

It requires the broadest literary and classical education of boyhood to counteract the necessarily narrowing influence of the professional studies of manhood; and it demands the largest possible infusion of purely scientific teaching, during professional pupilage, to correct the matter-of-fact influence of the practice. . . .

It is by . . . early restriction of thought and action within the narrow grooves of life's future pursuits that a merchant so often loses all power to enjoy the fruit of his toil, a physician is unknown beyond the sick room, a surgeon contributes nothing to the cause of science, and a dentist holds no social position.

The Principles and Practice of Dentistry

Thomas Huxley [1825–1895]

Education is the instruction of the intellect in the laws of Nature, under which name I include not merely

things and their forces, but men and their ways.

A Liberal Education

Perhaps the most valuable result of all education is the ability to make yourself do the thing you have to do, when it ought to be done, and whether you like it or not; it is the first lesson to be learned; and, however early a man's training begins, it is probably the last lesson that he learns thoroughly.

Technical Education

Theodor Billroth [1829–1894]

The future of a school is based on the work of the pupils, as is the future of a country on the work of its citizens.

Inaugural lecture, Second Surgical Department, Vienna, October 11, 1867

Can there be a better preparatory school for the physician than the study of the natural sciences? I think not!

The Medical Sciences in the German Universities, Pt. II, Ch. 2

There is only one way to train capable university teachers — one way that has been practically tested — and that is to secure for the universities the services of the most distinguished men of science, and to furnish them with the necessary equipment for their teaching.

Ibid., Pt. IV, "The Teaching Staff"

It is not the men of formal medical pedagogy that attract students; contrariwise, scientists are the magnets for these schools.

John Shaw Billings [1838–1913]

The education of the doctor which goes on after he has his degree is, after all, the most important part of his education.

Boston Medical and Surgical Journal 131:140, 1894

[1] Cf. Oliver Wendell Holmes, p. 602b.

Sir William Osler [1849–1919]

Undoubtedly the student tries to learn too much, and we teachers try to teach him too much — neither, perhaps, with great success. The existing evils result from neglect on the part of the teacher, student and examiner of the great fundamental principle laid down by Plato — that education is a life-long process, in which the student can only make a beginning during his college course. The system under which we work asks too much of the student in a limited time. To cover the vast field of medicine in four years is an impossible task. We can only instil principles, put the student in the right path, give him methods, teach him how to study, and early to discern between essentials and non-essentials. Perfect happiness for student and teacher will come with the abolition of examinations, which are stumbling blocks and rocks of offence in the pathway of the true student.

> *Aequanimitas, with Other Addresses,* "After Twenty-Five Years"

To study the phenomena of disease without books is to sail an uncharted sea, while to study books without patients is not to go to sea at all.

> *Ibid.,* "Books and Men"

In what may be called the natural method of teaching the student begins with the patient, continues with the patient, and ends his studies with the patient, using books and lectures as tools, as means to an end.

> *Ibid.,* "The Hospital as a College"

We expect too much of the student and we try to teach him too much. Give him good methods and a proper point of view, and all other things will be added, as his experience grows.

> *Idem*

There are many problems and difficulties in the education of a medical student, but they are not more difficult than the question of the continuous education of the general practitioner. . . . No class of men needs to call to mind more often the wise comment of Plato that education is a life-long business.

> *Ibid.,* "On the Educational Value of the Medical Society"

Given the sacred hunger and proper preliminary training, the student-practitioner requires at least three things with which to stimulate and maintain his education, a notebook, a library, and a quinquennial braindusting.

> *Ibid.,* "The Student Life"

The hardest conviction to get into the mind of a beginner is that the education upon which he is engaged is not a college course, not a medical course, but a life course, for which the work of a few years under teachers is but a preparation.

> *Idem*

Post-graduation study has always been a characteristic feature of our profession.

> *Lancet* 2:73, 1900

"Cabined, cribbed, confined" within the four walls of a hospital practising the fugitive and cloistered virtues of a clinical monk, how shall he, forsooth, train men for a race the dust and heat of which he knows nothing and — this is a possibility! — cares less? I cannot imagine anything more subversive to the highest ideal of a clinical school than to hand over young men who are to be our best practitioners to a group of teachers who are *ex officio* out of touch with the conditions under which these young men will live.

> Letter to Ira Remsen, President of the Johns Hopkins University, 1911

By the neglect of the study of the humanities, which has been far too general, the profession loses a very precious quality.

> *Montreal Medical Journal* 26: 186, 1897

Welch, it is lucky that we get in as professors; we could never enter as students.[1]

> Quoted by William H. Welch in Harvey Cushing's *The Life of Sir William Osler*, Ch. 15

The important thing is to make the lesson of each case tell on your education.

William H. Welch [1850–1934]

Medical education is not completed at the medical school: it is only begun. Hence it is not only the quantity of knowledge which the student takes with him from school which will help him in his future work: it is also the quality of mind, the disciplined habit of correct reasoning, the methods of work, the way of looking at medical problems, the estimate of the value of evidence.

> *Bulletin of the Harvard Medical School Association* 3:55, 1892

Let us not forget that a university or a medical college may have large endowments, palatial buildings, modern laboratories, and still the breath of life may not be in it. The vitalizing principle is in the men — both teachers and students — who work within its walls. Without this element of life, this bond between teacher and taught, these things are but outward pomp and show. But let these greater opportunities receive the breath of life from the inspiration of great teachers and they then become the mighty instruments of higher education and scientific progress.

> *Medical News* 65:63, 1894

It has been stated, and accurately so, that it is impossible to impart the entire contents of medical and surgical science to the student. You cannot even impart the contents of a single subject in the curriculum. The most you can expect is to give to the student a fair knowledge of the principles of the fundamental subjects in medicine, and the power to use the instruments and methods of his profession; the right attitude toward his patients and his fellow-members in the profession; above all, to put him in the position to carry on his education, because his education is only begun in the medical school. . . . The student does not go out a trained practitioner, a trained pathologist, or a trained anatomist, or a surgeon. Looked at from the point of view of mere knowledge, he has only a smattering.

> *Bulletin of the American Academy of Medicine* 11:720, 1910

Stephen Paget [1855–1926]

To be ill, or to undergo an operation, is to be initiated into the mystery of nursing, and to learn the comforts and discomforts of an invalid's life; the unearthly fragrance of tea at daybreak, the disappointment of rice-pudding when you thought it was going to be orange-jelly, and the behaviour of each constituent part of the bedclothes. You know, henceforth, how many hours are in a sleepless night; and what unclean fancies will not let us alone when we are ill; and how illness may blunt anxiety and fear, so that the patient is dull, but not unhappy or worried; and how we cling to life, not from terror of death, nor with any clear desire for the remainder of life, but by nature, not by logic. In brief, you learn from your own case many facts which are not in text-books and lectures: and your pa-

---

[1] In reference to the entrance standards originally set for the Johns Hopkins Medical School.

tients, in the years to come, will say that they prefer you to the other doctor, because you seem to understand exactly how they feel. I wish you therefore, young man, early in your career, a serious illness, or an operation, or both. For thus, and thus alone, may you complete your medical education, and crown your learning with the pure gold of experience.

Confessio Medici, Ch. 7

Karl Garré [1857–1928]

Fitting students and misfits, well trained and poorly trained people crowd our lecture rooms, people of visual and people of auditory perception. They will not become physicians unless we teach observation, yes, but also an understanding of natural events and the logic of the laws of physiology and pathology. In addition, however, the ethics of the profession must be taught. . . . Is our physician-to-be aware of the psychological problems of those who are ill? Is he aware of man's mind? Dutifully, he has attended courses about the reproduction of cryptograms and about the three pairs of gill-combs of the axolotl, but he has no idea about man's emotions, about the structure of the soul of the very object to whom he intends to devote the rest of his life.

Textbook on Surgery, Preface (tr. by Max Samter)

Friedrich von Müller [1858–1941]

The relentless logic of Latin is a stern apprenticeship for intellectual efforts. It teaches us to think clearly, more effectively so than any other language or discipline, including mathematics, which requires talent rather than labor.

Quoted by Johanna Haarer in *Die Welt des Arztes* (tr. by Max Samter)

Sir Arthur Conan Doyle [1859–1930]

Education never ends, Watson. It is a series of lessons with the greatest for the last.

His Last Bow, "The Adventure of the Red Circle"

William J. Mayo [1861–1939]

One of the chief defects in our plan of education in this country is that we give too much attention to developing the memory and too little to developing the mind; we lay too much stress on acquiring knowledge and too little on the wise application of knowledge.

Collected Papers of the Mayo Clinic and Mayo Foundation 25:1105, 1933

Sir Charles Sherrington [1861–1952]

Paradoxical though it may sound, the more skilfully a demonstration experiment is performed the less from it do some students learn.

Mammalian Physiology, Preface

Alfred North Whitehead [1861–1947]

There can be no adequate technical education which is not liberal and no liberal education which is not technical.

The Aims of Education, Ch. IV

W. F. R. Phillips [1863– ?]

The best educational preparation to bring to the study of medicine is the study of everything else than that which one will study specifically in the medical school.

Southern Medical Journal 11:322, 1918

Sir Andrew MacPhail [1864–1938]

I am well aware that in these days, when a student must be converted into a physiologist, a physicist, a chemist, a biologist, a pharmacologist, and an electrician, there is no time to make a physician of him. That consummation can only come after he has gone out in the world of sickness and suffering, unless indeed his mind is so bemused, his instincts so dulled, his sympathy so blunted by the long process of education in those sciences, that he is forever excluded from the art of medicine, which was to Hippocrates "the art" of all arts. In that case he is destined for the laboratory, the professor's chair, or the consultant's office. What would have happened to Sydenham had he been put through this machinery is a problem in infinity which no human intelligence is competent to solve.

> *British Medical Journal* 1:443, 1933

Charles H. Mayo [1865–1939]

One of the signs of a truly educated people, and a broadly educated nation, is lack of prejudice.

> *Collected Papers of the Mayo Clinic and Mayo Foundation* 18:1093, 1926

There are two objects of medical education: To heal the sick, and to advance the science.

> *Idem*

Abraham Flexner [1866–1959]

Medical education is a technical or professional discipline; it calls for the possession of certain portions of many sciences arranged and organized with a distinct practical purpose in view. That is what makes it a "profession." Its point of view is not that of any one of the sciences as such.

> *Medical Education, a Comparative Study*

Harvey Cushing [1869–1939]

We are tending to become a standardized country, and it is perhaps on standardization that industrial progress is founded. But standardization of

our educational systems is apt to stamp out individualism and defeat the very ends of education by leveling the product down rather than up. The qualities that really count in this world are quite beyond pigeonholing, quite beyond measurement by scales, tape, or mental tests, quite beyond rating by any known system of examination, all of which fail in giving us an estimate of that most precious of all qualities, personality.

The capacity of the man himself is only revealed when, under stress and responsibility, he breaks through his educational shell, and he may then be a splendid surprise to himself no less than to his teachers.

> *Consecratio Medici,* Ch. 1

Stephen B. Leacock [1869–1944]

In only one respect has there been a decided lack of progress in the domain of medicine, that is in the time it takes to become a qualified practitioner. In the good old days a man was turned out thoroughly equipped after putting in two winter sessions at a college and spending his summers in running logs for a sawmill. Some of the students were turned out even sooner. Nowadays it takes anywhere from five to eight years to become a doctor. Of course, one is willing to grant that our young men are growing stupider and lazier every year. This fact will be corroborated at once by any man over fifty years of age. But even when this is said it seems odd that a man should study eight years now to learn what he used to acquire in eight months.

> *Literary Lapses,* "How to Be a Doctor"

Fielding H. Garrison [1870–1935]

The future of American medical education is, like all other higher developments, simply in the hands of the only aristocracy we strive for — the aristocracy of an enlightened public opinion.

> *Introduction to the History of Medicine* (2nd ed.), Ch. 12

Harlan Fiske Stone [1872–1946]

Professional training . . . is in very real danger from a kind of competitive zeal which has for some years adversely affected undergraduate education. . . . The desire to do something distinctive, to give some evidence of originality, to attract public attention, or to secure patronage, has led from time to time to the presentation to the public of numerous educational nostrums as improvements.

> Annual Report of the Dean of the School of Law, Columbia University, November 3, 1923

Wilson Mizner [1876–1933]

I respect faith but doubt is what gets you an education.

Hans Zinsser [1878–1940]

We have been living in an era of science. And it is not unnatural that our university administrators should have given the scientific departments a disproportionate degree of encouragement and support to the neglect of the humanities. Yet there are growing indications that the tide is turning; and men in leading positions are beginning to realize that the backbone of intellectual training lies in liberal education and in the adjustment of the content of the humanities to modern conditions. In this maturing of our hard-pressed democratic civilization the classicist, the historian, the philosopher, and all those other devoted disciples of the learning called useless in this era of national adolescence, will come into their own again. And when this happens, and the mass of the high-school and college graduates go back into industrial and political life in ever increasing numbers as educated people, there may be hope of the

eventual triumph of humane civilization.

> *As I Remember Him,* Ch. 18, Sect. 2

Martin H. Fischer [1879–1962]

A good teacher must know the rules; a good pupil, the exceptions.

> Quoted by Howard Fabing and Ray Marr in *Fischerisms*

Education! Why say it is a stimulant when it has become a narcotic?

> *Idem*

The beginning of education lies in imitation — wherefore pick someone worth imitating.

> *Idem*

The great doctors all got their education off dirt pavements and poverty — not marble floors and foundations.

> *Idem*

The new appears as a minority point of view, and hence is unpopular. The function of a university is to give it sanctuary.

> *Idem*

Francis Weld Peabody [1881–1927]

It is probably fortunate that most systems of education are constantly under the fire of general criticism, for if education were left solely in the hands of teachers the chances are good that it would soon deteriorate. Medical education, however, is less likely to suffer from such stagnation, for whenever the lay public stops criticizing the type of modern doctor, the medical profession itself may be counted on to stir up the stagnant pool and cleanse it of its sedimentary deposit.

> *The Care of the Patient*

Vannevar Bush [1890–   ]

This great medical-school system has two faults: it does not train enough doctors, and it is a far cry from our ideal of equality of educational opportunity.

> *Modern Arms and Free Men,* Ch. XVI

Alan Gregg [1890–1957]

A good education should leave much to be desired.

C. Sidney Burwell [1893–1967]

My students are dismayed when I say to them, "Half of what you are taught as medical students will in ten years have been shown to be wrong, and the trouble is, none of your teachers knows which half."

> Quoted by G. W. Pickering in *British Medical Journal* 2:113, 1956

W. Russell, Lord Brain [1895–1966]

As each new specialty came of age it demanded a front door key to medical education, and a roof of its own in the curriculum and the examinations. . . . The curriculum should not be that of a honeycomb in which individual bees add cell to cell, but rather that of the cerebral cortex in which all the cells are functionally interrelated.

> *Canadian Medical Association Journal* 83:349, 1960

Dickinson W. Richards [1895–]

Socrates, you will remember, asked all the important questions, — but he never answered any of them.

> *Transactions of the American Clinical and Climatological Association* 65:91, 1953

C. C. Okell [fl. 20th Cent.]

One thing seems certain — if we taught and examined less, our students would learn more. If we add anything further to the medical curriculum let it be spare time.

> *Lancet* 1:107, 1938

Sir Robert Platt [1900–]

Given a few lectures and diagrams the principles of lung function could be grasped by anyone with a scientific background. Given three lectures on the violin, with suitable illustrations, the student wouldn't be able to play a note. (Of course, if university departments of music ever did stoop to such irrelevances as actually teaching people how to play, they would start with a year's instruction in physics and mathematics.)

> *British Medical Journal* 2:551, 1965

The first staggering fact about medical education is that after two and a half years of being taught on the assumption that everyone is the same, the student has to find out for himself that everyone is different, which is really what his experience has taught him since infancy. And the second staggering fact about medical education is that after being taught for two and a half years not to trust any evidence except that based on the measurements of physical science, the student has to find out for himself that all important decisions are in reality made, almost at unconscious level, by that most perfect and complex of computers the human brain, about which he has as yet learnt almost nothing, and will probably go on learning nothing to the end of his course — this computer which can take in and analyse an incredible number of data in an extremely short time. And the data are mostly not of the hard crude type with which that simple fellow the scientist has to deal, but are of a much more subtle, human, and interesting character, each tinted in its own colours of personality and emotion. All this the student has to discover for himself while his teachers strangely pretend to believe that the secrets of medicine are revealed only to those whose biochemical background is beyond reproach.

> *Idem*

If [clinical scientists] . . . leave the social medicine department to teach students the importance of environment and look upon psychological symptoms either as an inconvenient irrelevance or as a matter for the psychiatrist, then I fear I am not with them.

Universities Quarterly 17:327, 1963

The persistence of the archaic belief that an educated man is one who has been brought up on the classics has been an impediment to progress in the last 100 years.

Idem

Yale Kneeland, Jr. [1901–   ] **and Robert F. Loeb** [1895–   ]

One of the most valuable experiences the student may have from a pedagogical point of view is to be required to perform a complete physical examination on a patient under the eye of a senior instructor.

Martini's Principles and Practice of Physical Diagnosis, Ch. 7

Charles D. O'Malley [1907–   ]

One year they [teachers of medicine in Paris, 1533] were required to teach the "natural subjects" — anatomy, physiology, and botany — and the "non-natural" — hygiene and regimen. The following year instruction was given in subjects "contrary to nature" — pathology and therapeutics.

Andreas Vesalius of Brussels, 1514–1564, Ch. 4

George T. Harrell [1908–   ]

The physician's continuing education, whether he is a scientist practicing in a medical school or a general practitioner practicing in some rural area, is largely a process within himself, one he pursues on his own. He may have some help from his professional colleagues in the county medical society or in a research group, but most of

his true learning — the part that sticks with him — is what he does for himself, by himself.

Journal of Medical Education 33 (October, Pt. II):217, 1958

EMOTION

Chuang-tse [fl. 4th Cent. B.C.]

For just as joined toes are but useless lumps of flesh, and extra fingers but useless growths, so are the many artificial developments of the natural sentiments of men and the extravagances of charitable and dutiful conduct but so many superfluous uses of intelligence.

Joined Toes (tr. by Lin Yutang in *The Wisdom of China and India*)

Michel de Montaigne [1533–1592]

All passions that allow themselves to be savored and digested are only mediocre.

Essays, Bk. I, Ch. 2, "Of Sadness" (tr. by Donald M. Frame)

Blaise Pascal [1623–1662]

The heart has its reasons, which reason knows not.[1]

Pensées, Sect. IV (tr. by C. Kegan Paul)

Claude Bernard [1813–1878]

When it is said that great thoughts come from the heart, it means that they come from the feelings, for our feelings, which have their physiological origin in the nerve-centers, act upon the heart like peripheral sensations.

Sir William Osler [1849–1919]

Fed on the dry husk of facts, the human heart has a hidden want which science cannot supply.

Science and Immortality

[1] Le coeur a ses raisons, que la raison ne connaît point.

Otto Weininger [1880–1903]

With the woman, thinking and feeling are identical, for man they are in opposition.

Sex and Character, Pt. II, Ch. 3

Sir Robert Platt [1900–　]

There is a side to human behavior in health and disease which is not a thing of the intellect, which is irrational and emotional but important. It is the main spring of most of what we do and a great deal of what we think. It is being explored by psychiatry but is in danger of being neglected by clinical science.

Universities Quarterly 17:327, 1963

Jacques Barzun [1907–　]

There is nothing more injurious to the character and to the intellect than the suppression of generous emotion. . . . Cramp this emotion, and you will have a half-dead man, whose children will be less well-nourished than himself.

Irish Proverb

Seeing's believing — but feeling is God's own truth.

EMPIRICISM

See also EXPERIENCE, THEORY AND PRACTICE

Celsus [25 B.C.–A.D. 50]

Those who are called 'Empirici' because they have experience, do indeed accept evident causes as necessary; but they contend that inquiry about obscure causes and natural actions is superfluous, because nature is not to be comprehended. . . . Even in its beginnings, they add, the Art of Medi-cine was not deduced from such questionings, but from experience.

De Medicina, Prooemium (tr. by W. G. Spencer)

It was afterwards, . . . when the remedies had already been discovered, that men began to discuss the reasons for them: the Art of Medicine was not a discovery following upon reasoning, but after the discovery of the remedy, the reason for it was sought out.

Idem

Sir Francis Bacon [1561–1626]

Empirics and old women are more happy many times in their cures than learned physicians, because they are more exact and religious in holding to the composition and confection of tried medicines.

The Advancement of Learning, Bk. IV, Ch. II

Celsus . . . tells us that the experimental part of medicine was first discovered, and that afterwards men philosophised about it, and hunted for and assigned causes; and not by an inverse process that philosophy and the knowledge of causes led to the discovery and development of the experimental part.

Novum Organum, "Aphorisms," LXXIII

George Crabbe [1754–1832]

Habit with him was all the test of truth,
"It must be right: I've done it from my youth."

The Borough, Letter III

Benjamin Waterhouse [1754–1846]

I am indeed so disgusted with learned quackery, that I take some interest in honest, humane and strong-minded empiricism; for it has done more for our art, in all ages and in all countries, than all the universities since the time of Charlemagne. Where, for goodness

sake, did Hippocrates study? — air, earth and water — man, and his kindred vegetables — diseases and death and all casualties and concomitants of humanity, were the pages he studied — everything that surrounds and nourishes us, were the objects of his attention and study. In a word, he read diligently and sagaciously the Great Book of Nature . . . instead of the books of man.
> Letter to Dr. Samuel L. Mitchill, December 19, 1825

Peter Mere Latham [1789–1875]

In medical science, the only materials of our knowledge are those things which are referable to our sensations and perceptions: matters of fact.
> *Lectures on Clinical Medicine,* Lect. V

John Shaw Billings [1838–1913]

One hundred years ago the practice of medicine, and measures to preserve health, so far as these were really efficacious, were in the main empirical — that is, certain effects were known to follow the giving of certain drugs, or the application of certain measures, but why or how these effects were produced was unknown. They sailed then by dead-reckoning, in several senses of this phrase.
> *Boston Medical and Surgical Journal* 124:349, 1891

Martin H. Fischer [1879–1962]

Don't despise empiric truth. Lots of things work in practice for which the laboratory has never found proof.
> Quoted by Howard Fabing and Ray Marr in *Fischerisms*

ENDOCRINES

George Barger [1878–1939] and **Sir Henry Dale** [1875–   ]
The distinction drawn between the ac-

tion of a hormone, and that of a compound foreign to the body but producing similar effects, breaks down inevitably when a continuous series is available.
> *Journal of Physiology* 41:19, 1910

William Boyd [1885–   ]

It would indeed be rash for a mere pathologist to venture forth on the uncharted sea of the endocrines, strewn as it is with the wrecks of shattered hypotheses, where even the most wary mariner may easily lose his way as he seeks to steer his bark amid the glandular temptations whose siren voices have proved the downfall of many who have gone before.
> *Pathology for the Surgeon* (7th ed.), Ch. 32

Christopher Morley [1890–1957]

New York, the nation's thyroid gland.[1]
> *Shore Leave*

ENVIRONMENT

Christoph Wilhelm Hufeland [2] [1762–1836]

Meteorological phenomena exert their influence, I believe, on living matter as well as on the heavens. We cannot explain northern lights, meteors, or even the change in weather, and yet we know that they exist: the same applies to the effects of magnetism on man. It seems possible that the rational basis for these phenomena might forever elude us, and that they might never fit into an order which we can recognize.

---

[1] Morley, in editing the 12th edition of Bartlett's *Familiar Quotations,* included this saying, "If it isn't familiar, it will be."
[2] Hufeland was a compassionate and well-rounded German practitioner, a fascinating synthesis of the art and science of medicine, whose eclecticism was anathema to the fundamentalists of his time.

Charles Dickens [1812–1870]

If I be a miserable child, born and nurtured in the same wretched place, and tempted, in these better times, to the Ragged School, what can a few hours' teaching that I get there do for me, against the noxious, constant, ever-renewed lesson of my whole existence?
> Address to Metropolitan Sanitary Association, May 10, 1851

Homer W. Smith [1895–1962]

All samples of the fossil record . . . suggest that some death-dealing enemy, swift, merciless and irresistable, lurked in every corner of the world. This enemy, we believe, was the medium in which the early vertebrates were undergoing evolution: it was an enemy they could not see but one that pursued them every minute of the day and night, one from which there was no escape though they deployed from Spitsbergen to Colorado — the physical-chemical danger inherent in their new environment: their fresh-water home.
> *From Fish to Philosopher*, Ch. III

EPIDEMICS

See also INFECTION, PLAGUE, SWEATING SICKNESS

Juvenal [60?–140?]

Contagion has this illness widely spread;
And, I feel sure, will farther spread it yet;
As in the fields one scabby sheep the flock
Destroys, and one infected pig the stock.
> *Satires*, II.78

William Farr [1807–1883]

The curve of an epidemic at first ascends rapidly, then slopes up slowly to a maximum, to fall more rapidly than it mounted.
> *Farr's Law*

Sir William Withey Gull [1816–1890]

The diseases of the young are in large part preventable diseases. Epidemics carry off in great proportion the healthy members of a community.
> Address to the British Medical Association, 1868

Frank (Kin) Hubbard [1868–1930]

Some people are so sensitive they feel snubbed if an epidemic overlooks them.
> *Abe Martin's Broadcast*

Franklin D. Roosevelt [1882–1945]

When an epidemic of physical disease starts to spread, the community approves and joins in a quarantine of the patients in order to protect the health of the community against the spread of the disease.
> Address at Chicago, October 5, 1937

René and Jean Dubos [1901–] [1918–]

Epidemics have often been more influential than statesmen and soldiers in shaping the course of political history, and diseases may also color the moods of civilizations.
> *The White Plague*, Ch. V

EPILEPSY

See SEIZURES

EPITAPHS

See also LAST WORDS

Tutankhamen [d. 1343 B.C.]

Death will come on swift wings to

him who disturbs the sleep of the Pharaoh.
Inscription on his tomb

Empedocles [fl. 455 B.C.]

PAUSANIAS — not so named without a cause,
As one who oft has giv'n to pain a *pause* —
Blest son of Aesculapius, good and wise,
Here, in his native Gela, buried lies;
Who many a wretch once rescu'd by his charms
From dark Persephone's constraining arms.
Epitaph on the physician Pausanias (tr. by Merivale)

William Shakespeare [1564–1616]

Good frend, for Jesus sake forbeare,
To digg the Dust encloased heare!
Bleste be the Man that spares thes stones,
And curst be he that moves my bones.[1]
At Stratford-on-Avon

Thomas Fuller [1608–1661]

"Fuller's earth." [2]
Epitaph on himself

Isaac de Benserade [1613–1691]

Here lies one, who laid others low,
A most learned doctor
Of that art so fatal to the living.
Say paternosters for him.
Many through him have their inheritance.
They and their heirs gladly say them.

He waged war on every age and sex,

[1] John Dowdall, in a letter to Edward Southwell on April 10, 1693, records the tradition that this epitaph was "made by himself a little before his death"; there is another early tradition, however, that these lines were merely chosen by Shakespeare, not composed by him.
[2] This has also been attributed to Thomas Fuller [1654–1734].

With his bleedings and poisoned draughts.
He is now with a multitude of the dead
Dispatched by his means.

Health fled like a hare,
In front of him she doubled the pace;
Death was the only end
He put to a fever;
Greater foe was he to quinine
Than Augustus to Cinna.

A true basilisk, he killed with a look,
And cut the threads of the best lives;
He would not have spared his mule,
If the mule had been ill,
Or if he had not himself been struck down.
Epitaph on a Doctor

William Symons [1673–1753]

Here lies my corpse, who was the man
That loved a sop in the dripping pan;
But now believe me I am dead,
See here the pan stands at my head.
Still for sops till the last I cried,
But could not eat, & so I died.
My neighbours, they perhaps will laugh,
When they do read my epitaph.[1]
Near Newmarket, England

Messenger Monsey [1693–1788]

Here lie my old bones; my vexation now ends;
I have lived much too long for myself and my friends.
As to churches and churchyards, which men may call holy,
'Tis a rare piece of witchcraft, and founded on folly.
What the next world may be never troubled my pate;
And be what it may, I beseech you, O fate,
When the bodies of millions rise up in a riot,

[1] An iron dish is affixed to the gravestone, according to the instructions of the deceased.

To let the old carcass of Monsey be quiet.
> Epitaph on himself

Benjamin Franklin [1706–1790]

The body of Benjamin Franklin, printer, (like the cover of an old book, its contents torn out and stript of its lettering and gilding), lies here, food for worms; but the work shall not be lost, for it will (as he believed) appear once more in a new and more elegant edition, revised and corrected by the Author.
> Epitaph on himself, probably written in 1728

John Keats [1795–1821]

Here lies one whose name was writ in water.[1]
> Quoted by Joseph Severn in a letter to Charles Brown, February 8–14, 1821

Sir Robert Jones [1858–1933]

Here lies in honour all that can die of a pioneer in orthopaedia: Sir Robert Jones.
> On a plaque in Liverpool Cathedral

Victor Plarr [1863–1929]

Stand not uttering sedately
Trite oblivious praise above her!
Rather say you saw her lately
Kissing her last lover. . . .

Oh, for it would be a pity
To o'erpraise her or to flout her:
She was wild, and sweet, and witty —
Let's not say dull things about her.
> *In the Dorian Mood,* "Epitaphium Citharistriae"

John McCrae [1872–1918]

Here begynneth ye Booke of ye Deade, wherein is fayrely set foorth ye last state of four Hundred and seventeene

[1] On February 14, 1821, Keats asked his friend Severn to have these words inscribed on his gravestone. He died on February 23.

persones tht have departed this lyfe; wherein be tabled diverse straunge and fearsome condicions tht have ledde to ye same final ende: God have them of His Grace.
> Inscribed by Dr. McCrae, pathologist at Montreal General Hospital (1902–1904), in an autopsy book

Dorothy Parker [1893–1967]

Excuse my dust.
> Proposed epitaph on herself

Anonymous

A multitude of physicians have destroyed me.[1]
> Quoted by Pliny the Elder in *Natural History,* XXIX.v.11

These are the duties of a physician: First . . . to heal his mind and to give help to himself before giving it to anyone else.
> Epitaph of an Athenian doctor, A.D. 2 (Quoted in *Journal of the American Medical Association* 189:989, 1964)

Stay·Passenger·And·Viow·This·Stone
For·Under·It·Lyis·Such·A·One
Who·Cuired·Many·Whill·He·Lieved
Soe·Gracious·He·Noe·Man·Grieved
Yea·When·His·Phisicks·Force·Oft· Failed
His·Plesant·Purpose·Then·Prevailed
For·Of·His·God·He·Got·The·Grace
To·Live·In·Mirth·And·Die·In·Peace
Heavin·Hes·His·Soul·His·Corps·This· Stone
Sigh·Passinger·And·Soe·Be·Gone
> Epitaph of Peter Lowe, Glasgow Cathedral, ca. 1610 (Quoted in *Journal of the American Medical Association* 195:143, 1966)

[1] This quotation, cited by Pliny as "that gloomy inscription on monuments," has been attributed to Alexander the Great [356–323 B.C.] and Menander [343?–291 B.C.]; the Emperor Hadrian [76–138] directed these words to be carved on his tomb.

Two Great Physicians first
My loving husband tried,
　To cure my pain —
　In vain,
At last he got a third,
And then I died.
> Epitaph of Molly Dickie, Cheltenham, England

Here lies the body of Mary Ann
　Lowder,
She burst while drinking a seidlitz
　powder;
Called from this world to her heavenly
　rest,
She should have waited till it effervesced.
> At Burlington, Massachusetts

Grim death took me without any
　warning;
I was well at night, and dead at nine
　in the morning.
> At Sevenoaks, Kent, England

Man's life is like a Winter's day:
Some only breakfast and away;
Others to dinner stay and are full fed,
The oldest man but sups and goes to
　bed.
Long is his life who lingers out the
　day,
Who goes the soonest has the least to
　pay.
> At Barnwell, near Cambridge, England

Pain was my portion;
　Physic was my food;
Groans my devotion;
　Drugs did me no good.
> At Oldbury on Severn, England

Here lies one who for med'cines would
　not give
A little gold, and so his life he lost;
I fancy now he'd wish again to live,
　Could he but guess how much his
　funeral cost.

I was well
Wished to be better

Took physic
Here I am.

[Newspaper headline:] John Longbottom, Aged 3 Mos., Dies
[*Punch* comment:] Ars longa, vita brevis.

ERROR

Huang Ti (The Yellow Emperor) [2697–2597 B.C.]

Poor medical workmanship is neglectful and careless and must therefore be combatted, because a disease that is not completely cured can easily breed new disease or there can be a relapse of the old disease.
> *Nei Ching Su Wên*, Bk. 4, Sect. 13 (tr. by Ilza Veith in *The Yellow Emperor's Classic of Internal Medicine*)

Hippocrates [460?–377? B.C.]

Mistakes, no less than benefits, witness to the existence of the art; for what benefited did so because correctly administered, and what harmed did so because incorrectly administered. Now where correctness and incorrectness each have a defined limit, surely there must be an art. For absence of art I take to be absence of correctness and of incorrectness; but where both are present art cannot be absent.
> *The Art,* V (tr. by W. H. S. Jones)

I would give great praise to the physician whose mistakes are small, for perfect accuracy is seldom to be seen.
> *On Ancient Medicine,* IX (tr. by Francis Adams)

Ar-Rumi [836–896]

The blunders of a doctor are felt not by himself but by others.

Leonardo da Vinci [1452–1519]

Experience is not at fault; it is only our judgment that is in error in promising itself from experience things which are not within her power. Wrongly do men cry out against innocent experience, accusing her often of deceit and lying demonstrations!

> *Codice Atlantico*, 154 (tr. by Edward MacCurdy in *The Notebooks of Leonardo da Vinci*, Vol. I, Ch. I)

Marcellus Palingenius [16th Cent.]

Let them learn their art properly or cease to practise it. A mistake in other professions is tolerable, but this is full of danger if its practitioners are not perfect. It ravages like a hidden domestic plague.

> *The Zodiac of Life*, Bk. IV, "Leo"

Duc François de La Rochefoucauld [1613–1680]

Everyone complains of his memory, none of his judgment.

> *Maxims*, No. 89 (tr. by Constantine FitzGibbon)

Théodore Tronchin [1709–1781]

In medicine, sins of commission are mortal, sins of omission venial.

> Quoted by F. H. Garrison in *Bulletin of the New York Academy of Medicine* 5:155, 1929

Jean François Marmontel [1723–1799]

In the realm of error, the truth is only a point.

Peter Mere Latham [1789–1875]

In medicine (what men are scarcely aware of until they become somewhat severely practical), it requires as much labour and time fairly to lay hold of an error, and uproot it, and have done with it, as to learn and settle a truth, and abide by it.

> *General Remarks on the Practice of Medicine*, Ch. V

It takes as much time and trouble to pull down a falsehood as to build up a truth.

> *Ibid.*, Ch. VI

It is no easy task to pick one's way from truth to truth through besetting errors.

> *Ibid.*, Ch. VIII, Pt. 2

Amid many possibilities of error, it would be strange indeed to be always in the right.

> *Ibid.*, "The Heart and Its Affections," Ch. IV

Alonzo Clark [1807–1887]

The medical errors of one century constitute the popular faith of the next.

Charles Darwin [1809–1882]

False facts are highly injurious to the progress of science, for they often long endure; but false views, if supported by some evidence, do little harm, as every one takes a salutary pleasure in proving their falseness.

> *The Descent of Man*, Ch. 21

Thomas Huxley [1825–1895]

Irrationally held truths may be more harmful than reasoned errors.

> *Darwiniana*, "The Coming of Age of the *Origin of Species*"

Next to being right in this world, the best of all things is to be clearly and definitely wrong. If you go buzzing about between right and wrong, vibrating and fluctuating, you come out nowhere; but if you are absolutely and thoroughly and persistently wrong, you must, some of these days, have the extreme good fortune of knocking your head against a fact, and that sets you all straight again.

> *Science and Education,* "Science and Art and Education"

William Snowden Battles [1827–1895?]

And thus I dreamt that round me stood
The victims of disease,
The patients I had failed to cure,
Though some had paid my fees.

One said, "It is a happy place,
My bliss is unalloyed;
Through your mistakes just ten years more
Of Heaven I have enjoyed." . . .

Another made this queer complaint;
"I'm prematurely sent;
The bungling doctors got me here
Before development." . . .

I got here shaky in my shoes,
And asked if they'd attack us,
And raise a rumpus in these courts,
With questions of malpractice.
> *The Doctor's Dream*

Joseph, Lord Lister [1827–1912]

Next to the promulgation of the truth, the best thing I can conceive that a man can do is the public recantation of an error.

Sir Clifford Allbutt [1836–1925]

Another source of fallacy is the vicious circle of illusions which consists on the one hand of believing what we see, and on the other in seeing what we believe.

Sir William Osler [1849–1919]

Use the knife and the cautery to cure the intumescence and moral necrosis which you will feel in the posterior parietal region, in Gall and Spurzheim's centre of self-esteem, where you will find a sore spot after you have made a mistake in diagnosis.

> *Aequanimitas, with Other Addresses,* "The Student Life"

Errors in judgment must occur in the practice of an art which consists largely in balancing probabilities.

> *Ibid.,* "Teacher and Student"

J. Chalmers Da Costa [1863–1933]

The Master of Trinity is correct: "None of us infallible, not even the youngest of us."

> *The Trials and Triumphs of the Surgeon,* Ch. 1

What we call experience is often a dreadful list of ghastly mistakes.

> *Idem*

Charles Nicolle [1866–1936]

All method is imperfect. Error is all around it, and at the least opportunity invades it. . . . But what can we do? There is no other way.

> *Biologie de l'Invention,* Introduction

Martin H. Fischer [1879–1962]

It is a classic: the practical man is one who practices the mistakes of his forefathers.

> Quoted by Howard Fabing and Ray Marr in *Fischerisms*

Giuseppe Tomasi di Lampedusa [1896–1957]

Like clinics adept at treatment based on fundamentally false analyses of blood and urine which they are too lazy to rectify, the Sicilians of that time ended by killing off the patient.

> *The Leopard,* Ch. 3 (tr. by Archibald Colquhoun)

George Howard Bell [1905–   ]

In the practice of medicine more mistakes are made from lack of accurate

observation and deduction than from lack of knowledge.
Experimental Physiology

David D. Rutstein [1909–   ]

The commonest error in reports of clinical research results from unconscious selection; seek it carefully in reading reports of a study.
Quoted in *Clinical Aphorisms from the Harvard Medical School*

Anonymous

Today's facts are tomorrow's fallacies.

English Proverbs

Every age confutes old errors, and begets new.

Physicians' faults are covered with earth, and rich men's with money.[1]

Italian Proverb

A doctor's error, the will of God.

THE ESTABLISHMENT

Rhazes [850–923]

When Galen and Aristotle are unanimous in the expression of an opinion there lies absolute truth, but when they are at variance it is hard to decide, and we should arrive at the proper course of conduct by ratiocination. The skilled and experienced physician will act upon the promptings of his judgment.

Ambroise Paré [1517?–1590]

Antiquity and custom in such things as are performed by Art, ought not to have any sway, authority or place contrary to reason, as they oft-times have in civil affairs; wherefore let no man

[1] German Proverb: The doctor's errors are covered with earth, our own mistakes with love.

say unto us, that the Ancients have always done thus.
Works, Bk. 12, Ch. 24 (tr. by T. H. Johnson)

Richard Brinsley Sheridan [1751–1816]

I had rather follow you to your grave than see you owe your life to any but a regular-bred physician.
St. Patrick's Day, Act II, Sc. iv

Oliver Wendell Holmes [1809–1894]

It is so hard to get anything out of the dead hand of medical tradition!
Medical Essays, "Currents and Counter-Currents in Medical Science"

Sir William Osler [1849–1919]

We doctors have always been a simple trusting folk. Did we not believe Galen implicitly for 1500 years and Hippocrates for more than 2000?

James B. Herrick [1861–1954]

The paper [on the diagnosis of coronary thrombosis during life rather than only at autopsy] when read in 1912 before the Association of American Physicians . . . fell like a dud.
Memories of Eighty Years, Ch. XI

Sir Harold Gillies [1882–1960] and
D. Ralph Millard, Jr. [1919–   ]

London has its Harley Street, New York has Park Avenue, and few are immune to the snob value of having consulting-rooms on the chosen street.
The Principles and Art of Plastic Surgery, Vol. II, Ch. 20

James Howard Means [1885–1967]

They [organized doctors] forget perhaps that medicine is for the people, not for the doctors.
Daedalus 92:701, 1963

Dickinson W. Richards [1895–   ]

We may think in these days that in organized medicine we are good, but we are not that good. Until I wake up one morning and see on a fifty cent piece a statue of the President of the A.M.A. with a toga on one shoulder, waving across the coin at the Statue of Liberty — until I see this, I for one will not grant the A.M.A. even a minor place in the organized medicine of history.
> *Transactions of the Association of American Physicians* 75:1, 1962

Priesthood in medicine is, in fact, not a question of time, or of this particular institution or that. In its essence, priesthood is not an institution at all: it is a state of mind. If its traditionalism is less militant now than it used to be, it is more complex, and more insidious.
> *Idem*

Isaac Starr [1895–   ]

Too much emphasis on standards is a cause of decay; often it is a psychological defense mechanism set up by persons no longer productive. The organizations which become more and more exclusive tend to die of dry rot.
> *Journal of Clinical Investigation* 19:765, 1940

René J. Dubos [1901–   ]

Official academies are more likely to exhibit enthusiasm over the improvements of the commonplace than to recognize the unexpected when it is first brought to them.
> *Louis Pasteur, Free Lance of Science*, Ch. XII

Alan Jay Lerner [1918–   ]

Just think of the A.M.A. coming out *against* living in the past.
> *On a Clear Day You Can See Forever*

Donald H. Fleming [1923–   ]

Here Welch performed the ironic task of an Influential like himself, of denying full entry into the scientific consensus of the ideas of men greater than himself in research and inspiration.
> *William H. Welch and the Rise of Modern Medicine*, Ch. 10

John H. Knowles [1926–   ]

The A.M.A. operating from a platform of negative vigilance presents no solutions but busily fights each change and then loudly supports it against the next proposal.
> Speech to the Institute on Medical Center Problems, December 9, 1964

ETHICS

See also OATHS

Plato [427?–347 B.C.]

Life according to knowledge is not that which makes men act rightly and be happy, not even if all the sciences be included, but . . . this has to do with one science only, that of good and evil. For, let me ask you . . . whether, if you take away this science from all the rest, medicine will not equally give health? . . . And yet . . . none of these things will be well or beneficially done, if the science of the good be wanting.
> *Charmides*, 174.B (tr. by Benjamin Jowett)

Aristotle [384–322 B.C.]

It is easy to fly into a passion — anybody can do that — but to be angry with the right person and to the right extent and at the right time and with the right object and in the right way — that is not easy, and it is not everyone who can do it.
> *Nicomachean Ethics*, II.9 (tr. by J. A. K. Thomson)

We are told that a patient should call in a physician; he will not get better if he is doctored out of a book. . . . for the physician does nothing contrary to rule from motives of friendship; he only cures a patient and takes a fee. . . . And, indeed, if a man suspected the physician of being in league with his enemies to destroy him for a bribe, he would rather have recourse to the book. But certainly physicians, when they are sick, call in other physicians . . . as if they could not judge truly about their own case.

> *Politics,* III.xi.5 (tr. by Benjamin Jowett)

Thomas Sydenham [1624–1689]

Whoever takes up medicine should seriously consider the following points: firstly, that he must one day render to the Supreme Judge an account of the lives of those sick men who have been intrusted to his care. Secondly, that such skill and science as, by the blessing of Almighty God, he has attained, are to be specially directed toward the honour of his Maker, and the welfare of his fellow-creatures; since it is a base thing for the great gifts of Heaven to become the servants of avarice or ambition. Thirdly, he must remember that it is no mean or ignoble animal that he deals with. We may ascertain the worth of the human race, since for its sake God's Only-begotten Son became man, and thereby ennobled the nature that he took upon him. Lastly, he must remember that he himself hath no exemption from the common lot, but that he is bound by the same laws of mortality, and liable to the same ailments and afflictions with his fellows. For these and like reasons let him strive to render aid to the distressed with the greater care, with the kindlier spirit, and with the stronger fellow-feeling.

> *Medical Observations* (1st ed.), Preface (tr. by R. G. Latham in *Works*, Vol. I)

Richard Steele [1672–1729]

A wealthy Doctor, who can help a poor Man, and will not without a fee, has less Sense of Humanity than a poor Ruffian, who kills a rich Man to supply his Necessities. It is something monstrous to consider a Man of a liberal Education tearing out the Bowels of a poor Family, by taking for a Visit what would keep them a Week.

> *The Tatler,* Vol. II, No. 78 (October 6–8, 1709)

Sir William Blackstone [1723–1780]

Mala praxis is a great misdemeanor and offence at common law, whether it be for curiosity and experiment, or by neglect; because it breaks the trust which the party had placed in his physician, and tends to the patient's destruction.

> *Commentaries on the Laws of England,* Bk. III, Ch. 8

Thomas Percival [1740–1804]

In medical practice it is not an unfrequent occurrence, that a Physician is hastily summoned, through the anxiety of the family or the solicitation of friends, to visit a patient who is under the regular direction of another Physician, to whom notice of this call has not been given. Under such circumstances no change in the treatment of the sick person should be made, till a previous consultation with the stated Physician has taken place, unless the lateness of the hour precludes meeting, or the symptoms of the case are too pressing to admit of delay.

> *Medical Ethics,* Ch. 2

Johann Peter Frank [1745–1821]

[The professor] will teach everybody the necessity of keeping an inviolable silence on all the depositions of their patients and he will invite the greatest discretion toward those who must con-

fide in them their defects both physical and moral.

> Quoted by C. F. Wappler in
> *Plan d'école clinique, Vienna*
> (tr. by R. Baserga)

Sir Clifford Allbutt [1836–1925]

Unfortunately the game of medicine is
played with the cards under the table.
. . . In the intimacies of medical
counsels, . . . who is there to note
the significant glance, the shrug, the
hardly expressed innuendo of one or
other of our brethren? . . . Thus we
work not in the light of public opinion
but in the secrecy of the chamber; and
perhaps the best of us are apt at times
to forget the delicacies and sincerities
which under these conditions are essential to harmony and honour. But the
more careful we make ourselves of
these loyalties the less we shall suspect
others; the more candid and sincere
we become with our brethren the less
they will suspect us.

> *On Professional Education, with
> Special Reference to Medicine*

Hermann Nothnagel [1841–1905]

All knowledge attains its ethical value
and its human significance only by the
humane sense in which it is employed.
Only a good man can be a great physician.

Sir William Osler [1849–1919]

Nowadays that part of the Hippocratic
oath which enjoins secrecy as to the
things seen and heard among the sick,
should be administered to you at graduation.

Printed in your remembrance, written as headlines on the tablets of your
chatelaines, I would have two maxims: "I will keep my mouth as it
were with a bridle," and "If thou hast
heard a word let it die with thee."
Taciturnity, a discreet silence, is a
virtue little cultivated in these gar-
rulous days when the chatter of the
bander-log is every where about us.

> *Aequanimitas, with Other Ad-
> dresses,* "Nurse and Patient"

Sir W. Arbuthnot Lane [1856–1943]

The man whose first question after
what he considers to be a right course
of action has presented itself, is "What
will people say?" is not the man to do
anything at all.

> Quoted by W. E. Tanner in *Sir
> W. Arbuthnot Lane,* "Lane as
> I Knew Him"

Henry S. Pritchett [1857–1939]

By professional patriotism amongst
medical men I mean that sort of regard for the honor of the profession
and that sense of responsibility for its
efficiency which will enable a member
of that profession to rise above the
consideration of personal or professional gain.

> Introduction to Abraham Flex-
> ner's *Medical Education in the
> United States and Canada*

J. Chalmers Da Costa [1863–1933]

I have noticed a tendency on the part
of an occasional elderly and distinguished man to think that the rules of
medical ethics were meant for young
fellows just starting out, but not for
him.

> *The Trials and Triumphs of
> the Surgeon,* Ch. 1

Richard Clarke Cabot [1868–1939]

Ethics and Science need to shake
hands.

> *The Meaning of Right and
> Wrong,* Introduction

Edwin Arlington Robinson [1869–1935]

Like a physician who can do no good,
But knows how soon another would
  have his fee
Were he to tell the truth.

> *Avon's Harvest*

Richard Weil [1876–1917]

An ethical regard for the welfare of patients forbids the use of new and experimental remedies in cases which offer a hope of cure by . . . well tried methods.

Martin H. Fischer [1879–1962]

Only one rule in medical ethics needs concern you — that action on your part which best conserves the interests of your patient.

> Quoted by Howard Fabing and Ray Marr in *Fischerisms*

Sir Harold Gillies [1882–1960]
and
D. Ralph Millard, Jr. [1919–   ]

Medical ethics demand that we wait until we are consulted even when a case is screaming for treatment.

> *The Principles and Art of Plastic Surgery*, Vol. II, Ch. 20

Willard L. Sperry [1882–1954]

Once a doctor subordinates the claims of an individual patient under his care to the abstract claims of society in general, or the hypothetical claims of some possible alternate patient, he has sold the pass.

> *The Ethical Basis of Medical Practice*, Ch. 8

Sir F. M. R. Walshe [1888–   ]

The unchanging element in medicine that lifts it above the level of the natural sciences, namely, prudence, . . . the practical wisdom of the ancients, which belongs to the moral category and requires that we should always keep in view the highest good of our patients. . . . This aspect of medicine . . . I shall call humanism, not the secular humanism of the ancients but a humanism infused with the Christian ethic. Without this, medicine must degenerate into a chaos of techniques devoid of moral purpose.

> *Canadian Medical Association Journal* 67:397, 1952

Earle P. Scarlett [1896–   ]

Integrity and rectitude in our profession are paramount.

> *Archives of Internal Medicine* 118:603, 1966

We as doctors must never forget "the delicacies and sincerities" which are essential to medical honor and harmony.

> *Idem*

Alex Comfort [1918–   ]

It happens that the branch of science in which I was trained, medicine, is the only branch which not only has such a unified ethic but has had it for almost 6,000 years. The idea of the human responsibility of the doctor has been present since medicine was indistinguishable from magic.

> *The Listener*, November 29, 1951

Anonymous

Forasmuch as the lawe of God . . . allowes no man to touch the life or limme of any person except in a judicyall way, bee it hereby ordered and decreed, that no . . . physitians, chirurgians, midwives, or others, shall presume to exercise or putt forth any act contrary to the knowne rules of arte nor exercise any force, violence, or cruelty upon or towardes the bodyes of any, wether young or old . . . without the advice and consent of such as are skilfull in the same arte, if such may be had, or at least of the wisest and gravest then present, and consent of the patient or patients (if they be mentis compotes,) much lesse contrary to such advice and consent, upon such punishement as the nature of the fact may deserve; which lawe is not intended to discourage any from a lawfull use of their skill, but rather to encourage and direct them in the right use thereof, and to inhibit and strayne the presumptuous arrogance of such as through praesidence of their oune skill, or any other sinister respects, dare be bould to attempt to exercise any violence upon or towards the bodies of young or old, to the prejudice or hazard of the life or limme of men, woemen, or children.[1]

Law passed in the Massachusetts Bay Colony, May 3, 1649

Among physicians, tax law violators are few yet too many. Internal Revenue Service figures, recently released, show that federal judges pronounced sentences and fines on 1,024 tax offenders in 1962 and that 23 of them — more than 2 per cent — were physicians.

Tufts Folia Medica 9:61, 1963

Proverb

Happy the man whom the dangers to others make cautious.

EUGENICS

See also GENETICS, HEREDITY

Plato [427?–347 B.C.]

The bride and bridegroom should consider that they are to produce for the state the best and fairest specimens of children which they can.

Laws, VI.783 (tr. by Benjamin Jowett)

The best of either sex should be united with the best as often, and the inferior with the inferior, as seldom as possible.

Republic, V.459.D (tr. by Benjamin Jowett)

William Shakespeare [1564–1616]

We marry
A gentler scion to the wildest stock

[1] This was the first law on medical practice passed in the colonies.

And make conceive a bark of baser kind
By bud of nobler race. This is an art
Which does mend nature — change it rather; but
The art itself is nature.

The Winter's Tale, IV, iv, 92

Luther Burbank [1849–1926]

It would, if possible, be best absolutely to prohibit in every State in the Union the marriage of the physically, mentally and morally unfit.

The Training of the Human Plant, Ch. VI

Logan Clendening [1884–1945]

Men are not going to embrace eugenics. They are going to embrace the first likely, trim-figured girl with limpid eyes and flashing teeth who comes along, in spite of the fact that her germ plasm is probably reeking with hypertension, cancer, haemophilia, color blindness, hay fever, epilepsy, and amyotrophic lateral sclerosis.

J. B. S. Haldane [1892–1964]

Illiteracy in England is mainly determined by congenital weak-mindedness, in India by parental poverty.

Possible Worlds, "Eugenics and Social Reform"

Civilization stands in real danger of overproduction of "undermen."

Idem

EUTHANASIA

Sir Thomas More [1478–1535]

But yf the disease be not onelye uncurable, but also full of contynuall payne and anguishe; then the priestes and the magistrates exhort the man, seinge he is not hable to doo anye dewtye of lyffe, and by overlyvinge his owne deathe is noysome and irkesome to other, and grevous to him-

selfe: that he wyl determine with himselfe no longer to cheryshe that pestilent and peineful disease. And seinge
his lyfe is to him but a tormente, that
he wyl not bee unwillinge to dye, but
rather take a good hope to him, and
either dispatche himselfe out of that
payneful lyffe, as out of a prison, or
a racke of tormente, or elles suffer himselfe wyllingle to be rydde oute of it
by other. And in so doinge they tell
him he shall doo wysely, seing by his
deathe he shall lose no commoditye,
but ende his payne.

> *Utopia*, Bk. II, Ch. 7 (tr. by
> R. Robinson)

Thomas Fuller [1608–1661]

When he [the good physician] can
keep life no longer in, he makes a fair
and easie passage for it to go out.

> *The Holy State*, Ch. XVII

William Heberden [1710–1801]

Lord Verulam [1] blames physicians for
not making the euthanasia a part of
their studies: and surely though the
recovery of the patient be the grand
aim of their profession, yet where that
cannot be attained, they should try to
disarm death of some of its terrors,
and if they cannot make him quit his
prey, and the life must be lost, they
may still prevail to have it taken away
in the most merciful manner.

> *Commentaries on the History
> and Cure of Diseases*, Ch. 51

William Lamb, Lord Melbourne [1779–1848]

If they get the habit of doing such a
thing when a person is in a hopeless
state, why, they *may* do it when a
person is *not* in a hopeless state.

> Quoted by Queen Victoria in
> her diary (*The Girlhood of
> Queen Victoria*), February 13,
> 1838

[1] Sir Francis Bacon [1561–1626].

Arthur Hugh Clough [1819–1861]

Thou shalt not kill; but need'st not
  strive
Officiously to keep alive.[1]
> *The Latest Decalogue*

Thomas, Lord Horder [1871–1955]

The two extremes of dying in pain and
being killed do not exhaust the possibilities for the stricken patient, because there is the middle position
created by a kindly and skilful doctor
who gives assistance to an equally
kindly Nature, and that is what is at
present implicit in the patient's question: "You will stand by me, won't
you?" and the doctor's assurance:
"Yes, I will."

> Speech in the House of Lords,
> December 1936

It is the duty of a doctor to prolong
life. It is not his duty to prolong the
act of dying.

Warfield T. Longcope [1877–1953]

Why ward off death if in the attempt
we kill the living?
> *Bulletin of the Johns Hopkins
> Hospital* 50:4, 1932

Wilder Penfield [1891–   ]

There are times when compassion
should prompt us to forego prolonged
and costly treatment. If a man must
die, he has the right to die in peace,
as he would prefer to do if asked.
Positive action to take a life is not
permitted. But the negative decisions
that ease and shorten suffering have
always been ours to make.

> *The Second Career*, "A Doc-
> tor's Philosophy"

[1] This very "familiar" medical quotation
almost invariably is taken literally, probably
because it expresses the moral conviction of
those who quote it. That Clough was engaging in irony in "The Latest Decalogue" is
apparent from a reading of the other nine
commandments. Cf. Richard Asher, p. 673a.

Joseph Fletcher [1905–   ]

Having determined that a condition is hopeless, I cannot agree that it is either prudent or fair to physicians as a fraternity to saddle them with the onus of deciding whether to let the patient go.

> *Tufts Folia Medica* 8:30, 1962

EVOLUTION

Aristotle [384–322 B.C.]

Nature proceeds little by little from things lifeless to animal life in such a way that it is impossible to determine the exact line of demarcation, nor on which side thereof an intermediate form should lie.

> *Historia Animalium,* VIII.1 (tr. by D. W. Thompson)

Ennius [239–169 B.C.]

How like us is that ugly brute, the ape!

> Quoted by Cicero in *On the Nature of the Gods,* I.xxxv.97 (tr. by H. Rackham)

Plutarch [46?–120?]

Those descended from Hellen of old have also sacrificed to 'patriarchal Poseidon,' believing as the Syrians do that man developed from the moist element. So they also revere the fish, as being one with us in race and nurture, which is more reasonable as philosophy than Anaximander's theory. He affirms, not that men and fish were developed in the same environment, but that men were first engendered and nourished inside fish, as dog-fishes are, and when they were mature enough to look out for themselves, at that point they came out and took to the land.

> *Moralia,* VIII.viii.730 (tr. by Edwin L. Minar, Jr.)

William Congreve [1670–1729]

I confess freely to you, I could never look long upon a Monkey, without very Mortifying Reflections.

> Letter to John Dennis, July 10, 1695

Charles Darwin [1809–1882]

We must however acknowledge, as it seems to me, that man with all his noble qualities . . . still bears in his bodily frame the indelible stamp of his lowly origin.

> *The Descent of Man,* Ch. 21

I have called this principle, by which each slight variation, if useful, is preserved, by the term of Natural Selection, in order to mark its relation to man's power of selection. (The expression often used by Mr. Herbert Spencer of the Survival of the Fittest is more accurate, and is sometimes equally convenient.)

> *The Origin of Species,* Ch. 3

From the war of nature, from famine and death, the most exalted object which we are capable of conceiving, namely, the production of the higher animals, directly follows. There is grandeur in this view of life.

> *Ibid.,* Ch. 14

Natural selection . . . implies that the individuals which are best fitted for the complex, and in the course of ages changing conditions to which they are exposed, generally survive and procreate their kind.

> *The Variation of Animals and Plants Under Domestication,* Ch. 20

Walt Whitman [1819–1892]

In due time the evolution theory will have to abate its vehemence, cannot be allow'd to dominate every thing else, and will have to take its place as a segment of the circle, the cluster —

as but one of many theories, many thoughts, of profoundest value — and re-adjusting and differentiating much, yet leaving the divine secrets just as inexplicable and unreachable as before — maybe more so.

> *Notes Left Over,* "Darwinism — (Then Furthermore)"

Herbert Spencer [1820–1903]

Evolution . . . is — a change from an indefinite incoherent homogeneity to a definite coherent heterogeneity, accompanying the dissipation of motion and integration of matter.

> *First Principles,* Ch. 16, Sect. 138

Survival of the fittest.

> *Principles of Biology,* Pt. III, Ch. 12, Sect. 164

Sir Francis Galton [1822–1911]

The conditions that direct the order of the whole of the living world around us, are marked by their persistence in improving the birthright of successive generations. They determine, at much cost of individual comfort, that each plant and animal shall, on the general average, be endowed at its birth with more suitable natural faculties than those of its representative in the preceding generation.

> *Inquiries Into Human Faculty and Its Development,* "The Observed Order of Events"

Alfred R. Wallace [1823–1913]

The Darwinian theory, even when carried out to its extreme logical conclusion, not only does not oppose, but lends a decided support to, a belief in the spiritual nature of man. It shows us how man's body may have been developed from that of a lower animal form under the law of natural selection; but it also teaches us that we possess intellectual and moral faculties which could not have been so devel-

oped, but must have had another origin.

> *Darwinism,* Ch. 15

Thomas Huxley [1825–1895]

This hypothesis [natural selection] may or may not be sustainable hereafter; it may give way to something else, and higher science may reverse what science has here built up with so much skill and patience, but its sufficiency must be tried by the tests of science *alone,* if we are to maintain our position as the heirs of Bacon and the acquitters of Galileo.

> Letter to the *Times,* London, December 26, 1859

It is an error to imagine that evolution signifies a constant tendency to increased perfection. That process undoubtedly involves a constant remodelling of the organism in adaptation to new conditions; but it depends on the nature of those conditions whether the direction of the modifications effected shall be upward or downward.

> *Social Diseases and Worse Remedies,* "The Struggle for Existence in Human Society"

August Weismann [1834–1914]

Every individual alive today, the highest as well as the lowest, is derived in an unbroken line from the first and lowest forms.

> *Die Dauer des Lebens*

Sir William S. Gilbert [1836–1911]

I am, in point of fact, a particularly haughty and exclusive person, of pre-Adamite ancestral descent. You will understand this when I tell you that I can trace my ancestry back to a protoplasmal primordial atomic globule.

> *The Mikado,* Act I

Darwinian Man, though well-behaved, At best is only a monkey shaved!

> *Princess Ida,* Act II

W. Winwood Reade [1838–1875]

It is . . . [a] shabby-genteel senti-ment . . . which makes men prefer to believe that they are degenerated an-gels, rather than elevated apes.
> *The Martyrdom of Men,* Ch. III

William G. Sumner [1840–1910]

Darwin was as much of an emancipator as was Lincoln.
> *The Forgotten Man's Almanac,* February 12

Oliver Wendell Holmes, Jr. [1841–1935]

When one thinks coldly I see no reason for attributing to man a significance different in kind from that which be-longs to a baboon or to a grain of sand.
> *Holmes-Pollock* [1] *Letters,* August 30, 1907

Friedrich Nietzsche [1844–1900]

Species do not evolve toward perfec-tion, but quite the contrary. The weak, in fact, always prevail over the strong, not only because they are in the ma-jority, but also because they are the more crafty.
> *The Twilight of the Idols*

Elbert G. Hubbard [1856–1915]

The probable fact is that we are de-scended not only from monkeys but from monks.
> *A Thousand and One Epigrams*

William H. Carruth [1859–1924]

Some call it Evolution
And others call it God.
> *Each in His Own Tongue*

William Jennings Bryan [1860–1925]

What shall we say of the intelligence, not to say religion, of those who are so particular to distinguish between

[1] Sir Frederick Pollock [1845–1937].

fishes and reptiles and birds, but put a man with an immortal soul in the same circle with the wolf, the hyena, and the skunk? What must be the impression made upon children by such a degradation of man?
> Statement issued in Dayton, Tennessee, July 28, 1925 [1]

William (Billy) Sunday [1862–1935]

If a minister believes and teaches evo-lution, he is a stinking skunk, a hypo-crite, and a liar.
> Statement to the press, 1925

Oliver Herford [1863–1935]

Child-ren, be-hold the Chim-pan-zee;
He sits on the an-ces-tral tree
From which we sprang in ag-es gone.
I'm glad we sprang: had we held on,
We might, for aught that I can say,
Be horrid Chim-pan-zees to-day.
> *A Child's Primer of Natural History,* "The Chimpanzee"

Rudyard Kipling [1865–1936]

We are very slightly changed
From the semi-apes who ranged
   India's prehistoric clay.
> *General Summary*

Arthur Guiterman [1871–1943]

Recall from Time's abysmal chasm
That piece of primal protoplasm
The First Amoeba, strangely splendid,
From whom we're all of us descended.
> *Gaily the Troubadour,* "Ode to the Amoeba"

Sarah N. Cleghorn [1876–1959]

"The unfit die — the fit both live and
   thrive."
Alas, who say so? — They who do sur-vive.
> *The Survival of the Fittest*

[1] This statement was issued by Mrs. Bryan two days after the death of her husband, just after the close of the famous Scopes trial.

Lawrence J. Henderson
[1878–1942]

Darwinian fitness is compounded of a mutual relationship between the organism and the environment. Of this, fitness of environment is quite as essential a component as the fitness which arises in the process of organic evolution; and in fundamental characteristics the actual environment is the fittest possible abode of life.
> *The Fitness of the Environment*, Preface

J. B. S. Haldane [1892–1964]

I am quite sure that our views on evolution would be very different had biologists studied genetics and natural selection before and not after most of them were convinced that evolution had occurred.

Aldous Huxley [1894–1963]

A poor degenerate from the ape,
Whose hands are four, whose tail's a limb,
I contemplate my flaccid shape
And know I may not rival him.
> *Leda*, "First Philosopher's Song"

Konrad Lorenz [1903–   ]

Man appears to be the missing link between anthropoid apes and human beings.
> Quoted by John Pfeiffer in *The New York Times Magazine*, April 11, 1965

Maurice B. Strauss [1904–1974]

In the beginning the abundance of the sea
Led to profligacy.
The ascent through the brackish waters of the estuary
To the salt-poor lakes and ponds
Made immense demands
Upon the glands.
Salt must be saved, water is free.

In the never-ending struggle for security,
Man's chiefest enemy,
According to the bard of Stratford on the Avon,
The banks were climbed and life established on dry land
Making the incredible demand
Upon another gland
That water, too, be saved.
> *Body Water in Man*, "Salt and Water"

Tennessee Legislature

It shall be unlawful for any teacher in any of the Universities, Normals, and all other public schools of the State which are supported in whole or in part by the public school funds of the State, to teach any theory that denies the story of the Divine Creation of man as taught in the Bible, and to teach instead that man has descended from a lower order of animals.[1]
> Act of the Legislature, March 21, 1925, Sect. 1

Proverb

An ape is ne'er so like an ape
As when he wears a doctor's cape.

EXAMINATION

Archimathaeus [ca. 1100]

The fingers should be kept on the pulse at least until the hundredth beat in order to judge of its kind and character; the friends standing round will be all the more impressed because of the delay, and the physician's words will be received with just that much more attention.
> *The Coming of a Physician to His Patient* (tr. by J. J. Walsh)

William J. Mayo [1861–1939]

The examining physician often hesi-

---

[1] Repealed May 17, 1967.

tates to make the necessary examination because it involves soiling the finger.
Journal-Lancet 35:339, 1915

Russell John Howard
[1875–1942]

More mistakes are made from want of a proper examination than for any other reason.
Quoted by F. G. St. Clair Strange in *The Hip*, Ch. 5

Francis Weld Peabody
[1881–1927]

Of course, I shall examine the patient and listen to his chest; although I have auscultated thousands of lungs I have never heard two which sounded alike.[1]
Quoted by David Seegal in *Journal of Chronic Diseases* 16:441, 1963

Sir F. M .R. Walshe [1888–   ]

The more resources we have, and the more complex they are, the greater are the demands upon our clinical skill. These resources are calls upon judgment and not substitutes for it. Do not, therefore, scorn clinical examination; learn it sufficiently to get from it all it holds, and gain in it the confidence it merits.
Canadian Medical Association Journal 67:395, 1952

Dickinson W. Richards
[1895–   ]

One might appropriately consider the stethoscope as a symbol of another skill or set of skills, that appears to be fast disappearing from our medical scene. This is the use of our five senses, the use of simple perception, or ob-

servation. A certain old-timer, who is addicted in this way, and has not yet learned how to confine his attention to the ten channels of an electronic recorder — this old-timer made the curious suggestion not long ago that there might be founded a brand new society, a new society with an old objective, the Society for the Preservation of the Use of the Five Senses.
Transactions of the Association of American Physicians 75:1, 1962

David Seegal [1899–   ]

One of the unexpected and disturbing results of the development of increasingly precise and useful diagnostic measures in the laboratory and x-ray departments is a significant and often alarming decrease in emphasis on the training of the medical student to perform with excellence the average comprehensive physical examination.
Journal of the American Medical Association 180:476, 1962

EXERCISE

Hippocrates [460?–377? B.C.]

Fat people who want to reduce should take their exercise on an empty stomach and sit down to their food out of breath. . . . Thin people who want to get fat should do exactly the opposite and never take exercise on an empty stomach.
A Regimen for Health, IV (tr. by John Chadwick and W. N. Mann)

Cicero [106–43 B.C.]

Exercise and temperance can preserve something of our early strength even in old age.
On Old Age, X.34 (tr. by James Logan)

[1] A house officer, trying to conserve the strength of Dr. Peabody, then in the last stages of malignant disease, had suggested that he might pass by the next patient, who had a "typical" right-lower-lobe pneumonia. This was the response.

Desiderius Erasmus [1466?–1536]

Before Supper, take a little Walk, and do the same after supper.
> *Colloquies,* "Of the Method of Study" (tr. by N. Bailey)

John Dryden [1631–1700]

By Chace our long-liv'd Fathers earn'd their Food;
Toil strung the Nerves, and purifi'd the Blood:
But we, their Sons, a pamper'd Race of Men,
Are dwindl'd down to threescore Years and ten.
Better to hunt in Fields, for Health unbought,
Than fee the Doctor for a nauseous Draught.
The Wise, for Cure, on Exercise depend;
God never made his Work, for Man to mend.
> *Fables Ancient and Modern,* "To John Driden of Chesterton"

George Cheyne [1671–1743]

In short, your total Case is Scurbutico Nervose from a sedentary studious Life. I wonder you get not the Chamber-horse which is now so universally known and practiced in all the studious Professions in London. It is certainly admirable and has all the good and beneficial Effects of a hard Trotting Horse except the fresh Air.
> Letter to Samuel Richardson, April 20, 1740

Joseph Addison [1672–1719]

Exercise ferments the Humours, casts them into their proper Channels, throws off Redundancies, and helps Nature in those secret Distributions, without which the Body cannot subsist in its Vigour, nor the Soul act with Chearfulness.
> *The Spectator,* Vol. II, No. 115 (July 12, 1711)

John Gay [1685–1732]

Rosie-complexion'd health thy steps attends,
And exercise thy lasting youth defends.
> *Trivia,* Bk. I

Benjamin Franklin [1706–1790]

Use now and then a little exercise a quarter of an hour before meals, as to swing a weight, or swing your arms about with a small weight in each hand; to leap, or the like, for that stirs the muscles of the breast.
> *Poor Richard's Almanack,* 1742

Thomas Jefferson [1743–1826]

Not less than two hours a day should be devoted to exercise.
> Letter to Thomas M. Randolph, Jr., August 27, 1786

The sovereign invigorator of the body is exercise, and of all exercises walking is the best.
> *Idem*

Edward Stanley, Earl of Derby [1826–1893]

Those who think they have not time for bodily exercise will sooner or later have to find time for illness.
> *The Conduct of Life,* address at Liverpool College, December 20, 1873

Chauncey Depew [1834–1928]

I get my exercise acting as a pallbearer to my friends who exercise.

George Santayana [1863–1952]

He found escape . . . above all in bodily exercise. This was destined to be his sovereign medicine and sheet-anchor throughout his short life.
> *The Last Puritan,* Pt. II, Ch. VI

Logan Clendening [1884–1945]

Immature faddists are continuously proclaiming the value of exercise: four people out of five are more in need of rest than exercise.

> *Modern Methods of Treatment,*
> Ch. 1

John F. Kennedy [1917–1963]

The Greeks understood that mind and body must develop in harmonious proportions to produce a creative intelligence. And so did the most brilliant intelligence of our earliest days — Thomas Jefferson — when he said, not less than two hours a day should be devoted to exercise.

If the man who wrote the Declaration of Independence, was Secretary of State, and twice President, could give it two hours, our children can give it ten or fifteen minutes.

> Address to the National Football Foundation, December 5, 1961

The Bible

Bodily exercise profiteth little.

> *I Timothy* 4:8

Anonymous

I have two doctors — my left leg and my right.

The secret of my abundant health is that whenever the impulse to exercise comes over me, I lie down until it passes away.

> Quoted by J. P. McEvoy in *American Mercury,* December 1938, "Young Man Looking Backwards"

English Proverb

After dinner sit awhile, after supper walk a mile.

German Proverb

He who goes often for a walk shortens the way to his grave.

Hindu Proverb

Walking makes for a long life.

EXPERIENCE

See also EMPIRICISM

Paracelsus [1493?–1541]

Not even a dog-killer can learn his trade from books, but only from experience. And how much more is this true of the physician! . . . The art of medicine cannot be inherited, nor can it be copied from books.

> *Selected Writings,* Pt. II (tr. by Norbert Guterman)

Sir Francis Bacon [1561–1626]

The best demonstration by far is experience, if it go not beyond the actual experiment. For if it be transferred to other cases which are deemed similar, unless such transfer be made by a just and orderly process, it is a fallacious thing.

> *Novum Organum,* "Aphorisms," LXX

William Shippen, Jr. [1736–1808]

Experience is the mother of truth; and by experience we learn wisdom.

> Quoted by Betsy C. Corner in *William Shippen, Jr.*

Benjamin Rush [1745?–1813]

I now saw that men do not become wise by the experience of other people. Subsequent observations taught me that even our own experience does not always produce wise conduct though the lessons for that purpose are sometimes repeated two or three times.

> *Autobiography,* "Travels Through Life," Ch. V

Peter Mere Latham [1789–1875]

Truly do I wish that I could live a few past years again, and carry back with me my present experience, for the sake of treating again some cases . . . and of treating them better. . . . I cannot carry my experience backward, but you

may carry it forward. And it is in the hope of some practical good to come from it, that I have thus analyzed and exposed it.
> *Diseases of the Heart,* Lect. XII

Nothing is so difficult to deal with as man's own Experience, how to value it according to its amount, what to conclude from it, and how to use it and do good with it.
> *General Remarks on the Practice of Medicine,* Ch. XIII

We physicians had need be a self-confronting and a self-reproving race; for we must be ready, without fear or favour, to call in question our own Experience and to judge it justly; to confirm it, to repeal it, to reverse it, to set up the new against the old, and again to reinstate the old and give it preponderance over the new.
> *Idem*

Sir William Osler [1849–1919]

[We are] constantly misled by the ease with which our minds fall into the ruts of one or two experiences.
> *Aequanimitas, with Other Addresses,* "Teacher and Student"

Stephen Paget [1855–1926]

The crown of experience is like the crown of Lombardy, a band of iron set in a band of gold: and it is believed, even now, by some people, that the iron of that crown is more valuable than the gold.
> *Confessio Medici,* "The Spirit of Practice"

George Bernard Shaw [1856–1950]

Men are wise in proportion, not to their experience, but to their capacity for experience.
> *Man and Superman,* "Maxims for Revolutionists"

William J. Mayo [1861–1939]

Experience is the great teacher; unfortunately, experience leaves mental scars, and scar tissue contracts.
> *Journal of the American Medical Association* 77:597, 1921

J. Chalmers Da Costa [1863–1933]

Each one of us, however old, is still an undergraduate in the school of experience. When a man thinks he has graduated he becomes a public menace.
> *The Trials and Triumphs of the Surgeon,* Ch. 1

What we call experience is often a dreadful list of ghastly mistakes.
> *Idem*

Wilfred Trotter [1872–1939]

An event experienced is an event perceived, digested, and assimilated into the substance of our being, and the ratio between the number of cases seen and the number of cases assimilated is the measure of experience.
> *Collected Papers,* "Art and Science in Medicine," Sect. 6

Alan Gregg [1890–1957]

In all circumstances I have relied too much on others, and not been at the breasts of Experience myself.
> Aphorism (Quoted by Wilder Penfield in *The Difficult Art of Giving,* Appendix A)

Proverb

Experience is the mother of science.

EXPERIMENTAL MEDICINE

See also RESEARCH

Elisha Bartlett [1804–1855]

Remarks . . . may be made in regard

to the effects of the articles of the materia medica upon animals. The action of these substances upon the human body, in a state of health, is not to be positively inferred from their action upon the bodies of other animals in a state of health.

> *Philosophy of Medical Science,*
> Pt. II, Ch. 8

When the law that we are in search of is that of the effects of any given plan of treatment, upon any given disease, considered nosologically, or as a whole, *every case of the disease that presents itself,* should be taken into account, whatever may be its stage, its degree of severity, or its complications.

> *Ibid.,* Ch. 11

The number of cases, necessary to the determination of the actual or relative value of these different methods of treatment, is much less in certain diseases than in others.

> *Idem*

Claude Bernard [1813–1878]

Medicine includes real experiments which are spontaneous, and not produced by physicians.

> *An Introduction to the Study of Experimental Medicine,* Pt. I, Ch. 1, Sect. i (tr. by H. C. Greene)

Experiment is fundamentally only induced observation.

> *Ibid.,* Sect. v

Among the experiments that may be tried on man, those that can only harm are forbidden, those that are innocent are permissible, and those that may do good are obligatory. . . . If it is immoral, then, to make an experiment on man when it is dangerous to him, even though the result may be useful to others, it is essentially moral to make experiments on an animal, even though painful and dangerous to him, if they may be useful to man.

> *Ibid.,* Pt. II, Ch. 2, Sect. iii

Experimental medicine is not a new system of medicine, but on the contrary is the negation of all systems. . . . A science that halted in a system would remain stationary and would be isolated, because systematization is really a scientific encysting, and every encysted part of an organism ceases to take part in the organism's general life.

> *Ibid.,* Pt. III, Ch. 4, Sect. iv

Ivan Pavlov [1849–1936]

Only by passing through the fire of experiment will medicine as a whole become what it should be, namely, a conscious and, hence, always purposefully acting science.

> *Experimental Psychology and Other Essays,* Pt. X, Essay 3 (tr. by S. Belsky)

Béla Schick [1877–1967]

It is too bad that we cannot cut the patient in half in order to compare two regimens of treatment.

> Quoted by I. J. Wolf in *Aphorisms and Facetiae of Béla Schick,* "Early Years"

Franklin D. Roosevelt [1882–1945]

It is common sense to take a method and try it: If it fails, admit it frankly and try another. But above all, try something.

> Address at Oglethorpe University, May 22, 1932

Latin Proverb

Let the experiment be made on a worthless body.

EYE

See also BLINDNESS, SIGHT

Socrates [470?–399 B.C.]

People may injure their bodily eye by observing and gazing on the sun during an eclipse, unless they take the precaution of only looking at the image reflected in the water, or in some similar medium.

> Quoted by Plato in *Phaedo*, 99.D (tr. by Benjamin Jowett)

Dio Chrysostom [40?–115?]

Men with sore eyes . . . find the light painful, while the darkness, which permits them to see nothing, is restful and agreeable.

> *Eleventh (Trojan) Discourse*, II (tr. by J. W. Cohoon)

Paul of Aegina [ca. 615–690]

All those, therefore, who have cataract see the light more or less, and by this we distinguish cataract from amaurosis and glaucoma; for persons affected with these complaints do not perceive the light at all.

> *Works*, Bk. 6, "On Cataracts" (tr. by Francis Adams)

Leonardo da Vinci [1452–1519]

Who would believe that so small a space could contain the images of all the universe? O mighty process! What talent can avail to penetrate a nature such as these? What tongue will it be that can unfold so great a wonder? Verily, none! This it is that guides the human discourse to the considering of divine things.

> *Codice Atlantico*, 345 (tr. by Edward MacCurdy in *The Notebooks of Leonardo da Vinci*, Vol. I, Ch. IX)

William Shakespeare [1564–1616]

This is the foul fiend Flibbertigibbet. . . . He gives the web and the pin, squints the eye, and makes the harelip.
> *King Lear*, III, iv, 120

I remember thine eyes well enough. Dost thou squiny at me?
> *Ibid.*, IV, vi, 139

Get thee glass eyes
And, like a scurvy politician, seem
To see the things thou dost not.
> *Ibid.*, IV, vi, 174

Thou green sarcenet flap for a sore eye.
> *Troilus and Cressida*, V, i, 35

And all eyes
Blind with the pin and web but theirs
— theirs only,
That would unseen be wicked?
> *The Winter's Tale*, I, ii, 290

Alexander Pope [1688–1744]

Why has not Man a microscopic eye?
For this plain reason, Man is not a Fly.
Say, what the use, were finer Opticks giv'n,
T' inspect a Mite, not comprehend the Heav'n?
> *An Essay on Man*, Epistle I

Georg Christoph Lichtenberg [1742–1799]

How is it that animals do not squint? Is this another prerogative of the human species?
> *Reflections*

William Blake [1757–1827]

The Eye altering alters all.
> *The Mental Traveller*

Sir John Bland-Sutton [1855–1936]

The lemurs are pretty animals and very liable to suffer from cataract. I was very much attached to a ring-tailed lemur with a cataract in each eye, and asked A. D. Bartlett, the Superintendent, to allow me to remove them. He asked me if I had removed a cataract from a Man's eye successfully. I replied "No." He said indignantly, "How can you expect me to let you operate on a lemur, if you have not operated

on a Man successfully! This lemur is worth £50."
The Story of a Surgeon, Ch. IX

The Bible

Leah was tender eyed; but Rachel was beautiful and well favoured.
Genesis 29:17

The hearing ear, and the seeing eye.
Proverbs 20:12

The eye is not satisfied with seeing.
Ecclesiastes 1:8

The light of the body is the eye.
Matthew 6:22

In the twinkling of an eye.
I Corinthians 15:52

The Talmud

If the physician is a long way off, the eye will be blind [before he arrives].
Baba Kamma, VIII.85a (tr. by E. W. Kirzner)

Anonymous

There was a man of Thessaly,
And he was wondrous wise,
He jumped into a bramble bush
And scratched out both his eyes.
And when he saw his eyes were out,
With all his might and main
He jumped into another bush
And scratched them in again.
The Oxford Book of Nursery Rhymes, No. 498

English Proverbs

A small hurt in the eye is a great one.

Never rub your eye but with your elbow.

FACE-LIFTING

See PLASTIC SURGERY

FACTS

See also HYPOTHESIS, RESEARCH, SCIENTIFIC METHOD, THEORY

Sydney Smith [1771–1845]

Oh, don't tell me of facts, I never believe facts: you know Canning said nothing was so fallacious as facts, except figures.
Quoted by Lady Holland in *A Memoir of the Rev. Sydney Smith,* Ch. 11

William Beaumont [1785–1853]

My opinions may be doubted, denied or approved, according as they conflict or agree with the opinions of each individual who may read them; but their worth will be best determined by the foundation on which they rest — the incontrovertible facts.
Experiments and Observations, Preface

Nicholas Maurice Arthus [1862–1945]

Seek facts and classify them and you will be the workmen of science. Conceive or accept theories and you will be their politicians.
De l'Anaphylaxie à l'immunité

Alphonse Raymond Dochez [1882–1964]

It is difficult, often impossible, to estimate the ultimate value of a new scientific fact.
Quoted in *P & S Quarterly* 11: 18, June 1966

Alan Gregg [1890–1957]

A statistical résumé of 1000 opinions about gravity before Newton's time would not have given us the law. You cannot always arrive at facts through other folks' opinions or observations.

> Aphorism (Quoted by Wilder Penfield in *The Difficult Art of Giving,* Appendix A)

Aldous Huxley [1894–1963]

Facts are ventriloquists' dummies. Sitting on a wise man's knee they may be made to utter words of wisdom; elsewhere, they say nothing, or talk nonsense, or indulge in sheer diabolism.

> Letter

Nathan S. Kline [1916–   ]

Factifuging, like vermifuging, is an unpleasant but sometimes necessary task and it should be done with clean and sanitary techniques, and with the least possible destruction of healthy tissue.

> *Lancet* 1:1396, 1962

Anonymous

Facts, details, ye ken, are just the vertebrae of the world.

> Quoted in *Archives of Internal Medicine* 116:455, 1965

Today's facts are tomorrow's fallacies.

Proverb

A single fact is worth a shipload of argument.

FAINTING

Hippocrates [460?–377? B.C.]

Persons who have had frequent and severe attacks of swooning, without any manifest cause, die suddenly.

> *Aphorisms,* II.41 (tr. by Francis Adams)

William Shakespeare [1564–1616]

Many will swoon when they do look on blood.

> *As You Like It,* IV, iii, 159

Why does my blood thus muster to my heart,
Making both it unable for itself
And dispossessing all my other parts
Of necessary fitness?
So play the foolish throngs with one that swounds —
Come all to help him, and so stop the air
By which he should revive.

> *Measure for Measure,* II, iv, 20

The Bible

If thou faint in the day of adversity, thy strength is small.

> *Proverbs* 24:10

FAITH

See also RELIGION

Alonzo Clark [1807–1887]

The medical errors of one century constitute the popular faith of the next.

Oliver Wendell Holmes [1809–1894]

So long as the body is affected through the mind, no audacious device, even of the most manifestly dishonest character, can fail of producing occasional good to those who yield it an implicit or even a partial faith.

> *Medical Essays,* "Homoeopathy and Its Kindred Delusions"

Rudolf Virchow [1821–1902]

Belief has no place as far as science reaches, and may be first permitted to take root where science stops.

> *Disease, Life, and Man,* "On Man" (tr. by L. J. Rather)

There can be no scientific dispute with respect to faith, for science and faith exclude one another.

> *Idem*

Sir William Osler [1849-1919]

Nothing in life is more wonderful than faith — the one great moving force which we can neither weigh in the balance nor test in the crucible.

British Medical Journal 1:1470, 1910

Santiago Ramón y Cajal [1852-1934]

That which enters the mind through reason can be corrected. That which is admitted through faith, hardly ever.

Charlas de Café

Finley Peter Dunne ("Mr. Dooley") [1867-1936]

I don't see why anny man who believes in medicine wud shy at th' faith cure.

Mr. Dooley's Philosophy, "Casual Observations"

René J. Dubos [1901-   ]

Profound faith is always a little intolerant.

Louis Pasteur, Free Lance of Science, Ch. V

Samuel H. Kraines [1906-   ]

If the patient believes strongly in a cure . . . by his very belief he at once obtains sufficient moral support to face all of his problems with some degree of equanimity.

The Therapy of Neuroses and Psychoses

The Bible

The prayer of faith shall save the sick.

James 5:15

Arabic Proverb

Have faith, though it be only in a stone, and you will recover.

FAME

See also SUCCESS

Sir Thomas Browne [1605-1682]

Who cares to subsist like *Hippocrates* Patients, or *Achilles* horses in *Homer,* under naked nominations, without deserts and noble acts, which are the balsame of our memories, the *Entelechia* and soul of our subsistences? . . . But the iniquity of oblivion blindly scattereth her poppy, and deals with the memory of men without distinction to merit of perpetuity.

Urne-Buriall, Ch. V

John Milton [1608-1674]

Fame is the spur that the clear spirit doth raise
(That last infirmity of Noble mind)
To scorn delights, and live laborious dayes.

Lycidas

Fame is no plant that grows on mortal soil.

Idem

John Wolcot ("Peter Pindar") [1738-1819]

What rage for fame attends both great and small!
Better be damn'd, than not be nam'd at all.

Lyric Odes to the Royal Academicians for 1783, Ode IX

Ewald Hering [1834-1918]

The conscious memory of man dies with his death; but the unconscious memory of nature is faithful and indestructible. Whoever has succeeded in impressing the vestiges of his work upon it, will be remembered forever.

On Memory

Sir William Osler [1849-1919]

It is strange how the memory of a

man may float to posterity on what he would have himself regarded as the most trifling of his works.
> Quoted by Harvey Cushing in *Life of Sir William Osler*

Santiago Ramón y Cajal [1852–1934]

Glory is nothing more than oblivion postponed.
> *Charlas de Café*

Sir Berkeley Moynihan [1865–1936]

Such men are gratefully remembered by posterity, not so much for the work which their own hands or minds have created or have modified; not for their written words which so soon seem to possess little more than an antiquarian interest; not for their spoken words which, though at the moment of their delivery they may walk up and down in the hearts of men and stir them to new thought or to great action, yet seem so frail and cold and lifeless when the morning comes; not for any of these, but for the spiritual legacy they bequeath to those inspired by their own zeal and trained in their own methods to seek the truth in eternal principles. It is this which gives post-humous life, the true immortality.
> *Addresses on Surgical Subjects,* "Hunter's Ideals and Lister's Practice"

Hugh Cabot [1872–1945]

When a man goes and they say that there will never be anyone to take his place, then that is immortality.
> Lecture

Martin H. Fischer [1879–1962]

The trouble is that somebody is going to discover me fifteen years after I'm dead; and great men are not discovered for fifty years.
> Quoted by Howard Fabing and Ray Marr in *Fischerisms*

FASTING

See also DIET, EATING, HUNGER

St. John Chrysostom [345?–407]

Fasting is a medicine.
> *Homilies on the Statutes,* Homily III (tr. by John H. Parker)

William Shakespeare [1564–1616]

Say, can you fast? Your stomachs are
> too young,
And abstinence engenders maladies.
> *Love's Labour's Lost,* IV, iii, 294

Immanuel Kant [1724–1804]

There is no virtue in . . . penance and fasting, which merely waste the body; they are fanatical and monkish virtues.
> *Lectures on Ethics,* "Duties Towards the Body Itself" (tr. by Louis Infield)

Mahatma Gandhi [1869–1948]

I am not aware during the whole of the fast of having suffered any pangs of hunger. . . . The only pain which the memory has stored is a feeling of nausea, creeping over me now and then, which was as a rule overcome by sipping water.
> *Young India,* Pt. I, "The Physical Effects of Fasting"

The Bible

When ye fast, be not, as the hypocrites, of a sad countenance.
> *Matthew* 6:16

FATIGUE

Alexander Pope [1688–1744]

Shut, shut the door, good John! fatigued, I said,

Tie up the knocker, say I'm sick, I'm dead.
> *Epistle to Dr. Arbuthnot*

Anonymous

When Helen was quite old and with more energy left than strength, I asked her what her idea of Heaven was. She replied, "Perpetual activity without fatigue."
> Quoted in *Archives of Internal Medicine* 114:557, 1964

FEAR

Michel de Montaigne [1533–1592]

The thing I fear most is fear.
> *Essays,* Bk. I, Ch. 18, "Of Fear" (tr. by Donald M. Frame)

Sir Philip Sidney [1554–1586]

Fear is more pain than is the pain it fears.
> *Arcadia,* Bk. V, "Musidorus' Song"

William Shakespeare [1564–1616]

Why do I yield to that suggestion
Whose horrid image doth unfix my hair
And make my seated heart knock at my ribs
Against the use of nature?
> *Macbeth,* I, iii, 134

I have a faint cold fear thrills through my veins
That almost freezes up the heat of life.
> *Romeo and Juliet,* IV, iii, 15

Wilfred Trotter [1872–1939]

The most influential obstacle to freedom of thought and to new ideas is fear, and fear which can with inimitable art disguise itself as caution or sanity or reasoned skepticism or on occasion even as courage.
> *Collected Papers,* "The Commemoration of Great Men"

Franklin D. Roosevelt [1882–1945]

The only thing we have to fear is fear itself.
> Inaugural address, March 4, 1933

William Sharpe [1882–   ]

Yes, to fear something and *not* have it — that frequently seems to have more serious effects upon the patient than having the condition itself. So why not tell the patient the truth if he wants to know it.
> *Brain Surgeon,* Ch. XXVII

John A. Ryle [1889–1950]

If every doctor, in whatever branch of medicine, would consciously and earnestly study pain and fear, both in a scientific and humane regard and with full profit of their literature, and would then set about to improve his understanding and management of cases on the basis of that study, the practice of medicine and the public health would win benefits, less spectacular maybe, but falling little short of those conferred by the discoveries of Pasteur and of Lister.
> *Fears May Be Liars,* Ch. 6

Aldous Huxley [1894–1963]

Love casts out fear; but conversely fear casts out love. And not only love. Fear also casts out intelligence, casts out goodness, casts out all thought of beauty and truth. . . . in the end fear casts out even a man's humanity.
> *Ape and Essence,* Ch. 2

French Proverb

He who fears to suffer, suffers from fear.

Scottish Proverb

There's nae medicine for fear.

FEES

See also ECONOMICS

Hammurabi [ca. 1955–1913 B.C.]

If a doctor has treated a gentleman for severe wound with a bronze lancet and has cured the man, or has opened an abscess of the eye for a gentleman with a bronze lancet and has cured the eye of the gentleman, he shall take ten shekels of silver.

If he (the patient) be the son of a poor man, he shall take five shekels of silver.

If he be a gentleman's servant, the master of the servant shall give two shekels of silver to the doctor.

If a doctor has cured the shattered limb of a gentleman or has cured the diseased bowel, the patient shall give five shekels of silver to the doctor.

If he be the son of a poor man, he shall give three shekels of silver.

If a gentleman's servant, the master of the slave shall give two shekels of silver to the doctor.

Code of Hammurabi

Pindar [522?–443 B.C.]

But alas! even the lore of leech-craft is enthralled by the love of gain.

Pythian Ode, III.54 (tr. by J. Sandys)

Heraclitus [fl. 513 B.C.]

Doctors cut, burn, and torture the sick, and then demand of them an undeserved fee for such services.

On the Universe (tr. by P. Wheelwright)

Hippocrates [460?–377? B.C.]

It is better to reproach a patient you have saved than to extort money from those who are at death's door.

Precepts, IV (tr. by W. H. S. Jones)

Seneca [4? B.C.–A.D. 65]

People pay the doctor for his trouble; for his kindness they still remain in his debt.

Pliny the Elder [23–79]

I mean not to say ought of their [physicians'] extreme avarice . . . nor how high they hold (as it were in open market) the easement and release of the sicke mans pains, whiles he is under their hands; ne yet what pawnes and pledges they take as earnest of the bargaine, to dispatch the poore Patient out of the way at once; and lastly of their hidden secrets and paradoxes, which forsooth they will not divulge abroad, but for some round summe of money.

Natural History, XXIX.viii.21 (tr. by Philemon Holland)

John of Salisbury [d. 1180]

Some who sell pseudo favor and who wish to appear quite just by refusing to receive a penny until the patient is convalescent are far from just, in that they ascribe to their own skill the kindly work of time — nay, the gift of the Lord, notwithstanding that he whom God and the recuperating power of nature restore would have been restored without the physician's effort. To be sure, nowadays there are a few doctors who constantly advise one another with the words "Take your fee while the patient is still in pain." [1]

Policraticus, Bk. II, Ch. 29 (tr. by J. Pike)

Leonardo da Vinci [1452–1519]

Every man desires to acquire wealth in order that he may give it to the doctors, the destroyers of life; therefore they ought to be rich.

Manuscript F, Library of the Institut de France (tr. by Edward MacCurdy in *The Notebooks of Leonardo da Vinci,* Vol. I, Ch. VIII)

[1] Cf. Proverb, p. 179a.

Desiderius Erasmus [1466?–1536]

Antiquity . . . both believed and proclaimed that no reward could be found worthy enough for a learned and faithful doctor.
Declamatio in laudem artis medicae

Euricius Cordus [1486–1535]

Three faces the Phisition hath:
first as an Angell he,
When he is saught: next when he helpes,
a God he semes to be.
And last of all when he hath made,
the sicke diseased well
And askes his guerdon, then he semes
an oughly Fiend of hell.
Of Physicians (tr. by Timothy Kendall in *Flowers of Epigrams*)

William Shakespeare [1564–1616]

Kill thy physician, and the fee bestow
Upon the foul disease.
King Lear, I, i, 166

Ben Jonson [1573?–1637]

When men a dangerous disease did 'scape,
Of old, they gave a cock to Aesculape;
Let me give two, that doubly am got free;
From my disease's danger, and from thee.
Epigrams, "To Doctor Empiric"

John Earle [1601?–1665]

The best Cure hee [the physician] has done is upon his own purse, which from a leane sicklinesse he hath made lusty, and in flesh.
Microcosmographie, Ch. 4

Daniel Defoe [1659?–1731]

As frighted Patients, when they want a Cure,
Bid any Price, and any Pain endure:
But when the Doctor's Remedies appear,
The Cure's too easy, and the Price too dear!
The True-Born Englishman, "Britannia"

John Gay [1685–1732]

Is there no hope? the sick Man said.
The silent doctor shook his head,
And took his leave, with signs of sorrow,
Despairing of his fee to-morrow.
Fables (Series I), Fable 27

Lady Mary Wortley Montagu [1689–1762]

A world of filthy doses and more filthy doctors' fees.
Letter to Lady Mar, May 1727

John Hunter [1728–1793]

I must go and earn this damned guinea or I shall be sure to want it to-morrow.
Quoted by S. R. Gloyne in *John Hunter*, Ch. 5

John Morgan [1735–1789]

The paying of a physician for attendance and the apothecary for his Medicines apart is certainly the most eligible mode of practice, both to patient and practitioner. The apothecary then, who is not obliged to spend his time in visiting patients, can afford to make up medicines at a reasonable price; and it is as desirable, as just in itself, that patients should allow fees for attendance, whatever it may be thought to deserve. They ought to know what it is they really pay for their Medicine, and what for physical advice and attendance.
A Discourse Upon the Institution of Medical Schools in America, Preface

Thomas Gisborne [1758–1846]

A physician ought to be extremely watchful against covetousness; for it is a vice imputed, justly or unjustly, to his Profession.
The Duties of Physicians

There have been Physicians, the disgrace of their profession, who seem to have considered themselves, in studying Medicine, as studying not a liberal science, but a mere art for the acquisition of money; and have thence been solicitous to acquire an insight rather into the humours than into the diseases of mankind.
Idem

David Hosack [1769–1835]

If the patient can abstain from unnatural indulgence he is readily cured by the means I have enumerated. — A ten dollar bill inclosed in your reply will be useful.
Letter to a patient, April 21, 1815

Pierre Bretonneau [1778–1862]

I only take money from sick people. [Comment to a hypochondriac.]
Quoted by F. H. Garrison in *Bulletin of the New York Academy of Medicine* 5:154, 1929

Oliver Wendell Holmes [1809–1894]

My terms for a lecture where I stay over night are these: Fifteen dollars and my expenses; a room with a fire in it in a public house, and a mattress to sleep on, not a feather bed. As you write in your individual capacity I tell you at once all my habitual exigencies. I am afraid to sleep in a cold room, I can't sleep on a feather bed, I will not go to private houses, and I have figured on the sum mentioned as what it is worth to *me* to go away for the night to places that can not pay more.
Letter to J. W. Porter, October 1852

Anthony Trollope [1815–1882]

A physician should take his fee without letting his left hand know what his right hand was doing; it should be taken without a thought, without a look, without a move of the facial muscles; the true physician should hardly be aware that the last friendly grasp of the hand had been made precious by the touch of gold.
Doctor Thorne, Ch. III

Henry Wheeler Shaw ("Josh Billings") [1818–1885]

When a doctor looks me square in the face and kant see no money in me, then i am happy.
Quoted by Donald Day in *Uncle Sam's Uncle Josh*, Ch. 9

Sir William Osler [1849–1919]

Speck in cornea, . . . 50¢. [Account-book entry, first fee as a practising physician.]
Quoted by Harvey Cushing in *Life of Sir William Osler*, Ch. 6

George Bernard Shaw [1856–1950]

It is not the fault of our doctors that the medical service of the community, as at present provided for, is a murderous absurdity. . . . to give a surgeon a pecuniary interest in cutting off your leg, is enough to make one despair of political humanity. . . . And the more appalling the mutilation, the more the mutilator is paid. He who corrects the ingrowing toe-nail receives a few shillings; he who cuts your inside out receives hundreds of guineas, except when he does it to a poor person for practice.
The Doctor's Dilemma, "Preface on Doctors"

Robert Tuttle Morris [1857–1945]

One must not count upon all of his patients being willing to steal in order to pay doctor's bills.
Doctors Versus Folks, Ch. 3

J. Chalmers Da Costa [1863–1933]

A fashionable surgeon, like a pelican, can be recognized by the size of his bill.
The Trials and Triumphs of the Surgeon, Ch. 1

The time during which a surgeon can charge large fees is brief. Very few people are able to pay large fees. Very few of those who are able to do so are willing. The surprise of a professional philanthropist when asked to make a personal contribution, the obstinacy of a government mule confronting a stream which must be forded, the indignation of a reformer when forced to be specific and to keep his promises, the wrath of a politician on discovering an impending split in the party, the horror of a superstitious colored man upon seeing a ghost in a graveyard, when all combined do not quite serve to represent the state of mind of the average millionaire when presented with a fair bill for having had his life saved by surgery.

Idem

Edwin Arlington Robinson [1869–1935]

Like a physician who can do no good,
But knows how soon another would
    have his fee
Were he to tell the truth.
Avon's Harvest

Damon Runyon [1880–1946]

My old man used to say that he guessed the percentage of scoundrels was less among doctors than any other class of men, professional or otherwise, in the world. . . . He said his own life had been saved several times by doctors and that he always paid the doctor first and let the other debts incurred during his illness wait. He said he figured that had the doctor not saved him and put him in action again, the others would never have been paid anyway.
The Brighter Side

Sir Harold Gillies [1882–1960] and
D. Ralph Millard, Jr. [1919–   ]

Most medical men are amateurs at fi-

nance, and what is learned comes through bitter experience.
The Principles and Art of Plastic Surgery, Vol. II, Ch. 20

Edwin P. Lehman [1888–1954]

It is asking more than human perfection to assume that a surgeon's judgment may not be influenced unconsciously by pressing financial need.
Surgery 28:595, 1950

In commenting upon the moral conflict between surgical indications and fee, one must remember that it affects only the conscientious practitioner of surgery. The so-called surgeon who practices primarily for the fee, who advises operation without adequate study, who removes a normal organ without indications, who makes an emergency out of almost every case, has no problem of morals, nor has the occasional general practitioner who undertakes procedures for which he is not trained or who does an incomplete operation for malignant disease so that at least some of the surgical fee will stay at home.
Idem

Sidney Kingsley [1906–   ]

A doctor shouldn't have to worry about money! That's one disease he's not trained to fight. It either corrupts him . . . or it destroys him.
Men in White, Act I, Sc. iv

The Talmud

A physician who heals for nothing is worth nothing.
Baba Kamma, VIII.85a (tr. by E. W. Kirzner)

Anonymous

When Physick's dearly bought,
    it doth much healing bring,
But when 'tis freely given,
    'tis ne'er a useful thing.
Quoted by John of Mirfeld in *Florarum Bartholomei,* "De Medicis"

Proverbs

Get your money when the patient is in pain.[1]

God heals, and the doctor takes the fee.

Physicians are costly visitors.

The physician owes all to the patient, but the patient owes nothing to him but a little money.

Who pays the physician does the cure.

African (Jukun) Proverb

In the midst of your illness you will promise a goat, but when you have recovered, a chicken will seem sufficient.

African (Transvaal) Proverb

If you are too smart to pay the doctor, you had better be too smart to get ill.

Arabic Proverb

When the cure is effected avarice sets in.

German Proverb

The purse of the patient protracts his cure.

Latin Proverb

A physician is an angel when employed, but a devil when one must pay him.

Polish Proverb

The doctor demands his fees whether he has killed the illness or the patient.

FETUS

See also PREGNANCY

Leonardo da Vinci [1452–1519]

Your order shall commence with the formation of the child in the womb, saying which part of it is formed first and so on in succession, placing its parts according to the times of pregnancy until the birth, and how it is nourished, learning in part from the eggs which hens make.

Quaderni d'Anatomia, Vol. I (tr. by Edward MacCurdy in *The Notebooks of Leonardo da Vinci,* Vol. I, Ch. III)

Samuel Taylor Coleridge [1772–1834]

The history of man for the nine months preceding his birth would, probably, be far more interesting and contain events of greater moment than all the threescore and ten years that follow it.

Miscellanies, Aesthetic and Literary

Enid Bagnold [1889–   ]

Hanging head downwards between cliffs of bone, was the baby, its arms all but clasped about its neck, its face aslant upon its arms, hair painted upon its skull, closed, secret eyes, a diver poised in albumen, ancient and epic, shot with delicate spasms, as old as a Pharaoh in its tomb.

The Door of Life, Ch. 2

FEVER

See also DELIRIUM

Plautus [254?–184 B.C.]

'Tis a portentous sign
When a man sweats, and at the same time shivers.

Asinaria, II.ii.289

St. John Chrysostom [345?–407]

By a superabundance of bile fever is produced.

Homilies on the Statutes, Homily X (tr. by John H. Parker)

---

[1] Cf. John of Salisbury, p. 175b.

William Shakespeare [1564–1616]

And what's a fever but- a fit of madness?
> *The Comedy of Errors*, V, i, 76

Home without boots, and in foul weather too?
How scapes he agues, in the devil's name?
> *Henry IV, Part I*, III, i, 68

The wretch, whose fever-weaken'd joints,
Like strengthless hinges, buckle under life,
Impatient of his fit, breaks like a fire
Out of his keeper's arms.
> *Henry IV, Part II*, I, i, 140

We are all diseas'd
And with our surfeiting and wanton hours
Have brought ourselves into a burning fever,
And we must bleed for it.
> *Ibid.*, IV, i, 54

An untimely ague
Stay'd me a prisoner in my chamber.
> *Henry VIII*, I, i, 4

He had a fever when he was in Spain,
And when the fit was on him, I did mark
How he did shake. 'Tis true, this god did shake.
His coward lips did from their colour fly,
And that same eye whose bend did awe the world
Did lose his lustre. I did hear him groan.
Ay, and that tongue of his that bade the Romans
Mark him and write his speeches in their books,
Alas, it cried, "Give me some drink, Titinius,"
As a sick girl!
> *Julius Caesar*, I, ii, 119

But now will canker-sorrow eat my bud
And chase the native beauty from his cheek,
And he will look as hollow as a ghost,
As dim and meagre as an ague's fit;
And so he'll die.
> *King John*, III, iv, 82

This fever that hath troubled me so long
Lies heavy on me. . . .
Ay me, this tyrant fever burns me up.
> *Ibid.*, V, iii, 3

There is so hot a summer in my bosom
That all my bowels crumble up to dust.
I am a scribbled form drawn with a pen
Upon a parchment, and against this fire
Do I shrink up.
> *Ibid.*, V, vii, 30

Here let them lie
Till famine and the ague eat them up.
> *Macbeth*, V, v, 3

But at this instant he is sick, my lord,
Of a strange fever.
> *Measure for Measure*, V, i, 151

My wind, cooling my broth,
Would blow me to an ague.
> *The Merchant of Venice*, I, i, 22

My love is as a fever, longing still
For that which longer nurseth the disease;
Feeding on that which doth preserve the ill,
Th' uncertain sickly appetite to please.
> *Sonnet CXLVII*

If all the wine in my bottle will recover him, I will help his ague.
> *The Tempest*, II, ii, 96

My heart beats thicker than a feverous pulse.
> *Troilus and Cressida*, III, ii, 38

And danger like an ague subtly taints
Even then when we sit idly in the sun.
Ibid., III, iii, 232

John Milton [1608–1674]

The feaver is to the Physitians, the eternal reproach.
The Reason of Church Government, Preface

Thomas Sydenham [1624–1689]

Why! the Fever itself is Nature's instrument.
Medical Observations, Sect. I, Ch. 5 (tr. by R. G. Latham in *Works,* Vol. I)

Isaac Watts [1674–1748]

So when a raging Fever burns
We shift from side to side by turns,
And 'tis a poor Relief we gain
To change the Place but keep the Pain.
Hymns and Spiritual Songs, Bk. II, CXLVI

Sydney Smith [1771–1845]

Our evils have been, want of rain, and scarlet-fever in our village, where, in three-quarters of a year, we have buried fifteen, instead of one, per annum. You will naturally suppose I have killed all these people by doctoring them; but scarlet-fever awes me, and is above my aim. I leave it to the professional and graduated homicides.
Letter to the Countess Grey, September 22, 1833

Honoré de Balzac [1799–1850]

Six weeks with fever is an eternity. Hours are like days. . . . then the nights are not lost.

Ralph Waldo Emerson [1803–1882]

Dr. Bigelow's formula was, that fevers are self-limiting; afterwards that all disease is so; therefore no use in treatment. Dr. Holmes said, No use in drugs. Dr. Samuel Jackson said, Rest, absolute rest, is the panacea.
Journal, 1860

Mary Baker Eddy [1821–1910]

Fevers are errors of various types. The quickened pulse, coated tongue, febrile heat, dry skin, pain in the head and limbs, are pictures depicted by a mortal's mind on the body.
Science and Health, Ch. XII

Sir William Osler [1849–1919]

Humanity has but three great enemies; Fever, famine and war; of these by far the greatest, by far the most terrible, is fever.
Journal of the American Medical Association 26:999, 1896

The fever in malaria from the outset is marked by remissions . . . of a grade rarely seen in typhoid until the late stages. Once the fastigium is reached, the fever in the latter presents a remarkable steadiness; the two-hour record may show for several days a variation of not more than a degree. The chart has a "Pennsylvania-Railway-like" directness, in marked distinction to the zigzag "Baltimore-and-Ohio-Railway" chart of aestivo-autumnal fever.
New York Medical Journal 70: 673, 1899

English Proverb

An ague in the Spring is physic for a king.

German Proverbs

Adam ate the apple and we still have the fever.[1]

Hussars pray for war, and the doctors for fever.

Italian Proverb

A quartan ague kills old men and heals young.

[1] Cf. Hungarian Proverb, p. 606a.

FEVER SORES

William Shakespeare [1564–1616]

She gallops night by night . . .
O'er ladies' lips, who straight on kisses
dream,
Which oft the angry Mab with blisters
plagues,
Because their breaths with sweetmeats
tainted are.
> *Romeo and Juliet*, I, iv, 70

FISTULA

William Shakespeare [1564–1616]

BERTRAM: What is it, my good lord,
the King languishes of?
LAFEW: A fistula, my lord.
> *All's Well That Ends Well*, I, i,
> 37

William Heberden [1710–1801]

A bad state of health is often joined
with a fistula ani, and the mischief,
after the cure of the ulcer, has many
times fallen upon other parts, and particularly the lungs, and has brought on
asthmas, spittings of blood, and consumptions.
> *Commentaries on the History
> and Cure of Diseases*, Ch. 40

FITNESS

See also HEALTH, HYGIENE,
REGIMEN

Peter Mere Latham [1789–1875]

The older we get, and the more conversant we have become with diseases,
patients, and remedies, the more stress
do we find ourselves laying upon a
man's constitution.
> *General Remarks on the Prac-
> tice of Medicine*, Ch. XVI

Finley Peter Dunne ("Mr.
Dooley") [1867–1936]

Me timp'rature is normal save whin I'm
asked f'r money. Me pulse bates siv-
inty to th' minyit an' though I have
patches on me pantaloons, I've ne'er a
wan on me intestines.
> *Mr. Dooley's Opinions*,
> "Thanksgiving"

John F. Kennedy [1917–1963]

Physical fitness goes with mental fitness. It goes with energy.
> Interview, January 13, 1961

English Proverb

As fit as a fiddle.

Welsh Proverb

Three things give hardy strength:
sleeping on hairy mattresses, breathing
cold air, and eating dry food.

FLATULENCE

Aristophanes [446–380 B.C.]

My wind exploded like a thunder-clap.
. . . Iaso blushed a rosy red
And Panacea turned away her head
Holding her nose: my wind's not frank-
incense.
> *Plutus*, 699 (tr. by Benjamin B.
> Rogers)

FOOD

See DIET, EATING, HUNGER,
VEGETARIANISM, VITAMINS

FOXGLOVE

William Shakespeare [1564–1616]

There with fantastic garlands did she
come
Of crowflowers, nettles, daisies, and
long purples,

That liberal shepherds give a grosser
name,
But our cold maids do dead men's fingers call them.[1]
   Hamlet, IV, vii, 170

Abraham Cowley [1618–1667]
The *Fox-Glove* on fair *Flora's* hand
is worn,
Lest while she gathers Flow'rs she
meet a Thorn.
   Of Plants, Bk. IV (tr. by
   Nahum Tate)

Sarah Hoare [1767–1855]
The Foxglove's leaves, with caution
giv'n,
Another proof of favouring Heav'n
Will happily display;
The rapid pulse it can abate;
The hectic flush can moderate;
And, blest by Him whose will is fate,
May give a lengthened day.
   *The Pleasures of Botanical Pur-
suits*, appended to Priscilla
Wakefield's *An Introduction to
Botany*

Sir Walter Scott [1771–1832]
The primrose pale, and violet flower,
Found in each cliff a narrow bower;
Fox-glove and night-shade, side by
side,
Emblems of punishment and pride,
Group'd their dark hues with every
stain
The weather-beaten crags retain.
   Lady of the Lake, Canto I

John Keats [1795–1821]
O Solitude! if I must with thee dwell,
   . . . let me thy vigils keep
'Mongst boughs pavillion'd, where
the deer's swift leap
Startles the wild bee from the fox-glove
bell.
   Sonnet

[1] "Long purples" and "dead men's fingers"
were popular terms for foxglove.

David Macbeth Moir [1] [1798–1851]
The foxglove with its stately bells
Of purple, shall adorn thy dells.
   The Birth of the Flowers

Geoffrey Johnson [1893–   ]
The spire of foxglove hung with bells
Swings in the light till day is done,
Unknowing whether her function is
Man's bane or benison,

Uncaring whether her essence kills
A rat or an only child,
Eases the worn-out heart of a saint,
Of the sot or the self-reviled,

Uncaring that out of her acid earth
Springs the medicinal thorn,
Or the viper's form as comely as hers
And as deadly too is born.

For hers is the primal innocence
Breathed into flower and tree
When Lucifer shone unfallen from
heaven
And Adam was yet to be.
   The New York Times, May 2,
   1961, "The Foxglove"

Anne Guthrie Bicknell
[fl. 20th Cent.]

Tritoma was an ugly joker,
Fiery as a red-hot-poker,
How he hated Dig-i-tal-is.
For both loved the wee Oxalis.
Nothing could his feelings balk.
He pulled the bells off the other's stalk,
And thus so frightened poor Oxalis,
As a dose for life she took — Digitalis.
   Foxglove–Tritoma–Oxalis

FRACTURES

See BONES

[1] Known as Δ (Delta), his signature to
essays and poems contributed to *Blackwood's
Magazine*.

FROSTBITE

Silius Italicus [25?–101]

Men leave arms and legs behind, severed by the frost, and the cruel cold cuts off the limbs already broken.
Punica, III.552 (tr. by J. D. Duff)

GASTROINTESTINAL TRACT

See also BOWELS, DIGESTION, DYSENTERY, INDIGESTION, STOMACH

Robert Browning [1812–1889]

Before breakfast, a man feels but queasily,
And a sinking at the lower abdomen
Begins the day with indifferent omen.
The Flight of the Duchess, Pt. XII

George S. Chappell ("Walter Traprock") [1877–   ]

Through the Alimentary Canal With Gun and Camera.
Title of a book

Henry E. Sigerist [1891–1957]

Hawi (fl. 2500 B.C.) . . . attended to both ends of the gastrointestinal tract by being both physician of the teeth and guardian of the anus.
A History of Medicine, Vol. I, Ch. 3

GENERAL PRACTITIONER

See also PHYSICIANS, PRACTICE

Sir Walter Scott [1771–1832]

There is no creature in Scotland that works harder and is more poorly re-quited than the country doctor, unless perhaps it may be his horse. Yet the horse is, and indeed must be, hardy, active, and indefatigable, in spite of a rough coat and indifferent condition; and so you will often find in his master, under an unpromising and blunt exterior, professional skill and enthusiasm, intelligence, humanity, courage, and science.
The Surgeon's Daughter, Ch. 1

Frank Kittredge Paddock [1841–1901]

A general practitioner can no more become a specialist than an old shoe can become a dancing slipper. Both have developed habits which are immutable.
Aphorism

Sir William Osler [1849–1919]

I would speak of [the general practitioner's] failure to realize *first,* the need of a lifelong progressive personal training, and *secondly,* the danger lest in the stress of practice he sacrifice that most precious of all possessions, his mental independence.
Aequanimitas, with Other Addresses, "Chauvinism in Medicine"

In no profession does culture count for so much as in medicine, and no man needs it more than the general practitioner.
Idem

Charles L. Dana [1852–1935]

The old fashioned family physician and general practitioner . . . was a splendid figure and useful person in his day; but he was badly trained, he was often ignorant, he made many mistakes, for one cannot by force of character and geniality of person make a diagnosis of appendicitis, or recognize streptococcus infection.
New York Medical Journal 97:1, 1913

Opie Read [1852–1939]

In every country the family doctor is a natural sprout from the soil. His profession is almost as old as the daybreak of time. He bled the ancient Egyptians, blistered the knights of the Middle Ages, and poisoned the arrows of the Iroquois. He has been preserved in fiction, pickled in the drama, and peppered in satire.

Don Marquis [1878–1937]

"I haven't got time to be sick!" he said. "People need me." For he was a country doctor, and he did not know what it was to spare himself.
Country Doctor

Walter B. Pitkin [1878–1953]

A country doctor needs more brains to do his work passably than the fifty greatest industrialists in the world require.
The Twilight of the American Mind, Ch. 10

Sir Henry Howarth Bashford ("Peter Harding") [1880–1961]

General practice is at least as difficult, if it is to be carried on well and successfully, as any special practice can be, and probably more so; for the G.P. has to live continually, as it were, with the results of his handiwork.
The Corner of Harley Street, Ch. 26

Dana W. Atchley [1892–   ]

No warm sympathetic person is frozen by research experience, nor is a cold tactless individual thawed by general practice.
Journal of Medical Education 34 (October, Pt. II):17, 1963

Robert P. Andrews [1935–   ]

It [general practice] is not for everybody, and especially not for romantic refugees from big city life.
Tufts Folia Medica 9:25, 1963

GENETICS

See also EUGENICS, HEREDITY

Leonardo da Vinci [1452–1519]

The black races in Ethiopia are not the product of the sun; for if black gets black with child in Scythia, the offspring is black; but if a black gets a white woman with child the offspring is grey. And this shows that the seed of the mother has power in the embryo equally with that of the father.
Quaderni d'Anatomia, Vol. III (tr. by Edward MacCurdy in *The Notebooks of Leonardo da Vinci*, Vol. I, Ch. III)

William Shakespeare [1564–1616]

But where the bull and cow are both milk-white,
They never do beget a coal-black calf.
Titus Andronicus V, i, 31

George Gordon, Lord Byron [1788–1824]

That they bred *in and in,* as might be shown,
Marrying their cousins — nay, their aunts, and nieces,
Which always spoils the breed, if it increases.
Don Juan, Canto I, Stanza 57

Rudolf Virchow [1821–1902]

Where a cell arises, there a cell must have previously existed (omnis cellula e cellula), just as an animal can spring only from an animal, a plant only from a plant.
Cellular Pathology, Lect. II (tr. by Frank Chance)

E. A. Hooton [1887–1954]

In medical science lies the only practicable control of human evolution and of biological progress. Medical science must cease to regard its function as

primarily curative and preventive. It must rid itself of its obsession that its chief responsibility is to the individual rather than to society. It must allocate to itself the function of discovering how the human animal body may be improved as a biological organism. The future of mankind does not depend upon political or economic theory, nor yet upon measures of social amelioration, but upon the production of better minds in sounder bodies.
> *Apes, Men and Morons,* Ch. 18

A. H. Sturtevant [1891–   ]

The possibilities of the genetic study of Drosophila were then just beginning to be apparent; we were at the right place at the right time.[1]
> *American Scientist* 53:303, 1965

GENIUS

Seneca [4? B.C.–A.D. 65]

No great genius has ever existed without some touch of madness.
> *De Tranquillitate Animi,* XVII (tr. by J. B. Basore)

Herbert Spencer [1820–1903]

Only when Genius is married to Science can the highest results be produced.
> *Education,* Ch. 1

Thomas A. Edison [1847–1931]

Genius is one per cent inspiration and ninety-nine per cent perspiration.
> Aphorism

Santiago Ramón y Cajal [1852–1934]

Genius, like the inhabitants of the depths of the sea, moves by its own light.
> *Charlas de Café*

[1] Referring to 1910–1911, when, as an undergraduate, he had a desk in T. H. Morgan's laboratory at Columbia University.

Otto Weininger [1880–1903]

Talent is hereditary; it may be the common possession of a whole family (e.g., the Bach family); genius is not transmitted; it is never diffused, but is strictly individual.
> *Sex and Character,* Pt. II, Ch. IV

Michael Polanyi [1891–   ]

Genius seems to consist in the power of applying the originality of youth to the experience of maturity.
> *The Study of Man,* Ch. 1

GLUTTONY

See EATING, INDIGESTION, INTEMPERANCE

GOUT

Hippocrates [460?–377? B.C.]

Eunuchs do not take the gout, nor become bald.
> *Aphorisms,* VI.28 (tr. by Francis Adams)

A woman does not take the gout, unless her menses be stopped.
> *Ibid.,* VI.29

A young man does not take the gout until he indulges in coition.
> *Ibid.,* VI.30

Hedylus [fl. 270 B.C.]

The daughter of limb-relaxing Bacchus and limb-relaxing Aphrodite is limb-relaxing Gout.
> *Greek Anthology,* XI.414 (tr. by W. R. Paton)

Plautus [254?–184 B.C.]

You are gouty, And in slow motion have outdone a snail.
> *Poenulus,* III.i.532

Cicero [106–43 B.C.]

I say that the highest pain — and I say "highest" even if there is another ten atoms worse — is not consequently short, and I can name a number of worthy men who, according to their own account, have suffered tortures of pain from gout for several years.

Tusculan Disputations, II.xix.45 (tr. by J. E. King)

Martial [fl. 1st Cent.]

Diodorus goes to law, and suffers, Flaccus, from gout in the feet. But he offers his advocate no fee: this is gout in the hand.

Epigrams, I.98 (tr. by W. C. A. Ker)

When he refused any longer to endure and put up with the various gaddings about, and the devious morning calls, and the pride and salutations of wealthy patrons, Caelius set up the pretence of gout. And while he was anxious to prove it was quite genuine, and plastered and swathed his sound feet, and got along with a labouring gait, Caelius — what potency has the exercise and cultivation of illness! — has ceased to pretend gout!

Ibid., VII.39

Of mullets, and hares, and sow's paps, this is the result — a bilious complexion and torturing feet.

Ibid., XII.48

Nicarchus [fl. 1st Cent.]

Must I not die? What care I if I go to Hades with gouty legs or in training for a race? I shall have many to carry me; so let me become lame, if I wish. As far as that goes, as you see, I am quite easy, and never miss a banquet.

Greek Anthology, V.39 (tr. by W. R. Paton)

Aretaeus of Cappadocia [81–138?]

There is a great wonder in regard to them [arthritis and gout]; there is not the slightest pain in them, although you cut or squeeze them; but if pained of themselves, no other pain is stronger than this.

On the Causes and Symptoms of Chronic Diseases, II.12 (tr. by Francis Adams)

Lucian of Samosata [fl. 2nd Cent.]

Goddess who hatest the poor, sole vanquisher of wealth, who ever knowest to live well, even though it is thy joy to sit on the feet of others, thou knowest how to wear felt, and thou art fond of ointments. A garland delights thee and draughts of Italian wine. These things are never found among the poor. Therefore thou fliest the brassless (penniless) threshold of poverty, and delightest to come to the feet of wealth.

Greek Anthology, XI.403, "To the Gout" (tr. by W. R. Paton)

O horrid Name! detested by the Gods!
Gout, ruefull Gout! of sad *Cocytus* born!
Whom in the mirky Caves of *Tartarus*
The Fiend *Megaera* in her Womb conceiv'd.

The Triumphs of the Gout (tr. by G. West)

Then unperceiv'd she [Podagra, the foot-torturess] drives her piercing Dart,
And Wounds the inmost Sense with secret Smart. . . .
Thro' ev'ry Joint the thrilling Anguish pours,
And gnaws, and burns, and tortures, and devours;
Till Length of Suff'ring the dire Pow'r appease,
And the fierce Torments at her bidding cease.

Idem

What and whence are ye, that so proudly dare
The Lists to enter with the mighty Gout,
Whose Pow'r not *Jove* himself can overcome?
>   *Idem*

Ammianus Marcellinus [325–391]

Late in the day has the gout found him who deserved it, him who deserved to be gouty a hundred years ago.
>   *Greek Anthology*, XI.229 (tr. by W. R. Paton)

Claudian [ca. 395]

Canst thou talk of feet? Dost blame my verses
and criticize my lines, thou whose own feet are
so weak? This couplet, you say, will scarcely stand:
the scansion is shaky. Dear friend, a gouty man
thinks nothing at all can stand.
>   *To a Gouty Critic* (tr. by Maurice Platnauer)

Aetios [fl. ca. 500]

In January, take a glass of pure wine every morning; February: eat no beets; March: mix sweets with eatables and drinkables; April: refrain from horse radish; May: eat no polypus fishes; June: take cold water every morning; July: abstain from venery; August: eat no mallows; September: eat and drink milk; October: garlic must be eaten; November: bathing is prohibited; December: eat no cabbage.[1]
>   *Tetrabiblon*, Sermo III, IV. xlviii

Geronimo Cardano (Jerome Cardan) [1501–1576]

What a man gout makes! devout, morally pure, temperate, circumspect, wakeful. No one is so mindful of God as the man who is in the clutches of the

---

[1] A regimen for the gout sufferer.

pains of gout. He who suffers gout cannot forget that he is mortal, because it affects him in every part of his being.
>   *Podagrae Encomium*

Michel de Montaigne [1533–1592]

One of our gentlemen who was wondrously subject to the gout, on being urged by the doctors to give up entirely the use of salt meats, used to answer them very humorously that in the agonies and torments of the illness he wanted to have something to blame, and by crying out and cursing now the sausage, now the ox tongue and the ham, he felt just that much relieved.
>   *Essays*, Bk. I, Ch. 4, "How the Soul Discharges Its Passions on False Objects When the True Are Wanting" (tr. by Donald M. Frame)

Nicholas Breton [1545?–1626?]

There is no paine like the Gowt.
>   *Crossing of Proverbs*

Thomas Cogan [1545?–1607]

Drink wine & have the gowte; drink none & have the gowt.[1]
>   *Haven of Health*, Dedication

William Shakespeare [1564–1616]

>   Yet am I better
Than one that's sick o' th' gout, since he had rather
Groan so in perpetuity than be cur'd
By th' sure physician, Death.
>   *Cymbeline*, V, iv, 4

A man can no more separate age and covetousness than 'a can part young limbs and lechery; but the gout galls the one, and the pox pinches the other.
>   *Henry IV, Part II*, I, ii, 256

A pox of this gout! or, a gout of this pox! for the one or the other plays the rogue with my great toe.
>   *Ibid.*, I, ii, 273

---

[1] Cf. Thomas Sydenham, p. 190a.

Thomas Nash [1567–1601]

And well observe Hippocrates old rule,
The onely medicine for the foote is
rest.

> *Summers Last Will and Testament*

Philip Barrow [fl. 1590]

This disease is engendred of continuall
crudities and drunkennesse, and of immoderate using of lechery, through
vehement and swift deambulations and
walkings, through long standing, or
often riding, by suppression and stopping of accustomed excretions and
fluxes, and through intermission of
familiar exercises. Sorrowes, cares,
watchings, and other perturbations of
the minde, do not onely ingender this
evill, but also do breed hurtfull and
corrupt humours. . . . But for the
most part, a disposition of this kinde
of disease proceedeth from the parents
to the children, and their posteritie.
Also universally abundance of all raw
humours is the cause of this disease.
The humours that do abound, and do
fasten themselves in the joynts, either
be sanguine, or cholericke, or fleg-
maticke, or melancholious. Also some-
time this evill is ingendred of commix-
tion of humours.

> *The Method of Physick,* Bk.
> III, Ch. LXVI

Herman Busschof [fl. 17th Cent.]

'Tis become a Proverbial saying, viz.
that he who undertakes to perform
something extraordinary, is like him
that pretends to Cure the Gout.

> *Of the Gout*

Thomas Sydenham [1624–1689]

Gout attacks such old men as, after
passing the best part of their life in
ease and comfort, indulging freely in
high living, wine and other generous
drinks, at length, from inactivity, the
usual attendant of advanced life, have
left off altogether the bodily exercises
of their youth. Such men have gener-

ally large heads, are of a full, humid,
and lax habit, and possess a luxurious
and vigorous constitution, with excellent vital stamina.

> *Works,* "A Treatise on Gout
> and Dropsy" (tr. by R. G.
> Latham)

The victim goes to bed and sleeps in
good health. About two o'clock in the
morning he is awakened by a severe
pain in the great toe; more rarely in
the heel, ankle, or instep. The pain
is like that of a dislocation, and yet
the parts feel as if cold water were
poured over them. . . . Now it is a
violent stretching and tearing of the
ligaments — now it is a gnawing pain,
and now a pressure and tightening. So
exquisite and lively meanwhile is the
feeling of the part affected, that it
cannot bear the weight of the bedclothes nor the jar of a person walking
in the room. The night is spent in
torture.

> *Idem*

Pain, lameness, and the long list of
enumerated symptoms are not all.
Gout produces calculus in the kidney.
. . . the patient has frequently to entertain the painful speculation as to
whether gout or stone be the worst
disease.

> *Idem*

For humble individuals like myself,
there is one poor comfort, which is
this, viz. that gout, unlike any other
disease, kills more rich men than poor,
more wise men than simple. Great
kings, emperors, generals, admirals,
and philosophers have all died of gout.
Hereby Nature shows her impartiality:
since those whom she favours in one
way she afflicts in another — a mixture
of good and evil pre-eminently adapted
to our frail mortality.

> *Idem*

The more closely I have thought upon
gout, the more I have referred it to

indigestion, or to the impaired concoction of matters, both in the parts and the juices of the body. Gouty patients are, generally, either old men, or men who have so worn themselves out in youth as to have brought on a premature old age — of such dissolute habits none being more common than the premature and excessive indulgence in venery, and the like exhausting passions.

Idem

As for a radical cure, one altogether perfect, and one whereby a patient might be freed from even the disposition to the disease — this lies, like Truth, *at the bottom of a well;* and so deep is it in the innermost recesses of Nature, that I know not when or by whom it will be brought forward into the light of day.

Idem

I confidently affirm that the greater part of those who are supposed to have died of gout, have died of the medicine rather than the disease — a statement in which I am supported by observation.

Idem

The old saw is that "if you drink wine you have the gout, and if you do not drink wine the gout will have you." [1]

Idem

Sir Richard Blackmore [1650?–1729]

See, colic, gout, and stone, a cruel train,
Oppos'd by all the healing race in vain,
Their various racks and lingering plagues employ,
Relieve each other, and by turns annoy,
And, tyrant like, torment, but not destroy. . . .

[1] Cf. Thomas Cogan, p. 188b.

Howe'er the cause phantastic may appear,
Th' effect is real, and the pain sincere.
Creation, Bk. V

This disease is not bred in Prisons and Work-houses, nor engendered in the Galley or the Mine; but owes its Production to the Table of the Epicure and the Abuse of delicious Wine. It is the dissolute and voluptuous Indulgence of sensual Appetites, that administer to the Blood the Seeds of the Gout.

Discourses on the Gout, a Rheumatism, and the King's Evil

Cotton Mather [1663–1728]

Now lett the gouty People that are *chastened with Pain on their Bed, and the Multitude of their Bones with strong Pain, fall* into serious and awful *Meditations* on the *Pain,* which will be the Portion of them, on whom an All-powerful GOD will make known the *Power of His Anger.*

The Angel of Bethesda, Ch. XII

Jonathan Swift [1667–1745]

Dear honest Ned is in the gout,
Lies rackt with pain, and you without:
How patiently you hear him groan!
How glad the case is not your own!
On the Death of Dr. Swift

Philip Stanhope, Lord Chesterfield [1694–1773]

I have now been here [at Bath] near a month, bathing and drinking the waters, for complaints much of the same kind as yours; I mean pains in my legs, hips, and arms. . . . I wish it were a declared gout, which is the distemper of a gentleman; whereas the rheumatism is the distemper of a hackney-coachman or chairman, who are obliged to be out in all weathers and at all hours.

Letter to his son, November 28, 1765

"Philander Misaurus" [fl. 1699]

You could say, That when the Almighty God had, out of rude *Chaos*, built this goodly, Frame of Nature, which we see, and form'd his Noble Creature, Man; he indulged the Devil to create some one Thing; and his damn'd Envy gave being to the *Gout*.

The Honour of the Gout [1]

And yet there is the Right Honourable Sir R. H. the *Gout* is so salutary to him, that those two *Swiss* Doctors can't dispatch him. What would a certain Lord give, that those two coagulating Spirits could remove his Honour's *Gout?* But say I, *Gout, hold thy own;* for Earth has more need of the Cripple, than Heaven of the Saint.

Idem

How welcome is a Guest, that knows when to be gone? But if his Stay be longer than ordinary, we are ready to thrust him out of Doors. For these, and the like Considerations, the Way of the *Gout's* dealing with his Patients can never be enough esteem'd.

Idem

I am perswaded, that if the fortunate Patient would be at the Pains to observe all the Motions of the *Gout*, in his pinching, smarting, galling Accesses; in his gnawing, stabbing, burning Paroxysms; in his evacuating, tender, remitting Recesses; he might quickly come to wind a Storm so long before, that in a short Time, no Owners would think their Ship safe, but with a *Gouty* Master; Nor would any experienc'd Seaman, that wanted a Ship, offer himself to the Merchants, but upon Crutches.

Idem

[1] *The Honour of the Gout* by "Philander Misiatrus" [sic], first published in 1699, is listed in the 1963 *British Museum Catalogue* as "author unknown."

Francis Spilsbury [fl. 18th Cent.]

His manner of attacking is different from other maladies; they often dart, and kill at once: some, indeed, make regular advances, and retire, leaving the patient a certificate as a pledge of their returning no more: but this invader displays his subtility, by first raising apprehensions to terrify the objects of his spleen into his toils, then leisurely fetters and confines them as state prisoners in their chambers: if they are indulged to go abroad his badge accompanies them.

Free Observations on the Scurvy, Gout, Diet, and Remedy

Gerard F. van Swieten [1700–1772]

Seeing men of learning, and those of chief eminence in the affairs of government, are so often tormented by the gout, it ought to be a rule with them to dispatch all important business in the morning; taking care, however, to reserve two hours or so before dinner, to be employed in bodily exercise. The hours after dinner let them dedicate to walking or riding out, or to the agreeable conversation of their friends; but in the evening they must not at all be concerned in any business that requires the least stretch of thought or attention.

Commentaries upon Boerhaave's Aphorisms, Vol. 13, Sect. 1275

James Thomson [1700–1748]

The sleepless Gout here counts the crowing cocks,
A wolf now gnaws him, now a serpent stings.

The Castle of Indolence, Canto I, Stanza 77

John Wesley [1703–1791]

Regard them not who say, the gout ought not to be cured. They mean, it cannot. I know it cannot by their regular prescriptions. But I have known it cured in many cases, without any ill effects following. I have cured myself several times.

Primitive Physic, Sect. 103

Benjamin Franklin [1706–1790]

Be temperate in wine, in eating, girls, and sloth, or the Gout will seize you and plague you both.

Poor Richard's Almanack, 1734

Henry Fielding [1707–1754]

It is with jealousy as with the gout. When such distempers are in the blood, there is never any security against their breaking out; and that often on the slightest occasions, and when least suspected.

Tom Jones, Bk. II, Ch. 3

William Cullen [1710–1790]

This disease seldom attacks eunuchs; and when it does, they seem to be those who happen to be of a robust habit, to lead an indolent life, and to live very full.

First Lines of the Practice of Physic, Pt. I, Bk. II, Ch. 14

William Heberden [1710–1801]

Various distempers in certain ages and countries have had the fashion on their side, and have been thought reputable and desirable: others, on the contrary, have been reckoned scandalous and dreadful. . . . Some maladies have been esteemed honourable, because they have accidentally attacked the great, or because they usually belong to the wealthy, who live in plenty and ease. We have all heard of the courtiers who mimicked the wry neck of Alexander the Great; and when Lewis XIV happened to have a fistula, the French surgeons of that time complain of their being incessantly teased by people, who pretended, whatever their complaints were, that they proceeded from a fistula: and if there had been in

France a mineral water reputed capable of giving it them, they would perhaps have flocked thither as eagerly as Englishmen resort to Bath in order to get the gout. For this seems to be the favourite disease of the present age in England; wished for by those who have it not, and boasted of by those who fancy they have it, though very sincerely lamented by most who in reality suffer its tyranny. Hence, by a peculiar fate, more pains seem to be taken at present to breed or produce the gout, than to find out its remedy.

Commentaries on the History and Cure of Diseases, Ch. 9

The gout most usually begins with a pain in the first joint of the great toe, which soon looks very red, and after a little while begins to swell. The violence of the first pain seldom lasts twenty-four hours; but before it has quite ceased, another begins in the same, or some other part, where it continues as long. A succession of similar pains makes up a whole fit of the gout.

Idem

There will at first be an interval of two or three years, or more, between the fits; but after some time they will be repeated once or twice every year. The attacks of an old gout are less painful, but of longer continuance, and are attended with a greater and more lasting weakness. Most gouts continue to return to the end of life. I never knew a certain instance of their beginning before the years of puberty.

Idem

The gout affords a striking proof of the long experience and wary attention necessary to find out the nature of diseases and their remedies. For though this distemper be older than any medical records, and in all ages so common; and besides, according to Sydenham, chiefly attacks men of sense and reflexion, who would be able, as well as willing, to improve every hint which reason or accident might throw in their way; yet we are still greatly in the dark about its causes and effects, and the right method in which it should be treated.

Idem

The pains . . . are for the most part transmitted to the descendants of those who have suffered in any considerable degree.

Idem

William Cadogan [1711–1797]

The gout is so common a disease, that there is scarcely a man in the world, whether he has had it or not, but thinks he knows perfectly what it is. So does a cook-maid think she knows what fire is as well as Sir Isaac Newton.

A Dissertation on the Gout, and All Chronic Diseases, Jointly Considered

David Garrick [1717–1779]

I am tight in my Limbs, better in my head, & my belly is as big as Ever — I cannot quit Peck [1] & Booze — What's Life without Sack & Sugar! my lips were made to be lick'd, & if the Devil appears to me in the Shape of Turbot & Claret, my Crutches are forgot, & I laugh & Eat till my Navel rosebud is as full blown as a Sun flower.

Letter to the Rev. Doctor John Hoadly, May 9, 1771

Horace Walpole [1717–1797]

Another plague is, that everybody that ever knew anybody that had it, are so good as to come with advice, and direct me how to manage it — that is, how to continue to have it for a great many years. I am very refractory — I say to the gout, as great personages do to the executioner, "Friend, do your work as quick as you can."

Letter to George Montagu, August 12, 1760

[1] Peck = food.

It is very hard, when you can plunge over head and ears in Irish claret and not have even your heel vulnerable by the gout, that such a Pythagorean as I am, should yet be subject to it!

Ibid., May 14, 1762

The gout they tell me is to ensure me a length of years and health, but as I fear I must now and then renew the patent at the original expense, I am not much flattered by so dear an annuity.

Letter to Sir Horace Mann, July 12, 1765

I have one great blessing, there is drowsiness in all the square hollows of the red-hot bars of the gridiron on which I lie, so that I scream and fall asleep by turns like a babe that is cutting its first teeth.

Letter to Countess of Upper Ossory, December 27, 1784

You may imagine that I have made observations in plenty on the gout: yes, yes, I know its ways and its jesuitic evasions.

Letter to Sir Horace Mann, August 26, 1785

Since I must be old and have the gout, I have long turned those disadvantages to my own account, and plead them to the utmost when they will save me from doing anything I dislike.

Ibid., October 30, 1785

A finger of each hand has been pouring out a hail of chalk-stones and liquid chalk; and the first finger, which I hoped exhausted, last week opened again and threw out a cascade of the latter, exactly with the effort of a pipe that bursts in the streets.

Ibid., February 13, 1786

From the little finger of my left, through all that hand, wrist, and elbow, I am a line of gout, Madam.

Letter to Countess of Upper Ossory, December 11, 1795

Tobias Smollett [1721–1771]

An old officer, whose temper, naturally impatient, was, by repeated attacks of gout, which had almost deprived him of the use of his limbs, sublimated into a remarkable degree of virulence and perverseness.

> *The Adventures of Peregrine Pickle*, Ch. 70

William Cowper [1731–1800]

O may I live exempted (while I live
Guiltless of pamper'd appetite obscene)
From pangs arthritic that infest the toe
Of libertine Excess! The Sofa suits
The gouty limb, 'tis true; but gouty limb,
Though on a Sofa, may I never feel.

> *The Task*, Bk. I

Thomas Jefferson [1743–1826]

We have been for some days in much inquietude for the Count de Vergennes. He is very seriously ill. Nature seems struggling to decide his disease into a gout. A swelled foot, at present, gives us a hope of this issue.

> Letter to John Jay, February 1, 1787

Benjamin Rush [1745?–1813]

Solomon places all wisdom, in the management of human affairs, in finding out the proper times for performing certain actions. Skill in medicine consists in an eminent degree in timing remedies. . . . In a word, the cure of the gout depends wholly upon two things, viz. *proper* remedies, in their proper *times*, and *places*.

> *Medical Inquiries and Observations*, Vol. II, Ch. 7

Let not superstition say here, that the gout is the just punishment of folly and vice, and that the justice of Heaven would be defeated by curing it.

> *Idem*

I shall take leave of this disease, by comparing it to a deep and dreary cave in a new country, in which ferocious beasts and venomous reptiles, with numerous ghosts and hobgoblins, are said to reside. . . . At length a school boy, careless of his safety, ventures to enter this subterraneous cavern, when! to his great delight, he finds nothing in it but the same kind of stones and water he left behind him upon the surface of the earth. In like manner, I have found no other principles necessary to explain the cause of the gout, and no other remedies necessary to cure it, than such as are admitted in explaining the causes, and in prescribing for the most simple and common diseases.

> *Idem*

John Ring [1752–1821]

In the happy moment of mirth and conviviality, and the mad career of dissipation, an epicure, or a voluptuary, little dreams of the gout; which hangs over his head, like the sword of Damocles, and threatens his destruction.

Amid the joys of wine, and the shouts of the Bacchanals, the still voice of reason is not heard; the sober dictates of discretion are disregarded; and the friendly warnings of the physician are either totally forgotten, or treated with ridicule and contempt.

> *A Treatise on the Gout*

R. Drake [fl. 1758]

The Gout affects the Rich as well as Poor. It destroys indeed more rich and eminent Men, than those of low Degree; which demonstrates the Justice and Impartiality of Providence, who abundantly supplies those that want some of the agreeable Pleasures and Conveniencies of Life, with Vigour, Health and Strength, Blessings most desirable, even with the attendant Hardships of despicable Poverty: While

to the Rich he sends Sickness as an Allay.
> *An Essay on the Nature and Manner of Treating the Gout*

When Mankind loved Temperance and Labour, there were few or no Diseases. Exercise kept the Juices sweet. But when Luxury, Intemperance, and Indolence, came in Fashion, Diseases sprang up and multiplied; and it is past all doubt, from Experiment, that rich Foods, high Sauces, and generous Wines, are the Source of this Distemper.
> *Idem*

John Abernethy [1764–1831]

"Pray, Mr. Abernethy, what is a cure for gout?" was the question of an indolent and luxurious citizen. "Live upon sixpence a day — and earn it," was the cogent reply.
> Quoted by Thomas J. Pettigrew in *Medical Portrait Gallery*, Vol. II

Sydney Smith [1771–1845]

I am concerned to hear of Lord Holland's gout. I observe that gout loves ancestors and genealogy; it needs five or six generations of gentlemen or noblemen to give it its full vigour.
> Letter to Lady Holland, November 8, 1816

What a very singular disease gout is! It seems as if the stomach fell down into the feet. The smallest deviation from right diet is immediately punished by limping and lameness, and the innocent ankle and blameless instep are tortured for the vices of the nobler organs. The stomach having found this easy way of getting rid of inconveniences, becomes cruelly despotic, and punishes for the least offences. A plum, a glass of champagne, excess in joy, excess in grief, — any crime, however small, is sufficient for

redness, swelling, spasms, and large shoes.
> Letter to the Countess of Carlisle, September 5, 1840

We are tolerably well here; the gout is never far off, though not actually present; it is the only enemy that I do not wish to have at my feet.
> Letter to the Countess Grey, August 24, 1841

Oh! when I have the gout, I feel as if I was walking on my eyeballs.
> Quoted by Lady Holland in *A Memoir of the Rev. Sydney Smith*, Ch. 11

I find the power of colchicum so great, that if I feel a little gout coming on, I go into the garden, and hold out my toe to that plant, and it gets well directly.
> *Idem*

George Gordon, Lord Byron [1788–1824]

Just as old age is creeping on apace,
    And clouds come o'er the sunset of our day,
They kindly leave us, though not quite alone,
But in good company — the gout or stone.
> *Don Juan*, Canto III, Stanza 59

John Bell [1796–1872]

Great eaters, free drinkers of fermented liquors, the idle and the luxurious, are the foremost candidates for the articulation badges of "chalk-stones".
> *Lectures on the Theory and Practice of Physic*, Lect. CLXVII

Of the two forms of *arthritis* or articular inflammation, rheumatism is the tax most frequently paid by the vulgar dram and grog drinker; gout, that in-

curred by the genteel and sometimes the literary wine-bibber.
Idem

Thomas Hood [1799–1845]

Full soon the sad effect of this [port wine]
His frame began to show,
For that old enemy the gout
Had taken him in *toe!*
Lieutenant Luff

Nathaniel Hawthorne [1804–1864]

If gentlemen love the pleasant titillation of the gout, it is all one to the Town Pump.
Twice-Told Tales, "A Rill from the Town Pump"

Robert Browning [1812–1889]

Doctor once dubbed — what ignorance shall baulk
Thy march triumphant? Diagnose the gout
As cholic, and prescribe it cheese for chalk —

No matter! All's one: cure shall come about
And win thee wealth — fees paid with such a roar
Of thanks and praise alike from lord and lout.
Dramatic Idyls (Second Series), "Doctor ———"

Henry Wheeler Shaw ("Josh Billings") [1818–1885]

There is plenty ov happiness in this life if we only knu it: and one way tew find it iz, when we hav got the old rumatiz tew thank Heaven that it aint the old gout.
Works, "Tadpoles"

James Russell Lowell [1819–1891]

I do not find that there is any specific for the gout, but, on the *similia-similibus* principle, I eat "tomarters" daily.

The disease derives its name (like *mons a non movendo*) from the patient's inability to *go out.* The ordinary derivation from *gutta* is absurd — for not only is the German form *Gicht* deduced from *gehen,* but the persons incident to the malady are precisely those who themselves (or their ancestors for them) have kept just this side of the gutter. I never heard that my great-grandfather died insolvent, but I am obliged to *foot* some of his bills for port. I can't help thinking that I shall be worse if I indulge any longer in this kind of thing — so I shall stop.
Letter to Miss Norton, August 30, 1858

The gout hardly tolerates any distraction on the part of those it visits, and the material for a letter accumulates slowly.
Letter to Mrs. Edward Burnett, July 8, 1888

My neighbor, Mr. Warner, came in last evening and tells me the doctors pronounce it [your attack] to be inflammatory rheumatism. But from his account of it I am sure it was acute gout. *Experto crede Roberto,* as our old friend Democritus Junior used to say. Three more than intolerable days, and then a gradual relaxation of the vise, one turn at a time, but each a foretaste of Elysium — *that's* gout and nothing else. Our doctors don't know gout.
Letter to E. R. Hoar, June 1, 1891

I call *my* gout the unearned increment from my good grandfather's Madeira, and think how excellent it must have been, and sip it cool from the bin of fancy, and wish he had left me the cause instead of the effect. I dare say he would, had he known I was coming and was to be so unreasonable.
Idem

Sir Alfred Baring Garrod
[1819–1907]

There is no truth in medicine better established than the fact that the use of fermented liquors is the most powerful of all the predisposing causes of gout; nay, so powerful, that it may be a question whether gout would ever have been known to mankind had such beverages not been indulged in.
> *Gout and Rheumatic Gout*, Ch. 8

It is stated that in the case of the Emperor Galba, his hands and feet were so much distorted that he could neither wear a shoe, nor even hold a small book; and he is reported to have said, "When I stand in need of eating I have no hands; when walking is necessary I have no feet; but when I am to be tormented, then feet and hands are all ready."
> *Ibid.*

Sir William S. Gilbert [1836–1911]

A taste for drink combined with gout,
  Had doubled him up forever.
> *The Gondoliers*, Act I

Ambrose Bierce [1842–1914?]

GOUT, n. A physician's name for the rheumatism of a rich patient.
> *The Devil's Dictionary*

Henri Huchard [1844–1910]

Gout is to the arteries what rheumatism is to the heart.
> Quoted by D. Evan Bedford in *Lancet* 1:164, 1967

Havelock Ellis [1859–1939]

There is, however, a pathological condition which occurs so often, in such extreme forms, and in men of such pre-eminent intellectual ability, that it is impossible not to regard it as having a real association with such ability. I refer to gout.
> *A Study of British Genius*, Ch. 8

James Gibbons Huneker
[1860–1921]

My corns ache, I get gouty, and my prejudices swell like varicose veins.
> *Old Fogy*, Ch. I

George Herman Ellwanger
[fl. 1897]

The very name, "Gout!" has a ferocious ferine sound, like the growl of some remorseless monster ready to fasten upon his prey.
> *Meditations on Gout*, "The Malady"

As opposed to the charges of high-living and intemperance made by vegetarians, Grahamites, and intemperate tea and water devotees, it is time that Gout should be clearly defined for what it really is in very many instances, — a perverse, ungrateful, maleficent malady, that delights upon the slightest pretext in assaulting vulnerable humanity at the most unseasonable hours and inconvenient times; an infliction that is especially prone to picket club-men, physicians, poets, and heads of official departments.
> *Idem*

Its poison comes by heritage, its venom lurks in the wine-cup, its seeds are sown at the gatherings of good-cheer.
> *Idem*

To think that a bottle of wine or a truffled pâté, or even a glass of beer, instead of being absorbed and eliminated by the system in the usual manner, should mine its way through the thighs, knees, calves, ankles, and instep, to explode at last in a fiery volcano in one's great toe, seems a mirth-provoking phenomenon to all but him who is immediately concerned.
> *Idem*

In vain your moans of anguish as the awl, the gimlet, and probe of the Inquisitor are thrust into your very bone and marrow. You might as well im-

plore mercy from the Iron Virgin of the *Burg* of Nürnberg, or seek flight if locked in the dungeon of Chillon.
Idem

"In our case," says the Frenchman, addressing the Englishman, "we have 'goût' for the taste; in your case, you have 'gout' for the result!"
Ibid., "The Theory"

The sufferer, in order to free himself from repeated onslaughts on the part of the enemy, must govern his palate with an iron hand, and enter into a solemn compact with that functionary to relinquish all serious flirting with the sirens of the kitchen and the *houris* of the wine-cellar. The stomach, above all things, must be propitiated, and its good graces obtained as nearly as may be.
Ibid., "The Regimen"

Burgandy is dangerous, and the wine of the Douro yet more so. Indeed, Petrarch never followed the footsteps of Laura, or Herrick the form of Anthea with greater devotion than Gout waits upon his favourite hand-maiden, Port.
Ibid., "The Proscribed Fluids"

It is obdurate and implacable. Once the precedent formed by the stomach of allowing alcoholic fluids and gravies to rush into the feet; once the enemy having been permitted to obtain a foothold — it is next to impossible to rout him effectually, whatever the means of defence adopted.
Ibid., "The Quandary"

A. Nathan Caplan [1902–   ]

Oh! That metabolic woe,
Pain and redness of the toe,
Scattered tophi in the skin,
Uric acid crystals spin,
— Weave a pattern in and out,
Stiffening joints — we call it gout.
Those who suffer so afflicted

Colchicined and Benemided,
Have my heartfelt sympathy;
Thanks to God it's them not me.
New England Journal of Medicine 275:664, 1966

The Bible

And Asa in the thirty and ninth year of his reign was diseased in his feet, until his disease was exceeding great: yet in his disease he sought not to the Lord, but to the physicians.
  And Asa slept with his fathers, and died in the one and fortieth year of his reign.
II Chronicles 16:12

Anonymous

Screw up the vise as tightly as possible — you have rheumatism; give it another turn, and that is gout.

Hebrew Proverb

That city is in a bad case whose Physician hath the gout.[1]

Italian Proverb

With respect to the gout, the physician is but a lout.

Spanish Proverb

Gout is cured by walling up the mouth.

HAND

William Heberden [1710–1801]

What are those little hard knobs, about the size of a small pea, which are frequently seen upon the fingers, particularly a little below the top, near the joint? They have no connexion with the gout, being found in persons who never had it: they continue for life; and being hardly ever attended with pain, or disposed to be-

[1] Indian (Hindi) Proverb: Woe to the city whose doctors have gouty feet.

come sores, are rather unsightly, than inconvenient, though they must be some little hindrance to the free use of the fingers.
> *Commentaries on the History and Cure of Diseases,* Ch. 28

Charles Lamb [1775–1834]

I am shocked sometimes at the shape of my own fingers, not for their resemblance to the ape tribe (which is something) but for the exquisite adaptation of them to the purposes of picking, fingering, etc. No one that is so framed, I maintain it, but should tremble.
> Letter to Bernard Barton, December 1, 1824

Ambrose Bierce [1842–1914?]

AMBIDEXTROUS, adj. Able to pick with equal skill a right-hand pocket or a left.
> *The Devil's Dictionary*

HAND, n. A singular instrument worn at the end of the human arm and commonly thrust into somebody's pocket.
> *Idem*

The Bible

Ehud the son of Gera, a Benjamite, a man lefthanded.
> *Judges* 3:15

There were seven hundred chosen men lefthanded; every one could sling stones at an hair breadth, and not miss.
> *Judges* 20:16

HARELIP

William Shakespeare [1564–1616]

This is the foul fiend Flibbertigibbet. . . . He gives the web and the pin, squints the eye, and makes the harelip.
> *King Lear,* III, iv, 120

HEADACHE

William Shakespeare [1564–1616]

When your head did but ache,
I knit my handkercher about your brows.
> *King John,* IV, i, 41

OTHELLO: I have a pain upon my forehead here.
DESDEMONA: Faith, that's with watching; 'twill away again.
Let me but bind it hard, within this hour
It will be well.
> *Othello,* III, iii, 284

Lord, how my head aches! What a head have I!
It beats as it would fall in twenty pieces.
> *Romeo and Juliet,* II, v, 49

William Heberden [1710–1801]

The hemicrania, or pain of one half of the head, was very early distinguished by medical writers from the other species of head-achs: but we have not yet advanced much in knowing how this differs from other pains of the head.
> *Commentaries on the History and Cure of Diseases,* Ch. 17

There is a dimness of sight in which dark spots float before the eyes, or only half, or some part of all objects appear, which continues for twenty or thirty minutes, and then is succeeded by a head-ach lasting for several hours, and joined sometimes with sickness.
> *Ibid.,* Ch. 66

Thomas Jefferson [1743–1826]

An attack of the periodical head-ach, which came on me about a week ago rendering me unable as yet either to write or read without great pain.
> Letter to Thomas M. Randolph, Jr., May 9, 1790

Johann Wolfgang von Goethe
[1749–1832]

Sweet things and spices and strong
drink, one after
The other he consumes with eager
speed
And then complains about his turbid
mind.
Torquato Tasso, Act V, Sc. i

Ralph Waldo Emerson
[1803–1882]

At fifty years, 'tis said, afflicted citi-
zens lose their sick headaches.
Society and Solitude, "Old
Age"

**Lewis Carroll (Charles L.
Dodgson)** [1832–1898]

"I'm very brave generally," he went
on in a low voice: "only to-day I
happen to have a headache."
Through the Looking Glass,
Ch. 4

Mark Twain (Samuel L. Clemens)
[1835–1910]

Do not undervalue the headache.
While it is at its sharpest it seems a
bad investment; but when relief be-
gins, the unexpired remainder is worth
$4 a minute.
Following the Equator, Vol. II,
Ch. 18, "Pudd'nhead Wilson's
New Calendar"

English Proverb

When the head aches, all the body is
the worse.

HEALING

See also CURES, REMEDIES,
TREATMENT

Hippocrates [460?–377? B.C.]

Healing is a matter of time, but it is

sometimes also a matter of oppor-
tunity.
Precepts, I (tr. by W. H. S.
Jones)

Diphilius [4th Cent. B.C.]

Time is a physician that heals every
grief.

Seneca [4? B.C.–A.D. 65]

Time heals what reason cannot.
Agamemnon, 130

Nicholas Culpepper [1616–1654]

This creation, though composed of
contraries, is one united body of which
man is the epitome, and he, therefore,
who would understand the mystery of
healing must look as high as the stars.
A Physicall Directory

Sir James Paget [1814–1899]

Let me suggest that the instances
of recovery from disease and injury
seem to be only examples of a law yet
larger than that within the terms of
which they may be comprised; a law
wider than the grasp of science; the
law that expresses our Creator's will
for the recovery of all lost perfection.
To this train of thought we are guided
by the remembrance that the healing
of the body, was ever chosen as the
fittest emblem of His work.
Lectures on Surgical Pathology,
Lect. 7

The Bible

And Jesus went about all Galilee,
teaching in their synagogues, and
preaching the gospel of the kingdom,
and healing all manner of sickness
and all manner of disease among the
people.
Matthew 4:23

The Bible: Apocrypha

For of the most High cometh healing.
Ecclesiasticus 38:2

HEALTH

See also FITNESS, HYGIENE,
HYPOCHONDRIA, REGIMEN

Huang Ti (The Yellow Emperor)
[2697–2597 B.C.]

The people of these regions [the West]
. . . become robust and energetic.
. . . Hence evil cannot injure their
external bodies, and if they get diseases they strike at the inner body.
These diseases are most successfully
cured with poison medicines.
> *Nei Ching Su Wên*, Bk. 4, Sect.
> 12 (tr. by Ilza Veith in *The
> Yellow Emperor's Classic of In-
> ternal Medicine*)

Simonides of Ceos [556–469 B.C.]

There's no joy even in beautiful Wisdom, unless one have holy Health.
> Quoted by Sextus Empiricus in
> *Against the Mathematicians*
> (tr. by J. M. Edmonds)

Hippocrates [460?–377? B.C.]

The body of man has itself blood,
phlegm, yellow bile, and black bile;
these make up the stuff of his body
and through these he feels pain and
enjoys health. Now he enjoys the most
perfect health when these elements are
duly proportioned to one another in respect of compounding, power and bulk,
that is, when they are perfectly mingled.
> *The Nature of Man*, IV (tr.
> by W. H. S. Jones)

A wise man ought to realize that
health is his most valuable possession.
> *A Regimen for Health*, 9 (tr.
> by John Chadwick and W. N.
> Mann)

Cicero [106–43 B.C.]

Guard your health.[1]
> *Epistolae ad Familiares*, VII.5

[1] Cura ut valeas. This is a closing phrase
in many Latin letters.

Can anyone have an assurance of what
his health will be, I don't say a year
hence, but this evening?
> *De Finibus*, II.xxviii.92 (tr. by
> H. Rackham)

Martial [fl. 1st Cent.]

Life is not living, but living in health.
> *Epigrams*, VI.70 (tr. by W. C.
> A. Ker)

Plutarch [46?–120?]

Each person ought neither to be unacquainted with the peculiarities of
his own pulse (for there are many individual diversities), nor ignorant of
any idiosyncrasy which his body has
in regard to temperature and dryness,
and what things in actual practice
have proved to be beneficial or detrimental to it. For the man has no
perception regarding himself, and is
but a blind and deaf tenant in his own
body, who gets his knowledge of these
matters from another, and must inquire of his physician whether his
health is better in summer or winter,
whether he can more easily tolerate
liquid or solid foods, and whether his
pulse is naturally fast or slow. For it
is useful and easy for us to know
things of this sort, since we have
daily experience and association with
them.
> *Moralia*, "Advice About Keep-
> ing Well" (tr. by F. C. Babbitt)

Health is not to be purchased by
idleness and inactivity, which are the
greatest evils attendant on sickness,
and the man who thinks to conserve
his health by uselessness and ease does
not differ from him who guards his
eyes by not seeing, and his voice by
not speaking. For a man in good
health could not devote himself to
any better object than to numerous
humane activities.
> *Idem*

Tacitus [55?–after 177]

The healing art . . . is very little in demand and makes very little progress in countries where people enjoy good health and strong constitutions.
Dialogue on Orators, 41 (tr. by M. Hutton)

Leonardo da Vinci [1452–1519]

Strive to preserve your health; and in this you will the better succeed in proportion as you keep clear of the physicians, for their drugs are a kind of alchemy concerning which there are no fewer books than there are medicines.
Dell' Anatomia, Fogli A (tr. by Edward MacCurdy in *The Notebooks of Leonardo da Vinci*, Vol. I, Ch. VIII)

François Rabelais [1494?–1553]

Without health life is no life; it is unlivable. . . . Without health, life spells but languor and an image of death.
Pantagruel, Bk. IV, Prologue (tr. by Jacques Le Clercq)

Michel de Montaigne [1533–1592]

Health is a precious thing, and the only one, in truth, which deserves that we employ in its pursuit not only time, sweat, trouble, and worldly goods, but even life; inasmuch as without it life comes to be painful and oppressive to us. . . . As far as I am concerned, no road that would lead us to health is either arduous or expensive.
Essays, Bk. II, Ch. 37, "Of the Resemblance of Children to Fathers" (tr. by Donald M. Frame)

Sir Francis Bacon [1561–1626]

In sickness, respect health principally; and in health, action. For those that put their bodies to endure in health, may in most sicknesses, which are not very sharp, be cured only with diet and tendering.
Essays, "Of Regiment of Health"

There is a wisdom in this beyond the rules of physic: a man's own observation, what he finds good of, and what he finds hurt of, is the best physic to preserve health.
Idem

John Donne [1573–1631]

There is no health; Physitians say that wee,
At best, enjoy but a neutralitie.
An Anatomie of the World, "The First Anniversary"

Ben Jonson [1573?–1637]

O health! health! the blessing of the rich! the riches of the poor! who can buy thee at too deare a rate, since there is no enjoying this world, without thee?
Volpone, Act II, Sc. ii

Robert Burton [1577–1640]

Health indeed is a pretious thing, to recover and preserve which, we undergo any misery, drink bitter potions, freely give our goods: restore a man to his health, his purse lies open to thee.
The Anatomy of Melancholy, Pt. III, Sect. 1, Memb. 2, Subsect. 1

John Webster [1580?–1625?] and Thomas Dekker [1572?–1632?]

Gold that buys health can never be ill spent.
Westward Hoe, Act V

Francis Beaumont [1584–1616] and John Fletcher [1579–1625]

Health and an able body are two jewels.
The Wild-Goose Chase, Act II, Sc. 1

Robert Herrick [1591–1674]

Health is no other (as the learned hold)
But a just measure both of Heat and Cold.
    Hesperides, "Health"

Izaak Walton [1593–1683]

Look to your health: and if you have it, praise God, and value it next to a good conscience; for health is the second blessing that we mortals are capable of; a blessing that money cannot buy.
    The Compleat Angler, Pt. I, Ch. 21

René Descartes [1596–1650]

As soon as I had acquired some general notions respecting Physics . . . I perceived it to be possible to arrive at knowledge highly useful in life . . . especially for the preservation of health, which is without doubt, of all the blessings of this life, the first and fundamental one.
    Discours de la Méthode, Pt. VI (tr. by John Veitch)

Duc François de La Rochefoucauld [1613–1680]

To preserve one's health by too strict a regime is in itself a tedious malady.
    Maxims, No. 623 (tr. by Constantine FitzGibbon)

Joseph Addison [1672–1719]

Health and Chearfulness mutually beget each other.
    The Spectator, Vol. V, No. 387 (May 24, 1712)

John Gay [1685–1732]

Nor love, nor honour, wealth nor power
Can give the heart a cheerful hour,
When health is lost.
    Fables (Series I), Fable 31

James Thomson [1700–1748]

Health is the vital principle of bliss,
And exercise of health.
    The Castle of Indolence, Canto II, Stanza 57

Samuel Johnson [1709–1784]

Among the innumerable follies, by which we lay up in our youth repentance and remorse for the succeeding part of our lives, there is scarce any against which warnings are of less efficacy, than the neglect of health.
    The Rambler, No. 48 (September 1, 1750)

Denis Diderot [1713–1784]

Doctors are always working to preserve our health and cooks to destroy it, but the latter are the more often successful.

Laurence Sterne [1713–1768]

Grant me but health, thou great Bestower of it, and give me but this fair goddess as my companion — and shower down thy mitres . . . upon those heads which are aching for them!
    A Sentimental Journey, Bk. II, Ch. 3

O blessed health! . . . thou art above all gold and treasure. . . . He that has thee, has little more to wish for; and he that is so wretched as to want thee, wants everything with thee.
    Tristram Shandy, Bk. V, Ch. 33

William Shenstone [1714–1763]

Health is beauty, and the most perfect health is the most perfect beauty.
    Essays on Men and Manners, "On Taste"

Horace Walpole [1717–1797]

I am in a moment of prettywellness.
    Letter to Countess of Upper Ossory, January 14, 1792

John Leake [1720–1792]

The poor female cottager, who uses exercises in the open air, who eats the coarse, but wholesome bread of industry, and drinks from the cooling stream, is seldom troubled with those maladies which afflict the rich and indolent, undone by the abuse of plenty.

> *Practical Observations towards the Prevention and Cure of Chronic Diseases peculiar to Women*

Arthur Murphy [1727–1805]

Chearfulnes, Sir, is the principal Ingredient in the Composition of Health.

> *The Apprentice* (1764), Act II, Sc. iv

James Beattie [1735–1803]

From labour health, from health contentment springs.

> *The Minstrel,* Bk. I

John Morgan [1735–1789]

Health is that choice seasoning which gives a relish to all our enjoyments.

> *A Discourse Upon the Institution of Medical Schools in America*

Georg Christoph Lichtenberg [1742–1799]

The feeling of health is acquired only through sickness.

> *Aphorismen* (1793–1799)

Thomas Jefferson [1743–1826]

Health is the first requisite after morality.

> Letter to Peter Carr, August 10, 1787

Health is worth more than learning.

> Letter to John Garland Jefferson, June 11, 1790

I have been more fortunate than my friend in the article of health. So free from catarrhs that I have not had one, (in the breast, I mean) on an average of eight or ten years through life. I ascribe this exemption partly to the habit of bathing my feet in cold water every morning, for sixty years past. A fever of more than twenty-four hours I have not had above two or three times in my life. A periodical headache has afflicted me occasionally, once, perhaps, in six or eight years, for two or three weeks at a time, which seems not to have left me; and except on a late occasion of indisposition, I enjoy good health; too feeble, indeed, to walk much, but riding without fatigue six or eight miles a day, and sometimes thirty or forty.

> Letter to Dr. Vine Utley, March 21, 1819

Jeremy Bentham [1748–1832]

Health is the absence of disease, and consequently of all those kinds of pain which are among the symptoms of disease. A man may be said to be in a state of health when he is not conscious of any uneasy sensations, the primary seat of which can be perceived to be anywhere in his body.

> *The Principles of Morals and Legislation,* Ch. VI

Jean Paul Richter [1763–1825]

Sleep, riches, and health, to be truly enjoyed, must be interrupted.

> *Flower, Fruit and Thorn Pieces,* Ch. 8

Sir Walter Scott [1771–1832]

All health is better than wealth.

> *Familiar Letters,* Letter to C. Carpenter, August 4, 1812

William Ellery Channing [1780–1842]

Health is the working-man's fortune, and he ought to watch over it, more than the capitalist over his largest investments. Health lightens the efforts of body and mind. It enables a man to crowd much work into a narrow compass. Without it little can be earned, and that little by slow, exhausting toil.

> *Lectures on the Elevation of the Labouring Portion of the Community*

Charles C. Colton [1780?–1832]

The poorest man would not part with health for money, but the richest would gladly part with all their money for health.

> *Lacon,* Vol. I, Ch. CCXXV

Leigh Hunt [1784–1859]

The ground-work of all happiness is health.

> *The Indicator,* No. XXXI, "On the Realities of the Imagination"

Peter Mere Latham [1789–1875]

Perfect health, like perfect beauty, is a rare thing; and so, it seems, is perfect disease.

> *General Remarks on the Practice of Medicine,* Ch. X, Pt. 2

Thomas Carlyle [1795–1881]

The healthy know not of their health, but only the sick: this is the Physician's Aphorism.

> *Characteristics*

Ill-health, of body or of mind, is *defeat.* . . . health alone is victory. Let all men, if they can manage it, contrive to be healthy!

> *Sir Walter Scott*

Ralph Waldo Emerson [1803–1882]

Give me health and a day, and I will make the pomp of emperors ridiculous.

> *Nature,* Ch. 3

Samuel Bartlett Parris [1806–1827]

> With how much speed
> Doth health her smiles upon his count'nance spread,
> And breathe again her influence round his head;
> Roused by her touch, he wakes to life once more,
> With pleasures which he never felt before.
> (For who, that has not felt the loss of health,
> Can measure its inestimable wealth?)
>
> *Anticipations and Recollections,* Pt. I

John Greenleaf Whittier [1807–1892]

> Beneath her torn hat glowed the wealth
> Of simple beauty and rustic health.
>
> *Maud Muller*

Henry David Thoreau [1817–1862]

Measure your health by your sympathy with morning and spring. If there is no response in you to the awakening of nature, — if the prospect of an early morning walk does not banish sleep, if the warble of the first bluebird does not thrill you, — know that the morning and spring of your life are past. Thus may you feel your pulse.

> *Journal,* February 25, 1859

Herbert Spencer [1820–1903]

The preservation of health is a duty. Few seem conscious that there is such a thing as physical morality.

Henri Amiel [1821–1881]

Health is the first of all liberties, and happiness gives us the energy which is the basis of health.

> *Journal Intime,* April 3, 1865
> (tr. by Mrs. Humphrey Ward)

Gustave Flaubert [1821–1880]

HEALTHY: Too much health, the cause of illness.
> *Dictionary of Accepted Ideas*
> (tr. by Jacques Barzun)

George William Curtis [1824–1892]

Happiness lies, first of all, in health.
> *Lotus-Eating*, Ch. IV

Robert G. Ingersoll [1833–1899]

If I had my way I'd make health catching instead of disease.

Sir John Lubbock, Baron Avebury [1834–1913]

Plain living and high thinking will secure health for most of us.
> *The Use of Life*, Ch. 3

Samuel Butler [1835–1902]

It was a monotonous life, but it was very healthy; and one does not much mind anything when one is well.
> *Erewhon*, Ch. I

Mark Twain (Samuel L. Clemens) [1835–1910]

He had had much experience of physicians, and said "the only way to keep your health is to eat what you don't want, drink what you don't like, and do what you'd druther not."
> *Following the Equator*, Vol. II, Ch. 13, "Pudd'nhead Wilson's New Calendar"

Sir Clifford Allbutt [1836–1925]

It is steadily forgotten that health is a diathesis as much as is scrofula or syphilis, and that each of these is a mode of growth.

Robert Bridges [1844–1930]

> Is it foolish, hoping for a rescue,

First to appeal to the strong, for health to the healthy amongst us?
> *Now in Wintry Delights*

Robert Louis Stevenson [1850–1894]

It is better to lose health like a spendthrift than to waste it like a miser.
> *Virginibus Puerisque*, Ch. V

Ella Wheeler Wilcox [1850–1919]

Talk health. The dreary, never-ending tale
Of mortal maladies is worn and stale;
You cannot charm or interest or please
By harping on that minor chord, disease.
Say you are well, or all is well with you,
And God shall hear your words and make them true.
> *Speech*

Oscar Wilde [1854–1900]

She is very much interested in her own health.
> *A Woman of No Importance*, Act III

George Bernard Shaw [1856–1950]

Use your health, even to the point of wearing it out. That is what it is for. Spend all you have before you die; and do not outlive yourself.
> *The Doctor's Dilemma*, "Preface on Doctors"

Claude Bragdon [1866–1946]

Health and disease, thought and emotion, are communicable, contagious.

Sir Robert Hutchison [1871–1960]

Health, like happiness, is to be found, if at all, by the wayside, and the more you pursue it, the more it flees from you.

Harry Emerson Fosdick
[1878–   ]

The roster of the world's real persons is astonishingly inconsiderate of sound physical health.
On Being a Real Person, Ch. 1

H. L. Mencken [1880–1956]

The health of a President is watched very carefully, not only by the Vice-President but also by medical men detailed for the purpose by the Army or Navy. These medical men have high-sounding titles, and perform the duties of their office in full uniform, with swords on one side and stethoscopes on the other. The diet of their imperial patient is rigidly scrutinized. If he eats a few peanuts they make a pother; if he goes in for a dozen steamed hard crabs at night, washed down by what passes in Washington for malt liquor, they complain to the newspapers. Every morning they look at his tongue, take his pulse and temperature, determine his blood pressure, and examine his eye-grounds and his knee-jerks. The instant he shows the slightest sign of being upset they clap him into bed, post Marines to guard him, put him on a regimen fit for a Trappist, and issue bulletins to the newspapers.
Baltimore Evening Sun, August 17, 1931

Franklin P. Adams (F.P.A.)
[1881–1960]

Health is the thing that makes you feel that now is the best time of the year.

Jules Romains [1885–   ]

This epigraph, that I attributed to Claude Bernard: "Healthy people are sick people who don't know it."
Knock, Act I, Sc. i

T. S. Eliot [1888–1965]

We're all of us ill in one way or another:

We call it health when we find no symptom
Of illness. Health is a relative term.
The Family Reunion, Pt. I, Sc. iii

Lin Yutang [1895–   ]

Eventually we have to come to a conception of health and disease by which the two merge into each other.
The Importance of Living, Ch. IX, Sect. vii

David Seegal [1899–   ]

The physician would be quick to admit that sometimes he has less certainty in certifying the normal than the abnormal state of an organ or system. The early recognition of the transition from the healthy to the diseased condition may be difficult, if not impossible.
Journal of the American Medical Association 182:1031, 1962

The Bible

Beloved, I wish above all things that thou mayest prosper and be in health, even as thy soul prospereth.
III John:2

The Bible: Apocrypha

Health and good estate of body are above all gold, and a strong body above infinite wealth.
There is no riches above a sound body, and no joy above the joy of the heart.
Ecclesiasticus 31:15

Proverbs

Health and sickness surely are men's double enemies.

Health is not valued till sickness comes.[1]

___
[1] Spanish (Catalan) Proverb: From the bitterness of disease man learns the sweetness of health.

Health is the poor man's riches and the rich man's bliss.

English Proverb

Health is better than wealth.

French Proverbs

Good health or bad makes our philosophy.

More wealth, less health.[1]

Gaelic Proverb

Every healthy man is king.

Italian Proverb

Health without wealth is half a sickness.

Russian Proverb

One can always be healthy so long as one is not ill.

HEARING

See also DEAFNESS, EAR, SENSES

Epictetus [60?–120?]

Nature has given man one tongue, but two ears, that we may hear twice as much as we speak.
> *Fragments,* VI (tr. by E. Carter)

Abraham Coles [1813–1891]

Within a bony labyrinthean cave,
Reached by the pulse of the aërial wave
This sibyl, sweet, and mystic Sense is found —
Muse, that presides o'er all the Powers of Sound.
> *The Microcosm,* "Hearing — Powers of Sound — Music of Nature"

[1] Bulgarian Proverb: Riches do not buy health, yet they take health away.

Elizabeth Corbett [1887–   ]

Its principal disadvantage [of a hearing aid worn behind the ear] is that the microphone faces to the rear and picks up sounds behind the wearer with greater efficiency than sounds coming towards him. Socially, at least, the latter are likely to be the more important.
> *Atlantic Monthly,* October 1965

A sudden improvement in hearing [by means of a hearing aid] is not always an unmixed blessing, as many an older person living in a household full of noisy grandchildren has discovered.
> *Idem*

HEART

See also ANGINA, BLOOD, CIRCULATION

Huang Ti (The Yellow Emperor) [2697–2597 B.C.]

The heart is the root of life and causes the versatility of the spiritual faculties. The heart influences the face and fills the pulse with blood.
> *Nei Ching Su Wên,* Bk. 3, Sect. 9 (tr. by Ilza Veith in *The Yellow Emperor's Classic of Internal Medicine*)

The heart is in accord with the pulse. The complexion of a person shows when the heart is in a splendid condition. The heart rules the kidneys.
> *Ibid.,* Sect. 10

When man is serene and healthy the pulse of the heart flows and connects, just as pearls are joined together or like a string of red jade — then one can speak of a healthy heart.
> *Ibid.,* Bk. 5, Sect. 18

St. John Chrysostom [345?–407]

The heart is the most noble of all the members in our body.
>*Homilies on the Statutes,* Homily XI (tr. by John H. Parker)

Leonardo da Vinci [1452–1519]

The heart . . . moves of itself and does not stop unless for ever.
>*Dell' Anatomia,* Fogli B (tr. by Edward MacCurdy in *The Notebooks of Leonardo da Vinci,* Vol. I, Ch. III)

The heart in itself is not the beginning of life; but it is a vessel formed of thick muscle, vivified and nourished by the artery and vein as are the other muscles.
>*Idem*

William Shakespeare [1564–1616]

My heart,
Where either I must live or bear no life,
The fountain from the which my current runs
Or else dries up.
>*Othello,* IV, ii, 57

The canker gnaw thy heart.
>*Timon of Athens,* IV, iii, 49

I have tremor cordis on me; my heart dances.
>*The Winter's Tale,* I, ii, 110

O, cut my lace, lest my heart, cracking it,
Break too!
>*Ibid.,* III, ii, 174

William Harvey [1578–1657]

When I first gave my mind to vivisection, as a means of discovering the motions and uses of the heart, and sought to discover these from actual inspection, and not from the writings of others, I found the task so truly arduous, so full of difficulties, that I was almost tempted to think with Fracas-torius, that the motion of the heart was only to be comprehended by God.
>*On the Motion of the Heart and Blood in Animals,* Ch. 1 (tr. by Robert Willis)

Thus nature, ever perfect and divine, doing nothing in vain, has neither given a heart where it was not required, nor produced it before its office had become necessary; but by the same stages in the development of every animal, passing through the forms of all, as I may say (ovum, worm, foetus), it acquires perfection in each.
>*Ibid.,* Ch. 17

Peter Mere Latham [1789–1875]

It would be difficult to overrate the value, as guides to practice, of the signs which declare themselves through the medium of the lungs in every case of unsound heart.
>*Diseases of the Heart,* Lect. XXXV

Mark Twain (Samuel L. Clemens) [1835–1910]

I had to swallow suddenly, or my heart would have got out.
>*Roughing It,* Vol. II, Ch. 37

Martin H. Fischer [1879–1962]

The heart is the only organ that takes no rest. That is why it is so good.
>Quoted by Howard Fabing and Ray Marr in *Fischerisms*

Sir Thomas Lewis [1881–1945]

Many ultimately fail to know this murmur [mitral stenosis] through persisting in the effort to time, instead of learning to know it as one learns to know a dog's bark.
>*Diseases of the Heart,* Ch. 14

William Boyd [1885–   ]

Of all the ailments which may blow out life's little candle, heart disease is the chief.
>*Pathology for the Surgeon*

The Bible

A sound heart is the life of the flesh.
Proverbs 14:30

Anonymous

Everywhere he feels his Heart because its vessels run to all his limbs.
The Ebers Papyrus, Ch. XX, "The Beginning of the Secret Book of the Physician" (tr. by Cyril P. Bryan) [1]

HEREDITY

See also EUGENICS, GENETICS

Euripides [484–406 B.C.]

For they which share one father's blood shall oft
By many a bodily likeness kinship show.
Electra, 522 (tr. by A. S. Way)

Noble fathers have noble children.
Fragment

Horace [65–8 B.C.]

Gallant sons spring from the gallant and good. Good blood tells even in bullocks and horses, nor do bold eagles breed the timid dove.
Odes, IV.iv.31 (tr. by E. C. Wickham)

Asaph ben Berachiah [fl. 6th Cent.]

The humor and illnesses are already on the sperm and are transmitted to the embryo.
Quoted by Maxime Laignel-Lavastine in *Histoire Générale de la Médecine*, Vol. II

William Clowes [1544–1604]

It is true saying, the best apple will

[1] See note, p. 59a.

grow to be a crab unless some good fruit be grafted on the stock.
Treatise on Struma (ed. by F. N. L. Poynter in *Selected Writings of William Clowes*, Ch. 4)

William Shakespeare [1564–1616]

'Tis as like you
As cherry is to cherry.
Henry VIII, V, i, 168

Good wombs have borne bad sons.
The Tempest, I, ii, 120

Alas, our frailty is the cause, not we!
For such as we are made of, such we be.
Twelfth Night, II, ii, 32

Thomas Middleton [1570?–1627]
and
William Rowley [1585?–1642?]

Wise men begets fools, and fools are the fathers
To many wise children; *hysteron proteron,*
A great scholar may beget an idiot,
And from the plough-tail may come a great scholar.
A Fair Quarrel, Act I, Sc. i

Joseph Hall [1574–1656]

Brag of thy father's faults: they are thine own.
Virgidemiae, Bk. IV, Satire iii

Henry Peacham [1576?–1643?]

As for the most part, wee see children of Noble Personages to beare the lineaments and resemblance of their Parents: so in like manner, for the most part, they possesse their vertues and Noble dispositions, which even in their tenderest yeeres will bud forth, and discover it selfe.
The Compleat Gentleman, Ch. 1

Claude Quillet [1602–1661]

But he, who judges right of what is Fair,

With healthy Sons will healthy Daughters Pair.
As unperforming, useless *Drones,* will drive,
The *Weak* and *Sickly* from the *Marriage Hive.*
Whether a Man by frequent Visits feel
The gnawing Torments of the *Gouty Ill.*
Or, sudden *Epilepsies* seize his Mind,
Or, *bilious Cholic* rack his *Breast* with Wind.
Or, on his wasted *Lungs* an *Ulcer* prey,
Or, a Consumption, lingringly Betray
His pining Life, and Murder by Delay.

For, Man's new curious System to compose,
An equal Portion every Limb bestows,
From every Nerve collected Nature flows.
Whence by Traduction from the Father run,
Ill Habitudes intail'd upon the Son.
> *Callipaedia: The Art of Getting Beautiful Children,* Bk. I (tr. by Nicholas Rowe)

Edmund Waller [1606–1687]

The sap which at the root is bred
In trees, thro' all the boughs is spread;
But virtues which in parents shine,
Make not like progress thro' the line.
> *To Zelinda*

Aphra Behn [1640–1689]

She's a Chick of the old Cock.
> *Sir Patient Fancy,* Act IV, Sc. iv

Alain René Lesage [1668–1747]

We come into the world with the mark of our descent, and with our characters about us.
> *The Adventures of Gil Blas de Santillana*

Joseph Addison [1672–1719]

What a figure is the young heir likely to make, who is a dunce both by father and mother's side?
> *The Guardian,* No. 155 (September 8, 1713)

Frederick II (the Great) of Prussia [1712–1786]

Men are born with an indelible character.
> Letter to d'Alembert, August 13, 1777 (tr. by Thomas Holcroft)

Edmund Burke [1729–1797]

People will not look forward to posterity, who never look backward to their ancestors.
> *Reflections on the Revolution in France*

He was not merely a chip of the old 'block,' but the old block itself.[1]
> Speech in the House of Commons, February 26, 1781

Andrew Combe [1797–1847]

What we desire our children to become, we must endeavour to be before them.
> *Physiological and Moral Management of Infancy*

Ralph Waldo Emerson [1803–1882]

Men resemble their contemporaries even more than their progenitors.
> *Representative Men,* "Uses of Great Men"

What can I do against the influence of Race, in my history? What can I do against heredity and constitutional habits, against scrofula, lymph, impotence?
> *Ibid.,* "Montaigne; or, The Sceptic"

---

[1] Referring to William Pitt the Younger [1759–1806] on the occasion of his first speech.

Edward Bulwer-Lytton
[1803–1873]

A man's ancestry is a positive property to him. How much, not only of acres, but of his constitution, his temper, his conduct, character and nature he may inherit from some progenitor ten times removed!
The Caxtons, Pt. XI, Ch. VII

Oliver Wendell Homes
[1809–1894]

I go (always, other things being equal) for the man who inherits family traditions and the cumulative humanities of at least four or five generations.
The Autocrat of the Breakfast Table, Sect. I

John Ruskin [1819–1900]

The greatness or smallness of a man is, in the most conclusive sense, determined for him at his birth, as strictly as it is determined for a fruit whether it is to be a currant or an apricot.
Modern Painters, Pt. IV, Ch. III

Samuel Butler [1835–1902]

Was there nothing which I could say to make them feel that the constitution of a person's body was a thing over which he or she had had at any rate no initial control whatever, while the mind was a perfectly different thing, and capable of being created anew and directed according to the pleasure of its possessor? Could I never bring them to see that while habits of mind and character were entirely independent of initial mental force and early education, the body was so much a creature of parentage and circumstances, that no punishment for ill-health should be ever tolerated save as a protection from contagion, and that even where punishment was inevitable it should be attended with compassion?
Erewhon, Ch. XIV

Oliver Wendell Holmes, Jr.
[1841–1935]

Three generations of imbeciles are enough.
Buck v. Bell in *U.S. Reports,* Vol. 274 (1927)

Victor C. Vaughan [1851–1929]

Rare is the tree whose every bud develops into perfect fruit and if there be such a family tree I find no adequate evidence of it.
A Doctor's Memories, Ch. 1

Otto Weininger [1880–1903]

Talent is hereditary; it may be the common possession of a whole family (e.g., the Bach family); genius is not transmitted; it is never diffused, but is strictly individual.
Sex and Character, Pt. II, Ch. IV

Edwin Carleton MacDowell
[1887–   ]

Heredity sets limits, environment decides the exact position within these limits.

David Seegal [1899–   ]

The beginnings of all genotypic diseases of man are established at conception. Without prejudice to the romantic relationship of the honeymoon, it is a truism that the penetration of the sperm into the ovum will often result in offspring stigmatized by a wide variety of heredital disorders.
Journal of Pediatrics 63:685, 1963

Elizabeth N. Munger [1924–   ]

The match fell through, my dear, specifically,
after they measured scientifically
the selective factors that brought them together,
in order to determine for their children whether

they'd be bright enough, on examination,
for the top one per cent of the population.

Well, believe me, they matched like
two peas in a pod —
he, Phi Beta Kappa, and she from
Cape Cod;
they would have gone through with
the wedding dutifully,
their I.Q.'s and profiles combining so
beautifully
to improve the breed with such high
probability —
but his income scored lower than her
patibility.
> *Perspectives in Biology and
> Medicine* 5:390, 1962

The Bible

As is the mother, so is her daughter.
> *Ezekiel* 16:44

A good tree cannot bring forth evil
fruit, neither can a corrupt tree bring
forth good fruit.
> *Matthew* 7:18

Proverbs

He's a chip of [off] the old block.

Like father, like son.

Like hen, like chicken.

What is bred in the bone will never
come out of the flesh.

French Proverb

He shames his mother who does not
resemble his father.

Irish Proverb

A wild goose never laid a tame egg.

Italian Proverb

What is born of a hen will scrape.

Scottish Proverb

An ill cow may have a good calf.[1]

HERNIA

Ben Jonson [1573?–1637]

He has a rupture, hee has sprung a
leake.
> *The Staple of News,* Act I,
> Sc. ii

HICCUP

Hippocrates [460?–377? B.C.]

Sneezing coming on, in the case of a
person afflicted with hiccup, removes
the hiccup.
> *Aphorisms,* VI.13 (tr. by Fran-
> cis Adams)

HISTORY

Thomas Sydenham [1624–1689]

As no man can say who it was that
first invented the use of clothes and
houses against the inclemency of the
weather, so also can no investigator
point out the origin of Medicine —
mysterious as the source of the Nile.
There has never been a time when it
was not.
> *Medical Observations* (1st ed.),
> Preface (tr. by R. G. Latham
> in *Works,* Vol. I)

Auguste Comte [1798–1857]

To understand a science it is necessary
to know its history.
> *Positive Philosophy*

Emile Littré [1801–1881]

If the science of medicine is not to be
lowered to the rank of a mere mechan-

[1] A good cow may have an ill calf.

ical profession it must pre-occupy itself with its history. The pursuit of the development of the human mind, this is the role of the historian.

Alfred Stillé [1813–1900]

Medicine, like all knowledge, has a past as well as a present and a future, and . . . in that past is the indispensable soil out of which improvement must grow.

Medical News 44:433, 1884

Charles Daremberg [1817–1872]

The besetting vice of the histories of medicine, one which afflicts them almost all with sterility, is the circumstance that in these works our discipline, be such taken as a whole or in its details, is considered as an isolated invention without either relations or consanguinity with the other creations of the human spirit: "Proles sine matre creata." [1]

Histoire des sciences médicales, Ch. 1

Hermann von Helmholtz [1821–1894]

The history of [medicine] claims, therefore, a very special interest in the history of the development of the human mind. None other is, perhaps, more fitted to show that a true criticism of the sources of cognition is also practically an exceedingly important object of true philosophy.

Das Denken in der Medizin (tr. by E. Atkinson in *Popular Lectures on Scientific Subjects*)

Sir William Osler [1849–1919]

In the continual remembrance of a glorious past individuals and nations find their noblest inspiration.

Aequanimitas, with Other Addresses, "The Leaven of Science"

[1] Offspring created without a mother.

Karl Sudhoff [1853–1938]

The development of human thought and achievement, as a whole, has not been, as commonly supposed, a continual upward progression, nor even the equivalent of a continuous series of ascertained results. . . . The intuition of the true investigator and pathfinder of today and tomorrow must find its own way to new guiding principles from the work of yesterday, before yesterday, and the distant past.

Sir John Bland-Sutton [1855–1936]

It is difficult to see the past in true perspective: the years seem almost on one plane like images in a kaleidoscope.

The Story of a Surgeon, Ch. I

James G. Mumford [1863–1914]

The history of medicine does not depart from the history of the people.

Charles N. Camac [1868–1940]

In other branches of science, as physics and chemistry, in law and in art, the teachings of great authorities are familiarly quoted and used as guides. There is no reason why in medicine such familiarity should not be considered requisite to a proper education.

Imhotep to Harvey: Backgrounds of Medical History

Fielding H. Garrison [1870–1935]

The history of medicine is, in fact, the history of humanity itself, with its ups and downs, its brave aspirations after truth and finality, its pathetic failures. The subject may be treated variously as a pageant, an array of books, a procession of characters, a succession of theories, an exposition of human ineptitudes, or as the very bone and marrow of cultural history.

Introduction to the History of Medicine, Preface

William Warner Bishop
[1871–1955]

Without a sense of the historic setting of his work a man is almost as hopeless as is the man who lacks a sense of humor! You cannot argue with the one or the other. In fact, I dare go further and affirm that only by the combination of the historical and the experimental methods can any work of first rate importance be produced in any field of knowledge.

Henry E. Sigerist [1891–1957]

The very popular hunting for "Fathers" of every branch of medicine and every treatment is, therefore, rather foolish; it is unfair not only to the mothers and ancestors but also to the obstetricians and midwives.
> *A History of Medicine*, Vol. I,
> Introduction

Medical history teaches us where we came from, where we stand in medicine at the present time, and in what direction we are marching. It is the compass that guides us into the future. If our work is not to be haphazard but to follow a well-laid plan, we need the guidance of history, and it is not by accident that all great medical leaders were fully aware of the value of historical studies.

André F. Cournand [1895–   ]

Is it of benefit to revive the knowledge of the past? In unfolding the common patrimony which unites successive generations of inquiring men, in meeting them as individuals, in attempting to understand the problems they had to face, the intellectual climate in which their investigations were pursued, and the historical and social conditions under which they lived, it is my belief that a sharper consciousness of our own nature is brought forth, and the continuous doubt of the truths which we are build-

ing is revealed as our main motivation.
> *Circulation of the Blood* (ed.
> by A.P. Fishman and D.W.
> Richards), Pt. I, Ch. I

Earle P. Scarlett [1896–   ]

The history of medicine is more than "an addendum to the history of science." The great central highway along which medical-scientific progress has moved is firmly based on probity of teaching and learning, integrity in professional conduct, service to society, and the pursuit of knowledge. . . . in spite of all its shortcomings medical history is in a sense the history of civilization.
> *Archives of Internal Medicine*
> 118:603, 1966

Félix Martí-Ibáñez [1915–   ]

The physician must have a thorough knowledge of the history of the world and of the society in which he lives, and he must also know the links between the past and his present duties. For without history nothing has a full meaning.
> *Ariel,* "The Fabric and Creation of a Dream"

The history of medicine is a study not only of man's health and diseases throughout history, including the geographic, economic, and other conditions in time and space that may have affected health and caused disease as well as what the physician and society at any given time in history did to fight disease or prevent its spread, but also the history of all human activities connected directly or indirectly with the pursuits of medicine.
> *Idem*

HISTORY TAKING

Sir Francis Bacon [1561–1626]
The deficiencies [in medicine] which I think good to note . . . I will enu-

merate. . . . The first is the discontinuance of the ancient and serious diligence of Hippocrates, which used to set down a narrative of the special cases of his patients, and how they proceeded, and how they were judged by recovery or death.
> *The Advancement of Learning,* Bk. II

Giovanni Lancisi [1655–1720]

Poor patients are usually questioned with too little attention by physicians; and the patients themselves are equipped with too untrained intelligence and likewise estimate and describe their troubles with too little accuracy.
> *Aneurysms,* Ch. III, Proposition xxi (tr. by Wilmer C. Wright)

Martin H. Fischer [1879–1962]

Nowadays the clinical history too often weighs more than the man.
> Quoted by Howard Fabing and Ray Marr in *Fischerisms*

David Seegal [1899–   ]

The medical student has a better understanding of the educational continuum when he is convinced that the history he constructs is his signature and professional image to his colleagues. He learns that the history is a living document and not some inert words on paper to be added to the reams of dusty files in the record room.
> *Journal of Medical Education* 39:1033, 1964

Although the perfect history has never been taken by any physician, his careful, sympathetic, and discerning questions frequently yield information from the sick person which enlarges the doctor's horizon of knowledge and experience as well as presenting him with unexpected examples of the dramatic or bizarre.
> *The Pharos of Alpha Omega Alpha* 26:7, 1963

Paul Hamilton Wood [1907–1962]

The best history taker is he who can best interpret the answer to a leading question.
> *Diseases of the Heart and Circulation*

Anonymous

A doctor who cannot take a good history and a patient who cannot give one are in danger of giving and receiving bad treatment.
> Quoted by Paul Dudley White in *Clues in the Diagnosis and Treatment of Heart Diseases* (2nd ed.), Introduction

HOBBIES

Sir William Osler [1849–1919]

No man is really happy or safe without [a hobby], and it makes precious little difference what the outside interest may be — botany, beetles or butterflies, roses, tulips or irises; fishing, mountaineering or antiquities — anything will do so long as he straddles a hobby and rides it hard.
> *British Medical Journal* 2:925, 1909

You will be a better man and not a worse practitioner for an avocation.
> *The Student Life*

Sir Winston Churchill [1874–1965]

Muscles may relax, and feet and hands slow down; the nerve of youth and manhood may become less trusty. But painting is a friend who makes no undue demands, excites to no exhausting pursuits, keeps faithful pace with feeble steps, and holds her canvas as a screen between us and the envious eyes of Time or the surly advance of Decrepitude.
> *Painting as a Pastime*

Anonymous

Among the performing arts, the Old Doctor's Almanac rates music highest because it (a) tends to silence or even remove family and friends, (b) requires little practice or exertion to effect (a), and (c) can be made with other doctors.
Tufts Folia Medica 8:112, 1963

HOMESICKNESS

Benjamin Rush [1745?–1813]

The NOSTALGIA, . . . or the *homesickness*, was a frequent disease in the American army, more especially among the soldiers of the New England states.
An Account of the Influence of the Military and Political Events of the American Revolution upon the Human Body

Witter Bynner [1881–   ]

Name me no names for my disease,
  With uninforming breath;
I tell you I am none of these,
  But homesick unto death.
Selected Poems, "The Patient to the Doctors"

HOPE

Theocritus [3rd Cent. B.C.]

While there is life there's hope; the dead, I ween,
Are hopeless.
The Swains, 42 (tr. by M. J. Chapman)

Ovid [43 B.C.–A.D. 17?]

Oft has a man been abandoned by the skill and care of physicians, but hope leaves him not though his pulses fail.
Pontic Epistles, I.vi.35 (tr. by A. L. Wheeler)

Galen (fl. 2nd Cent.]

Confidence and hope do be more good than physic.

Ambroise Paré [1517?–1590]

Always give the patient hope, even when death seems at hand.

Robert Burton [1577–1640]

Hope and Patience are two soveraigne remedies for all, the surest reposals, the softest cushions to lean on in adversity.
The Anatomy of Melancholy, Pt. II, Sect. iii, Memb. 3

Samuel Taylor Coleridge [1772–1834]

He is the best physician who is the best inspirer of hope.
Table Talk

Sir Frederick Treves [1853–1923]

In the fact of misfortune it is merciless to blot out hope.

Proverb

While there's life there's hope.

Irish Proverb

Hope is the physician of each misery.

HOSPITALS

See also INSANITY: INSANE ASYLUMS

Sir Thomas Browne [1605–1682]

But if the example of the Mite bee not onely an act of wonder, but an example of the noblest charity, surely poore men may also build Hospitals.
Religio Medici, Pt. II, Sect. 13

John Milton [1608–1674]

A Lazar-house it seemd, wherein were laid

Numbers of all diseas'd, all maladies
Of ghastly Spasm, or racking torture,
    qualmes
Of heart-sick Agonie, all feavorous
    kinds,
Convulsions, Epilepsies, fierce Ca-
    tarrhs,
Intestin Stone and Ulcer, Colic pangs,
Daemoniac Phrenzie, moaping Melan-
    cholie,
And Moon-struck madness, pining
    Atrophie,
Marasmus, and wide-wasting Pesti-
    lence,
Dropsies, and Asthma's, and Joint-
    racking Rheums.
Dire was the tossing, deep the groans,
    despair
Tended the sick busiest from Couch to
    Couch.
            Paradise Lost, Bk. XI

Benjamin Franklin [1706–1790]

In the Year of Christ
MDCCLV
George the Second Happily Reigning
(For He Sought the Happiness of His
    People)
Philadelphia Flourishing
(For Its Inhabitants Were Publick
    Spirited)
This Building
By the Bounty of the Government
And of Many Private Persons
Was Piously Founded
For the Relief of the
Sick and Miserable;
May the God of Mercies
Bless the Undertaking.

Inscription for the cornerstone
of the University of Pennsylvania Hospital, Philadelphia

Thomas Jefferson [1743–1826]

Their situation too, when sick, in the
family of a good farmer, where every
member is emulous to do them kind
offices, where they are visited by all
the neighbors, who bring them the little
rarities which their sickly appetites
may crave, and who take by rotation

the nightly watch over them, when
their condition requires it, is without
comparison better than in a general
hospital, where the sick, the dying and
the dead are crammed together in the
same rooms, and often in the same
beds. The disadvantages, inseparable
from general hospitals, are such as can
never be counterposed by all the reg-
ularities of medicine and regimen. Nature and kind nursing save a much
greater proportion in our plain way, at
a smaller expense, and with less abuse.
One branch only of hospital institution
is wanting with us; that is, a general
establishment for those laboring under
difficult cases of chirurgery. The aids
of this art are not equivocal. But an
able chirurgeon cannot be had in every
parish. Such a receptacle should therefore be provided for those patients;
but no others should be admitted.
        Notes on the State of Virginia,
        Query XIV

Chammousset [fl. 1762]

How can one understand that civilized
nations have not yet agreed to treat
hospitals as sanctuaries of humanity
which the victor must respect and protect?

Comment made as superintendent of French military hospitals

James Jackson [1777–1867] **and**
John Collins Warren [1778–1856]

A hospital is an institution absolutely
essential to a medical school, and one
which would afford relief and comfort
to thousands of the sick and miserable.
On what other objects can the super-
fluities of the rich be so well bestowed?

Fund-raising letter, August 20,
1810

Daniel Drake [1785–1852]

The laboratory is not more necessary
for the study of chemistry, or a garden
of plants for the study of botany, than

a hospital for the study of practical medicine and surgery.

> Introductory lecture, Medical College of Ohio, 1849

Johns Hopkins [1795–1873]

The indigent sick of this city and its environs, without regard to sex, age or color, who may require surgical or medical treatment, and who can be received into the Hospital without peril to the other inmates, and the poor of this city and State, of all races, who are stricken down by any casualty, shall be received into the Hospital, without charge, for such periods of time and under such regulations as you may prescribe.

> Letter to the first Trustees of the Johns Hopkins Hospital, March 1873

Elizabeth Barrett Browning [1806–1861]

How sick we must be, ere we make men just!
I think it frets the saints in heaven to see
How many desolate creatures on the earth
Have learnt the simple dues of fellowship
And social comfort, in a hospital.
> *Aurora Leigh*, Bk. III

Massachusetts General Court [1811]

The Hospital [Massachusetts General], thus established, is intended to be a receptacle for . . . persons of every age and sex, . . . those in indigent circumstances, who, while in health, can gain by their labour a subsistence for themselves and their families but, when assailed by disease, are deprived of the ordinary comforts of life. . . . These are among that wretched portion of the community, for whom it is intended to open a tranquil and comfortable asylum.
> *Report of Legislative Committee*

John Fisher Murray [1811–1865]

"She says, if you please, sir, she only wants to be let die in peace."
"What! and the whole class to be disappointed, impossible! Tell her she can't be allowed to die in peace; it is against the rules of the hospital!"
> *The World of London*

Florence Nightingale [1820–1910]

It may seem a strange principle to enunciate as the very first requirement in a Hospital that it should do the sick no harm.
> *Notes on Hospitals*, Preface

Charles Baudelaire [1821–1867]

Life is a hospital in which every patient is possessed by the desire to change his bed.
> *Small Poems in Prose*, "Anywhere Out of the World" (tr. by Arthur Symons)

John Shaw Billings [1838–1913]

It has been considered from the point of view of the hygienist, the physician, the architect, the tax-payer, the superintendents, and the nurse, but of the several hundred books, pamphlets, and articles on the subject with which I am acquainted, I do not remember to have seen one from the point of view of the patient.
> *Public Health Reports* 2:384, 1874–75

A hospital is a living organism, made up of many different parts having different functions, but all these must be in due proportion and relation to each other, and to the environment, to produce the desired general results. The stream of life which runs through it is incessantly changing; patients and nurses and doctors come and go, today it has to do with the results of an epidemic, tomorrow with those of an explosion or a fire, the reputation of its physicians or surgeons attracts those suffering from a particular form of disease, and as the one changes so do the others. Its work is never done; its equipment is never complete; it is always in need of new means of diagnosis, of new instruments and medicines; it is to try all things and hold fast to that which is good.

> Address on the opening of the Johns Hopkins Hospital, May 7, 1889

As regards the external appearance of the building [the Johns Hopkins Hospital], opinions will, of course, differ. I will only say that it has been planned from within outward, which is the reason why it looks like a laboratory and not like a castle or a cathedral; and there is very little useless exterior decoration.[1]

> *Medical News* 60:230, 1892

William Ernest Henley
[1849–1903]

And lo, The Hospital, grey, quiet, old, Where Life and Death like friendly chafferers meet.

> *In Hospital,* "Enter Patient"

Sir William Osler [1849–1919]

The work of an institution in which there is no teaching is rarely first class. There is not that keen interest, nor the thorough study of the cases, nor amid the exigencies of the busy life is the hospital physician able to escape clinical slovenliness unless he teaches and in turn is taught by assistants and students. It is, I think, safe to say that in a hospital with students in the wards the patients are more carefully looked after, their diseases are more fully studied and few mistakes made.

> *Aequanimitas, with Other Addresses,* "The Hospital as a College"

[1] Billings was the designer of this and other hospitals of his day.

Charles H. Mayo [1865–1939]

The sooner patients can be removed from the depressing influence of general hospital life the more rapid their convalescence.

> *Journal-Lancet* 36:1, 1916

E. O. Laughlin ("Eolus")
[1867– ?]

Within these gray walls Life begins and ends,
Here, in this harbor, worn, sea-weary ships
Drop anchor, as the fading sun descends,
And new-launched vessels start their outbound trips.

> *Collected Poems,* "Inscription for a Hospital"

W. Somerset Maugham
[1874–1965]

The impression [of an Out-Patient Department] was neither of tragedy nor of comedy. . . . It was manifold and various; there were tears and laughter, happiness and woe; it was tedious and interesting and indifferent; it was as you saw it: it was tumultuous and passionate; it was grave; it was sad and comic; it was trivial; it was simple and complex; joy was there and despair. . . . There was neither good nor bad there. There were just facts. It was life.

> *Of Human Bondage,* Ch. LXXXI

Albert Schweitzer [1875–1965]

Here, at whatever hour you come, you will find light and help and human kindness.

> Inscribed on the lamp outside his jungle hospital at Lambaréné

Frank Patch [1878–1953]

Walk softly and think deeply here, gentlemen, for these are the hallowed

halls wherein the ghost of Osler walks.
Address to the interns at
Montreal General Hospital,
1936

Will Rogers [1879–1935]

In Yellowstone Park they've got signs
saying "Don't Feed Bear," and they
have got a hospital for them that do.

Nathaniel Faxon [1880–   ]

[The purpose of a teaching hospital
is] to advance knowledge, to train
doctors, and to set an example of
practice.
Quoted by F. M. R. Walshe in
Teachers of Medicine

Franklin D. Roosevelt [1882–1945]

I now propose for the consideration of
the Congress a program for the construction of small hospitals in needy
areas of the country, especially in
rural areas, not now provided with
them. Hospitals are essential to physicians in giving modern medical service
to the people. . . . The provision of
hospitals in the areas to which I refer
will greatly improve existing health
services, attract competent doctors and
raise the standards of medical care in
these communities. The new hospitals
should serve the additional purpose
of providing laboratory and other
diagnostic facilities for the use of
local physicians, as well as accom-
modations for local health departments. . . . Treatment in such a hospital would, of course, be available to
men, women and children who literally
can afford to contribute little or nothing toward their treatment.
Message to Congress, January
30, 1940

Henry E. Sigerist [1891–1957]

Hospitals are the temples of medicine.
What may not always be possible in
private practice must be possible in
a hospital. Accidents and delays which
might be forgiven in private practice
are inexcusable in the hospital.
American Medicine, Ch. 7 (tr.
by Hildegard Nagel)

The hospital is developing into the
center of all therapeutic activity,
where medicine is organized and co-
ordinated. Hospitals will come to extend their functions, till they include
prophylaxis, and grow to be veritable
centers for the preservation and restoration of the health of the community.
Idem

Stephen Vincent Benét [1898–1943]

As he often did, when he waked up,
he had a sense of the whole big mechanism of the hospital, cut off from the
rest of the world, yet self-sufficient,
like a boat or a train. That was a
hang-over from the dreams after the
operation. But it made an amount of
sense. There was a routine, with fixed
stops, and you saw a great deal of
people you would probably never see
again. Sometimes you didn't even see
them — just knew them as you knew
his neighbor, No Visitors, from a card
stuck in a door and a radio heard
through the wall.
Tales of Our Time, "No Visitors"

So it was all modern and scientific and
well-arranged. You could die very
nearly as privately in a modern hospital as you could in the Grand Central
Station, and with much better care.
Idem

Sir George W. Pickering [1904–   ]

Medicine is an advancing science and
the best hospitals in the world are not
those which merely use new knowledge,
but those which create it.

Walsh McDermott [1909–   ]

A medical center is one of the few places — perhaps the only place — where one can see the entire exciting process of the mind of man working at its best from start to finish. . . . the birth of an idea; the establishment of its validity; the placing it in a usable concept; the teaching of it to others; the testing it for practical utility; the careful weighing of the moral and ethical questions that inevitably arise concerning its use; and its discriminating application for the benefit of a particular human being.
Journal of Chronic Diseases 16:108, 1963

Anonymous

Patients may not swear, curse, get drunk, behave rudely or indecently on pain of expulsion after the first admonition. There shall be no card playing or dicing and such patients as are able shall assist in nursing others, washing and ironing linen and cleaning the rooms and such other services as the matron may require.
Regulations of the Philadelphia General Hospital, 1790

HOUSE STAFF

Lloyd Roberts [1835–1920]

If you want to be on the staff of a hospital, lad, pretend you're a fool till you're on it.
Quoted in *Lancet* 2:766, 1920

William Stewart Halsted [1852–1922]

The interne suffers not only from inexperience, but also from over-experience. He has in his short term of service responsibilities which are too great for him; he becomes accustomed to act without preparation and he acquires a confidence in himself and a self-complacency which may be useful in times of emergency, but which tend to blind him to his inadequacy and to warp his career.
Bulletin of the Johns Hopkins Hospital 15:267, 1904

Anonymous

Poverty is a virtue greatly exaggerated by physicians no longer forced to practice it.[1]

HUMILITY

Sir Thomas Browne [1605–1682]

Guide not the Hand of God, nor order the Finger of the Almighty, unto thy will and pleasure; but sit quiet in the soft showers of Providence, and Favorable distributions in this World, either to thy self or others. And since not only Judgments have their Errands, but Mercies their Commissions, snatch not at every Favour, nor think thy self passed by, if they fall upon thy Neighbour. . . . If thou doest not anoint thy Face, yet put not on sackcloth at the felicities of others.
Christian Morals, Pt. III, Sect. 5

Where there is an obscurity too deep for our reason, 't is good to sit down with a description, periphrasis, or adumbration.
Religio Medici, Pt. I, Sect. 10

Claude Bernard [1813–1878]

Our feelings lead us at first to believe that absolute truth must lie within our realm; but study takes from us, little by little, these chimerical conceits.
An Introduction to the Study of Experimental Medicine, Pt. II, Ch. 1, Sect. ix (tr. by H. C. Greene)

Science increases our power in proportion as it lowers our pride.

[1] In reference to the pay of house staff.

Sir William Osler [1849–1919]

The Art of Detachment, the Virtue of Method, and the Quality of Thoroughness may make you students, in the true sense of the word, successful practitioners, or even great investigators; but your characters may still lack that which can alone give permanence to power — the *Grace of Humility*.
> *Aequanimitas, with Other Addresses,* "Teacher and Student"

Walter B. Cannon [1871–1945]

The only reasonable attitude for the seeker after truth is that of true humility.
> *The Way of an Investigator,* "Fitness for the Enterprise"

Sir Henry Howarth Bashford ("Peter Harding") [1880–1961]

After all, we are merely the servants of the public, in spite of our M.D.'s and our hospital appointments.
> *The Corner of Harley Street,* Ch. 8

Howard, Lord Florey [1898–1968]

I don't think I am too optimistic in thinking that this is a very promising line.[1]
> Quoted by R. B. Fosdick in *Rockefeller Foundation Review for 1943*

HUNGER

See also DIET, EATING, FASTING

Homer [ca. 850 B.C.]

There is nothing in the world more shameless than this cursed belly! It

[1] Letter to the Rockefeller Foundation requesting financial support for his work on penicillin, which won him the Nobel prize for medicine in 1945 with Sir Alexander Fleming and Ernst B. Chain.

forces a man to remember it, in spite of dire distress and sorrow of heart.
> *Odyssey,* VII.215 (tr. by W. H. D. Rouse)

All deaths are hateful to miserable mortals, but the most pitiable death of all is to starve.
> *Ibid.,* XII.341

Hippocrates [460?–377? B.C.]

When in a state of hunger, one ought not to undertake labor.
> *Aphorisms,* II.16 (tr. by Francis Adams)

Drinking strong wine cures hunger.
> *Ibid.,* II.21

Horace [65–8 B.C.]

Only a stomach that seldom feels hunger scorns things common.
> *Satires,* II.ii.38 (tr. by H. R. Fairclough)

Thomas Tusser [1524?–1580]

Make hunger thy sauce, as a medcine for helth.
> *Five Hundred Pointes of Good Husbandrie,* Ch. 10

Francis Beaumont [1584–1616] and John Fletcher [1579–1625]

Hunger is sharper than the sword.
> *The Honest Man's Fortune,* Act I, Sc. ii

Izaak Walton [1593–1683]

The belly has no ears when hunger comes upon it.
> *The Compleat Angler,* Pt. I, Ch. VIII

Matthew Henry [1662–1714]

They that die by famine die by inches, and feel themselves die.
> *An Exposition on the Old and New Testament,* "Psalms 59: 15"

George Gordon, Lord Byron
[1788–1824]

Famish'd people must be slowly nurst,
And fed by spoonfuls, else they always
burst.
> *Don Juan,* Canto II, Stanza
> 158

William Cooper Brann
[1855–1898]

No man can be a patriot on an empty
stomach.
> *Brann, the Iconoclast,* "Old
> Glory," July 4, 1893

Mahatma Gandhi [1869–1948]

To a man with an empty stomach
food is God.
> Quoted by Edgar Snow in
> *Journey to the Beginning,* Ch. 8

The Bible

They that be slain with the sword
are better than they that be slain
with hunger: for these pine away,
stricken through for want of the fruits
of the field.
> *Lamentations* 4:9

I was an hungred, and ye gave me
meat.
> *Matthew* 25:35

Proverbs

Hunger is not dainty.

Hunger is the best sauce.

The belly hates a long sermon.

Italian Proverb

Who goes to bed supperless, all night
tumbles and tosses.

Scottish Proverb

A sharp stomach makes short devotion.

HYDROTHERAPY

William Shakespeare [1564–1616]

And grew a seething bath, which yet
men prove
Against strange maladies a sovereign
cure.
> *Sonnet CLIII*

Tobias Smollett [1721–1771]

There is always a great shew of the
clergy at Bath; none of your thin,
puny, yellow, hectic figures, exhausted
with abstinence and hardy study,
labouring under the *morbi eruditorum;*
but great overgrown dignitaries and
rectors, with rubicund noses and gouty
ankles, or broad bloated faces, drag-
ging along great swag bellies, the emblems of sloth and indigestion.
> *The Expedition of Humphry
> Clinker,* Letter 26

Georg Christoph Lichtenberg
[1742–1799]

If one would keep a record of patients who have not been helped by
certain springs and spas with the same
care with which one records the opposite, no one would go there any
longer, at least no one who is ill.
> *Ideen, Maximen und Einfälle*
> (tr. by Max Samter)

Thomas Jefferson [1743–1826]

Staid at Aix long enough to prove the
inefficacy of the waters.
> Letter to John Jay, May 4,
> 1787

There are several medicinal springs,
some of which are indubitably efficacious, while others seem to owe their
reputation as much to fancy and
change of air and regimen, as to their
real virtues. None of them having undergone a chemical analysis in skilful
hands, nor been so far the subject of
observations as to have produced a

reduction into classes of the disorders which they relieve; it is in my power to give little more than an enumeration of them.

> *Notes on the State of Virginia,* Query VI

The *Hot spring* is about six miles from the Warm, is much smaller, and has been so hot as to have boiled an egg. Some believe its degree of heat to be lessened. It raises the mercury in Farenheit's thermometer to 112 degrees, which is fever heat. It sometimes relieves where the Warm fails.

> *Idem*

Charles Lamb [1775–1834]

The first water cure was the Flood, and it killed more than it cured.

HYGIENE

See also HEALTH, PREVENTIVE MEDICINE, REGIMEN

Huang Ti (The Yellow Emperor) [2697–2597 B.C.]

There was temperance in eating and drinking. Their hours of rising and retiring were regular and not disorderly and wild. By these means the ancients kept their bodies united with their souls, so as to fulfill their allotted span completely, measuring unto a hundred years before they passed away.

> *Nei Ching Su Wên,* Bk. 1, Sect. 1 (tr. by Ilza Veith in *The Yellow Emperor's Classic of Internal Medicine*)

The sages followed the laws [of nature] and therefore their bodies were free from strange diseases; they did not lose anything (which they had received by nature) and their spirit of life was never exhausted.

> *Ibid.,* Sect. 2

The ancient sages practiced not to undertake any worldly affairs, and in their pleasures and joys they were dignified and tranquil. They followed their own desires and they never directed their will and ambition toward the protection of a purpose that was empty of meaning. Thus their allotted span of life was without limit, like Heaven and Earth. This was the way the ancient sages controlled and conducted themselves.

> *Ibid.,* Bk. 2, Sect. 5

Aristotle [384–322 B.C.]

Whatever is pleasant is good, unless it can be shown that in the long run it is harmful or, in other words, not pleasant but unpleasant.

Chu Hui Weng

To avoid sickness, eat less; to prolong life, worry less.

> Quoted by F. H. Garrison in *Bulletin of the New York Academy of Medicine* 4:985, 1928

Plutarch [46?–120?]

A man ought to handle his body like the sail of a ship, and neither lower and reduce it much when no cloud is in sight, nor be slack and careless in managing it when he comes to suspect something is wrong.

> *Moralia,* "Advice About Keeping Well" (tr. by Frank Cole Babbitt)

Moses ben Maimon (Maimonides) [1135–1204]

It is obligatory upon man to avoid things which are detrimental to the body and acclimatize himself to things which heal and fortify it. These are as follows: A person should never eat except when he is hungry nor drink unless he is thirsty. He should not postpone his eliminations for even a single moment; rather, every time that micturition or defecation become necessary, he should respond thereto immediately.

> *Mishneh Torah,* "Hilchoth De'oth," Ch. IV, No. 1 (tr. by Fred Rosner in *Annals of Internal Medicine* 62:372, 1965)

The manner of [correct] bathing is for a person to enter the bathhouse [and bathe] every seven days. One should not enter [the bath] immediately after eating nor when one is hungry but when the food begins to be digested. He should wash his entire body with hot water that will not scald the body and the head alone [may be washed] with water hot enough to scald the body. Then he should wash his body with lukewarm water and then with tepid water [and so on] until he washes with cold water. Over his head he should not pour either lukewarm or cold water. In the rainy [winter] season, one should not bathe in cold water. . . . as soon as one perspires and the body becomes supple, one should rinse [the body] and leave [the bath].

> *Ibid.,* No. 16

When a person leaves the bath, he should put his clothes on and cover his head in the outer chamber [of the bathhouse] so that he should not be caught in a cold draft. Even in the summer one must be careful [in this regard]. After he leaves, he should wait until his soul has settled, his body has rested, and the warmth [from the bath] dissipated and then he may eat. If he should sleep a little after leaving the bath before eating, this is excellent. He should not drink cold water upon leaving the bath and certainly not while in the bath. If he is thirsty upon leaving the bath and cannot restrain himself [from drinking], he should mix water in wine or in honey and then drink it. If, in the winter, he anoints himself with oil in the bath after [the final] rinsing, this is beneficial.

> *Ibid.,* No. 17

I guarantee anyone who conducts himself according to the directions we have laid down that he will not be afflicted with illness all the days of his life until he ages greatly and expires. He will not require a physician, and his body will be complete and remain healthy all his life unless his body was defective from the beginning of his creation, or unless he became accustomed to one of the bad habits from the onset of his youth, or unless the plague of pestilence or the plague of drought comes onto the world.

> *Ibid.,* No. 20

All these helpful rules which we have presented should be followed only by a healthy [individual]. However, an ill person or someone in whom one of his organs is ailing or someone who has accustomed himself to a bad habit for many years, for each of these there are different directions and rules [to follow] according to [the nature of] his illness, as is expounded in the book[s] on medicine: "A change in one's living habits is the beginning of illness."

> *Ibid.,* No. 21

No disciple of a Sage should reside in a city that does not possess the ten following things, and these are a physician, a surgeon, a bathhouse, a lavatory, a water supply such as a river or well, a synagogue, a school teacher, a scribe, a charity treasurer, and a court of law [with authority] to punish with lashes and imprisonment.

> *Ibid,* No. 23

John Florio [1553?–1625]

Cloathe warme, eate little, drink wel, so shalt thou lyve.

> *First Frutes,* Folio 34

William Shakespeare [1564–1616]

Bid them wash their faces
And keep their teeth clean.
Coriolanus, II, iii, 67

Friedrich von Logau [1604–1655]

Joy and Temperance and Repose
Slam the door on the doctor's nose.
*Deutscher Sinngedichte Drei-
tausend* (tr. by Henry Wadsworth Longfellow in *Poetic
Aphorisms*, "The Best Medicines")

John Locke [1632–1704]

Narrow Breasts, short and stinking
Breath, ill Lungs, and Crookedness, are
the Natural and almost constant Effects of *hard Bodice, and Cloths that
pinch.* That way of making slender
Wastes, and fine Shapes, serves but the
more effectually to spoil them.
*Some Thoughts Concerning Ed-
ucation*, Sect. 12

St. Jean Baptiste de la Salle
[1651–1719]

It belongs to decency to wash the
hands before sitting down to table,
and it is even considered indispensably
necessary.
*The Rules of Christian Man-
ners and Civility*, Ch. II

Alexander Pope [1688–1744]

Healthy by temperance, and by exercise.
Epistle to Dr. Arbuthnot

Benjamin Franklin [1706–1790]

Keep your mouth wet, feet dry.
Poor Richard's Almanack, 1733

Temperance, Employment and a
chearful Spirit, are the great Preservers
of Health.
Ibid., 1760

Ralph Waldo Emerson
[1803–1882]

A Frenchman may possibly be clean:
an Englishman is conscientiously clean.
English Traits, Ch. VI

Richard D. Arnold [1808–1876]

The best quarantine is Hygiene.
Letter to Meredith Clymer, October 11, 1871

Peter L. Panum [1820–1885]

When a physician is called to work in
a place where climate and dietary conditions are different from those to
which he has been accustomed, his
first problem is to study the hygienic
potentialities which affect the state of
health of the inhabitants.
*Observations Made During the
Epidemic of Measles on the
Faroe Islands in the Year 1846*
(tr. by Ada S. Hatcher)

Robert G. Ingersoll [1833–1899]

Above all things, keep clean. It is
not necessary to be a pig in order to
raise one.
Lectures, "About Farming in
Illinois"

Sir William S. Gilbert [1836–1911]

Beauty will fade and perish, but personal cleanliness is practically undying,
for it can be renewed whenever it discovers symptoms of decay.
The Sorcerer, Act II

Charles H. Mayo [1865–1939]

The object of all health education is
to change the conduct of individual
men, women and children by teaching
them to care for their bodies well, and
this instruction should be given
throughout the entire period of their
educational life.
Minnesota Medicine 15:40,
1932

Samuel Hopkins Adams
[1871–1958]

Hygienic law, like martial law, supersedes rights in crises.
The Health Master, Ch. I

"What you don't know won't hurt you." It's a poor principle in matters of hygiene.
Idem

Arthur Guiterman [1871–1943]

And each imbibes his rations from a
　　Hygienic Cup —
The Bunny and the Baby and the
　　Prophylactic Pup.
　　　The Laughing Muse, "Strictly
　　　Germ-Proof"

George Sacks [20th Cent.]

Europe, unlike Gaul, may be divided into two parts. In one the bidet is universal. In the other it is regarded as a highly immoral contraption. Yet hospital and nursing home architects would be well-advised to allow for them in their designs.
　　*Central African Journal of
　　Medicine* 2:160, 1956

Hilary Koprowski [1916–　]

Continue washing your hands between patients and before meals, and advise others to follow this archaic custom. I would guess that even in your time, environmental sanitation cannot be replaced by the best of the antibiotics.
　　Man and His Future (ed. by
　　Gordon Wolstenholme), "Future of Infectious and Malignant Diseases"

The Koran

Truly Allah . . . loveth those who have a care for cleanness.
　　Sûrah, II.222

The Talmud

Whoever eats bread without previously washing the hands is as though he had intercourse with a harlot.
　　Sotah, I.4b (tr. by I. Epstein)

Anonymous

Cleanliness is a fine life-preserver.

One keep-clean is better than ten make-cleans.

Proverbs

Cleanliness is next to godliness.

Our fathers, which were wondrous wise,
Did wash their throats, before they
　　wash'd their eyes.

English Proverb

Wash your hands often, your feet seldom, and your head never.

Indian (Hindustani) Proverb

Bathe early every day and sickness will avoid you.

Spanish Proverb

Dine with little, sup with less, sleep high, and thou wilt live.

Swedish Proverb

Fear less, hope more;
Eat less, chew more;
Whine less, breathe more;
Hate less, love more;
And all good things are yours.

West African Proverb

A butcher who does not bathe is not patronized.

HYPOCHONDRIA

See also NEUROSIS, PSYCHO-
SOMATICS

Plato [427?–347 B.C.]

Excessive care of the body, when

carried beyond the rules of gymnastic, is most inimical to the practice of virtue . . . and, what is most important of all, irreconcilable with any kind of study or thought or self-reflection — there is a constant suspicion that headache and giddiness are to be ascribed to philosophy, and hence all practicing or making trial of virtue in the higher sense is absolutely stopped; for a man is always fancying that he is being made ill, and is in constant anxiety about the state of his body.

> *Republic,* III.407.B (tr. by Benjamin Jowett)

Joseph Addison [1672–1719]

Multitudes of Imaginary Sick Persons . . . break their Constitutions by Physick, and throw themselves into the Arms of Death, by endeavoring to escape it. This Method is not only dangerous, but below the practice of a Reasonable Creature. . . . To consult the Preservation of Life, as the only End of it, To make our Health our Business, To engage in no Action that is not part of a Regimen, or course of Physic; are Purposes so abject, so mean, so unworthy human Nature, that a generous Soul would rather die than submit to them.

> *The Spectator,* Vol. I, No. 25 (March 29, 1711)

Benjamin Franklin [1706–1790]

Nothing is more fatal to *Health,* than an *over Care* of it.

> *Poor Richard's Almanack,* 1760

William Cullen [1710–1790]

It is said to be the manner of hypochondriacs to change often their physician; and indeed they often do it consistently: For a physician who does not admit the reality of the disease cannot be supposed to take much pains to cure it, or to avert the danger of which he entertains no apprehension.

> *First Lines of the Practice of Physic,* Pt. II, Bk. II, Ch. 3

William Heberden [1710–1801]

This state [which] I call the hypochondriac affection in men, and the hysteric in women . . . is a sort of waking dream, which, though a person be otherwise in sound health, makes him feel symptoms of every disease; and, though innocent, yet fills his mind with the blackest horrors of guilt.

> *Commentaries on the History and Cure of Diseases,* Ch. 49

Hypochondriac complaints resemble the gout, and madness, and consumptions, in their not appearing before the age of puberty.

> *Idem*

Laurence Sterne [1713–1768]

People who are always taking care of their health are like misers, who are hoarding a treasure which they have never spirit enough to enjoy.

Tobias Smollett [1721–1771]

I have had an hospital these fourteen years within myself, and studied my own case with the most painful attention.

> *The Expedition of Humphry Clinker,* Letter 11

Charles Churchill [1731–1764]

The surest road to health, say what they will,
Is never to suppose we shall be ill.
Most of those evils we poor mortals know
From doctors and imagination flow.

> *Night*

Arthur Schopenhauer [1788–1860]

Hypochondria torments us not only with causeless irritation with the things of the present; not only with ground-less anxiety on the score of future misfortunes entirely of our own man-ufacture; but also with unmerited self-reproach for our own past actions.

> *Parerga und Paralipomena*, Vol. II, Ch. 26, Sect. 322

Karl F. H. Marx [1796–1877]

Physicians see many "diseases" which have no more real existence than an image in a mirror.

> Quoted by F. H. Garrison in *Bulletin of the New York Acad-emy of Medicine* 4:1001, 1928

Henry Wheeler Shaw ("Josh Billings") [1818–1885]

I never knu a man yet who was allwuss watching his helth, to die enny whare near az soon az he expected to.

> *Farmer's Allminax*, March 1876

Sir Clifford Allbutt [1836–1925]

A neuralgic woman seems thus to be peculiarly unfortunate. However bitter and repeated may be her visceral neuralgias, she is either told she is hysterical or that it is all uterus. In the first case she is comparatively fortunate, for she is only slighted; in the second case she is entangled in the net of the gynaecologist, who finds her uterus, like her nose, is a little on one side, or again, like that organ, is running a little, or it is flabby as her biceps, so that the unhappy viscus is impaled upon a stem, or perched upon a prop, or is painted with carbolic acid every week in the year except during the long vacation when the gynaecologist is grouse-shooting, or salmon-catching, or leading the fashion in the Upper Engadine. Her mind thus fastened to a more or less nasty mystery becomes newly apprehensive and physically introspective and the morbid chains are riveted more strongly than ever. Arraign the uterus, and you fix in the woman the arrow of hypochondria, it may be for life.

> *Lancet* 1:459, 1884

William J. Mayo [1861–1939]

To a considerable extent we leave reassurance to the quack and the cultist, and if we are unable to find physical disease we say that a patient needs no medical attention, although he may be urgently in need of reas-surance and mental comfort.

> *Proceedings of the Staff Meet-ings of the Mayo Clinic* 2:167, 1927

E. B. White [1899–   ]

The imaginary complaints of inde-structible old ladies.

> *Harper's Magazine*, November 1941

HYPOTHESIS

See also RESEARCH, SCIEN-TIFIC METHOD, THEORY

Thomas Percival [1740–1804]

The invention of an hypothesis is a work of no difficulty to a lively imag-ination; and the fiction, by its tinsel glitter, never fails to dazzle the igno-rant and vulgar. But to watch with close attention the operations of na-ture, to treasure up a store of useful facts, to learn, by accurate observa-tion, the diagnostics of diseases, and by unbiassed experience, the true method of cure, requires unwearied labour, assiduity, and patience, at the same time that it admits of no pomp-ous display of wit or knowledge.

> *Essays Medical, Philosophical, and Experimental*, Vol. I, "The Empiric"

Thomas Jefferson [1743–1826]

The adventurous physician goes on, & substitutes presumption for knowl-edge. From the scanty field of what is known, he launches into the bound-less region of what is unknown. He establishes for his guide some fanciful theory of corpuscular attraction, of chemical agency, of mechanical powers, of stimuli, of irritability accumulated or exhausted, of depletion by the lancet & repletion by mercury, or some other ingenious dream, which lets him into all nature's secrets at short hand.

> Letter to Dr. Caspar Wistar, June 21, 1807

It is in this part of medicine that I wish to see a reform, an abandonment of hypothesis for sober facts, the first degree of value set on clinical observation, and the lowest on visionary theories.

> *Idem*

Benjamin Rush [1745?–1813]

I have formerly said that there was but one fever in the world. Be not startled, Gentlemen, follow me and I will say there is but one disease in the world.

> *Lectures on the Practice of Physic*, I, No. 31

Sir Humphry Davy [1778–1829]

Hypothesis should be considered merely as an intellectual instrument of discovery, which at any time may be relinquished for a better instrument. It should never be spoken of as truth; its highest praise is verisimility. Knowledge can only be acquired by the senses; nature has an archetype in the human imagination; her empire is given only to industry and action, guided and governed by experience.

> Quoted by John Davy in *Life of Sir Humphry Davy*, Vol. I, Ch. 3

Peter Mere Latham [1789–1875]

There are subjects upon which the most sober and practical minds cannot help speculating a little beyond what they know.

> *General Remarks on the Practice of Medicine*, Ch. II

Elisha Bartlett [1804–1855]

The restless and inquisitive mind, from its very constitution insatiable, and ever unsatisfied with its actual and absolute possessions, endeavors to imagine the phenomena, which it cannot demonstrate; it struggles to overleap the boundary, whose inexorable circumference cages it in; and, failing to do this, it fills the infinite and unknown regions, beyond and without it, with its own creations.

> *Philosophy of Medical Science*, Pt. I, Ch. 4

The very existence of ultimate molecules, or atoms, with the qualities which we so confidently assign to them, is a matter of the purest conjecture; it is entirely a fiction of the mind.

> *Idem*

This utter and absolute ignorance in which we are placed, of the ultimate constitution of matter, and of the relations which may exist between its elementary constituents, ought at least to teach us caution in the construction of theories, or hypotheses, founded on an assumed condition of this constitution, and of these relations, and modesty in the promulgation and defence of such theories, or hypotheses.

> *Idem*

Under all circumstances, amongst all nations, in every stage and phasis of human progress, under the reign of all philosophies, and all religions; in all times, and everywhere, within the range of civilization, has medical science been attended with its protean hosts of hypotheses.

> *Ibid.*, Pt. II, Ch. 12

In order to interpret, and account for, the appreciable phenomena and relationships of morbid actions, certain properties and conditions of the body, wholly unknown and imaginary, are assumed; then, these supposed prop-

erties and conditions, by a second assumption, are said to be connected with certain obvious states of the skin, and the natural outlets of the body, and, through this connexion, susceptible of being ascertained; and, finally, by a process of *à priori* reasoning, the treatment of all diseases, thus ascertained, is made to consist in the removal of these assumed and imaginary conditions; the therapeutics of the methodists naturally, necessarily, and rationally, as it is called, flowing from their pathology. Such, I say, when analyzed, and reduced to its actual elements, is the character of all medical hypotheses.
> *Idem*

One of the first and most inevitable effects of a belief in any *à priori* system of medicine is an utter disqualification of the mind for correct and trustworthy observation. No man with one of these hypothetical crotchets in his brain is to be trusted. Every object about him is discolored and distorted by this doctrinal medium through which he sees it. His intellectual vision is neither true nor achromatic. He will always find what he expects to find; and he will always fail to discover what he has concluded beforehand will not be present.
> *Idem*

Let us be careful how we mistake for the rational indications and the sober teachings of philosophy, the golden day-dreams and the fairy imaginations of a speculative optimism.
> *Ibid.*, Ch. 16

Charles Darwin [1809–1882]

I have steadily endeavoured to keep my mind free so as to give up any hypothesis, however much beloved (and I cannot resist forming one on every subject) as soon as facts are shown to be opposed to it.
> Quoted by Francis Darwin in
> *Charles Darwin*, Ch. 2

Claude Bernard [1813–1878]

A scientific hypothesis is merely a scientific idea, preconceived or previsioned. A theory is merely a scientific idea controlled by experiment.
> *An Introduction to the Study of Experimental Medicine*, Pt. I, Ch. 1, Sect. vi (tr. by H. C. Greene)

Paul Broca [1824–1880]

The least questioned assumptions are often the most questionable.
> *Quelques propositions sur les tumeurs dites cancéreuses*

Thomas Huxley [1825–1895]

The great tragedy of Science — the staying of a beautiful hypothesis by an ugly fact.
> *Collected Essays*, Ch. VIII, "Biogenesis and Abiogenesis"

Hughlings Jackson [1835–1911]

We have multitudes of facts, but we require, as they accumulate, organisations of them into higher knowledge; we require generalisations and working hypotheses.

Alfred North Whitehead [1861–1947]

It is more important that a proposition be interesting than that it be true.
> *Adventures of Ideas*, Ch. XVI

Martin H. Fischer [1879–1962]

Don't confuse *hypothesis* and *theory*. The former is a possible explanation; the latter, the correct one. The establishment of theory is the very purpose of science.
> Quoted by Howard Fabing and Ray Marr in *Fischerisms*

René J. Dubos [1901–   ]

In medicine even more than in other fields of science, theories and practice have always been under the sway of *à priori* philosophical attitudes and rationalized beliefs. The social forces that have influenced medical history range from the primitive fear of demons to the current wave of faith healing, from Rousseau's assertion that "hygiene is less a science than a virtue" to the modern illusion that diseases can be conquered by drugs.

Among all the medical utopias that have flourished in the course of time, none has blossomed so constantly and in so many forms as the belief that disease can be entirely eliminated from the earth. At the present time this illusion is based on an uncritical faith in the magic power of experimental science.

> *The Dreams of Reason,* Ch. IV

W. I. B. Beveridge [1908–   ]

There is an interesting saying that no one believes an hypothesis except its originator but everyone believes an experiment except the experimenter. Most people are ready to believe something based on experiment but the experimenter knows the many little things that could have gone wrong in the experiment. For this reason the discoverer of a new fact seldom feels quite so confident of it as do others. On the other hand other people are usually critical of an hypothesis, whereas the originator identifies himself with it and is liable to become devoted to it. It is as well to remember this when criticising someone's suggestion, because you may offend and discourage him if you scorn the idea. A corollary to this observation that an hypothesis is a very personal matter, is that a scientist usually works much better when pursuing his own than that of someone else. It is the originator who gets both the personal satisfaction and most of the credit if his idea is proved correct, even if he does not do the work himself. A man working on an hypothesis which is not his own often abandons it after one or two unsuccessful attempts because he lacks the strong desire to confirm it which is necessary to drive him to give it a thorough trial and think out all possible ways of varying the conditions of the experiment.

> *The Art of Scientific Investigation,* Ch. V

Anonymous

We must discover the laws on which our profession rests, and not invent them.

HYSTERIA

See HYPOCHONDRIA, NEUROSIS

IDEAS

See also HYPOTHESIS, THEORY

Claude Bernard [1813–1878]

Our ideas are only intellectual instruments which we use to break into phenomena; we must change them when they have served their purpose, as we change a blunt lancet that we have used long enough.

> *An Introduction to the Study of Experimental Medicine,* Pt. I, Ch. 2, Sect. iv (tr. by H. C. Greene)

Thomas Huxley [1825–1895]

Whatever practical people may say, this world is, after all, absolutely governed by ideas, and very often by the wildest and most hypothetical ideas.

> *Science and Education,* "On the Study of Biology"

Sir Clifford Allbutt [1836–1925]

A critical and flexible judgement comes of a familiarity with, and an apprecia-

tion of, the relative values of ideas, present and past.
> *British Medical Journal* 2:407, 1922

Wilfred Trotter [1872–1939]

If mankind is to profit freely from the small and sporadic crop of the heroically gifted it produces, it will have to cultivate the delicate art of handling ideas.
> *Collected Papers,* "The Commemoration of Great Men"

The mind likes a strange idea as little as the body likes a strange protein, and resists it with similar energy. It would not be too fanciful to say that a new idea is the most quickly acting antigen known to science. If we watch ourselves honestly we shall often find that we have begun to argue against a new idea before it has been completely stated.
> *Ibid.,* "Has the Intellect a Function?"

William E. Tanner [1889–   ]

Ideas lead to action, but equally action leads to ideas.
> *Sir W. Arbuthnot Lane,* Epilogue

IDLENESS

Celsus [25 B.C.–A.D. 50]

Too idle a life is inexpedient, because there may come up some necessity for labour.
> *De Medicina,* I.iii.3 (tr. by W. G. Spencer)

Leonardo da Vinci [1452–1519]

Iron rusts from disuse; stagnant water loses its purity and in cold weather becomes frozen; even so does inaction sap the vigour of the mind.
> *Codice Atlantico,* 289 (tr. by Edward MacCurdy in *The Notebooks of Leonardo da Vinci,* Vol. I, Ch. II)

Samuel Johnson [1709–1784]

It is certain that any wild wish or vain imagination never takes such firm possession of the mind as when it is found empty or unoccupied. . . . To be idle is to be vicious.
> *The Rambler,* No. 85 (January 8, 1751)

Sir William Osler [1849–1919]

By nature man is the incarnation of idleness, which quality alone, amid the ruined remnants of Edenic characters, remains in all its primitive intensity.
> *Aequanimitas, with Other Addresses,* "Teacher and Student"

IGNORANCE

Samuel Johnson [1709–1784]

Nothing has more retarded the advancement of learning than the disposition of vulgar minds to ridicule and vilify what they cannot comprehend.
> *The Rambler,* No. 117 (April 30, 1751)

Johann Wolfgang von Goethe [1749–1832]

Nothing is more terrible than to see ignorance in action.
> *Maxims and Reflexions,* I (tr. by John Stuart Blackie in *The Wisdom of Goethe*)

Armand Trousseau [1801–1867]

We do not know the mode of action of almost all remedies. Why therefore fear to confess our ignorance? In truth, it seems that the words "I do not know" stick in every physician's throat.

> *Bulletin de l'Académie Impériale de Médecine* 25:733, 1860

Sir William Osler [1849–1919]

The greater the ignorance the greater the dogmatism.

> *Aequanimitas, with Other Addresses*, "Chauvinism in Medicine"

W. Somerset Maugham [1874–1965]

If you are hidebound with prejudice, if your temper is sentimental, you can go through the wards of a hospital and be as ignorant of man at the end as you were at the beginning.

> *The Summing Up*, Sect. xix

Wilder Penfield [1891–   ]

In spite of all these disquieting triumphs in the field of natural science, it's astonishing how little man has learned about himself, and how much there is to learn. How little we know about this brain which made social evolution possible, and of the mind. How little we know of the nature and spirit of man and God. We stand now before this inner frontier of ignorance. If we could pass it, we might well discover the meaning of life and understand man's destiny.

> Dartmouth Convocation on *The Great Issues of Conscience in Modern Medicine* (1960), Third Panel Discussion

ILLEGITIMACY

William Shakespeare [1564–1616]

Peace is . . . a getter of more bastard children than war's a destroyer of men.

> *Coriolanus*, IV, v, 238

She grew round-womb'd, and had indeed, sir, a son for her cradle ere she had a husband for her bed.

> *King Lear*, I, i, 14

Judge Leon R. Yankwich [1888–   ]

There are no illegitimate children — only illegitimate parents.

> Decision in *Zipkin v. Mozon,* California, June 1928

English Proverb

God gave him no children; but the devil furnished him with abundance of bastards.

IMAGINATION

A. C. Bradley [1851–1935]

Research, though toilsome, is easy; imaginative vision, though delightful, is difficult.

> *Oxford Lectures on Poetry*, "Shakespeare's Theatre and Audience"

John Dewey [1859–1952]

Every great advance in science has issued from a new audacity of imagination.

> *The Quest for Certainty*, Ch. 11

W. I. B. Beveridge [1908–   ]

Other things being equal, the person with a fertile imagination makes a better leader than someone with a purely logical mind, for the former is more inspiring as well as more useful in providing ideas.

> *The Art of Scientific Investigation*, Ch. X

IMPOTENCE

See also SEX

Rutherford Morison [1853–1939]

The functional form of impotence fills the coffers of the quacks, and swells the list of suicides.

> Quoted in *The Practitioner*, October 1965

Dr. Dunlop [fl. early 20th Cent.]

You notice that the tabetic has the power of holding water for an indefinite period. He also is impotent — in fact two excellent properties to possess for a quiet day on the river.

> Teaching at Charing Cross Hospital, London

Fuller Albright [1900–   ]

A patient who complains of lifelong impotence or lack of libido does not suffer from hormonal lack; a patient with real endocrine insufficiency, e.g., eunuchoidism, has impotence and absent libido, but does not complain of them, but of something more trivial, such as being mistaken for a girl over the telephone.

> *Textbook of Medicine* (8th ed. by Russell L. Cecil and Robert F. Loeb), "Diseases of the Ductless Glands," Introduction

INCURABLE

Sushruta [5th Cent.? B.C.]

Diseases affecting a Bráhmana well versed in the Vedas, or a king, or a woman, or an infant, or an old man, or a timid person, or a man in the royal service, or a cunning man, or a man who pretends to possess a knowledge of the science of medicine, or a man who conceals his disease, or a man of an excessively irascible temperament, or a man who has no control over his senses, or a man in extremely indigent circumstances of life or without any one to take care of him, are apt to run into an incurable type though appearing in a common or curable form at the outset. The physician, who practices his art with a regard to these facts, acquires piety, wealth, fame and all wished for objects in life.

> *Sushruta-Samhitá,* "Sutrasthánam," Ch. 10 (tr. by K. K. L. Bhishagratna)

Hippocrates [460?–377? B.C.]

If a man demand from an art a power over what does not belong to the art, or from nature a power over what does not belong to nature, his ignorance is more allied to madness than to lack of knowledge. For in cases where we may have the mastery through the means afforded by a natural constitution or by an art, there we may be craftsmen, but nowhere else. Whenever therefore a man suffers from an ill which is too strong for the means at the disposal of medicine, he surely must not even expect that it can be overcome by medicine.

> *The Art,* VIII (tr. by W. H. S. Jones)

Pien Ch'iao [fl. 255 B.C.]

Six reasons on the incurability of a disease . . . are: to lead a life of dissipation, to value money more than health, to lack proper food and clothing, to suffer from a fatal illness, to be so emaciated as not to be able to swallow medicine, and to believe in sorcerers instead of doctors.

> Quoted by K. C. Wong and Wu Lien-teh in *History of Chinese Medicine,* Bk. I, Ch. 5

Ovid [43 B.C.–A.D. 17?]

'Tis not always in a physician's power to cure the sick; at times the disease is stronger than trained art. You see how the blood emitted from a tender lung

leads by an unerring path to the waters of the Styx. Let the Epidaurian [1] in person bring holy herbs, he will have no skill with which to heal wounds in the heart. The healing art knows not how to remove crippling gout, it helps not the fearful dropsy.
> *Pontic Epistles*, I.iii.17 (tr. by A. L. Wheeler)

Seneca [4? B.C.–A.D. 65]

Not even medicine can master incurable diseases.
> *Moral Epistles to Lucilius*, XCIV (tr. by Richard M. Gummere)

What can't be cured were best endured.[2]
> *Ibid.*, CVII.9

Sir Thomas More [1478–1535]

Such as be sicke of incurable diseases they comforte with sittinge by them, with talkinge with them, and to be shorte with all maner of helpes that may be.
> *Utopia*, Bk. II, Ch. 7 (tr. by R. Robinson)

Michael Drayton [1563–1631]

Past cure, past care.
> *Englands Heroicall Epistles*, "Richard the Second to Queene Isabel"

William Shakespeare [1564–1616]

I say, we must not
So stain our judgment or corrupt our hope
To prostitute our past-cure malady
To empirics, or to dissever so
Our great self and our credit to esteem
A senseless help, when help past sense we deem.
> *All's Well That Ends Well*, II, i, 122

---

[1] Aesculapius.
[2] Optimum est pati, quod emendare non possis.

Past cure is still past care.
> *Love's Labour's Lost*, V, ii, 28

IAGO: What, are you hurt, Lieutenant?
CASSIO: Ay, past all surgery.
> *Othello*, II, iii, 259

Your master will be dead ere you return.
There's nothing can be minist'red to nature
That can recover him.
> *Pericles*, III, ii, 7

Hermann Boerhaave [1668–1738]

A good Doctor can foresee the fatal outcome of an incurable illness: when he cannot help, the experienced Doctor will take care not to aggravate the sick person's malady by tiring but injurious efforts; and in an impossible case he will not frustrate himself further with ineffective solicitude.
> *Atrocis, nec Descripti Prius, Morbi Historia* (tr. in *Bulletin of the Medical Library Association* 43:217, 1955)

Johann Stieglitz [1767–1840]

I have often thought it would be important to instruct physicians how to behave in cases of incurable disease; not so much to tell them what to do, but rather what not to do.
> Letter to Dr. Karl F. H. Marx, December 15, 1826

Jacob Bigelow [1786–1879]

When we know that a case is self-limited or incurable, we are to consider how far it is in our power to palliate or diminish sufferings which we are not competent to remove.
> *Nature in Disease*, Ch. 2

Peter Mere Latham [1789–1875]

In truth, the amount of irremediable disease in the world is enormous.
> *General Remarks on the Practice of Medicine*, Ch. VI

Matthew Arnold [1822–1888]

Nor bring, to see me cease to live,
Some doctor full of phrase and fame,
To shake his sapient head and give
The ill he cannot cure a name.
New Poems, "A Wish"

Simon Baruch [1840–1921]

There are no such things as incurable,
there are only things for which man
has not found a cure.[1]
> Quoted by Bernard Baruch in
> an address to the President's
> Committee on Employment of
> the Physically Handicapped,
> April 30, 1954

Robert Louis Stevenson [1850–1894]

Even if the doctor does not give you
a year, even if he hesitates about a
month, make one brave push and see
what can be accomplished in a week.
Virginibus Puerisque, Ch. V

Hilaire Belloc [1870–1953]

Physicians of the Utmost Fame
Were called at once; but when they
came
They answered, as they took their
Fees,
"There is no cure for this disease."
Cautionary Tales for Children,
"Henry King"

Warfield T. Longcope [1877–1953]

When a cure is impossible, it is the
duty of the physician to bring contentment, comfort or even happiness to his
patients to lighten their affliction. But
this does not mean necessarily that he
should limit living to prolong life.
*Bulletin of the Johns Hopkins
Hospital* 50:4, 1932

---

[1] Simon Baruch, Bernard's father, was a
pioneer surgeon and the father of scientific
hydrotherapy in the United States.

Arabic Proverb

He has an incurable disease who believes all he hears.

English Proverb

If Physic do not work, prepare for the
kirk.

German Proverb

Where there is no hope of a cure one
saves the medicine.

INDIGESTION

See also EATING, DIGESTION

Seneca [4? B.C.–A.D. 65]

Drinking and sweating, — it's the life
of a dyspeptic! [1]
Moral Epistles to Lucilius, XV
(tr. by Richard M. Gummere)

Juvenal [60?–140?]

Here, too, sick people die for lack of
sleep,
their illness the result of food gone
sour.
Satires, III.232 (tr. by J.
Mazzaro)

William Shakespeare [1564–1616]

Unquiet meals make ill digestions.
The Comedy of Errors, V, i, 73

Oft the teeming earth
Is with a kind of colic pinch'd and
vex'd
By the imprisoning of unruly wind
Within her womb.
Henry IV, Part I, III, i, 28

A surfeit of the sweetest things
The deepest loathing to the stomach
brings.
A Midsummer Night's Dream,
II, ii, 137

---

[1] Bibere et suadere vita cardiaci est.

Samuel Pepys [1633–1703]

About the middle of the night I was very ill — I think with eating and drinking too much — and I was forced to call the mayde, who pleased my wife and I in her running up and down so innocently in her smock.
    Diary

Tobias Smollett [1721–1771]

This sudden change from his former way of life agreed so ill with his disposition that, for the first time, he was troubled with flatulencies and indigestion, which produced anxiety and dejection of spirits.
    The Adventures of Peregrine Pickle, Ch. 95

Sydney Smith [1771–1845]

The longer I live, the more I am convinced that the apothecary is of more importance than Seneca; and that half the unhappiness in the world proceeds from little stoppages, from a duct choked up, from food pressing in the wrong place, from a vext duodenum, or an agitated pylorus.
    Quoted by Lady Holland in *A Memoir of the Rev. Sydney Smith,* Ch. 6

James Jackson [1777–1867]

Dyspepsy and cheerfulness do not go together.
    Letter to Anna C. Lowell, November 12, 1843

William Hazlitt [1788–1830]

An indigestion is an excellent common-place for two people that never met before.
    Literary Remains, "The Fight"

R. H. Barham ("Thomas Ingoldsby") [1788–1845]

'Tis not *her* coldness, father,
That chills my labouring breast;

It's that confounded cucumber
I've eat and can't digest.
    The Ingoldsby Legends, "The Confession"

George Gordon, Lord Byron [1788–1824]

    Indigestion is — that inward fate
Which makes all Styx through one small liver flow.
    Don Juan, Canto IX, Stanza 15

Thomas Carlyle [1795–1881]

I lead a most dyspeptic, solitary, self-shrouded *life:* consuming, if possible in silence, my considerable daily allotment of *pain.*
    Letter to Ralph Waldo Emerson, February 8, 1839

Victor Hugo [1802–1885]

Indigestion is charged by God with enforcing morality on the stomach.
    Les Misérables, "Fantine," Bk. III, Ch. 7 (tr. by C. E. Wilbour)

Robert G. Ingersoll [1833–1899]

Many people think they have religion when they are troubled with dyspepsia.
    Liberty of Man, Woman and Child, Sect. 3

Ambrose Bierce [1842–1914?]

INDIGESTION, n. A disease which the patient and his friends frequently mistake for deep religious conviction and concern for the salvation of mankind. As the simple Red Man of the western wild put it, with, it must be confessed, a certain force: "Plenty well, no pray; big bellyache, heap God."
    The Devil's Dictionary

Robert Louis Stevenson [1850–1894]

He sows hurry and reaps indigestion.
    Virginibus Puerisque, Ch. III

INFECTION

See also ANTISEPSIS, DIS-
EASE, EPIDEMICS, MI-
CROBES, PLAGUE

Tung-su Pai

A dirty cook gives diarrhoea quicker
than rhubarb.

> Quoted by F. H. Garrison in
> *Bulletin of the New York
> Academy of Medicine* 4:979,
> 1928

Ovid [43 B.C.–A.D. 17?]

What timid man does not avoid contact with the sick, fearing lest he contract a disease so near?

> *Pontic Epistles,* III.ii.13 (tr.
> by A. L. Wheeler)

Juvenal [60?–140?]

This plague has come upon us by infection, and it will spread still further,
just as in the fields the scab of one
sheep, or the mange of one pig, destroys an entire herd.

> *Satires,* II.78 (tr. by G. G.
> Ramsay)

William Shakespeare [1564–1616]

Pursue him to his home and pluck him
thence,
Lest his infection, being of catching
nature,
Spread further.

> *Coriolanus,* III, i, 309

Men take diseases, one of another.
Therefore let men take heed of their
company.

> *Henry IV, Part II,* V, i, 85

'Tis time to give 'em physic, their
diseases
Are grown so catching.

> *Henry VIII,* I, iii, 36

It is not for your health thus to
commit
Your weak condition to the raw cold
morning.

> *Julius Caesar,* II, i, 235

Sickness is catching.

> *A Midsummer Night's Dream,*
> I, i, 186

All the infections that the sun sucks
up
From bogs, fens, flats, on Prosper fall
and make him
By inchmeal a disease!

> *The Tempest,* II, ii, 1

Jacob Bigelow [1786–1879]

Our lot is cast in a perilous age. . . .
But where shall we fly to escape from
east winds and dogdays, from pestilences that come and pestilences that
do not come, from ships that bring us
yellow fever and quarantines that
nourish and cultivate it, from cattle
diseases that can only be exterminated
by exterminating the cattle, from lead
pipes for water contrived to kill everybody except the animalcules, from
fraudulent food and deleterious physic,
from drugs that are poisonous and
poisons that are adulterated, from infectious patients whose pulses must
be felt with a pair of tongs and their
chests explored with a tarred stethoscope?

> Address at the Fourth National
> Quarantine and Sanitary Con-
> vention, 1860

Claude Bernard [1813–1878]

A few days ago, two surgeons came
to give me a cystic examination. . . .
both of them washed their instruments
and their hands. Gosselin washed his
after, but your pupil, Guyon, *before*
this small operation.[1]

> Quoted by J. M. D. Olmsted in
> *Claude Bernard, Physiologist,*
> Ch. 8

[1] From a conversation between Bernard
and Louis Pasteur around 1877, when
Pasteur had been severely attacked for his
views on infection.

Robert Koch [1843–1910]

It is certainly a one-sided opinion — even though generally adopted at the moment — that all infectious agents which are still unknown must be bacteria. Why should not other microorganisms just as well be able to exist as parasites in the body of animals?
> *Zur Untersuchung von pathogenen Organismen,* 1881 (tr. by Max Samter) [1]

Charles V. Chapin [1856–1941]

As it takes two to make a quarrel, so it takes two to make a disease, the microbe and its host.
> *Papers,* "The Principles of Epidemiology"

Luigi Pirandello [1867–1936]

Though none of them was aware of it, the instrument of death was there all the time — still there and so small that it could hardly be noticed. It was a fly on the wall close by. It seemed to be quite still, but if one looked closely at it one could see that sometimes it stretched out its little proboscis and sucked, whilst at others it rapidly cleaned its two slender forelegs, rubbing them together with apparent satisfaction.
> *The Fly*

A. A. Milne [1882–1956]

They wondered
If wheezles
Could turn
Into measles,
If sneezles
Would turn
Into mumps. . . .
All sorts and conditions
Of famous physicians
Came hurrying round
At a run.
> *Now We Are Six,* "Sneezles"

[1] This work precedes the more widely quoted paper on the etiology of tuberculosis which appeared in 1882.

René J. Dubos [1901–   ]

Throughout nature, infection without disease is the rule rather than the exception.
> *Man Adapting,* Ch. VII

Anonymous (R. B. P.)

Staphylococcus Aureus,
　By Gram and Koch he swore
He would invade new regions
　Unconquered heretofore —
By Gram and Koch he swore it,
　To take a patient's life,
And called the Cocci, young and old,
From all his colonies of gold
　To aid him in the strife.
> *St. Bartholomew's Hospital Journal* 17:13, 1909, "The Battle of Furunculus"

Proverb

Let an ill man lie in thy straw, and he looks to be thy heir.

INFLUENZA

Philip Stanhope, Lord Chesterfield [1694–1773]

There reigns an epidemical distemper, called by the genteel name of *l'influenza.* It is a little fever, of which scarcely any body dies: and it generally goes off with a little looseness.
> Letter to his son, July 9, 1767

George Bernard Shaw [1856–1950]

During the first great epidemic of influenza towards the end of the nineteenth century a London evening paper sent round a journalist-patient to all the great consultants of that day, and published their advice and prescriptions: a proceeding passionately denounced by the medical papers as a breach of confidence of these eminent physicians. The case was the same; but the prescriptions were different, and so was the advice.
> *The Doctor's Dilemma,* "Preface on Doctors"

INSANITY

See also MIND, NEUROSIS,
PSYCHIATRY, PSYCHOANAL-
YSIS, PSYCHOLOGY, PSYCHO-
THERAPY

I. GENERAL

Homer [ca. 850 B.C.]

Zeus the counsellor hath utterly robbed
him of his wits.
> *Iliad,* IX.377 (tr. by A. T.
> Murray)

The gods have made thee mad.
> *Odyssey,* XXIII.11

Lycurgus [396?–323? B.C.]

When the wrath of the gods would
strike a mortal, they first stifle the
noble voice of reason in him.[1]
> *Against Leocratus,* XXI.92

Plautus [254?–184 B.C.]

Can it be that they are mad themselves
since they call me mad? [2]
> *Menaechmi,* V.v.962

Cicero [106–43 B.C.]

Saneness of mind has for its basis a
certain tranquillity and self-consis-
tency. The state of mind that lacks
these qualities they [philosophers]
term "insanity" because in a disturbed mind, as in a disturbed body,
sanity can not be.
> *Tusculan Disputations,* III.iv.9
> (tr. by A. P. Peabody)

Horace [65–8 B.C.]

Anger is short-lived madness.
> *Epistles,* I.ii.62 (tr. by H. R.
> Fairclough)

[1] Lycurgus is here quoting one version of
an idea often repeated by the classical
authors. Cf. Latin Proverb, p. 247a.
[2] Cf. Latin Proverb, p. 247a.

Ovid [43 B.C.–A.D. 17?]

He who can counterfeit sanity will be
sane.
> *The Remedies of Love,* 504 (tr.
> by J. H. Mozley)

Avicenna [980–1037]

The different sorts of madness are
innumerable.

Geoffrey Chaucer [1340?–1400]

Wood [1] . . . as an hare.
> *The Canterbury Tales,* "The
> Friar's Tale"

Sir Francis Bacon [1561–1626]

Lucid intervals and happy pauses.
> *The History of the Reign of
> King Henry VII*

William Shakespeare [1564–1616]

Lord Hamlet, with his doublet all
    unbrac'd,
No hat upon his head, his stockings
    foul'd,
Ungart'red, and down-gyved to his
    ankle;
Pale as his shirt, his knees knocking
    each other,
And with a look so piteous in purport
As if he had been loosed out of hell
To speak of horrors — he comes before
    me.
> *Hamlet,* II, i, 78

      For, to define true madness,
What is't but to be nothing else but
    mad?
> *Ibid.,* II, ii, 93

That he is mad, 'tis true: 'tis true 'tis
    pity;
And pity 'tis 'tis true.
> *Ibid.,* II, ii, 97

And he . . .
Fell into a sadness, then into a fast,
Thence to a watch, thence into a weak-
    ness,

[1] Wood = mad.

Thence to a lightness, and, by this declension,
Into the madness wherein now he raves.
Ibid., II, ii, 146

Though this be madness, yet there is method in't.
Ibid., II, ii, 208

I am but mad north-north-west. When the wind is southerly I know a hawk from a handsaw.
Ibid., II, ii, 396

O, what a noble mind is here o'er-thrown!
The courtier's, scholar's, soldier's, eye, tongue, sword,
Th' expectancy and rose of the fair state,
The glass of fashion and the mould of form,
Th' observ'd of all observers — quite, quite down!
And I . . .
Now see that noble and most sovereign reason,
Like sweet bells jangled, out of tune and harsh;
That unmatch'd form and feature of blown youth
Blasted with ecstasy.
Ibid., III, i, 158

There's something in his soul
O'er which his melancholy sits on brood;
And I do doubt the hatch and the disclose
Will be some danger.
Ibid., III, i, 172

Alas, how is't with you,
That you do bend your eye on vacancy,
And with th' incorporal air do hold discourse?
Forth at your eyes your spirits wildly peep;
And, as the sleeping soldier in th' alarm,

Your bedded hairs, like life in excrements,
Start up and stand on end.
Ibid., III, iv, 116

HAMLET: Ay, marry, why was he sent into England?
CLOWN: Why, because 'a was mad. 'A shall recover his wits there; or, if 'a do not, 'tis no great matter there.
HAMLET: Why?
CLOWN: 'Twill not be seen in him there. There the men are as mad as he.
Ibid., V, i, 163

Infirmity doth still neglect all office
Whereto our health is bound. We are not ourselves
When nature, being oppress'd, commands the mind
To suffer with the body.
King Lear, II, iv, 107

That way madness lies.
Ibid., III, iv, 21

A foolish extravagant spirit, full of forms, figures, shapes, objects, ideas, apprehensions, motions, revolutions. These are begot in the ventricle of memory, nourished in the womb of pia mater.
Love's Labour's Lost, IV, ii, 68

Infected minds
To their deaf pillows will discharge their secrets.
More needs she the divine than the physician. . . .
Remove from her the means of all annoyance,
And still keep eyes upon her.
Macbeth, V, i, 80

MACBETH: How does your patient, doctor?
DOCTOR: Not so sick, my lord,
As she is troubled with thick-coming fancies
That keep her from her rest.
MACBETH: Cure her of that!
Canst thou not minister to a mind diseas'd,

Pluck from the memory a rooted
  sorrow,
Raze out the written troubles of the
  brain,
And with some sweet oblivious antidote
Cleanse the stuff'd bosom of that per-
  ilous stuff
Which weighs upon the heart?
DOCTOR: Therein the patient
Must minister to himself.
MACBETH: Throw physic to the dogs,
  I'll none of it!
      Ibid., V, iii, 37

Lovers and madmen have such seething brains,
Such shaping fantasies, that apprehend
More than cool reason ever comprehends.
      A Midsummer Night's Dream,
      V, i, 4

This music mads me. Let it sound no
  more;
For though it have holp madmen to
  their wits,
In me it seems it will make wise men
  mad.
      Richard II, V, v, 61

This closing with him fits his lunacy.
Whate'er I forge to feed his brainsick
  humours
Do you uphold and maintain in your
  speeches.
      Titus Andronicus, V, ii, 70

One of thy kin has a most weak pia
mater.
      Twelfth Night, I, v, 122

Why, this is very midsummer madness.
      Ibid., III, iv, 61

Henry More [1614–1687]

Running about like mad.
      An Antidote against Atheisme,
      Bk. III, Ch. 7

Blaise Pascal [1623–1662]

Whence comes it that a cripple does
not irritate us, and a crippled mind

does irritate us? Because a cripple recognizes that we go straight, and a
crippled spirit says that it is we who
limp; were it not for this we should
have pity for him and not anger.
      Pensées, Sect. II

John Dryden [1631–1700]

                    There is a pleasure, sure,
In being mad, which none but madmen
  know!
      The Spanish Friar, Act II, Sc.
      ii

Joseph Addison [1672–1719]

There is not a Sight in Nature so mortifying as that of a Distracted Person,
when his Imagination is troubled, and
his whole Soul disordered and confused.
      The Spectator, Vol. VI, No. 421
      (July 3, 1712)

Samuel Johnson [1709–1784]

All power of fancy over reason is a degree of insanity.
      Rasselas, Ch. XLIV

William Heberden [1710–1801]

Great anxiety of mind, whatever may
have been its origin, is a principal
cause of insanity, that is, a disordered
understanding with a quiet pulse and
without any acute illness. It has been
the consequence of some diseases, particularly of worms, and epileptic fits,
and of many affections of the head, as
dropsies of the ventricles of the brain,
and scirrhous tumors, and also of
blows.
      *Commentaries on the History
      and Cure of Diseases,* Ch. 53

Tobias Smollett [1721–1771]

I think for my part onehalf of the nation is mad — and the other not very
sound.
      *The Adventures of Sir Launce-
      lot Greaves,* Ch. 6

Christoph Wilhelm Hufeland [1762–1836]

Someone may be perfectly rational, yet commit manslaughter, adultery, theft: he will easily find a physician who testifies that the action must be credited to temporary insanity. In the past, proof of insanity during a crime required proof of irrational behavior before the act was committed; now, the opposite seems to be true. Some time ago . . . a lawyer who defended a thief claimed that the exaggerated "thieving area" of the defendant's skull suggested an irresistible urge to steal; and that he could thus not be held responsible for the theft. "One more reason to hang him," replied the judge, "since it is obvious that he will steal again, sooner or later."
> *Neue Auswahl kleiner medizinischen Schriften I*, 1834

Heinrich Heine [1797–1856]

Ordinarily he is insane, but he has lucid moments when he is only stupid.
> Comment about Savoye, appointed ambassador to Frankfurt by Lamartine, 1848

Nathaniel Hawthorne [1804–1864]

The sick in mind . . . are rendered more darkly and hopelessly so, by the manifold reflection of their disease, mirrored back from all quarters, in the deportment of those about them; they are compelled to inhale the poison of their own breath, in infinite repetition.
> *The House of the Seven Gables*, Ch. 9

Oliver Wendell Holmes [1809–1894]

Insanity is often the logic of an accurate mind overtasked.
> *The Autocrat of the Breakfast Table*, Sect. II

Charles Baudelaire [1821–1867]

I cultivated my hysteria with joy and terror. Now I am always dizzy, and today, January 23, 1862, I experienced a singular premonition, I felt pass over me a breath of wind from the wings of madness.
> *Journeaux Intimes*, "Fusées," XVI

Emily Dickinson [1830–1886]

Much Madness is divinest Sense —
To a discerning Eye —
Much Sense — the starkest Madness —
> *Poems*, "Much Madness Is Divinest Sense"

Ambrose Bierce [1842–1914?]

All are lunatics, but he who can analyze his delusion is called a philosopher.
> *Epigrams*

Friedrich Nietzsche [1844–1900]

Insanity in individuals is something rare — but in groups, parties, nations, and epochs it is the rule.
> *Beyond Good and Evil*, Ch. IV (tr. by Helen Zimmern)

George Bernard Shaw [1856–1950]

I'm going clean off my chump.
> *Heartbreak House*, Act II

Frederick Peterson [1859–1938]

Through his misshapen soul and brain
No thought has passed and left its trace,
And all that brings man joy and pain,
Finds in his heart no dwelling-place;
His life is the world's stain.

The horrid vacant visage leers
And shows its heritage of woe,
Its scars — the sins of ancient years.
Could any love or hate it? — No!
Pity may give her tears.
> *The Idiot*

O. Henry (William Sydney Porter) [1862–1910]

Crazy as a loon.
> *A Blackjack Bargainer*

Eden Phillpotts [1862–1960]

His father's sister had bats in the belfry and was put away.
>   *Peacock House and Other Mysteries,* "My First Murder"

Rudyard Kipling [1865–1936]

Every one is more or less mad on one point.
>   *Plain Tales from the Hills,* "On the Strength of a Likeness"

Thomas Mann [1875–1955]

For lunacy undoubtedly in many cases meant the kind of self-abandonment which was the refuge of a weak nature against extreme distress, a defence against such overwhelming blows of destiny as it felt itself, when in its right mind, unable to cope with.
>   *The Magic Mountain,* Ch. VI, "Operationes Spirituales" (tr. by H. T. Lowe-Porter)

Martin H. Fischer [1879–1962]

An insane man is a sick man. Please don't forget that, gentlemen.
>   Quoted by Howard Fabing and Ray Marr in *Fischerisms*

If you are physically sick, you can elicit the interest of a battery of physicians; but if you are mentally sick, you are lucky if the janitor comes around.
>   *Idem*

When a man lacks mental balance in pneumonia he is said to be delirious. When he lacks mental balance without the pneumonia, he is pronounced insane by all smart doctors.
>   *Idem*

T. S. Eliot [1888–1965]

Where does one go from a world of insanity?
Somewhere on the other side of despair.
>   *The Family Reunion,* Pt. II, Sc. ii

Ernest Hemingway [1899–1961]

He is crazy as a bedbug.
>   *For Whom the Bell Tolls*

Mary Jane Ward [1905–   ]

This is something to remember when you are sorry for men on account of their dull way of dressing. When they lose their minds they look less lost than women.
>   *The Snake Pit,* Ch. 5, Pt. iv

Abraham A. Ribicoff [1910–   ]

Let us evaluate our thinking about mental illness and how we have dealt with it. Let us ask ourselves — are even the modest advances we have made in recent years on the right track? Or do we need an entirely new point of departure? Are we exploring every possibility and innovation — psychological, social, and biological? . . . Are we using our hospitals — the places where the patients are — as the logical place for constructive research? Are we as individuals ready to accept an act on the findings provided for us?
>   Address to the Mental Health Institute, Washington, D.C., May 3, 1961

John F. Kennedy [1917–1963]

We cannot afford to postpone any longer a reversal in our approach to mental affliction. For too long the shabby treatment of the many millions of the mentally disabled in custodial institutions and many millions more now in communities needing help has been justified on grounds of inadequate funds, further studies and future promises. We can procrastinate no more. The national mental health program and the national program to combat mental retardation herein proposed warrant prompt congressional attention.
>   *Message to Congress on Mental Health,* February 5, 1963

Don D. Jackson [1920–   ]

The term "schizophrenia" in medical circles carries almost as much of a ring of authenticity as "diabetic" or "tubercular." Yet it is actually nearly as much a fiction as that lovely legal appellation a "reasonable man."

The Etiology of Schizophrenia,
Introduction

Legal Phrases

A madman has no free will.
[Furiosi nulla voluntas est.]

Not of sound mind.
[Non compos mentis.]

Proverb

One mad action is not enough to prove a man mad.

English Proverbs

As mad as a hatter.[1]

As mad as a March hare.

Latin Proverbs

Every madman thinks all other men mad.[2]

Whom fate wishes to ruin she first makes mad.[3]

II. INSANE ASYLUMS

See also HOSPITALS

Philippe Pinel [1745–1826]

In all public asylums as well as in prisons and hospitals, the surest, and, perhaps, the only method of securing health, good order, and good manners, is to carry into decided and habitual execution the natural law of bodily labour, so contributive and essential to human happiness.

A Treatise on Insanity, Sect. 94
(tr. by D. D. Davis)

Dorothea Dix [1802–1887]

The *present* state of insane persons, confined within this Commonwealth, in *cages, closets, cellars, stalls, pens! Chained, naked, beaten with rods,* and *lashed* into obedience.

Memorial to the Legislature of Massachusetts, January 1843

I have myself seen *more than nine thousand idiots, epileptics, and insane, in these United States . . .* bound with galling chains, bowed beneath fetters and heavy iron balls attached to drag-chains, lacerated with ropes, scourged with rods.

Memorial to the Senate and House of Representatives, June 23, 1848

Havelock Ellis [1859–1939]

The place where optimism most flourishes is the lunatic asylum.

The Dance of Life, Ch. 3

Had there been a Lunatic Asylum in the suburbs of Jerusalem, Jesus Christ would infallibly have been shut up in it at the outset of his public career.

Impressions and Comments,
Series III, January 5, 1922

INSOMNIA

See SLEEP: INSOMNIA

INSTRUMENTS

Johann Wolfgang von Goethe [1749–1832]

Microscopes and telescopes, properly

---

[1] Hatters exposed to the mercuric nitrate employed in matting felt developed "hatter's shakes," characterized by tremors, extreme lack of coordination, delusions, and hallucinations.

[2] Cf. Plautus, p. 242a.

[3] Cf. Lycurgus, p. 242a.

considered, put our human eyes out of their natural, healthy, and profitable point of view.

> *Wilhelm Meisters Wanderjahre,* "Betrachtungen im Sinne der Wanderer," No. 63

Victor Hugo [1802–1885]

Where the telescope ends, the microscope begins. Which of the two has the grander view?

> *Les Misérables,* "Saint Denis," Bk. III, Ch. 3 (tr. by C. E. Wilbour)

Sir James Mackenzie [1853–1925]

The seeming exactness of a mechanical device appeals much more strongly to certain minds than a process of reasoning.

> Quoted by R. McNair Wilson in *The Beloved Physician,* Ch. 12

Oliver St. John Gogarty [1878–1957]

The telescope, the microscope and the test-tube have made sceptics of us all. We have changed wisdom for an exact knowledge of stains, precipitants, reactions and refractions, and put it, for this generation at least, beyond recall.

> *I Follow Saint Patrick,* Ch. 15

David Seegal [1899–   ]

An increasing worship of the instrument for its own sake sometimes leads to enslavement by it.

> *Journal of Medical Education* 39:321, 1964

William T. Salter [1901–1952]

As he picks up his beautiful new tool, however, it is well for the modern biologist to remind himself how subtly and completely a fascination for gadgets can betray sound sense.

> *Science* 109:453, 1949

INTEMPERANCE

See also ALCOHOL, EATING, INDIGESTION, TEMPERANCE

Huang Ti (The Yellow Emperor) [2697–2597 B.C.]

Afflicted are those who dissipate; they become nervous and startled. But those who are aware of their needs and desires are encouraged, and as an expression of this encouragement they become peace-loving and virtuous.

> *Nei Ching Su Wên,* Bk. 3, Sect. 8 (tr. by Ilza Veith in *The Yellow Emperor's Classic of Internal Medicine*)

Edmund Burke [1729–1797]

Men of intemperate minds cannot be free. Their passions forge their fetters.

> *A Letter to a Member of the National Assembly*

Oscar Wilde [1854–1900]

Moderation is a fatal thing. . . . Nothing succeeds like excess.

> *A Woman of No Importance,* Act III

German Proverb

Intemperance is the doctor's wetnurse.

INTESTINES

See BOWELS, GASTRO-INTESTINAL TRACT

INVALID

See also PATIENTS

Plato [427?–347 B.C.]

He [Herodicus] had a mortal disease

which he perpetually tended, and as recovery was out of the question, he passed his entire life as a valetudinarian; he could do nothing but attend upon himself, and he was in constant torment whenever he departed in anything from his usual regimen, and so dying hard, by the help of science he struggled on to old age.

> *Republic*, III.406.A (tr. by Benjamin Jowett)

Pierrard Poullet [fl. 1590]

He dies every day who lives a lingering life.

> *La Charité*

Cotton Mather [1663–1728]

Let not the Patients be (as I have said once already) too soon, or too much, confined unto their Beds.

> *The Angel of Bethesda*, Ch. 20 (In Otho T. Beall, Jr., and Richard H. Shryock's *Cotton Mather, First Significant Figure in American Medicine*)

Tobias Smollett [1721–1771]

The inconveniences [1] which I overlooked in the highday of health, will naturally strike with exaggerated impression on the irritable nerves of an invalid, surprised by premature old age, and shattered with longsuffering.

> *The Expedition of Humphry Clinker*, Letter 14

Charles Lamb [1775–1834]

He lies pitying himself, honing and moaning to himself; he yearneth over himself; his bowels are even melted within him, to think what he suffers; he is not ashamed to weep over himself.

> *The Last Essays of Elia*, "The Convalescent"

Nicholas I of Russia [1796–1855]

We have on our hands a sick man — a very sick man.[1]

> *Parliamentary Papers*, "Accounts and Papers," Vol. LXXI, Pt. 5

Henrik Ibsen [1828–1906]

Oh, one soon makes friends with invalids; and I need so much to have someone to live for.

> *Hedda Gabler*, Act IV (tr. by M. Meyer)

Friedrich Nietzsche [1844–1900]

The sick man is a parasite of society. In certain cases it is indecent to go on living. To continue to vegetate in a state of cowardly dependence upon doctors and special treatments, once the meaning of life, the right to life has been lost, ought to be regarded with the greatest contempt by society.

> *The Twilight of the Idols*, "Skirmishes in a War with the Age" (tr. by Anthony M. Ludovici)

Thomas Mann [1875–1955]

A human being who is first of all an invalid is *all* body; therein lies his inhumanity and his debasement.

> *The Magic Mountain*, Ch. IV, "Necessary Purchases" (tr. by H. T. Lowe-Porter)

The pity the well person felt for the sick — a pity that almost amounted to awe, because the well person could not imagine how he himself could possibly bear such suffering — was very greatly exaggerated. The sick person had no real right to it. It was, in fact, the result of an error in thinking, a sort of hallucination; in that the well man

---

[1] At Bath, where he plans to visit the mineral waters after a long absence.

[1] Referring to the dying Ottoman Empire of the Turks.

attributed to the sick his own emotional equipment, and imagined that the sick man was, as it were, a well man who had to bear the agonies of a sick one — than which nothing was further from the truth. For the sick man was — precisely that, a sick man: with the nature and modified reactions of his state.

> *Ibid.*, Ch. VI, "Operationes Spirituales"

Katherine Mansfield [1888–1923]

It is a fearful thing to have to lie in bed. To be sent to bed, to be commanded to stay there — to gaze from a little valley of humiliation, up, up, up to that ineffable brow that, wreathed with the mists of discretion and vacancy, bends over one. . . . To pipe, "When shall I be allowed to get up again?", and to be answered by, "We had rather postpone our answer for the present." These are moments which set the soul yearning to be taken suddenly, snatched out of the very heart of some fearful joy, and set before its Maker hatless, dishevelled and gay, with its spirit unbroken. For it is impossible to go condemned to bed in our grown-uppishness without recalling how favorite a remedy it was with our parents and nurses for a spirit that wanted breaking.

> Letter, 1920

Richard Asher [1912–   ]

Look at a patient lying long in bed. What a pathetic picture he makes! The blood clotting in his veins, the lime draining from his bones, . . . the flesh rotting from his seat . . . and the spirit evaporating from his soul.

> *British Medical Journal* 2:967, 1947

German Proverb

Invalids live longest.

INVESTIGATORS

See also RESEARCH, SCIENTISTS

François Magendie [1783–1855]

I am a mere street scavenger of science. With hook in hand and basket on my back, I go about the streets of science collecting whatever I find.

John Henry, Cardinal Newman [1801–1890]

It is a matter of primary importance in the cultivation of those sciences, in which truth is discoverable by the human intellect, that the investigator should be free, independent, unshackled in his movements; that he should be allowed and enabled to fix his mind intently, nay exclusively, on his special object, without the risk of being distracted every other minute in the process and progress of his inquiry, by charges of temerariousness, or by warnings against extravagance or scandal.

> *Christianity and Scientific Investigation*

Rudolf Virchow [1821–1902]

If only people would finally stop finding points of disagreement in the personal characteristics and external circumstances of investigators! It does not matter at all whether someone is a professor of clinical medicine or of theoretical pathology, whether he is a practitioner or a hospital physician, if only he possesses material for observation. In addition, it is not of decisive significance whether he confronts an overwhelming or a modest amount of material, if only he understands how to exploit it. And to do this he must know what he wants and how he can achieve what he wants: in other words, he must be in a position to put the right questions and to find the right methods for answering them.

> *Disease, Life, and Man,* "Cellular Pathology" (tr. by L. J. Rather)

Sir James M. Barrie [1860–1937]

Those hateful persons called Original Researchers.

> *My Lady Nicotine,* Ch. 13

William M. Bayliss [1860–1924]

It is not going too far to say that the greatness of a scientific investigator does not rest on the fact of his having never made a mistake, but rather on his readiness to admit that he has done so, whenever the contrary evidence is cogent enough.

> *Principles of General Physiology,* Preface

Alan Gregg [1890–1957]

Most of the knowledge and much of the genius of the research worker lie behind his selection of what is worth observing. It is a crucial choice, often determining the success or failure of months of work, often differentiating the brilliant discoverer from the . . . plodder.

> *The Furtherance of Medical Research*

David Seegal [1899–   ]

It is no forced extrapolation to state that every physician is perforce also a potential clinical investigator when he soundly fulfills his responsibilities for each patient.

> *The Pharos of Alpha Omega Alpha* 26:7, 1963

Sir Robert Platt [1900–   ]

The conventional picture of the research worker is that of a rather austere man in a white coat with a background of complicated glassware. My idea of a research worker, on the other hand, is a man who brushes his teeth on the left side of his mouth only so as to use the other side as a control and see if tooth-brushing has any effect on the incidence of caries.

> *British Medical Journal* 1:577, 1953

W. I. B. Beveridge [1908–   ]

People in most other walks of life can allow themselves the indulgence of fixed ideas and prejudices which make thinking so much easier, . . . but the research worker must try to keep his mind malleable and avoid holding set ideas in science. We have to strive to keep our mind receptive and to examine suggestions made by others fairly and on their own merits, seeking arguments for as well as against them. We must be critical, certainly, but beware lest ideas be rejected because an automatic reaction causes us to see only the arguments against them. We tend especially to resist ideas competing with our own.

> *The Art of Scientific Investigation,* Ch. VII

When Simon Flexner was planning the Rockefeller Institute he was asked "are you going to allow your men to make fools of themselves at your Institute?" The implication was that only those who would risk doing so were likely to make important discoveries.[1]

> *Ibid.,* Ch. XI

ITCH

See also SCRATCHING

Sir Francis Bacon [1561–1626]

Itch . . . also be pleasing to the touch.

> *A Natural History,* Century VII, No. 694

[1] Cf. Rudolf Virchow, p. 669b.

William Shakespeare [1564–1616]

What's the matter, you dissentious
  rogues
That, rubbing the poor itch of your
  opinion,
Make yourselves scabs?
  Coriolanus, I, i, 168

My elbow itch'd! I thought there
would a scab follow.
  Much Ado About Nothing, III,
  iii, 106

I would thou didst itch from head to
foot and I had the scratching of thee.
I would make thee the loathsom'st
scab in Greece.
  Troilus and Cressida, II, i, 29

Chang Ch'ao [ca. 1676]

It is easy to stand a pain, but difficult
to stand an itch.
  Sweet Dream Shadows (tr. by
  Lin Yutang in *The Importance
  of Living,* Ch. X, Sect. vii)

Anonymous

Have faith in the Lord but use sulphur
for the itch.

'Tis better than riches
To scratch when it itches.

Proverb

Itch is more intolerable than smart.

English Proverb

As old as the itch.

JAUNDICE

Lucretius [96?–55 B.C.]

Jaundiced persons see everything a
greenish-yellow, because many seeds of
this greenish-yellow colour stream out
from their bodies to meet the images
of things, and besides many are mingled in their own eyes which by their
contact paint everything with lurid
hues.
  On the Nature of Things,
  IV.333 (tr. by W. H. D. Rouse)

William Shakespeare [1564–1616]

What grief hath set these jaundies o'er
  your cheeks?
  Troilus and Cressida, I, iii, 2

Alexander Pope [1688–1744]

All looks yellow to the jaundic'd eye.
  An Essay on Criticism, Pt. II

William Heberden [1710–1801]

A violent itching of the skin without
any eruption is familiar to the jaundice,
and adds sometimes to the discomforts of old age.
  *Commentaries on the History
  and Cure of Diseases,* Ch. 23

Percy Bysshe Shelley [1792–1822]

Surely the bile-suffused cheek of
Buonaparte, his wrinkled brow, and
yellow eye, the ceaseless inquietude of
his nervous system, speak no less
plainly the character of his unresting
ambition than his murders and his
victories.
  Queen Mab, Notes

Sir William Osler [1849–1919]

Jaundice is the disease that your
friends diagnose.
  Quoted by William B. Bean in
  Sir William Osler: Aphorisms,
  Ch. 5

KIDNEY

See also URINE

Huang Ti (The Yellow Emperor)
[2697–2597 B.C.]

The kidneys are like the officials who

do energetic work, and they excel through their ability and cleverness.
Nei Ching Su Wên, Bk. 3, Sect. 8 (tr. by Ilza Veith in *The Yellow Emperor's Classic of Internal Medicine*)

The kidneys crave the salty flavor.
Ibid., Sect. 10

William Shakespeare [1564–1616]

A man of my kidney!
The Merry Wives of Windsor, III, v, 117

William Heberden [1710–1801]

The most dangerous ischuria is that, in which the kidneys secrete no urine from the blood.
Commentaries on the History and Cure of Diseases, Ch. 55

Richard Bright [1789–1858]

I have never yet examined the body of a patient dying with dropsy attended by coagulable urine, in whom some obvious derangement was not discovered in the kidneys. . . . In all the cases in which I have observed the albuminous urine, it has appeared to me that the kidney has itself acted a more important part, and has been more deranged both functionally and organically than has generally been imagined.
Reports of Medical Cases, 1827

John Punnett Peters [1887–1955]

A large proportion of the phenomena termed uremic are, as Volhardt and Foster pointed out almost 40 years ago, vascular in origin, consequences of hypertension, arterial disease, and heart failure. Others are results, not of retention of waste products, but of failure of the conservative functions of the kidneys. If their true nature were more frequently analyzed in detail and corrective measures instituted for each, therapy would be greatly advanced. The term uremia has a defeatist ring that fosters complacency or routine procedures rather than thoughtful action.
Yale Journal of Biology and Medicine 26:179, 1953

Too much attention has been paid to the excretory offices of the kidney to the neglect of its conservative services.
Idem

Homer W. Smith [1895–1962]

Superficially, it might be said that the function of the kidneys is to make urine; but in a more considered view one can say that the kidneys make the stuff of philosophy itself.
From Fish to Philosopher, Ch. I

It is no exaggeration to say that the composition of the blood is determined not by what the mouth takes in but by what the kidneys keep.
Idem

Bones can break, muscles can atrophy, glands can loaf, even the brain can go to sleep, without immediately endangering our survival; but should the kidneys fail . . . neither bone, muscle, gland, nor brain could carry on.
Idem

Anonymous

Doctor Richard Bright of Guy's
Had several patients large in size.
Their legs were swollen as could be;
Their eye so puffed they could not see.
To this oedema Bright objected,
And so he had them venesected.
He took a teaspoon by the handle,
Held it above a tallow candle,
And boiled some urine o'er the flame
(As you or I might do the same).
To his surprise, we find it stated,
The urine was coagulated.
Alas, his dropsied patients died.
Our thoughtful doctor looked inside:
He found their kidneys large and white,
The capsules were adherent quite.

So that is why the name of Bright is Associated with nephritis.

> Quoted by the Editors of *St. Bartholomew's Hospital Journal* in *Round the Fountain*

KNOWLEDGE

See also EDUCATION, LEARNING, LOGIC, TEACHING, WISDOM

Plato [427?–347 B.C.]

We shall be better and braver and less helpless if we think that we ought to inquire, than we should have been if we indulged in the idle fancy that there was no knowledge and no use in seeking to know what we do not know.

Leonardo da Vinci [1452–1519]

The acquisition of any knowledge whatever is always useful to the intellect, because it will be able to banish the useless things and retain those which are good. For nothing can be either loved or hated unless it is first known.

> *Codice Atlantico*, 226 (tr. by Edward MacCurdy in *The Notebooks of Leonardo da Vinci*, Vol. I, Ch. II)

All our knowledge originates in our sensibilities.

> *Codice Trivulziano*, 41 (*ibid.*, Ch. I)

Great love is born of great knowledge of the objects one loves. If you do not understand them you can only admire them lamely or not at all — and if you only love them on account of the good you expect from them, and not because of the sum of their qualities, then you are as the dog that wags his tail to the person who gives him a bone. Love is the daughter of knowledge and love is deep in the same degree as the knowledge is sure — love conquers all things.

> *Treatise on Painting*, Ch. 80 (tr. by McMahon)

Sir Francis Bacon [1561–1626]

I have taken all knowledge to be my province.

> Letter to My Lord Treasurer Burghley, 1592

Sir Thomas Browne [1605–1682]

I envy no man that knowes more than my selfe, but pity those that know less.

> *Religio Medici*, Pt. II, Sect. 3

Duc François de La Rochefoucauld [1613–1680]

For true understanding, comprehension of detail is imperative. Since such detail is wellnigh infinite, our knowledge is always superficial and imperfect.

> *Maxims*, No. 106 (tr. by Constantine FitzGibbon)

Thomas Jefferson [1743–1826]

The state of medicine is worse than that of total ignorance. Could we divest ourselves of everything we suppose we know in it, we should start from a higher ground and with fairer prospects.

Peter Mere Latham [1789–1875]

There is nothing so captivating as NEW knowledge.

> *Diseases of the Heart*, Lect. IV

A small overweight of knowledge is often a sore impediment to the movements of common sense.

> *General Remarks on the Practice of Medicine*, Ch. V

Knowledge may be an incumbrance as well as a help. Many men know more than they are able to wield. There is a point (I believe) in the acquisition of knowledge (and this point varies

infinitely in different individuals), beyond which, if more be acquired, the whole mass becomes useless to its possessor.
> *Lectures on Clinical Medicine,*
> Lect. I

Charles Augustin Sainte-Beuve [1804–1869]

It is with medicine as with mathematics: we should occupy our minds only with what we continue to know; what we once knew is of little consequence.

Oliver Wendell Holmes [1809–1894]

The best part of our knowledge is that which teaches us where knowledge leaves off and ignorance begins. Nothing more clearly separates a vulgar from a superior mind, than the confusion in the first between the little that it truly knows, on the one hand, and what it half knows and what it thinks it knows on the other.
> *Medical Essays,* "Border Lines of Knowledge in Some Provinces of Medical Science"

Our American atmosphere is vocal with the flippant loquacity of half knowledge. We must accept whatever good can be got out of it, and keep it under as we do sorrel and mullein and witchgrass, by enriching the soil, and sowing good seed in plenty; by good teaching and good books, rather than by wasting our time in talking against it. Half knowledge dreads nothing but whole knowledge.
> *Ibid.,* "Medical Libraries"

All systematic knowledge involves much that is not practical, yet it is the only kind of knowledge which satisfies the mind, and systematic study proves, in the long-run, the easiest way of acquiring and retaining facts which are practical. There are many things which we can afford to forget, which yet it was well to learn.
> *Ibid.,* "The Young Practitioner"

It is the province of knowledge to speak and it is the privilege of wisdom to listen.
> *The Poet at the Breakfast Table,* Sect. X

Claude Bernard [1813–1878]

It is that which we do know which is the great hindrance to our learning that which we do not know.
> *An Introduction to the Study of Experimental Medicine*

Rudolf Virchow [1821–1902]

Humanism, therefore, is neither atheistic nor pantheistic, for it knows only one formula for everything lying beyond the bounds of knowledge: I do not know.
> *Disease, Life, and Man,* "On Man" (tr. by L. J. Rather)

Thomas Huxley [1825–1895]

Indeed, if a little knowledge is dangerous, where is the man who has so much as to be out of danger?
> *Collected Essays,* Vol. III, "On Elementary Instruction in Physiology"

S. Weir Mitchell [1829–1914]

The largest knowledge finds the largest excuses.

Cyrus Fogg Brackett [1833–1915]

Facts in books, statistics in encyclopedias, the ability to use them in men's heads!
> Quoted by Fred B. Rogers in *Help-Bringers*

Samuel Gee [1839–1911]

A comprehensive dogmatic system . . . requires the science systematized to be at a standstill, not to say dead. Knowl-

edge is a ferment, expanding on all sides so much and so rapidly as during the past hundred years, [and] must speedily burst the old bottle of any dogmatic system.
> *Medical Lectures,* Ch. 14

William Stewart Halsted [1852–1922]

We can hardly understand in these days that surgeons who were at the same time anatomists and physiologists could have accepted for so many centuries, almost without remonstrance, Galen's views. Our inability to comprehend their state of mind with reference to this problem illustrates particularly well the difficulty experienced when we attempt to transport ourselves to other times, to obtain the point of view which subjugated our forefathers of centuries ago. It is now, as it was then and as it may ever be; conceptions from the past blind us to facts which almost slap us in the face.
> *Surgical Papers,* Vol. II, "The Training of the Surgeon"

Sir Arthur Conan Doyle [1859–1930]

A man should keep his little brain attic stocked with all the furniture that he is likely to use, and the rest he can put away in the lumber-room of his library, where he can get it if he wants it.
> *The Adventures of Sherlock Holmes,* "Five Orange Pips"

Alfred North Whitehead [1861–1947]

Knowledge does not keep any better than fish.
> *The Aims of Education,* Sect. III, Ch. VII

Aristotle discovered all the half-truths which were necessary to the creation of science.
> *Dialogues,* Dialogue XLII, September 11, 1945

The doctrines which best repay critical examination are those which for the longest period have remained unquestioned.

Edward Archibald [1872–1945]

To gather knowledge and to find out new knowledge is the noblest occupation of the physician. To apply that knowledge . . . with sympathy born of understanding, to the relief of human suffering, is his loveliest occupation.

Wilfred Trotter [1872–1939]

All knowledge comes from noticing resemblances and recurrences in the events that happen around us.
> *Collected Works,* "Has the Intellect a Function?"

Martin H. Fischer [1879–1962]

Knowledge is a process of piling up facts; wisdom lies in their simplification.
> Quoted by Howard Fabing and Ray Marr in *Fischerisms*

Albert Szent-Györgyi [1893–   ]

Knowledge is a sacred cow, and my problem will be how we can milk her while keeping clear of her horns.
> *Science* 146:1278, 1964

Sir Robert Platt [1900–   ]

New knowledge is not generally very difficult to use. Those of us who lived and practised before the days of antibiotics and even of sulphonamides did not have to go back to the university to study organic chemistry or pharmacology in order to know how to use them.
> *British Medical Journal* 2:551, 1965

René J. Dubos [1901–   ]

Medical statesmanship cannot thrive only on scientific knowledge, because exact science cannot encompass all the

human factors involved in health and in disease. Knowledge and power may arise from dreams as well as from facts and logic. Utopias are often but the memory of Arcadias.
> *Mirage of Health,* Ch. VI

Anonymous

The forward sweep of medical science has brought a kind of "instant obsolescence" in medical knowledge.
> *Report of the President's Commission on Heart Disease, Cancer and Stroke,* Vol. II, Report of the Subcommittee on Communications

LAST WORDS

See also EPITAPHS

Socrates [470?–399 B.C.]

Crito, I owe a cock to Aesculapius; will you remember to pay the debt?
> Quoted by Plato in *Phaedo,* 118

Alexander the Great [356–323 B.C.]

I die by the help of too many physicians.
> Comment on his deathbed

Germanicus Caesar [15 B.C.–A.D. 19]

I end a life of consummate misery by a death most revolting.
> Comment on his deathbed in Antioch

Sir Thomas More [1478–1535]

Pluck up thy spirits, man, and be not afraid to do thine office. My neck is very short; take heed therefore thou strike not awry, for saving of thine honesty.[1]
> Comment to the executioner on the scaffold (Quoted by William Roper in *The Life of Sir Thomas More, Knight*)

[1] honesty = professional reputation.

Duc Anne de Montmorency [1493–1567]

Father, do you believe that a man who knew how to live for nearly eighty years with honor does not know how to die for a quarter of an hour?
> Comment while dying of a wound received at the battle of St. Dénis, November 11, 1567

François Rabelais [1494?–1553]

I am going to seek a great Perhaps.[1]
> Spoken about two days before his death

Sir Walter Raleigh [1552?–1618]

I thank my God heartily, that he hath brought me into the light to die, and hath not suffered me to die in the dark prison of the Tower.
> Speech on the scaffold, October 29, 1618

'Tis a sharp remedy, but a sure one for all ills. [Feeling the edge of the ax before his execution.]
> Quoted by David Hume in *The History of England,* Ch. 48

Thomas Hobbes [1588–1679]

I am about to take my last voyage, a great leap in the dark.
> Comment on his deathbed, December 4, 1679 (Quoted by John Watkins in *Anecdotes of Men of Learning*)

Oliver Cromwell [1599–1658]

My desire is to make what haste I may to be gone.

Sir Henry Vane [1613–1662]

Death is but a little word, but 'tis a great work to die.
> Speech on the scaffold (Quoted by John Willcock in *The Life of Sir Henry Vane the Younger,* Ch. 19)

[1] Je vais querir un grand *Peut-être.*

Charles II of England [1630–1685]

Let not poor Nelly [1] starve.
> Quoted by Bishop Gilbert Burnet in *History of His Own Time*, Bk. III

Louis XIV of France [1638–1715]

I have always heard that it is difficult to die; I who am on the brink of this moment, so dreaded by men, I do not find it so fearful.
> Comment on his deathbed to Madame de Maintenon

Cotton Mather [1663–1728]

Is this dying? Is this all? Is this all that I feared, when I prayed against a hard death? Oh, I can bear this! I can bear it! I can bear it!

Joseph Addison [1672–1719]

See in what peace a Christian can die.
> Comment to his stepson, Lord Warwick, June 17, 1719

George II of England [1683–1760]

Your eyes look like those of a calf that has just had its throat cut.
> To his wife, Caroline, at her deathbed, November 15, 1737

John Gay [1685–1732]

Where there is life, there's hope, he cry'd;
Then why such haste? so groan'd and dy'd.
> *Fables* (First Series), Fable 27

Alexander Pope [1688–1744]

Here am I dying of a hundred good symptoms.[2]
> Comment to George Lyttleton, May 15, 1744 (Quoted by Rev. Joseph Spence in *Anecdotes, Observations and Characters*, Sect. VIII)

[1] Nell Gwyn, his favorite mistress.
[2] Spence notes, "This was just after Dr. T. had been telling him that he was glad to find that he breathed so much easier; that his pulse was good; and several other encouraging things." Pope died on May 30.

Benjamin Franklin [1706–1790]

A dying man can do nothing easy.

Frederick II (the Great) of Prussia [1712–1786]

We are over the hill, we shall go better now.
> Quoted by Thomas Carlyle in *History of Frederick the Great*, Bk. XXI, Ch. 9

Jean Jacques Rousseau [1712–1778]

See how pure the sky is, there is not a single cloud. Don't you see that God is waiting for me?

William Hunter [1718–1783]

If I had the strength to hold a pen, I would write how easy and pleasant a thing it is to die.
> Quoted by S. R. Gloyne in *John Hunter*, Ch. 10

Oliver Goldsmith [1728–1774]

[When asked if his mind was at rest:] No, it is not.
> Quoted by James Prior in *Life of Oliver Goldsmith*, Vol. II, Ch. XXV

George Washington [1732–1799]

Doctor, I die hard, but I am not afraid to go.

Joseph II of Austria [1741–1790]

I would have engraven on my tomb, "Here lies a sovereign, who with the best intentions never carried a single project into execution."
> Quoted by William Coxe in *History of the House of Austria*, Vol. III, Ch. CXXX

Major John André [1751–1780]

It will be but a momentary pang.
> Last words on scaffold (Quoted by Alexander Hamilton in a letter to Henry Laurens, September 1780)

John Quincy Adams [1767–1848]

This is the last of earth! I am content!
> Comment on his deathbed,
> February 23, 1848

Maréchal Michel Ney [1769–1815]

Soldiers, aim straight at my heart!
> At his execution, December 7,
> 1815

John Keats [1792–1821]

O! I can feel the cold earth upon me
— the daisies growing over me — . . .
how long will this posthumous life of
mine last? [1]
> Quoted by Joseph Severn in a
> letter to John Taylor, March 6,
> 1821

Benjamin Disraeli, Lord Beaconsfield [1804–1881]

Mitchell Bruce, who with Sir Richard
Quain attended Lord Beaconsfield in
his last illness, told me that to the
end he was a little theatrical. "Let me
see," he said to his doctors, "the
bulletin which will delight or alarm
the British public to-morrow morning."
"I have suffered much," he said in
reply to some inquiry. "If I had been
a Nihilist I should have confessed all."
When the nurse came into the bedroom
with a bed-pan, he waved his hand,
and with a look of horror, exclaimed:
"No! No! take that away; it's too
like a pantomime."
> Quoted by Sir James Crichton-
> Browne in *The Doctor's After-
> Thoughts*

I had rather live, but I am not afraid
to die.
> Quoted by Moneypenny in *Life
> of Disraeli*, Bk. IV, Ch. XVI

Thomas (Stonewall) Jackson [1824–1863]

Let us cross over the river, and rest
under the shade of the trees.

Charles J. Guiteau [1841–1882]

Glory hallelujah! Glory hallelujah! I
am with the Lord! Glory, ready, go.[1]
> Last words on the scaffold, June
> 30, 1882

Cecil Rhodes [1853–1902]

So little done, so much to do.
> Comment made a few hours be-
> fore his death

Sir David Bruce [1855–1913]

If any notice is taken of my scientific
work when I am gone, I should like
it to be known that Mary [2] is entitled
to as much credit as I am.
> Quoted in *Annals of Internal
> Medicine* 115:351, 1965

Charles Frohman [1860–1915]

Why fear death? It is the most beautiful adventure in life.
> Comment before going down in
> the *Lusitania*, May 7, 1915

LEANNESS

See also BODY, OBESITY

William Shakespeare [1564–1616]

Yond Cassius has a lean and hungry
look;
He thinks too much. Such men are
dangerous.
> *Julius Caesar*, I, ii, 194

Tobias Venner [1577–1660]

Men of a lean habit of body are commonly a long time healthy, having good
appetites and strong stomachs for digestion.
> *Via recta ad vitam longam*

---

[1] Keats spoke these words to his friend
Severn four days prior to his death on
February 23, 1821.

[1] Guiteau, the assassin of President James
A. Garfield, also read on the scaffold a
poem he had composed for the occasion.
[2] His wife.

Anthelme Brillat-Savarin
[1755–1826]

For women, however, it is a frightful
evil, for with them beauty is more
than life, and beauty consists especially in the roundness of limbs and
figure, in the gracefully curved out-
lines.
>*La Physiologie du Goût*, Ch. 23
>(tr. by R. E. Anderson as *Gas-*
>*tronomy as a Fine Art*)

Welsh Proverb

Thin women live long.

LEARNING

See also EDUCATION, KNOWL-
EDGE, LOGIC, TEACHING,
WISDOM

Confucius [551–478 B.C.]

Learning without thinking is useless.
Thinking without learning is dangerous.
>*Analects*, Bk. II, Ch. XV (tr.
>by William E. Soothill)

Epictetus [60?–120?]

It is impossible for any one to begin
to learn what he thinks he already
knows.
>*Discourses*, II.xvii (tr. by E.
>Carter)

Sir Francis Bacon [1561–1626]

Learning . . . disposeth the constitution of the mind not to be fixed or
settled in the defects thereof, but still
to be capable and susceptible of growth
and reformation.
>*The Advancement of Learning*,
>Bk. I

John Hunter [1728–1793]

Man is born or comes into the world
ignorant; but he is furnished with the
senses, so as to be impressed with the
properties of things; by which means
he gradually, of himself, acquires a
degree of knowledge. But Man goes
farther, he has the power of receiving
information of things that never impressed his senses; and, if he has that
power, it is natural to suppose that
one Man has the power of communi-
cating his knowledge of things to another, each giving and receiving recip-
rocally; which we find to be the case.
>*Essays and Observations*, Vol.
>I, "Introduction to Natural
>History"

William Lamb, Lord Melbourne
[1779–1848]

Nobody ever learns anything by experience; everybody does the same
thing over and over again.
>Quoted by David Cecil in *The*
>*Young Melbourne*, Ch. IX

Peter Mere Latham [1789–1875]

People do not come to read by being
taught the philosophy of reading, but
simply by doing the thing itself, simply
by reading.
>*Collected Works*, Vol. II, "A
>Word or Two on Medical Ed-
>ucation"

Oliver Wendell Holmes
[1809–1894]

The easiest and surest way of acquiring
facts is to learn them in groups, in
systems, and systematized knowledge
is science. You can very often carry
two facts fastened together more
easily than one by itself, as a house-
maid can carry two pails of water with
a hoop more easily than one without
it.
>*Medical Essays*, "Scholastic and
>Bedside Teaching"

Jean Martin Charcot [1825–1893]

Why do we have to go over the same
set of symptoms twenty times before

we understand them? Why does the first statement of a new fact always leave us cold? Because our minds have to take in something which deranges our original set of ideas, but we are all like that in this miserable world.

Joseph, Lord Lister [1827–1912]

You must always be students, learning and unlearning till your life's end, and if, gentlemen, you are not prepared to follow your profession in this spirit, I implore you to leave its ranks and betake yourself to some third-class trade.

Sir William Osler [1849–1919]

That man can interrogate as well as observe nature was a lesson slowly learned in his evolution.
> *Transactions of the Congress of American Physicians and Surgeons* 7:1, 1907

It is always best to do a thing wrong the first time.
> Comment as he showed a medical student the correct way to perform an autopsy

Charles H. Mayo [1865–1939]

Once you start studying medicine you never get through with it.
> *University of Toronto Medical Journal*, April 1928

Martin H. Fischer [1879–1962]

It is not hard to learn more. What is hard is to unlearn when you discover yourself wrong.
> Quoted by Howard Fabing and Ray Marr in *Fischerisms*

David Seegal [1899–   ]

"The way to learn is to teach" is a cliché which is far from threadbare. It may be that the way to learn doubly is to teach the student not only to learn but to teach.
> *Journal of Medical Education* 39:1030, 1964

Carl Sagan [1934–   ]

It is of interest to note that while some dolphins are reported to have learned English — up to 50 words used in correct context — no human has been reported to have learned dolphinese.
> *The Christian Science Monitor*, November 15, 1965

LECTURE

See also EDUCATION, TEACHING

Hippocrates [460?–377? B.C.]

If for the sake of a crowded audience you do wish to hold a lecture, your ambition is no laudable one, and at least avoid all citations from the poets, for to quote them argues feeble industry.
> *Precepts*, XII (tr. by W. H. S. Jones)

Samuel Johnson [1709–1784]

Lectures were once useful; but now, when all can read, and books are so numerous, lectures are unnecessary.
> Quoted by James Boswell in *Life of Samuel Johnson*, April 15, 1781

Peter Mere Latham [1789–1875]

Lectures . . . are a temptation to the more contemplative mind to learn diseases by the study of models, rather than of the things themselves. They tend to divorce him from the workshop and the chips and fragments and rude designs that lie about within it, and introduce him into a room swept and garnished and hung round with masterpieces for his contemplation. This may be all very well for gentlemen who patronise the arts; but this is not the way to make the artist.
> *Collected Works*, Vol. II, "A Word or Two on Medical Education"

Oliver Wendell Holmes
[1809-1894]

My terms for a lecture where I stay over night are these: Fifteen dollars and my expenses; a room with a fire in it in a public house, and a mattress to sleep on, not a feather bed. As you write in your individual capacity I tell you at once all my habitual exigencies. I am afraid to sleep in a cold room, I can't sleep on a feather bed, I will not go to private houses, and I have figured on the sum mentioned as what it is worth to *me* to go away for the night to places that can not pay more.
> Letter to J. W. Porter, October 1852

Clark L. Hull [1884-1952]

His mind could scintillate in a brilliant fashion, but his approach to psychology was largely qualitative and literary. . . . He would sometimes lecture for five minutes at a time in perfectly good sentences, yet hardly say a thing.[1]
> *A History of Psychology in Autobiography*, Vol. IV, Ch. 7

Dickinson W. Richards
[1895-   ]

For our students, we have thrown the lecture into outer darkness, as an outworn remnant of an earlier pedagogic era; but for ourselves, we teachers continue to lecture to each other, almost incessantly. We dash all around the country, indeed half way around the world, winter and summer, spring and fall, leaving our appointed tasks — such as teaching students — and when we get there, what do we do? We sit down and listen to lectures, or, worse still, we stand up and give them.
> *Transactions of the American Clinical and Climatological Association* 65:91, 1953

[1] Referring to Joseph Jastrow [1863-1944], professor at the University of Wisconsin.

Anonymous

When two or three are gathered together, someone is sure to wish to lecture.

LEFT-HANDEDNESS

See HAND

LEPROSY

William Shakespeare [1564-1616]
> Itches, blains,
> Sow all th' Athenian bosoms, and their crop
> Be general leprosy!
> *Timon of Athens*, IV, i, 28

> This yellow slave [gold]
> Will . . .
> Make the hoar leprosy ador'd.
> *Ibid.*, IV, iii, 33

Paul W. Brand [1914-   ]

The greatest danger now is that we, who previously did nothing because we thought nothing could be done, will now do nothing because the little we can do seems so small compared with the size of the problem.
> *Rehabilitation Literature* 21: 238, 1960, "Life After Leprosy Through Rehabilitation"

The Bible

The leper in whom the plague is, his clothes shall be rent, and his head bare, and he shall put a covering upon his upper lip, and shall cry, Unclean, unclean.
> *Leviticus* 13:45

Jesus put forth his hand, and touched him, saying, . . . be thou clean. And immediately his leprosy was cleansed.
> *Matthew* 8:3

LIBRARIES

See also LITERATURE, READING

John Morgan [1735–1789]

The establishment of a medical library in this college [1] would prove another great benefit to students, and tend likewise to influence their resort hither.
> *A Discourse Upon the Institution of Medical Schools in America*

Sir William Osler [1849–1919]

For the general practitioner a well-used library is one of the few correctives of the premature senility which is so apt to overtake him.
> *Aequanimitas, with Other Addresses,* "Books and Men"

Santiago Ramón y Cajal [1852–1934]

Libraries are successively the cradles and the sepulchres of the human mind.
> *Charlas de Café*

Anonymous

Healing-place of the Soul.
> Inscription on the library at Thebes

Food for the soul.[2]
> Inscription on the State Library at Berlin

LIFE

See also LIFE AND DEATH, LONGEVITY, MAN

Huang Ti (The Yellow Emperor) [2697–2597 B.C.]

Man draws life from Earth, but his

---

[1] The University of Pennsylvania, which had the first medical school in the United States.
[2] Nutrimentum spiritus.

fate depends upon Heaven. Heaven and Earth unite to bestow life-giving vigor as well as destiny upon man.
> *Nei Ching Su Wên,* Bk. 8, Sect. 25 (tr. by Ilza Veith in *The Yellow Emperor's Classic of Internal Medicine*)

Lao-tzu [604–531 B.C.]

Those who flow as life flows know
They need no other force:
They feel no wear, they feel no tear,
They need no mending, no repair.
> *The Way of Life* (tr. by Witter Bynner)

Herodotus [484–424 B.C.]

Misfortunes falling upon us and diseases disturbing our happiness make the time of life, though short indeed, seem long.
> *Histories,* VII.xlvi (tr. by Thomas Babington Macaulay)

Martial [fl. 1st Cent.)

In narrow means 'tis easy to despise life; he acts the strong man who is wretched and can endure.
> *Epigrams,* XI.56 (tr. by W. C. A. Ker)

Marcus Aurelius [121–180]

Altogether the interval is small (between birth and death); and consider with how much trouble, and in company with what sort of people, and in what a feeble body this interval is laboriously passed.
> *Meditations,* IV.50 (tr. by G. Long)

Leonardo da Vinci [1452–1519]

Movement is the cause of all life.
> Manuscript H, Library of the Institut de France (tr. by Edward MacCurdy in *The Notebooks of Leonardo da Vinci,* Vol. I, Ch. I)

William Harvey [1578–1657]

Ex ovo omnia.[1]
[All out of the egg.]
> *De Generatione* (1651), legend
> to title-page illustration

Abraham Cowley [1618–1667]

Life is an incurable Disease.
> *Pindarique Odes,* "To Dr.
> Scarborough," VI

Alexander Pope [1688–1744]

This long disease, my Life.
> *Epistle to Dr. Arbuthnot*

Samuel Johnson [1709–1784]

Surely life, if it be not long, is tedious,
since we are forced to call in the assistance of so many trifles to rid us of
our time, of that time which never can
return.
> Letter to Joseph Baretti, June
> 10, 1761

Human life is every where a state in
which much is to be endured, and
little to be enjoyed.
> *Rasselas,* Ch. XI

Jean Jacques Rousseau
[1712–1778]

Teach him to live rather than to avoid
death: life is not breath, but action,
the use of our senses, our mind, our
faculties, every part of ourselves which
makes us conscious of our being.
> *Émile,* Bk. I (tr. by Barbara
> Foxley)

Thomas Jefferson [1743–1826]

Life is of no value but as it brings us
gratifications. Among the most valuable of these is rational society. It informs the mind, sweetens the temper,
chears our spirits, and promotes health.
> Letter to James Madison, Feb-
> ruary 20, 1784

[1] Commonly misquoted since Wahlbom
wrote in 1746, "Harvey also long ago exclaimed *omne vivum ex ovo.*"

Peter Mere Latham [1789–1875]

It is often only when the powers of
medicine are pressed even to the verge
of destroying life, that life is saved.
> *Diseases of the Heart,* Lect. X

Life is only known as the complex of
many functions, and health as the integrity of these functions, each in itself, and their harmony among others.
> *General Remarks on the Prac-
> tice of Medicine,* Ch. XI

It is the great mystery of life itself
which is at the bottom of all the mysterious language we are obliged to
employ concerning it.
> *Ibid.,* Ch. XVI

Emile Deschamps [1791–1871]

That long and cruel malady which one
calls life.

Madame Jean Joseph Pasteur
[d. 1848]

Whatever happens to you, do not
grieve; nothing in life is more than a
chimera.
> Letter to her son Louis, Janu-
> ary 1, 1848

Thomas Lovell Beddoes
[1803–1849]

> If man could see
The perils and diseases that he elbows,
Each day he walks a mile; which catch
> at him,
Which fall behind and graze him as he
> passes;
Then would he know that Life's a
> single pilgrim,
Fighting unarmed amongst a thousand
> soldiers.
> *Death's Jest-Book,* Act IV,
> Sc. i

Oliver Wendell Holmes
[1809–1894]

Life is a fatal complaint, and an emi-
nently contagious one.
> *The Poet at the Breakfast
> Table,* Sect. XII

Claude Bernard [1813–1878]

If I had to define life in a single phrase, I should clearly express my thought by throwing into relief the one characteristic which, in my opinion, sharply differentiates biological science. I should say: life is creation.
An Introduction to the Study of Experimental Medicine, Pt. II, Ch. 2, Sect. i (tr. by H. C. Greene)

Sören Kierkegaard [1813–1855]

It is probably true, as philosophers say, that life must be understood backwards. But they forget the other proposition, that it must be lived forwards.
Journal

Herbert Spencer [1820–1903]

A living thing is distinguished from a dead thing by the multiplicity of the changes at any moment taking place in it.
Principles of Biology, Pt. I, Ch. 4, Sect. 25

Matthew Arnold [1822–1888]

This strange disease of modern life,
With its sick hurry, its divided aims.
The Scholar Gipsy

Samuel Butler [1835–1902]

Life is one long process of getting tired.
Note-Books, Ch. I, "Life"

William James [1842–1910]

For my own part, I do not know what the sweat and blood and tragedy of this life mean, if they mean anything short of this. If this life be not a real fight, in which something is eternally gained for the universe by success, it is no better than a game of private theatricals, from which one may withdraw at will. But it *feels* like a real fight, — as if there were something really wild in the universe which we, with all our idealities and faithfulnesses, are needed to redeem; and first of all to redeem our own hearts from atheisms and fears.
The Will to Believe and Other Papers, "Is Life Worth Living?"

Be not afraid of life. Believe that life *is* worth living, and your belief will help create the fact.
Idem

Robert Bridges [1844–1930]

Man's life is not the ease that a peace-loving generation has found it or thought to make it, but the awful conflict with evil which philosophers and saints have depicted.
The Spirit of Man, Preface

Friedrich Nietzsche [1844–1900]

He who has a *why* to live can bear with almost any *how*.
Twilight of the Idols, "Maxims and Missiles," 12

Manuel Acuna [1849–1873]

Life is a circle, and when measuring it
We do wrong in assigning to it
The cradle and the sepulcher for extremes.

For at the end of this transitory existence,
To which our anxiety so much adheres,
Matter, immortal as glory,
Changes in forms, but never can die.
Before a Corpse (tr. by E. S. Green and H. Von Lowenfels)

Sir William Osler [1849–1919]

While change is the law, certain great ideas flow fresh through the ages, and control us effectually as in the days of Pericles. Mankind, it has been said, is always advancing, man is always the same. The love, hope, fear and faith that make humanity, and the elemental passions of the human heart, remain unchanged, and the secret of inspiration in any literature is the capacity to touch the cord that vibrates in a sympathy that knows not time nor place.

The quiet life in day-tight compartments will help you to bear your own and others' burdens with a light heart. Pay no heed to the Batrachians who sit croaking idly by the stream. Life is a straight, plain business, and the way is clear, blazed for you by generations of strong men, into whose labours you enter and whose ideals must be your inspiration.

A Way of Life

Sigmund Freud [1856–1939]

It is the eternal changefulness of life that makes it so beautiful.

George Bernard Shaw [1856–1950]

Life is a disease; and the only difference between one man and another is the stage of the disease at which he lives.

Back to Methuselah, Pt. II, "Gospel of the Brothers Barnabas"

Jules Laforgue [1860–1887]

Oh, how daily life is! [1]

Les Complaintes, "Complainte sur certains ennuis"

George Santayana [1863–1952]

Sanity is a madness put to good uses; waking life is a dream controlled.

Interpretations of Poetry and Religion, Ch. X

Sir Andrew MacPhail [1864–1938]

Life and art become mean, poor, and debased when they lack control by some principle of unity. Life is never mean when it is lived at the proper level; and there is no poverty where there is no pretence. The soldier in his hut, the priest in his cubicle, the family in the cottage — none of these are poor so long as they live in subordination to their essential idea. They are artists seeking to express themselves with not how much but with how little.

The Master's Wife, Ch. 10

[1] Ah, que la vie est quotidienne!

Paul Valéry [1871–1945]

You must live as you think. If not, sooner or later you end up by thinking as you have lived.

Thomas Mann [1875–1955]

What then was life? It was warmth, the warmth generated by a form-preserving instability, a fever of matter, which accompanied the process of ceaseless decay and repair of albumen molecules that were too impossibly complicated, too impossibly ingenious in structure. It was the existence of the actually impossible-to-exist, of a half-sweet, half-painful balancing, or scarcely balancing, in this restricted and feverish process of decay and renewal, upon the point of existence. It was not matter and it was not spirit, but something between the two, a phenomenon conveyed by matter, like the rainbow on the waterfall, and like the flame.

The Magic Mountain, Ch. V, "Research" (tr. by H. T. Lowe-Porter)

What was life? No one knew. No one knew the actual point whence it sprang, where it kindled itself. Nothing in the domain of life seemed uncausated, or insufficiently causated, from that point on; but life itself seemed without antecedent. If there was anything that might be said about it, it was this: it must be so highly developed, structurally, that nothing even distantly related to it was present in the inorganic world. Between the protean amoeba and the vertebrate the difference was slight, unessential, as compared to that between the simplest living organism and that nature which did not even deserve to be called dead, because it was inorganic. For death was only the logical negation of life; but between life and inanimate nature yawned a gulf which research strove in vain to bridge.

Idem

Albert Schweitzer [1875–1965]

At the very moment when, at sunset, we were making our way through a herd of hippopotamuses, there flashed upon my mind, unforeseen and unsought, the phrase, "Reverence for Life." The iron door had yielded: the path in the thicket had become visible.
Out of My Life and Thought, Ch. 13 (tr. by C. T. Campion)

As in my will-to-live there is ardent desire for further life and for the mysterious exaltation of the will-to-live which we call pleasure, while there is fear of destruction and of that mysterious depreciation of the will-to-live which we call pain: so too are these in the will-to-live around me, whether it can express itself to me, or remains dumb. . . . The man who has become a thinking being feels a compulsion to give to every will-to-live the same reverence for life that he gives to his own. He experiences that other life in his own. He accepts as being good: to preserve life, to promote life, to raise to its highest value life which is capable of development; and as being evil: to destroy life, to injure life, to repress life which is capable of development.
Idem

The purpose of human life is to serve and to show compassion and the will to help others.
The Schweitzer Album

Austen Fox Riggs [1876–1940]

Worry is a complete circle of inefficient thought whirling about a pivot of fear. Accept the material of life. Do not criticize your part in the play. Study it, understand it, and then play it, sick or well, rich or poor, with courage, and with proper grace.
Notebooks

Otto Weininger [1880–1903]

He who is tired of life, for whom life has ceased to be of interest, is interesting to no one.
Sex and Character, Pt. II, Ch. 5

Sinclair Lewis [1885–1951]

Whether my life was happening to me or to somebody else.

Victor Robinson [1886–1947]

Life is a great experiment in physiology, in which we all take part; the unknown holds the protocols, and Death writes the conclusions. We do not know where the experiment is tending, nor can we control the outcome. There are gates we cannot open, and impassable roads without a guide-post.
Letter

Albert Szent-Györgyi [1893–   ]

What drives life is thus a little electric current, kept up by the sunshine. All the complexities of intermediary metabolism are but the lacework around this basic fact.
Introduction to Submolecular Biology, Ch. 3

Homer W. Smith [1895–1962]

If [man] wishes to know where life begins and ends, then he must study it, see how it works and what it is. Perhaps the perfect knowledge . . . may never come to him, for the stream of life may shift to some other bed before that time, and leave him a blind alley.
Kamongo, Ch. VI

Life is like a whirlpool in many ways. . . . When once set a-going it spins on and on. . . . In that tendency to spin on for ever there is life's purpose — to go on living.
Ibid., Ch. VII

Must we for ever be like children, seeking purpose in the fall of the rain, in the sweep of the wind, in the strike of the lightning! Why must we always

seek it in ourselves? . . . No, your life has no more purpose than that of any other beast. . . . It has no purpose except as you choose to give it one. I give you, in the very nature of life itself, in the momentum that keeps it spinning on its course, an unquenchable instinct for self-determination — if you wish to call it that; and in the flesh which life accumulates around itself I give you the capacity to learn by experience and to test your knowledge by experiment. Is that not enough? . . . But I cannot give you any personal, predetermined significance. You are only a branch of the stream that is flowing on, resisting the world about it, trying.
Ibid., Ch. VIII

René J. Dubos [1901–   ]

Complete freedom from disease . . . is almost incompatible with the process of living.
Mirage of Health, Ch. I

Louis Lasagna [1923–   ]

It would seem important to devote more of the energies of man to improving the quality of life, so that it may be joyous, or noble, or creative. Otherwise, existence is nothing but the bored molecular unwinding of a dismal biological clock. Should life be longer than it is? Yes — if it has charm, grace, purpose, or productivity. But what if it is empty, sullen, frustrated, ignoble? One can weep for the death of Christ or Schubert, but surely not for the end of Caligula or Hitler.
The Doctors' Dilemmas, Epilogue

Leston L. Havens [1924–   ]

The slow compromise, or even surrender, of our fondest hopes is a regular feature of normal human life.
New England Journal of Medicine 272:401, 1965

Persian Proverb

Life is a perpetual drunkenness — the pleasure passes, but the headache remains.

LIFE AND DEATH

See also BIRTH AND DEATH, DEATH, LIFE, SLEEP AND DEATH

Seneca [4? B.C.–A.D. 65]

Why is it surprising that a man should die when his whole life is nothing but a journey towards death?
Epistles, "To Polybius on Consolation," XI (tr. by J. W. Basore)

Before I became old I tried to live well; now that I am old, I shall try to die well; but dying well means dying gladly.
Moral Epistles to Lucilius, LXI (tr. by Richard M. Gummere)

Marcus Aurelius [121–180]

The act of dying too is one of the acts of life.
Meditations, VI.2 (tr. by C. R. Haines)

Leonardo da Vinci [1452–1519]

While I thought that I was learning how to live, I have been learning how to die.
Codice Atlantico, 252 (tr. by Edward MacCurdy in *The Notebooks of Leonardo da Vinci*, Vol. I, Ch. I)

Elizabeth I of England [1533–1603]

As for me, I assure you I find no great cause I should be fond to live. I take no such pleasure in it that I should

much wish it, nor conceive such terror in death that I should greatly fear it.[1]
> Speech to Parliament, November 24, 1586

Michel de Montaigne [1533–1592]

He who would teach men to die would teach them to live.
> *Essays*, Bk. I, Ch. 20, "That to Philosophize Is to Learn to Die" (tr. by Donald M. Frame)

William Shakespeare [1564–1616]

CLAUDIO: I have hope to live, and am prepar'd to die.
DUKE: Be absolute for death. Either death or life
Shall thereby be the sweeter.
> *Measure for Measure*, III, i, 4

Sir Thomas Browne [1605–1682]

The long habit of living indisposeth us for dying.
> *Urne-Buriall*, Ch. V

John Dryden [1631–1700]

Ev'ry Man who lives, is born to die,
And none can boast Sincere felicity.
With equal Mind, what happens, let us bear,
Nor joy, nor grieve too much for Things beyond our Care.
Like Pilgrims, to th' appointed Place we tend;
The World's an Inn, and Death the Journeys End.
> *Fables Ancient and Modern*, "Palamon and Arcite," Bk. III

Bishop Thomas Ken [1637–1711]

Teach me to live, that I may dread
The grave as little as my bed.
> *An Evening Hymn*

[1] This version is found in the British Museum, Lansdowne MS. 94, fol. 87, a printed text heavily amended in the Queen's hand. Another version of the quote is reported in William Camden's *Annals:* "As for me, I see no such great reason why I should either be fond to live, or fear to die."

Jean de La Bruyère [1645–1696]

There are but three events which concern man: birth, life, and death. They are unconscious of their birth, they suffer when they die, and they neglect to live.
> *Characters*, "Of Mankind" (tr. by Henri van Laun)

François de La Mothe-Fénelon [1651–1715]

Do not men die fast enough, without being destroyed by each other? Can any man be insensible of the brevity of life; and can he who knows it, think life too long?
> *Telemachus*, Bk. VII (VIII as tr. by John Hawkesworth)

Matthew Prior [1664–1721]

Life an ill whose only cure is death.
> *Epistle to Dr. Sherlock*

Joseph Addison [1672–1719]

The Preservation of Life should be only a secondary Concern, and the Direction of it our Principal. If we have this Frame of Mind, we shall take the best Means to preserve Life, without being over-sollicitous about the Event; and shall arrive at that Point of Felicity which *Martial* has mentioned as the Perfection of Happiness, of neither fearing nor wishing for Death.
> *The Spectator*, Vol. I, No. 25 (March 29, 1711)

Nicholas Rowe [1674–1718]

Death is the Privilege of human Nature,
And Life without it were not worth our taking.
> *The Fair Penitent*, Act V, Sc. i

Thomas Tickell [1686–1740]

There taught us how to live; and (oh! too high

The price for knowledge) taught us
   how to die.[1]
      To the Earl of Warwick, on the
      Death of Mr. Addison

Alexander Pope [1688–1744]

Oh let me live my own, and die so too!
(To live and die is all I have to do.)
      Epistle to Dr. Arbuthnot

Samuel Johnson [1709–1784]

Thus, not only in the slumber of sloth,
but in the dissipation of ill-directed
industry, is the shortness of life generally forgotten. As some men lose
their hours in laziness, because they
suppose, that there is time enough for
the reparation of neglect; others busy
themselves in providing that no length
of life may want employment; and it
often happens, that sluggishness and
activity are equally surprised by the
last summons, and perish not more
differently from each other, than the
fowl that received the shot in her
flight, from her that is killed upon
the bush.
      The Rambler, No. 71 (Novem-
      ber 20, 1750)

James Montgomery [1771–1854]

'Tis not the whole of life to live,
Nor all of death to die.

Heinrich Heine [1797–1856]

Death — it is still, cold night;
   Life — it is sultry day.
      Der Tod das ist die kühle Nacht
      (tr. by M. M. Bozman)

Elizabeth Barrett Browning
[1806–1861]

Knowledge by suffering entereth;
And Life is perfected by Death.
      A Vision of Poets

[1] Cf. Joseph Addison, p. 258a.

Alfred, Lord Tennyson
[1809–1892]

No life that breathes with human
   breath
Has ever truly long'd for death.
      The Two Voices

Robert Browning [1812–1889]

A man can have but one life and one
   death,
One heaven, one hell.
      In a Balcony

Giuseppe Verdi [1813–1901]

After all, death is all there is in life.
What else is there?
      Quoted by George Martin in
      Verdi, His Music, Life and
      Times

Herman Melville [1819–1891]

Born in throes, 't is fit that man should
live in pains and die in pangs!
      Moby Dick, Ch. 99

Edward H. Parker [1823–1896]

Life's race well run,
Life's work all done,
Life's victory won;
   Now cometh rest.
      New York Observer, May 13,
      1880

**Edward Bulwer-Lytton ("Owen
Meredith")** [1831–1891]

There's nothing certain in man's life
   but this:
That he must lose it.
      Clytemnestra, Pt. XX

Edwin Booth [1833–1893]

Why do not you look at this miserable
little life, with all its ups and downs,
as I do? At the very worst, 'tis but
a scratch, a temporary ill, to be soon
cured by that dear old doctor, Death

— who gives us a life more healthful and enduring than all the physicians, temporal or spiritual, can give.

Letter to William Winter, 1886

Samuel Butler [1835–1902]

The Erewhonians, therefore, hold that death, like life, is an affair of being more frightened than hurt.

Erewhon, Ch. XIII

The dead are often just as living to us as the living are, only we cannot get them to believe it. They can come to us, but till we die we cannot go to them. To be dead is to be unable to understand that one is alive.

Note-Books, Ch. XXIII

Henry van Dyke [1852–1933]

Many people are so afraid to die that they never begin to live.

Theodore Roosevelt [1858–1919]

No man has a right to live who has not in his soul the power to die nobly for a great cause.

Fear God and Take Your Own Part, Ch. IV

Sir Walter Langdon-Brown [1870–1946]

We may say then that death has been evolved for the good of the race, to remove worn out structures in favour of more active ones. And death being thus merely the servant of life, life ultimately attains the mastery over death.

Thus We Are Men, Pt. III, Ch. V

Marcel Proust [1871–1922]

Let an illness, a duel, a runaway horse make us see death face to face, how richly we should have enjoyed the life of pleasure, the travels in unknown lands which are about to be snatched from us. And no sooner is the danger past than what we find once again before us is the same dull life in which none of those delights had any existence for us.

The Sweet Cheat Gone, Ch. 1 (tr. by C. K. Scott-Moncrieff)

Oliver St. John Gogarty [1878–1957]

It adds a pleasant tang to life to know that it is fleeting. If I may be forgiven for employing a medical term: Death is Life's astringent.

Tumbling in the Hay, Ch. 6

Anonymous

Be happy while y'er leevin,
For y'er a lang time deid.

Scottish motto (Quoted in *Notes and Queries,* Series IX, No. 206, p. 469)

Life is a railway, the years are the stations, death the terminus, and doctors — the stokers.

The art of living consists of dying young — but as late as possible!

Time flies, and will not return. The wings of Man's life are plumed with the feathers of death.

From a petition addressed to Elizabeth I of England by a seaman, ca. 1587

French Proverbs

One dies of what another lives by.

We come and cry, and that is life; we cry and go, and that is death.

Latin Proverb

Live your own life, for you will die your own death.

Yiddish Proverb

Ever since dying came into fashion, life hasn't been safe.

LITERATURE

See also LIBRARIES, READ-
ING, WRITING

Hippocrates [460?–377? B.C.]

The power, too, to study correctly
what has been written I consider to
be an important part of the art of
medicine.
> *Epidemics,* III.XVI (tr. by
> W. H. S. Jones)

Sir Thomas Browne [1605–1682]

'T is not a melancholy *utinam* of my
own, but the desires of better heads,
that there were a general synod . . .
for the benefit of learning, to reduce
it, as it lay at first, in a few and solid
authors; and to condemn to the fire
those swarms and millions of rhapsodies, begotten only to distract and
abuse the weaker judgements of scholars, and to maintain the trade and
mystery of typographers.
> *Religio Medici,* Pt. I, Sect. 24

Alexander Pope [1688–1744]

Index learning turns no student pale,
Yet holds the eel of science by the tail.
> *The Dunciad,* Bk. I

René Laënnec [1781–1826]

I risked my life, but the book I am
going to publish will be, I hope, useful enough sooner or later to be worth
the life of a man.
> *De l'auscultation médiate,* Pref-
> ace

Peter Mere Latham [1789–1875]

A bad book is generally a very easy
book, having been composed by its
author with no labour of mind whatever; whereas a good book, though it
be not necessarily a hard one, yet,
since it contains important facts, duly
arranged, and reasoned upon with
care, must require from the reader
some portion of the same attention
and study to comprehend and profit by
it, as it required from the writer to
compose it.
> *Lectures on Clinical Medicine,*
> Lect. III

Never read any book that bears internal marks of being addressed more
to the public than to the profession.
They are all bad, and many dishonest.
> *Idem*

Karl F. H. Marx [1796–1877]

If an author's books die with him, it
shows them to be parasites, which
survived only through him, with no
independent life of their own.
> Quoted by F. H. Garrison in
> *Bulletin of the New York Acad-
> emy of Medicine* 4:1001, 1928

Edward Bulwer-Lytton
[1803–1873]

In science, read, by preference, the
newest works; in literature, the oldest.
> *Caxtoniana,* Essay X

Oliver Wendell Holmes
[1809–1894]

There is a dead medical literature,
and there is a live one. The dead is
not all ancient, the live is not all
modern. There is none, modern or
ancient, which, if it has no living
value for the student, will not teach
him something by its autopsy.
> *Medical Essays,* "Medical Li-
> braries"

The remarkable Discourse of Dr. Jacob
Bigelow upon Self-Limited Diseases
. . . has, I believe, done more than
any other work or essay in our own
language to rescue the practice of
medicine from the slavery to the drugging system which was a part of the
inheritance of the profession.
> *Ibid.,* "Some of My Early
> Teachers"

Sir William T. Gairdner
[1824–1907]

On various occasions it has happened to me, upon becoming interested in some particular subject, to find out from Dr. Billings' catalogue that I had written something on the subject twenty years before which had entirely escaped my memory.

> *Transactions of the Association of American Physicians* 6:257, 1891

Count Leo Tolstoy [1828–1910]

Printing, which is unquestionably useful for the vast masses of the little educated, has in the midst of the well-to-do people for a long time served as the chief instrument for the diffusion of ignorance, and not of enlightenment.

> Introduction to Wilhelm von Polenz's *Der Buttnerbauer* (tr. by Leo Weiner)

John Shaw Billings [1838–1913]

In medical literature, as in other departments, we find books and papers from men who are either constitutionally incapable of telling the simple literal truth as to their observations and experiments, although they may not write with fixed intention to deceive, or from men who seek to advertise themselves by deliberate falsehoods as to the results of their practice.

> *Our Medical Literature*

There is a vast amount of this effete and worthless material in the literature of medicine, and it is increasing rapidly. . . . our preparers of compilations and compendiums, big and little, acknowledged or not, are continually increasing the collection, and for the most part with material which has been characterized as "superlatively middling, the quintessential extract of mediocrity."

> *Idem*

Nine-tenths at least, of it, becomes worthless, and of no interest within ten years after the date of its publication, and much of it is so when it first appears.

> *Transactions of the Association of American Physicians* 2:57, 1887

They [indexers] have to handle much rubbish, for the proportion of what is both new and true is not much greater in medicine than it is in theology.

> *Ibid.*, 6:251, 1891

This probably is the last volume of the Index-Catalogue which will be issued under my personal supervision, and, in closing the work, I can only say that it has been to me a "labor of love." [1]

> *Index Catalogue of the Library of the Surgeon-General's Office* 16:v, 1895

Henry P. Bowditch [1840–1911]

The accumulated literature in every department of science is already so enormous and is increasing at such a rapid rate that any association or individual undertaking to contribute thereto should do so only under a sense of grave moral responsibility.

> *Proceedings of the American Association for the Advancement of Science* 35:237, 1887

Sir William Osler [1849–1919]

Let the old men read new books; you read the journals and the old books. . . . As a teacher you can never get *orientirt* without a knowledge of the Fathers, ancient and modern. And do not forget, above all things, the famous advice to Blackmore, to whom, when he first began the study of physic, and asked what books he should read, Sydenham replied, *Don Quixote*, mean-

[1] At a banquet in honor of Billings in 1895, Jacob M. Da Costa remarked, "This seems the most extraordinary pathologic development of the amorous instinct on record."

ing thereby, as I take it, that the only book of physic suitable for permanent reading is the book of Nature.

> *Aequanimitas, with Other Addresses,* "Internal Medicine as a Vocation"

What should attract us all is the study of the growth of the American mind in medicine since the starting of the colonies. As in a mirror this story is reflected in the literature of which you are the guardians and collectors — in letters, in manuscripts, in pamphlets, in books, and in journals. In the eight generations which have passed, the men who have striven and struggled . . . have made us what we are. With the irrevocable past into which they have gone lies our future, since our condition is the resultant of forces which, in these generations, have moulded the profession of a new and mighty empire.

> *Ibid.,* "Some Aspects of American Medical Bibliography"

It is much simpler to buy books than to read them, and easier to read them than to absorb their contents.

> *British Medical Journal* 2:925, 1909

William H. Welch [1850–1934]

I question whether America has made any larger contribution to medicine than that made by Dr. Billings in building up and developing the surgeon-general's library and in the publication of the Index Catalogue and the Index Medicus. That in my judgment is our greatest contribution to medicine, and we owe it to this extraordinary man.

> *Bulletin of the Johns Hopkins Hospital* 25:244, 1914

John Newport Langley [1852–1925]

Those who have occasion to enter into the depths of what is oddly, if generously, called the literature of a scientific subject, alone know the difficulty of emerging with an unsoured disposition. The multitudinous facts presented by each corner of Nature form in large part the scientific man's burden to-day, and restrict him more and more, willy-nilly, to a narrower and narrower specialism. But that is not the whole of his burden. Much that he is forced to read consists of records of defective experiments, confused statements of results, wearisome description of detail, and unnecessarily protracted discussion of unnecessary hypotheses. The publication of such matter is a serious injury to the man of science; it absorbs the scanty funds of his libraries, and steals away his poor hours of leisure.

> *Report of the British Association for the Advancement of Science,* 1899, "Presidential Address to the Physiology Section"

J. Chalmers Da Costa [1863–1933]

Now and then a very learned article or lecture, like the talk of the man mentioned in Wolfville, increases the sum total of human ignorance.

> *The Trials and Triumphs of the Surgeon,* Ch. 1

George Ade [1866–1944]

Only the more Rugged Mortals should attempt to Keep Up on Current Literature.

> *Fables in Slang,* "The Fable of the Man Who Didn't Care for Storybooks"

Arthur R. Cushny [1866–1926]

The growth in the literature of the kidney has been extraordinary since the time when you and I began to work on it, and this increase in bulk has not gone along with an improvement of quality, but rather the reverse.

> Communication to Ernest Henry Starling

Sir Robert Hutchison [1871–1960]

The amount of writings of a profession is a measure of its vitality and activity, whilst their quality is a rough indication of its intellectual state. Medical literature . . . is the currency or medium of exchange by which a man contributes to or borrows from the common stock of knowledge and experience, and the volume of this currency and the character of its metal are of the greatest importance to us all.

> *Lancet* 2:1059, 1939

Béla Schick [1877–1967]

After twenty years one is no longer quoted in the medical literature. Every twenty years one sees a republication of the same ideas.

> Quoted by I. J. Wolf in *Aphorisms and Facetiae of Béla Schick,* "Early Years"

Sir Thomas Lewis [1881–1945]

Reform, to be useful, must render the student of medicine discriminating in a world where a disquieting proportion of what is offered him in conversation and in the generality of journals and books is inaccurate, slovenly, or redundant.

> *Lancet* 1:619, 1944

Dame Rose Macaulay [1881–1958]

He felt about books as doctors feel about medicines, or managers about plays — cynical but hopeful.

> *Crewe Train,* Ch. VIII, Pt. 2

Alphonse Raymond Dochez [1882–1964]

Some of the papers presented at today's medical meetings tell us what we already know, but in a much more complicated manner.

> Quoted in *P & S Quarterly* 11:18, June 1966

Many clues to the unknowns in medicine are locked in the library, waiting for someone to open the right book at the right time.

> Comment to Dr. David Seegal, 1932

John Maddox [1925–]

In many laboratories reprints are displayed much as if they were campaign medals on show in a general's drawing room.

> *Rockefeller Institute Review,* February 1963

LIVER

Robert Greene [1560?–1592]

Wine and water is good against the heate of the liver.

> *A Quippe for an Upstart Courtier*

William Shakespeare [1564–1616]

I had rather heat my liver with drinking.

> *Antony and Cleopatra,* I, ii, 23

Let my liver rather heat with wine
Than my heart cool with mortifying groans.

> *The Merchant of Venice,* I, i, 81

If he were open'd, and you find so much blood in his liver as will clog the foot of a flea, I'll eat the rest of th' anatomy.

> *Twelfth Night,* III, ii, 65

Were my wive's liver
Infected as her life, she would not live
The running of one glass.

> *The Winter's Tale,* I, ii, 304

William Heberden [1710–1801]

In affections of the liver, haemorrhoidal bleedings are very common.

> *Commentaries on the History and Cure of Diseases,* Ch. 44

Men are more commonly affected with scirrhous livers than women, because they are more given to intemperate drinking, which is the principal cause of this disorder.

Ibid., Ch. 50

George Gordon, Lord Byron [1788–1824]

The liver is the lazaret of bile.

Don Juan, Canto II, Stanza 215

John Shaw Billings [1838–1913]

You cannot legislate a new layer of cortical gray matter into, or a cirrhosed liver out of, a man.

Boston Medical and Surgical Journal 131:125, 1894

Ambrose Bierce [1842–1914?]

LIVER, n. A large red organ thoughtfully provided by nature to be bilious with. . . . It was at one time considered the seat of life; hence its name — liver, the thing we live with.

The Devil's Dictionary

Merrill Moore [1903–1957]

You cannot undo Liver, you can take
A finger off, a leg; make and remake
The nose, the ear, the face; break and unbreak
A compensating heart, fake and refake
A joint disabled or a stomach-ache
But Liver (Hepar), Liver must go on
Importantly as fifth wheel in the machine
Playing its rôle for every body's sake:

I must be here in beady drops of bile
Liver says (its only way to talk):
Liver says *I will not run, I will walk*
In my predestined way and all the while
I plod for you, you may run many a mile,
But O your slowness if I ever balk!
　　　　Six Sides to a Man, "Surgery of the Liver"

Anonymous

A man's liver is his carburetor.

French Proverb

If you would live ever, you must wash milk from your liver.

LOGIC

See also REASON, THINKING

Sir Francis Bacon [1561–1626]

My plan is to proceed regularly and gradually from one axiom to another, so that the most general are not reached till the last: but then when you do come to them you find them . . . such as lie at the heart and marrow of things.

The Great Instauration, "The Plan of the Work"

The syllogism consists of propositions, propositions consist of words, words are symbols of notions. Therefore if the notions themselves (which is the root of the matter) are confused and over-hastily abstracted from the facts, there can be no firmness in the superstructure. Our only hope therefore lies in a true induction.

Novum Organum, "Aphorisms," XIV

Jacob Bigelow [1786–1879]

It is common error to infer that things which are consecutive in order of time have necessarily the relation of cause and effect.

Self-Limited Diseases

Peter Mere Latham [1789–1875]

No good ever comes from pretending to more precision than the thing itself admits of.

Diseases of the Heart, Lect. I

It is safest and best to fill up the gaps of our knowledge from analogy.
> *General Remarks on the Practice of Medicine,* Ch. II

Common sense is in medicine the master workman.
> *Ibid.,* Ch. V

It is safer to appeal to men's perceptions than to their logic.
> *Ibid.,* Ch. XIV

People in general have no notion of the sort and amount of evidence often needed to prove the simplest matter of fact.
> *Ibid.,* "The Heart and Its Affections," Ch. II

A premature desire to generalize, an eagerness to arrive at conclusions, and a readiness to rest in them, are very common infirmities, and they offer very serious hindrances to the right acquisition of facts.
> *Lectures on Clinical Medicine,* Lect. V

Bear in mind, then, that abstractions are *not facts;* and next bear in mind that *opinions* are not facts.
> *Idem*

Edward FitzGerald [1809–1883]

Myself when young did eagerly frequent
Doctor and Saint, and heard great argument
  About it and about: but evermore
Came out by the same door where in I went.
> *The Rubáiyát of Omar Khayyám* (3rd ed.), Stanza 27

Oliver Wendell Holmes [1809–1894]

The inveterate logical errors to which physicians have always been subject are chiefly these: —
  The mode of inference *per enumer-*

ationem simplicem, in scholastic phrase; that is, counting only their favorable cases. . . .
  The *post hoc ergo propter hoc* error; he got well after taking my medicine; therefore in consequence of taking it.
  The false induction from genuine facts of observation, leading to the construction of theories which are then deductively applied in the face of the results of direct observation. . . .
  And lastly, the error which Sir Thomas Browne calls giving "a reason of the golden tooth"; that is, assuming a falsehood as a fact, and giving reasons for it.
> *Medical Essays,* "Currents and Counter-Currents in Medical Science"

Sir William Jenner [1815–1898]

The invariable antecedent of any event is not necessarily its cause. Invariable antecedent and invariable consequent are not synonymous with cause and effect.
> *St. Bartholomew's Hospital Reports* 52:41, 1916

Sir Clifford Allbutt [1836–1925]

In medieval times, so fastidious were logic and abstraction that practice became a vulgarity, and he was the greatest teacher who carried his pupils furthest from things.

Sir W. Arbuthnot Lane [1856–1943]

If everyone believes a thing it is probably untrue!
> Quoted by W. E. Tanner in *Sir W. Arbuthnot Lane,* "Genesis"

Anonymous

No one appreciates the medical profession more highly than myself. Doctors are the most generous of men; but they are unwise when they represent doctoring either as an art or a science. . . . doctors would be better appreciated if they would frankly admit that doctoring is like logic.

More from a Lawyer's Notebook, "Doctors"

LONGEVITY

See also EUTHANASIA, LIFE, OLD AGE

Huang Ti (The Yellow Emperor) [2697–2597 B.C.]

In ancient times the people lived (through the years) to be over a hundred years, and yet they remained active and did not become decrepit in their activities.

Nei Ching Su Wên, Bk. 1, Sect. 1 (tr. by Ilza Veith in *The Yellow Emperor's Classic of Internal Medicine*)

Mimnermus [fl. late 7th Cent. B.C.]

Would that by no disease, nor cares opprest,
I in my sixtieth year were laid to rest.
Quoted by Diogenes Laertius in *Lives of Eminent Philosophers,* I.60 (tr. by R. D. Hicks)

Solon [638?–559? B.C.]

Surely a wiser wish were thus expressed,
At eighty years let me be laid to rest.[1]
Fragments, XXXVII

Seneca [4? B.C.–A.D. 65]

No man can have a peaceful life who thinks too much about lengthening it.
Moral Epistles to Lucilius, IV (tr. by Richard M. Gummere)

Leonardo da Vinci [1452–1519]

Life well spent is long.
Codice Trivulziano, 63 (tr. by Edward MacCurdy in *The Notebooks of Leonardo da Vinci,* Vol. I, Ch. I)

[1] This answer to Mimnermus is also quoted by Diogenes Laertius.

Michel de Montaigne [1533–1592]

Let the doctors excuse my liberty a bit. . . . The antipathy I have for their art is hereditary with me. My father lived seventy-four years, my grandfather sixty-nine, my great-grandfather nearly eighty, without having tasted any sort of medicine.
Essays, Bk. II, Ch. 37, "Of the Resemblance of Children to Fathers" (tr. by Donald M. Frame)

Sir Francis Bacon [1561–1626]

I will divide [medicine] into three parts, which I will term its three offices; the first whereof is the Preservation of Health, the second the Cure of Diseases, and the third the Prolongation of Life. But this last the physicians do not seem to have recognized as the principal part of their art, but to have confounded, ignorantly enough, with the other two. For they imagine that if diseases be repelled before they attack the body, and cured after they have attacked it, prolongation of life necessarily follows. . . . But the lengthening of the thread of life itself, and the postponement for a time of that death which gradually steals on by natural dissolution and the decay of age, is a subject which no physician has handled in proportion to its dignity.
The Advancement of Learning, Bk. IV, Ch. II

John Northbrooke [fl. 1568]

Among many evilles & naughty affections which folow the nature of man corrupted by sinne, none bringeth greater inconvenience than the inordinate hope of long life.
A Treatise Wherein Dicing, Dauncing, Vaine Playes . . . Are Reproved, "To the Christian and Faithful Reader"

Robert Burton [1577–1640]

Paracelsus may brag that he could make

a man live 400 years or more, if he might bring him up from his infancy, and diet him as he list; and some physicians hold, that there is no certain period of man's life; but it may still by temperance and physic be prolonged.

> *The Anatomy of Melancholy,* Pt. 1, Sect. 1, Memb. 1, Subsect. 2

John Dryden [1631–1700]

Of no distemper, of no blast he dy'd,
But fell like Autumn-Fruit that mellow'd long:
Ev'n wonder'd at, because he dropt no
    sooner.
Fate seem'd to wind him up for four-
    score years;
Yet freshly ran he on
Ten Winters more:
Till, like a Clock worn out with eating
    time,
The Wheels of weary life at last stood
    still.

> *Oedipus,* Act IV

Giorgio Baglivi [1669–1707?]

Length of life does not depend so much on a good physical constitution as it does on the best use of the six non-natural things,[1] which if we rule aright, we shall live long and healthy lives: to divide the day properly between sleep and waking; to adjust our air to the needs of the body; to take more or less food and drink according to our age, our temperament, and whether we live an active or inactive life; to take exercise or rest according to the quantity of our food and whether we are lean or fat; to know ourselves, and be able to rule our emotions, and subject them to our reason. Whoever handles

[1] In medieval medicine, the six "nonnatural" things (things which caused health or disease and were not actual parts of the human body) were meat and drink, retention and evacuation, air, exercise, sleep and waking, and passions of the mind. Baglivi mentions all but the second.

these wisely will live long and seldom need a doctor.

> *De Fibra Motrice,* Pt. II, Ch. VI

Benjamin Franklin [1706–1790]

It is recorded of Methusalem, who, being the longest liver, may be supposed to have best preserved his health, that he slept always in the open air; for when he had lived five hundred years, an angel said to him, "Arise, Methusalem, and build thee an house, for thou shalt live yet five hundred years longer." But Methusalem answered and said, "If I am to live but five hundred years longer, it is not worth while to build me an house; I will sleep in the air, as I have been used to do."

> *The Art of Procuring Pleasant Dreams*

Samuel Johnson [1709–1784]

Enlarge my life with multitude of days,
In health, in sickness, thus the suppliant prays;
Hides from himself his state, and shuns to know,
That life protracted is protracted woe.

> *The Vanity of Human Wishes*

Thomas Jefferson [1743–1826]

My only fear now is that I may live too long. This would be a subject of dread to me.

> Letter to Philip Mazzei, March 17, 1801

Oliver Wendell Holmes [1809–1894]

[Formula for longevity:] Have a chronic disease and take care of it.

Henry Thomas Buckle [1821–1862]

The diminution of pain is, looking at things in a large point of view, the least of the benefits derived from the soothing hand of the accomplished physician. His influence on the progress of civilization consists in being enabled to lengthen life.

> *Miscellaneous and Posthumous Works*, Vol. II, Fragment 7

Sir James Crichton-Browne [1840–1938]

There is no short-cut to longevity. To win it is the work of a lifetime, and the promotion of it is a branch of preventive medicine.

> *The Prevention of Senility*

Ambrose Bierce [1842–1914?]

LONGEVITY, n. Uncommon extension of the fear of death.

> *The Devil's Dictionary*

Santiago Ramón y Cajal [1852–1934]

Zoology is often very instructive. It is well known how extraordinary is the longevity of the crocodile and the elephant, animals of thick and almost impenetrable hide. From this we may infer that to attain long life, we should sheathe our spiritual skin, making it insensible to the pinpricks of rivals, of enemies and of the envious.

> *Charlas de Café*

George Bernard Shaw [1856–1950]

Do not try to live forever. You will not succeed.

> *The Doctor's Dilemma*, "Preface on Doctors"

Warfield T. Longcope [1877–1953]

As I grow older, I have less and less sympathy with the conscientious efforts merely to extend life in old age.

> *Bulletin of the Johns Hopkins Hospital* 50:4, 1932

George M. Piersol [1880–1966] and Edward L. Bortz [1896–   ]

The society which fosters research to save human life cannot escape responsibility for the life thus extended. It is for science not only to add years to life, but more important, to add life to the years.

> *Annals of Internal Medicine* 12:964, 1939

James Howard Means [1885–1967]

We have, inadvertently, trained our young doctors to consider it a virtue to prolong life for the sole purpose of prolonging it.

> *Daedalus* 92:701, 1963

Wilder Penfield [1891–   ]

It would seem that modern science has not really changed man's normal span of life. Nineteen hundred years ago, Pliny the Elder wrote that centenarians were common enough at that time in Rome. He even told of an actress who boasted that she had survived a hundred years. The change which we should recognize in this generation is that more men and women reach life's true goal, fulfilling the cycle set for us, bypassing the plagues and disease and famine.

> *The Second Career*, Ch. I

Louis Lasagna [1923–   ]

Medicine might . . . consider forsaking the worship of the goddess Longevity. Must we be ardent Methuselites, blindly adoring a giant hourglass on a sere and treeless plain? Is a mummy preserved for centuries preferable to the most briefly flowering crocus? Epicurus warned that most people spend their lives preparing to live. If existence is truly precious, man should grasp it in a fervent embrace, rather than waste his days as a lonely voyeur, peeping ineffectually at life from afar. Can the man whose life is not rich really profit from its extension?

> *The Doctors' Dilemmas*, Epilogue

The Bible

All the days of Methuselah were nine hundred sixty and nine years: and he died.

> *Genesis* 5:27

And all the days of Noah were nine hundred and fifty years: and he died.
Genesis 9:29

Moses was an hundred and twenty years old when he died: his eye was not dim, nor his natural force abated.
Deuteronomy 34:7

And he [King David] died in a good old age, full of days, riches, and honour.
I Chronicles 29:28

Anonymous Latin Poem [1st Cent.]

You that with powerful drugs defy our fate
And lengthen life beyond the appointed date.

Proverbs

All would live long, but none would be old.

He lives long that lives till all are weary of him.

Long life hath long misery.

Italian Proverb

He who would live long must sometimes change his way of living.

LOVE

Leonardo da Vinci [1452–1519]

Great love is born of great knowledge of the objects one loves. If you do not understand them you can only admire them lamely or not at all — and if you only love them on account of the good you expect from them, and not because of the sum of their qualities, then you are as the dog that wags his tail to the person who gives him a bone. Love is the daughter of knowledge and love is deep in the same degree as the knowledge is sure — love conquers all things.
Treatise on Painting, Ch. 80 (tr. by McMahon)

John Lyly [1554?–1606]

O ye gods, have ye ordained for every malady a medicine, for every sore a salve, for every pain a plaster, leaving only love remedyless?
Euphues

William Shakespeare [1564–1616]

My love is as a fever, longing still
For that which longer nurseth the disease;
Feeding on that which doth preserve the ill,
Th' uncertain sickly appetite to please.
Sonnet CXLVII

Abraham Cowley [1618–1667]

Come, doctor, use thy roughest art,
   Thou canst not cruel prove;
Cut, burn, and torture every part,
   To heal me of my *Love*.

There is no danger, if the pain
   Should me to 'a *Fever* bring;
Compar'd with *Heats* I now sustain,
   A *Feaver* is so *Cool* a thing,
   (Like *drink* which feaverish men desire)
That I should hope 'twould almost quench my *Fire*.
The Cure

George Gordon, Lord Byron [1788–1824]

Love's a capricious power: I've known it hold
   Out through a fever caused by its own heat,
But be much puzzled by a cough and cold,
   And find a quinsy very hard to treat;
Against all noble maladies he's bold,
   But vulgar illnesses don't like to meet,
Nor that a sneeze should interrupt his sigh,
Nor inflammation redden his blind eye.

But worst of all is nausea, or a pain
   About the lower region of the bowels;

Love, who heroically breathes a vein,
  Shrinks from the application of hot
  towels,
And purgatives are dangerous to his
  reign.
Sea-sickness death.
    Don Juan, Canto II, Stanza 22

Douglas Jerrold [1803–1857]

They say love's like the measles — all
the worse when it comes late in life.
    *Wit and Opinions of Douglas
    Jerrold, a Philanthropist*

Edward Bulwer-Lytton [1803–1873]

In all cases of heart-ache, the application of another man's disappointment
draws out the pain and allays the
irritation.
    The Lady of Lyons, Act I, Sc. ii

Henry Wheeler Shaw ("Josh Billings") [1818–1885]

Love iz like the meazels, we kant alwus
tell when we ketched it and ain't ap
tew hav it severe but onst, and then it
ain't kounted mutch unless it strikes
inly.
    Josh Billings: His Sayings, Ch.
    53

Henry Cuyler Bunner [1855–1896]

Now, the Doctor feared no foe, in
medicine or in love; but when a young
woman is inscrutable as to the state of
her affections, when the richest young
man in the county is devoting himself
to her, and when the young lady's
mother is backing the rich man, a
young country doctor may well feel
perplexed and anxious over his chance
of the prize.
    Short Sixes, "The Infidelity of
    Zenobia"

Jerome K. Jerome [1859–1927]

Love is like the measles; we all have to
go through it.
    *Idle Thoughts of an Idle
    Fellow*, "On Being in Love"

Marcel Proust [1871–1922]

Love is an incurable malady like those
diathetic states in which rheumatism
affords the sufferer a brief respite only
to be replaced by epileptiform headaches.
    The Captive, Pt. I, Ch. 1 (tr.
    by C. K. Scott-Moncrieff)

The beloved object is successively the
malady and the remedy that suspends
and aggravates it.
    Cities of the Plain, Pt. I, Ch. 2

Erich Fromm [1900–   ]

*The affirmation of one's own life, hap-
piness, growth, freedom is rooted in
one's capacity to love,* i.e., in care, respect, responsibility, and knowledge.
If an individual is able to love pro-
ductively, he loves himself too; if he
can love *only* others, he cannot love at
all.
    The Art of Loving, Ch. 2, Pt. 3,
    Sect. d

Childish love knows no bounds, it demands exclusive possession, is satisfied
with nothing less than all. But it has a
second characteristic: it has no real
aim; it is incapable of complete satisfaction and this is the principal reason
why it is doomed to end in disappointment and to give place to a hostile attitude.

Dame Kathleen Lonsdale [1903–   ]

Any scientist who has ever been in love
knows that he may understand everything about sex hormones but the actual experience is something quite
quite different.
    Quoted by Sir Robert Platt in
    Universities Quarterly 17:327,
    1963

Spanish Proverb

Love is like a sprain, a second time it
arrives more easily.

LUNGS

See also BREATHING,
TUBERCULOSIS

William Pitt, Earl of Chatham
[1708–1778]

The parks are the lungs of London.
> Quoted by William Windham in
> the House of Commons, June
> 30, 1808

Randolph S. Churchill [1911–   ]

My father [Sir Winston Churchill] was
only sent to Harrow because it was
quaintly thought at the time that he
suffered from some lung trouble and
that Harrow-on-the-Hill would be
better for him than Eton in the fog.
Actually lack of lung power has never
subsequently been detected in my
father, but perhaps it was the salu-
brious climate of Harrow which rid
him of this complaint.
> *Twenty-One Years,* Pt. I

MALARIA

William Shakespeare [1564–1616]

He is so shak'd of a burning quotidian
tertian that it is most lamentable to
behold.
> *Henry V,* II, i, 123

**Sir David Dalrymple, Lord
Hailes** [1726–1792]

Much are we beholden to physicians,
who only prescribe the bark of the
quinquina, when they might oblige
their patients to swallow the whole
tree.

Sir Ronald Ross [1857–1932]

I was tired, and what was the use?
I must have examined the stomachs of
a thousand mosquitoes by this time.

But the Angel of Fate fortunately laid
his hand on my head.
> *Memoirs,* Ch. 13

In this, O Nature, yield I pray to me.
I pace and pace, and think and think,
     and take
The fever'd hands, and note down all
     I see,
That some dim distant light may haply
     break.

The painful faces ask, can we not cure?
We answer, No, not yet; we seek the
     laws.
O God, reveal thro' all this thing ob-
     scure
The unseen, small, but million-murder-
     ing cause.
> *Philosophies,* "Indian Fevers"

This day relenting God
     Hath placed within my hand
A wondrous thing; and God
     Be praised. At His command,

Seeking His secret deeds
     With tears and toiling breath,
I find thy cunning seeds,
     O million-murdering death.

I know this little thing
     A myriad men will save.
O Death, where is thy sting?
     Thy victory, O Grave? [1]
> *Ibid,* "In Exile," Pt. VII

René J. Dubos [1901–   ]

DDT went further toward the eradication of malariologists than of mosquitoes.
> *Man Adapting,* Ch. XIV

West African Proverb

The back of a chicken does not mind
mosquitoes.[2]

---

[1] Written on August 20, 1897, when he
made his great discovery of the vector of
malaria.
[2] In parts of Europe, livestock were placed
near dwellings in an attempt to reduce malaria by drawing the mosquitoes away from
humans.

MALNUTRITION

See NUTRITION

MAN

See also LIFE, SEX

Euripides [484–406 B.C.]

No mortal is there but pain finds him
    out
And sickness; many must their chil-
    dren bury,
And sow fresh issue; death is end for
    all;
In vain do these things vex the race
    of men.
Earth must go back to earth: then
    life by all
Like crops is harvested. So must it be.
    Fragment from *Hypsipyla*, 757
    (tr. by J. E. King)

Terence [185–159 B.C.]

I am a man, and nothing human is
foreign to me.[1]
    Heauton Timorumenos, Act I

Seneca [4? B.C.–A.D. 65]

Man is a reasoning animal.
    Mortal Epistles to Lucilius,
    XLI (tr. by Richard M. Gum-
    mere)

Epictetus [60?–120?]

For I will assert of the foot as such
that it is natural for it to be clean, but
if you take it as a foot, and not as a
thing detached, it will be appropriate
for it to step into mud and trample
on thorns and sometimes to be cut off
for the sake of the whole body; otherwise it will no longer be a foot. We
ought to hold some such view also
about ourselves. What are you? A
man. Now if you regard yourself as

[1] Homo sum; humani nil a me alienum
puto.

a thing detached, it is natural for you
to live to old age, to be rich, to enjoy
health. But if you regard yourself as
a man and as a part of some whole, on
account of that whole it is fitting for
you now to be sick, and now to make
a voyage and run risks, and now to
be in want, and on occasion to die before your time. Why, then, are you
vexed? Do you not know that as the
foot, if detached, will no longer be a
foot, so you too, if detached, will no
longer be a man?
    Discourses, II.v.24 (tr. by W.
    A. Oldfather)

Pierre Charron [1541–1603]

The true science and the true study of
man is man.
    Traité de la Sagesse, Bk. I,
    Ch. 1

Sir Francis Bacon [1561–1626]

The World's a bubble; and the life of
    man
    Lesse than a span.
In his conception wretched; from the
    wombe,
    So to the tombe:
Curst from the cradle, and brought up
    to yeares,
    With cares and feares.
Who then to fraile Mortality shall
    trust,
But limmes the water, or but writes in
    dust.
    The World

John Donne [1573–1631]

No man is an *Iland*, intire of it selfe;
every man is a peece of the *Continent*,
a part of the maine.
    *Devotions Upon Emergent Oc-
    casions*, XVII

William Browne [1591–1643?]

What's he, born to be sick, so always
    dying,
That's guided by inevitable fate;
That comes in weeping, and that goes
    out crying;

Whose calendar of woes is still in date;
Whose life's a bubble, and in length
  a span;
A concert still in discords?
             'T is a man.
  Britannia's Pastorals, Bk. I,
  Song II

Sir Thomas Browne [1605–1682]

Thus are we men, and we know not
how; there is something in us, that
can be without us, and will be after
us, though it is strange that it hath
no history, what it was before us, nor
can tell how it entred in us.
  Religio Medici, Pt. I, Sect. 36

Henry Vaughan [1622–1695]

Man is the shuttle, to whose winding
  quest
And passage through these looms
God order'd motion, but ordain'd no
  rest.
  Man

John Dryden [1631–1700]

Men are but Children of a larger
  growth.
  All for Love, Act IV

Alexander Pope [1688–1744]

The proper study of Mankind is Man.
  An Essay on Man, Epistle II

Oliver Goldsmith [1728–1774]

Man wants but little here below,
Nor wants that little long.
  The Vicar of Wakefield, Ch. 8,
  "A Ballad"

Georg Christoph Lichtenberg
[1742–1799]

Man is essentially a bulb with many
thousands of roots. In him the nerves
alone feel; the rest serves to hold them
together and to move them about more
conveniently. What we see then is the
pot in which the man (the nerves) is
planted.
  Aphorismen (1764–1771)

Man is perhaps half spirit and half
matter, just as a polyp is half plant
and half animal. The strangest creatures are always found on the border-
lines.
      Ibid. (1772–1775)

Thomas Jefferson [1743–1826]

What a stupendous, what an incomprehensible machine is man! who can endure toil, famine, stripes, imprisonment
& death itself in vindication of his own
liberty, and the next moment be deaf
to all those motives whose power supported him thro' his trial, and inflict
on his fellow men a bondage, one hour
of which is fraught with more misery
than ages of that which he rose in
rebellion to oppose.
  *Observations on the Article
  "Etats-Unis" of M. de Meusnier
  Prepared for the Encyclopédie,*
  June 26, 1786

Benjamin Rush [1745?–1813]

A man's pictures and books are generally pretty correct copies of the intellectual and moral qualities of the
mind.
  Autobiography, "Travels
  Through Life," Ch. III

Sir Charles Bell [1774–1842]

I thought that all was right in the system of the universe — that consistent
with our desires and passions was the
shortness of our life and our being
liable to suffering and disease — that
without this we should have been inanimate, cold, and heartless creatures.

Thomas Carlyle [1795–1881]

No man who has once heartily and
wholly laughed can be altogether ir-
reclaimably bad.
  Sartor Resartus, Bk. I, Ch. 4

Oliver Wendell Holmes
[1809–1894]

Nothing but a cloud of elements organic,

C. O. H. N. Ferrum, Chlor. Flu. Sil.
Potassa,
Calc. Sod. Phosph. Mag. Sulphur,
Mang.(?)
Alumin.(?) Cuprum,(?)
Such as man is made of.
*The Professor at the Breakfast
Table,* Sect. I

Alfred, Lord Tennyson
[1809–1892]

I am a part of all that I have met.
Ulysses

Mary Baker Eddy [1821–1910]

Man is not matter — made up of
brains, blood, bones, and other material elements. The Scriptures inform
us that man is made in the image and
likeness of God. Matter is not that
likeness.
Science and Health, Ch. XIV

Thomas Huxley [1825–1895]

Men, my dear, are very queer animals,
a mixture of horse-nervousness, ass-
stubbornness, and camel-malice, with
an angel bobbing about unexpectedly
like the apple in the posset, and when
they can do exactly as they please,
they are very hard to drive.
Letter to Mrs. W. K. Clifford,
February 10, 1895

Mark Twain (Samuel L. Clemens)
[1835–1910]

Man is a museum of diseases, a home
of impurities; he comes today and is
gone tomorrow; he begins as dirt and
departs as stench.

Sir Clifford Allbutt [1836–1925]

The laws of the lawgiver are impotent
beside the laws of human nature as,
to his disillusion, many a lawgiver has
discovered.

David B. Henderson [1840–1906]

I took my medicine like a man.
Congressional Record, January
7, 1896

Oliver Wendell Holmes, Jr.
[1841–1935]

It seems to me probable that the only
cosmic significance of man is that he
is a part of the cosmos, but that seems
to me enough.
Letter to Sir Frederick Pollock,
May 26, 1919

Also as I see no reasons for attributing
cosmic importance to man, other than
that attaching to whatever is, I regard
him as I do the other species (except
that my private interests are with his)
having for his main business to live
and propagate, and for his main interest food and sex.
Letter to Harold J. Laski, January 11, 1929

William James [1842–1910]

How to gain, how to keep, how to
recover happiness, is in fact for most
men at all times the secret motive of
all they do, and of all they are willing
to endure.
*Varieties of Religious Experi-
ence,* Lect. IV

Friedrich Nietzsche [1844–1900]

The earth, said he, hath a skin; and
this skin hath diseases. One of those
diseases, for example, is called "man."
Thus Spake Zarathustra, Pt. II,
Ch. 40 (tr. by Oscar Levy)

Rudyard Kipling [1865–1936]

Man . . . might be defined as "An imperfectly denatured animal intermit-
tently subject to the unpredictable
reactions of an unlocated spiritual
area."
Surgeons and the Soul

Thomas Mann [1875–1955]

All interest in disease and death is
only another expression of interest in
life, as is proven by the humanistic
faculty of medicine, that addresses life
and its ails always so politely in Latin,

and is only a division of the great and pressing concern which, in all sympathy, I now name by its name: the human being, the delicate child of life, man, his state and standing in the universe.

> *The Magic Mountain*, Ch. VI, "Snow" (tr. by H. T. Lowe-Porter)

Abraham Myerson [1881–1948]

To me man is a thickened node in the web of a universe of forces which, ever repetitively and ever anew, flow in and out of him; he is part of an ecology that involves plants, animals, climate, soil, and all kinds of radiant forces and chemicals. He is united by the invisible strands of heredity to every form of life that ever lived; and his fundamental drives and compulsive activities go back to the first piece of life that ever appeared on earth. He is packed with chemical factories, his every cell a better chemist and physicist than all the Nobel prize laureates put together. He is immersed in age-old and ever changing social forces that compress, enhance, destroy, or deform his trends. At every step he is beset by conflict between his biology and his sociology. . . . Somehow there is a constant and shifting balance of forces in which hormones, ferments, enzymes, memories, ideas, emotions, and moods all play a part; and all of this is an unexplainable transit from conception to that catalytic dispersal, perhaps reassemblage, called death.

> *Speaking of Man*, Foreword

Baroness Karen Blixen ("Isak Dinesen") [1885–1962]

What is man, when you come to think upon him, but a minutely set, ingenious machine for turning, with infinite artfulness, the red wine of Shiraz into urine?

> *Seven Gothic Tales*, "The Dreamers"

Sir Julian Huxley [1887–   ]

The human race will be the cancer of the planet.

Christopher Morley [1890–1957]

A human being, he wrote, is a whispering in the steam pipes on a cold night; dust sifted through a locked window; one or the other half of an unsolved equation; a pun made by God; an ingenious assembly of portable plumbing.

> *Human Being*, Ch. 11

Sir James Calvert Spence [1892–1954]

We of this generation through the decline of the family are witnessing the most sudden biological change the human race has known.

> *The Purpose and Practice of Medicine*, Ch. 12

Homer W. Smith [1895–1962]

Because he is the highest vertebrate he can do what no other vertebrate can do: when, out of whatever desire and knowledge may be his, he makes a choice, he can say "I will." . . . And knowing how and why he says "I will," he comes to his own as a philosopher.

> *From Fish to Philosopher*, Ch. 13

In man the "self," the seemingly enduring spectator-director who commands the performance, is an impermanently sustained pattern of neural activity. Far from an entity enduring from day to day, it is a flickering image formed where the rays of sense are brought to focus in the conscious pattern; it forms and dissolves in successive instants, and never re-forms the same.

> *Idem*

René J. Dubos [1901–   ]

Among other living things, it is man's dignity to value certain ideals above comfort, and even above life. This

human trait makes of medicine a philosophy that goes beyond exact medical sciences, because it must encompass not only man as a living machine but also the collective aspirations of mankind.
Mirage of Health, Ch. VIII

Margaret Mead [1901–   ]

Our humanity rests upon a series of learned behaviors, woven together into patterns that are infinitely fragile and never directly inherited.
Male and Female, Ch. IX

Leon J. Saul [1901–   ]

Humans are children for so long that they never get over it.
Emotional Maturity, Pt. I

Arthur Miller [1915–   ]

He's not the finest character that ever lived. But he's a human being, and a terrible thing is happening to him. So attention must be paid. He's not to be allowed to fall into his grave like an old dog.
Death of a Salesman, Act I

French Proverb

We drink without being thirsty, and make love at any time; that is the only distinction between us and the other animals.

MARRIAGE

See also SEX, WIVES

Book of Common Prayer [1662]

To have and to hold from this day forward, for better, for worse, for richer, for poorer, in sickness and in health, to love and to cherish, till death us do part.
Solemnization of Matrimony

Samuel Johnson [1709–1784]

A gentleman who had been very unhappy in marriage, married immediately after his wife died: Johnson said, it was the triumph of hope over experience.
Quoted by James Boswell in
Life of Samuel Johnson, 1770

Honoré de Balzac [1799–1850]

No man should marry until he has studied anatomy and dissected at least one woman.
The Physiology of Marriage,
Meditation V, Aphorism 28

A husband should never go to sleep first or wake last.
Ibid., Aphorism 50 (tr. by G. Burnham Ives)

Lawrence S. Kubie [1896–   ]

Many marriages are contracted not on a basis of health, but on that of neurotic purposes. The story is all too familiar of maladjusted young people who try to escape their separate miseries by joining their problems in marriage. Since marriage never cured a neurosis, it usually ends up by being blamed for it; and presently the neurotic angers of both partners are pitted against each other in a merciless battle.
Practical and Theoretical Aspects of Psychoanalysis, "Psychoanalysis and Marriage"

C. D. Darlington [1903–   ]

A large proportion of mankind, like pigeons and partridges, on reaching maturity, having passed through a period of playfulness or promiscuity, establish what they hope and expect will be a permanent and fertile mating relationship. This we call marriage.
Genetics and Man, Ch. 16

French and Danish Proverb

A deaf husband and a blind wife are always a happy couple.

German Proverbs

Matrimony is a reversed fever, it starts with heat and ends with cold.

Matrimony is the hospital for love.

MATERNITY

See also CHILD HEALTH, CHILDREN, CONCEPTION, PARENTS, PREGNANCY

Aristotle [384–322 B.C.]

Mothers love their children more than fathers, because parenthood cost the mother more trouble [and the mother is more certain that the child is her own].
> *Nicomachean Ethics*, IX.vii (tr. by H. Rackham)

Menander [343?–291? B.C.]

A mother loves her child more than a father does, for she knows it's her own while he but thinks it's his.
> *Fragments*, 657 (tr. by F. G. Allinson)

Scevola de Sainte-Marthé [1526–1623]

'Twas a sage said it, and the saying's good,
The mother's milk's the only wholesome food.
Large meals upon the suckling babe bestow,
And freely let the snowy fountains flow.
> *The Art of Bringing Up Children*

Samuel Johnson [1709–1784]

As I wandered wrapped up in thought, my eyes were struck with the hospital for the reception of deserted infants, which I surveyed with pleasure, till, by a natural train of sentiment, I began to reflect on the fate of the mothers. For to what shelter can they fly? Only to the arms of their betrayer, which perhaps are now no longer open to receive them; and then how quick must be the transition from deluded virtue to shameless guilt, and from shameless guilt to hopeless wretchedness?
> *The Rambler*, No. 107 (March 26, 1751)

Oliver Wendell Holmes [1809–1894]

The woman about to become a mother, or with her new-born infant upon her bosom, should be the object of trembling care and sympathy wherever she bears her tender burden, or stretches her aching limbs. The very outcast of the streets has pity upon her sister in degradation, when the seal of promised maternity is impressed upon her. The remorseless vengeance of the law, brought down upon its victim by a machinery as sure as destiny, is arrested in its fall at a word which reveals her transient claim for mercy. The solemn prayer of the liturgy singles out her sorrows from the multiplied trials of life, to plead for her in the hour of peril. God forbid that any member of the profession to which she trusts her life, doubly precious at that eventful period, should hazard it negligently, unadvisedly, or selfishly!
> *Medical Essays*, "The Contagiousness of Puerperal Fever"

Count Leo Tolstoy [1828–1910]

My wife, who wanted herself to suckle and did suckle the last four children, was not in good health when the first baby was born. The doctors, who cynically undressed and felt her all over, for which I had to thank them and pay them money, — these charming doctors found that she must not herself nurse, and she was, during this first time, deprived of the only means

which would have saved her from coquetry.
>　*The Kreutzer Sonata,* Ch. XIV
>　(tr. by L. Weiner)

Ambrose Bierce [1842–1914?]

MAMMALIA, n. pl. A family of vertebrate animals whose females in a state of nature suckle their young, but when civilized and enlightened put them out to nurse, or use the bottle.
>　*The Devil's Dictionary*

Wilhelm Conrad Roentgen [1854–1923]

The question "What would your mother have said and done in this or that confused situation?" has often shown me the right way out of it. The maternal heart with its infinite store of love and her kind soul which is always ready to understand and to forgive lead us always to the proper road even if the mother is no longer alive.

Boris Pasternak [1890–1960]

For every one of them, God is in her child. Mothers of great men must have this feeling particularly, but then, at the beginning, all women are the mothers of great men — it isn't their fault if life disappoints them later.
>　*Doctor Zhivago,* Ch. 9, Sect. 3
>　(tr. by Max Hayward and
>　Manya Harari)

MATURITY

See also AGE, MIDDLE AGE, YOUTH

Samuel Pepys [1633–1703]

This day I am, by the blessing of God, 34 years old, in very good health and mind's content, and in condition of estate much beyond whatever my friends could expect of a child of theirs this day 34 years.
>　*Diary,* February 23, 1667

Samuel Johnson [1709–1784]

Ladies — stock and tend your Hive,
Trifle not at Thirty-five:
For howe'er we boast and strive,
Life declines from Thirty-five;
He that ever hopes to thrive
Must begin at Thirty-five.
>　*To Hester Thrale on Her 35th*
>　*Birthday*

George Gordon, Lord Byron [1788–1824]

The fair sex should be always fair; and
　no man
Till thirty, should perceive there's a
　plain woman.
>　*Don Juan,* Canto XIII, Stanza
>　3

Arthur Schopenhauer [1788–1860]

The intellectual powers are most capable of enduring great and sustained efforts in youth, up to the age of thirty-five at latest; from which period their strength begins to decline, though very gradually.
>　*Counsels and Maxims,* "The
>　Ages of Life" (tr. by T. B.
>　Saunders)

Ralph Waldo Emerson [1803–1882]

Men and women at thirty years, and even earlier, have lost all spring and vivacity, and if they fail in their first enterprizes they throw up the game.
>　*Papers from* The Dial, "The
>　Tragic"

Alexander Smith [1830–1867]

The man who has reached thirty, feels at times as if he had come out of a great battle. Comrade after comrade has fallen; his own life seems to have been charmed.
>　*Dreamthorp,* Ch. III

Sir William Osler [1849–1919]

Take the sum of human achievement in action, in science, in art, in literature — subtract the work of the men above forty, and while we should miss great treasures, even priceless treasures, we would practically be where we are today. . . . The effective, moving, vitalizing work of the world is done between the ages of twenty-five and forty.

> *Aequanimitas, with Other Addresses,* "The Fixed Period"

George Moore [1852–1933]

The knell of my thirtieth year has sounded; in three or four years my youth will be as a faint haze on the sea, an illusive recollection.

> *Confessions of a Young Man,* Ch. XVI

MEASLES

Avicenna [980–1037]

The physical signs of measles are nearly the same as those of smallpox, but nausea and inflammation is more severe, though the pains in the back are less. The rash of measles usually appears at once, but the rash of smallpox spot after spot.

> *The Canon,* Bk. IV

William Shakespeare [1564–1616]

As for my country I have shed my blood,
Not fearing outward force, so shall my lungs
Coin words till their decay against those measles
Which we disdain should tetter us, yet sought
The very way to catch them.

> *Coriolanus,* III, i, 76

Douglas Jerrold [1803–1857]

They say love's like the measles — all the worse when it comes late in life.

> *Wit and Opinions of Douglas Jerrold, a Philanthropist*

Henry Wheeler Shaw ("Josh Billings") [1818–1885]

Love iz like the meazels, we kant alwus tell when we ketched it and ain't ap tew hav it severe but onst, and then it ain't kounted mutch unless it strikes inly.

> *Josh Billings: His Sayings,* Ch. 53

Charles Farrar Browne ("Artemus Ward") [1834–1867]

Did you ever hav the measels, and if so how many?

> *Artemus Ward His Book,* "The Census"

Samuel Butler [1835–1902]

They are only more lenient towards the diseases of the young — such as measles, which they think to be like sowing one's wild oats — and look over them as pardonable indiscretions if they have not been too serious, and if they are atoned for by complete subsequent recovery.

> *Erewhon,* Ch. X

Eugene Field [1850–1895]

A Chicago Papa is so Mean he Wont let his Little Baby have More than One Measle at a time.

> *Nonsense for Old & Young,* "A Mean Man"

Jerome K. Jerome [1859–1927]

Love is like the measles; we all have to go through it.

> *Idle Thoughts of an Idle Fellow,* "On Being in Love"

Chinese Proverb

Starve the measles, and nourish the smallpox.

MECHANISM

See REDUCTIONISM

MEDICAL SCHOOLS

See also EDUCATION, STU-
DENTS, TEACHERS, TEACH-
ING

John Abernethy [1764–1831]
The Hospital is the only proper Col-
lege in which to rear a true disciple of
Aesculapius.
> Quoted by Thomas Pettigrew
> in *Biographical Memoirs*

Daniel Drake [1785–1852]
The establishment of medical schools
is a prolific source of discord in the
profession.
> *Practical Essays on Medical
> Education and the Medical
> Profession in the United States,*
> Essay VII

Johns Hopkins [1795–1873]
This estate . . . is to be the site of
a great university, a place where the
young men of coming generations will
have the opportunity which I have always longed for. Young men will study
great things here. . . . and yonder
. . . will be a great hospital. . . .
Like the man in the parable, I have
had many talents given to me and I
feel they are in trust; I shall not bury
them but give them to the lads who
long for a wide education and who
will do great things someday with the
knowledge they receive here in this
university.
> Quoted by Abraham Flexner in
> *Daniel Coit Gilman,* Ch. 3

Theodor Billroth [1829–1894]
The greatest happiness of my life was
founding a school that carries on my
aims of scientific and humanitarian
accomplishments.
> Letter to Wilhelm His, 1893

Philip A. Bruce [1856–1933]
Jefferson must have tacitly recognized,
although he never directly admitted
the fact, that one of the important deficiencies in the course of studies
which he had projected for the University was the entire absence of hospital
facilities. Without those facilities, a
medical school, independently of anatomy, must always remain principally
an historical school, a school of theory,
a descriptive rather than a practically
illustrative school.
> *History of the University of
> Virginia,* Fourth Period

Bernard De Voto [1897–1955]
The only places where American medicine can fully live up to its possibilities
are the teaching hospitals.
> *Harper's Magazine,* January
> 1951

Roy O. Greep [1905–   ]
Alumni Day — when the alumni return to have their consciences pricked
and their pockets picked.
> Comment at Class Day, Har-
> vard Medical School

MEDICARE

Anonymous
Show me a man who needs Medicare,
and I'll show you a sick old man.

MEDICINE

See also PHYSICIANS, PRAC-
TICE, PROFESSIONS

Hippocrates [460?–377? B.C.]
Life is short, and the Art long; the
occasion fleeting; experience fallacious,
and judgment difficult. The physician
must not only be prepared to do what

is right himself, but also to make the patient, the attendants, and externals co-operate.[1]

> *Aphorisms*, I.i (tr. by Francis Adams)

The art has three factors, the disease, the patient, the physician. The physician is the servant of the art. The patient must co-operate with the physician in combating the disease.

> *Epidemics*, I.XI (tr. by W.H.S. Jones)

In the cities there is no punishment connected with the practice of medicine (and with it alone) except disgrace, and that does not hurt those who are familiar with it.

> *Law*, I (tr. by Francis Adams)

Necessity itself made medicine to be sought out and discovered by men, since the same things when administered to the sick, which agreed with them when in good health, neither did nor do agree with them.

> *On Ancient Medicine*, III (tr. by Francis Adams)

We ought not to reject the ancient Art, as if it were not, and had not been properly founded, because it did not attain accuracy in all things, but rather, since it is capable of reaching to the greatest exactitude by reasoning, to receive it and admire its discoveries, made from a state of great ignorance, and as having been well and properly made, and not from chance.

> *Ibid.*, XII

I think that one cannot know anything certain respecting nature from any other quarter than from medicine; and that this knowledge is to be attained when one comprehends the whole subject of medicine properly, but not until then.

> *Ibid.*, XX

---

[1] Cf. Geoffrey Chaucer, p. 294b; Johann Wolfgang von Goethe, p. 297a.

Wherever the art of medicine is loved, there also is love of humanity.

> *Precepts*, VI

Plato [427?–347 B.C.]

The soul and body being two, have two arts corresponding to them: there is the art of politics attending on the soul; and another art attending on the body, of which I know no single name, but which may be described as having two divisions, one of them gymnastic, and the other medicine.

> *Gorgias*, 464.B (tr. by Benjamin Jowett)

Medicine is an art, and attends to the nature and constitution of the patient, and has principles of action and reason in each case.

> *Ibid.*, 501.A

And this is what the physician has to do, and in this the art of medicine consists: for medicine may be regarded generally as the knowledge of the loves and desires of the body, and how to satisfy them or not; and the best physician is he who is able to separate fair love from foul, or to convert one into the other; and he who knows how to eradicate and how to implant love, whichever is required, and can reconcile the most hostile elements in the constitution and make them loving friends, is a skilful practitioner.

> *Symposium*, 186.C (tr. by Benjamin Jowett)

Cicero [106–43 B.C.]

Nor do all sick persons get well, but that does not prove that there is no art of medicine.

> *On the Nature of the Gods*, II.iv.12 (tr. by H. Rackham)

Ovid [43 B.C.–A.D. 17?]

The art of medicine is my discovery. I am called Help-Bringer throughout the world, and all the potency of herbs is known to me. [Spoken by Apollo.]

> *Metamorphoses*, I.521 (tr. by F. J. Miller)

Celsus [25 B.C.–A.D. 50]

Just as agriculture promises nourishment to healthy bodies, so does the Art of Medicine promise health to the sick.

> *De Medicina*, Prooemium (tr. by W. G. Spencer)

The Art of Medicine is in need really of reasoning, . . . for this is a conjectural art. However, in many cases not only does conjecture fail, but experience as well.

> *Idem*

The Art of Medicine admits of scarcely any universal precepts.

> *Idem*

In medicine, rules may be absolute, but consequences are variable.

> *Ibid.*, VI.13

Pliny the Elder [23–79]

Is there any trade or occupation goeth beyond it for poisoning? What is the cause of more gaping and laying wait after wils and testaments, than this? What adulteries have been committed under the colour hereof, even in Princes and Emperors palaces?

> *Natural History*, XXIX.viii.20 (tr. by Philemon Holland)

It is striking that there is no art so incomprehensible or liable to change its methods oftener than medicine, as there is none other so lucrative.

Galen [fl. 2nd Cent.]

Those things which bring about health where it does not exist are called medicines and remedies, while those which maintain it where it exists are called healthy modes of living. Thus also, according to an old saying, medicine is the science of agencies healthful and harmful, the healthful being alike those which conserve existing health and those which restore it when deranged; while the harmful are the opposite of these.

> *De Sectis ad eos, qui introducuntur*, I

Decimus Magnus Ausonius [309?–394?]

My father practised medicine — the only one of all the arts which produced a god [Aesculapius].[1]

> *Idylls*, I.i.13

Rhazes [850–923]

Truth in medicine is an unattainable goal, and the art as described in books is far beneath the knowledge of an experienced and thoughtful physician.

> Quoted by Max Neuburger in *History of Medicine*, Vol. I

Geoffrey Chaucer [1340?–1400]

The lyf so short, the craft so long to lerne,
Th'assay so hard, so sharp the conquerynge.[2]

> *The Parliament of Fowls*

Sir Thomas More [1478–1535]

Thoughe there be almost no nation under heaven that hath lesse nede of Phisicke than they, yet this notwithstandyng, Phisicke is no where in greater honour; bycause they counte the knowledge of it among the goodlyeste, and most profytable partes of Philosophie.

> *Utopia*, Bk. II, Ch. 6 (tr. by R. Robinson)

Paracelsus [1493?–1541]

Internal medicine and surgery are based on philosophy and must not be separated except in practice; every

---

[1] His father, Julius Ausonius [287–377], was a celebrated doctor.
[2] Cf. Hippocrates, p. 293a; Johann Wolfgang von Goethe, p. 297a.

physician must be a doctor of both medicines.
Die grosse Wundarznei

Medicine is not only a science; it is also an art. It does not consist of compounding pills and plasters; it deals with the very processes of life, which must be understood before they may be guided.
Idem

Jean Fernel [1497–1558]

Is there a greater blessing vouchsafed to mankind than medicine is? Life is our dearest possession by which we breathe and enjoy the company of our fellow beings. Can any calling be worthier than that which preserves and maintains life itself? Is wealth or fortune in whatever measure, in the last resort, more estimable than is good health? Is any misfortune or disaster more grievous than ill health? He who succors the sufferer and the sick exercises a knowledge which deserves the admiration and affectionate regard of all men.
Quoted by Sir Charles Sherrington in *The Endeavor of Jean Fernel*, Pt. I

Sir Francis Bacon [1561–1626]

The poets did well to conjoin Music and Medicine in Apollo: because the office of medicine is but to tune this curious harp of man's body and to reduce it to harmony.
The Advancement of Learning, Bk. II

Sir Theodore Mayerne [1573–1655]

The King [James I] laughs at medicine and holds it so cheap that he declares physicians to be of very little use and hardly necessary. He asserts the art of medicine to be supported by mere conjectures and useless because uncertain.

René Descartes [1596–1650]

It is true that the science of Medicine, as it now exists, contains few things whose utility is very remarkable: but without any wish to depreciate it, I am confident that there is no one, even among those whose profession it is, who does not admit that all at present known in it is almost nothing in comparison of what remains to be discovered; and that we could free ourselves from an infinity of maladies of body as well as of mind, and perhaps also even from the debility of age, if we had sufficiently ample knowledge of their causes, and of all the remedies provided for us by Nature.
Discours de la Méthode, Pt. VI (tr. by John Veitch)

Gilles Ménage [1613–1692]

Medicine may be defined as the art or the science of keeping a patient quiet with frivolous reasons for his illness and amusing him with remedies good or bad until nature kills him or cures him.
Ménagiana, Pt. III

Thomas Sydenham [1624–1689]

The art of medicine was to be properly learned only from its practice and its exercise.
Medical Observations (3rd ed.), Dedicatory Epistle (tr. by R. G. Latham in *Works*, Vol. I)

Sir Richard Blackmore [1650?–1729]

The Art of Healing was, in the eldest Ages of Learning, but a tender Plant, sprung newly from the Ground; and notwithstanding it was cherished with Care, and cultivated by industrious Hands, acquired however but little Growth and Vigour during a long Series of Years, and could only boast of some green and unripe Fruit; tho', 'tis true, it was then adorned with Plenty of Leaves and Blossoms, that promised maturer and more generous Productions to come.

> *Discourses on the Gout, a Rheumatism, and the King's Evil*

Archibald Pitcairne [1652–1713]

The Art of Healing is of greater Antiquity than the Study of Philosophy; because when Men first began with Medicine, or Philosophy, as they were determined by their Regards to the Body or the Mind, the Reasons for the former they found perpetual, but for the latter only fortuitous and accidental. For they who in the beginning peopled the Earth, lived at first on its Produce, and then on Flesh, were exposed to the Inclemencies of the Air, and the Viscissitudes of Heat and Cold; that is, they ailed before they provided themselves with Houses or Clothing: Those were their first Grievances, and these their first remedies. . . . But Men began not to philosophize till they had experienced the Operations of Remedies, and till they could with Security, and at their Leisure, search into the Relations of things, and emulate each other in intellectual Endowments.

> *The Philosophical and Mathematical Elements of Physick*, Introduction

Jonathan Swift [1667–1745]

Apollo was held the god of physic and sender of diseases. Both were originally the same trade, and still continue.

> *Thoughts on Various Subjects, Moral and Diverting*

Giorgio Baglivi [1669–1707?]

Medicine is not a production bursting suddenly from the genius of man, but is the child of time.

> *Opera Omnia Medica*, Preface

Samuel Johnson [1709–1784]

Medicine is a profession which must, undoubtedly, claim the second place

amongst those which are of the greatest benefit to mankind.

Thomas Jefferson [1743–1826]

Harvey's discovery of the circulation of the blood was a beautiful addition to our knowledge of the animal economy, but on a review of the practice of medicine before and since that epoch, I do not see any great amelioration which has been derived from that discovery.[1]

> Letter to Edward Jenner, May 14, 1806 (Quoted by John Baron in *Life of Edward Jenner*, Vol. II, Ch. 3)

The only sure foundations of medicine are, an intimate knowledge of the human body, and observation on the effects of medicinal substances on that.

> Letter to Dr. Caspar Wistar, June 21, 1807

John Coakley Lettsom [1744–1815]

[Medicine] is not a lucrative profession. It is a divine one.

> Letter to a friend, September 6, 1791

Benjamin Rush [1745?–1813]

Medicine is an occupation for slaves.

> *Autobiography*

When that time [death] shall come, I shall relinquish many attractions to life, and among them a pleasure which has to me no equal in human pursuits; I mean that which I derive from studying, teaching and practising medicine.

> Letter to Dr. David Hosack

The art of healing is like an unroofed temple; uncovered at the top, and cracked at the foundation.

John Aikin [1747–1822]

Evils, no doubt, moral and natural, will remain as long as the world remains;

[1] See note, p. 26a.

but the certainty of the perpetual existence of vice, is no more an argument against attempting to correct it, than the same certainty with respect to disease, is a reason against exercising the art of medicine.

> Letters from a Father to his Son, Letter XX, "On the Inequality of Conditions"

Johann Wolfgang von Goethe [1749–1832]

Art is long, life short, judgment difficult, occasion transient.[1]

> Wilhelm Meister, Bk. VII, Ch. 9 (tr. by Thomas Carlyle)

Medicine absorbs the physician's whole being because it is concerned with the entire human organism.

Nicholas de Belleville [1753–1831]

The advantage that the practice of medicine has over surgery is, that if you do not know what the matter is, you can call it occult, and get off with credit, but as surgery is demonstrable, they hold you to the proof.

> Quoted by Fred B. Rogers in Help-Bringers, "Belleville"

Jean Nicolas Corvisart des Marets [1755–1821]

Medicine is a conjectural art.

Pierre Cabanis [1757–1808]

In order to study and practice medicine in a proper manner, it is necessary to be impressed with its importance; and to be truly impressed, we must believe in it.

> Du Degré de Certitude de la Médecine, Preface

Karl von Clausewitz [1780–1831]

The art of medicine for the most part, deals only with physical phenomena; it has to do with the animal organism,

which is subject to perpetual changes and is never quite the same for two moments. This makes its task very difficult and places the judgment of the physician above his knowledge; but how much more difficult is the case if a mental and moral effect comes in as well, and how much higher do we set the physician of the soul.

François Magendie [1783–1855]

Medicine is a science in the making.

Jacob Bigelow [1786–1879]

The death of medical men . . . reminds us, that we, in turn, are to become victims of the incompetency of our own art. It admonishes us, that the sphere of our professional exertions is limited, at last, by insurmountable barriers. It brings with it the humiliating conclusion, that while other sciences have been carried forward, within our own time and almost under our own eyes, to a degree of unprecedented advancement, Medicine, in regard to some of its professed and most important objects, is still an ineffectual speculation.

> Self-Limited Diseases

Peter Mere Latham [1789–1875]

Medicine is a strange mixture of speculation and action. We have to cultivate a science and to exercise an art. The calls of science are upon our leisure and our choice; the calls of practice are of daily emergence and necessity.

> Diseases of the Heart, Lect. XXXVII

A man need not have grown old in the practice of medicine to bear witness to its having undergone considerable changes.

> General Remarks on the Practice of Medicine, Ch. II

There are peculiar causes which will ever prevent medicine from arriving at

---

[1] Cf. Hippocrates, p. 293a; Geoffrey Chaucer, p. 294b.

the certainty of purely physical science.

> *Lectures on Clinical Medicine,*
> Lect. V

Henry McMurtrie [1793–1865]

Boys, don't study medicine. By the time you earn your bread, you will have no teeth left to eat it with.

> Quoted in *The Barnwell Bulletin* 18:22, October 1940

Karl F. H. Marx [1796–1877]

Medicine heals doubts as well as diseases.

> Quoted by F. H. Garrison in *Bulletin of the New York Academy of Medicine* 4:1001, 1928

For thousands of years, medicine has united the aims and aspirations of the best and noblest of mankind. To depreciate its treasures is to discount all human endeavour and achievement as naught.

> *Ibid.,* 5:156, 1929

He, who has no notion of the inconceivable wealth of proven experience and helpful wisdom which is in medicine, may censure it as fragmentary, under the delusion of extenuating his own ignorance.

> *Idem*

Ralph Waldo Emerson [1803–1882]

In the hands of the discoverer medicine becomes a heroic art. . . . Wherever life is dear he is a demigod.

> *Uncollected Lectures,* "Resources"

Elisha Bartlett [1804–1855]

The obligations of the world to the science and the art of medicine . . . are beyond all measurement or estimate. There is no process that can reckon up the amount of good which they have conferred upon the human race; there is no moral calculus that

can grasp and comprehend the sum of their beneficent operations. Ever since the first dawn of civilization and learning . . . they have been the true and constant friends of the suffering sons and daughters of men. . . . they have blunted the arrows of death, and rendered less rugged and precipitous the inevitable pathway to the tomb.

> *An Inquiry into the Degree of Certainty in Medicine*

Oliver Wendell Holmes [1809–1894]

The truth is, that medicine, professedly founded on observation, is as sensitive to outside influences, political, religious, philosophical, imaginative, as is the barometer to the changes of atmospheric density.

> *Medical Essays,* "Currents and Counter-Currents in Medical Science"

All a man's powers are not too much for such a profession as Medicine.

> *Ibid.,* "Scholastic and Bedside Teaching"

Heinrich Haeser [1811–1884]

Medicine is as old as the human race, as old as the necessity for the removal of disease.

> *Lehrbuch der Geschichte der Medizin,* Erste Periode

Alfred Stillé [1813–1900]

It behooves us to remember that medicine is, above all else, humane as well as human; that its beginning, middle, and end is to relieve suffering, and that whatever is outside this may indeed be science of some sort, but certainly is not medicine.

> *Medical News* 44:433, 1884

George Eliot (Marian Evans Cross) [1819–1880]

I should never have been happy in any profession that did not call forth the highest intellectual strain, and yet

keep me in good warm contact with my neighbors. There is nothing like the medical profession for that: one can have the exclusive scientific life that touches the distance, and befriend the old fogies in the parish too.
>   *Middlemarch*, Ch. 16

Henry Thomas Buckle [1821–1862]

Among the arts, medicine, on account of its eminent utility, must always hold the highest place.
>   *Miscellaneous and Posthumous Works*, Vol. II, Fragment 7

Gustave Flaubert [1821–1880]

MEDICINE: When in good health, make fun of it.
>   *Dictionary of Accepted Ideas* (tr. by Jacques Barzun)

Rudolf Virchow [1821–1902]

Practical medicine is never the same thing as scientific medicine but rather, even in the hands of the greatest master, an application of it.
>   *Disease, Life, and Man,* "Standpoints in Scientific Medicine" (tr. by L. J. Rather)

If popular medicine gave the people wisdom as well as knowledge, it would be the best protection for scientific and well-trained physicians.

Hermann von Helmholtz [1821–1894]

An old student, like myself, scarcely recognizes the somewhat matronly aspect of Dame Medicine, when he accidentally comes again in relation to her, so vigorous and so capable of growth has she become in the fountain of youth of the Natural Sciences.
>   *Das Denken in der Medizin* (tr. by E. Atkinson in *Popular Lectures on Scientific Subjects*)

Medicine was once the intellectual home in which I grew up, and even the emigrant understands and is best understood by his native land.
>   *Idem*

Andrew James Symington [1825– ?]

The medical profession is a noble and pleasant one, though laborious and often full of anxiety.

Theodor Billroth [1829–1894]

It is quite correct to distinguish between medical science and the physician's art.

A person may have acquired from books a vast amount of medical knowledge, he may even have memorized from books the technic of its application; such a person has much knowledge of medicine, and yet with it all he is no physician. He must see and hear a master's diagnosis, prognosis, and treatment of disease. He must witness the master's skill in action, in order himself to become a practitioner. The more he knows, the more he will be able to accomplish later. Now the object of our modern endeavor is to make the physician's skill independent of tradition, and by means of written records to conserve the art of healing for all time, so that it may be independent of the talent of the individual and may be reduced to an absolute science. All knowledge and skill are to be determined and controlled by means of the laws of arithmetic and logic in order to make everything absolute and permanent. How long have we been seeking absolute truth and absolute beauty? . . .

I doubt if this goal will ever be reached — at least in the art of healing. . . . The physician, like the artist, must constantly produce and reproduce. Disease processes and disease products which lie veiled before him must crystallize out of the many direct and indirect sense impressions in his mind into a picture which will become clearer and more nearly correct the more he knows about these disease processes and disease products. But this knowledge is of no value to him if he lacks imagination and the power of synthesis. The student can learn to develop this power, to practise it, to guard against errors, only by observing a master in action.

> *The Medical Sciences in the German Universities*, Pt. I, "The Early Universities"

Charles Dudley Warner
[1829–1900]

In the minds of the public, there is mystery about the practice of medicine.

Edward Berdoe [1836–1916]

Medicine now has no mysteries to conceal from the true student of nature.

Sir James Bryce [1838–1922]

Medicine [is] the only profession that labours incessantly to destroy the reason for its own existence.

> Address, March 23, 1914

Frank Payne [1840–1910]

This basis of medicine is sympathy and the desire to help others, and whatever is done with this end must be called medicine.

> *English Medicine in the Anglo-Saxon Times*

Robert Bridges [1844–1930]

Tho' MEDICINE makes not so plain an
    appeal to the vulgar,
Yet she lags not a whit: her pregnant
    theory touches
Deeper discoveries, her more complete
    revolution
Gives promise of wider benefits in
    larger abundance.
> *Now in Wintry Delights*

Nicholas Senn [1844–1908]

Superstition and medicine are incompatible neighbors. Science should precede — it certainly must accompany — progressive modern medicine.

> *American Medicine* 4:467, 1902

Sir William Osler [1849–1919]

The profession of medicine is distinguished from all others by its *singular beneficence*.

> *Aequanimitas, with Other Addresses*, "Chauvinism in Medicine"

Medicine is the only world-wide profession, following everywhere the same methods, actuated by the same ambitions, and pursuing the same ends.

> *Ibid.*, "Unity, Peace, and Concord"

Medicine is a science of uncertainty and an art of probability.

> Quoted by William B. Bean in *Sir William Osler: Aphorisms*, Ch. 5

Karl Sudhoff [1853–1938]

Medicine is a sacred calling, and he who makes it ridiculous is guilty of sacrilege.

George Bernard Shaw [1856–1950]

Medical science is as yet very imperfectly differentiated from common curemongering witchcraft.

> *The Doctor's Dilemma*, "Preface on Doctors"

John C. Hemmeter [1863–1931]

In the eighteenth and during the first part of the nineteenth century medicine was comparable to a sterile unproductive heath, in which some evil spirits drove about the speculating medical philosophers in a circle. Now we have gotten into an overfruitful swamp or jungle in which the facts grow so luxuriantly that they threaten to smother our thinking powers.

> *Master Minds in Medicine*, Ch. XII

Charles H. Mayo [1865–1939]

While medicine is a science, in many particulars it cannot be exact, so baffling are the varying results of varying conditions of human life.

> *Collected Papers of the Mayo Clinic and Mayo Foundation* 1:601, 1909

Medicine is about as big or as little in any community, large or small, as the physicians make it.

> *University of Toronto Medical Journal,* April 1928

Abraham Flexner [1866–1959]

From the earliest time, medicine has been a curious blend of superstition, empiricism, and that kind of sagacious observation, which is the stuff out of which ultimately science is made. Of these three strands — superstition, empiricism, and observation — medicine was constituted in the days of the priest-physicians of Egypt and Babylonia; of the same three strands it is still composed. The proportions have, however, varied significantly; an increasingly alert and determined effort, running through the ages, has endeavored to expel superstition, to narrow the range of empiricism, and to enlarge, refine, and systematize the scope of observation.

> *Medical Education, A Comparative Study,* Ch. 1

Samuel Hopkins Adams [1871–1958]

Medicine would be the ideal profession if it did not involve giving pain.

> *The Health Master,* Ch. III

Marcel Proust [1871–1922]

Medicine being a compendium of the successive and contradictory mistakes of medical practitioners, when we summon the wisest of them to our aid, the chances are that we may be relying on a scientific truth the error of which will be recognized in a few years' time. So that to believe in medicine would be the height of folly, if not to believe in it were not greater folly still, for from this mass of errors there have emerged in the course of time many truths.

> *The Guermantes Way,* Pt. I, "My Grandmother's Illness" (tr. by C. K. Scott-Moncrieff)

William D. Haggard [1872–1940]

The obligation of the profession in medicine, as well as in surgery, is a very sacred one. It must be our constant endeavor by the unwritten laws of custom, by the force of speech, by ethical regulation in the profession, by educational betterment and by statutory enactment, to safeguard the traditions and ideals of the profession and fulfill our highest obligation in caring for the lives, the health and the happiness of the people of this country.

> *Journal of the American Medical Association* 61:161, 1913

Wilfred Trotter [1872–1939]

[The medical career is one] in which it is possible for people — men or women — to pursue the dying ideal that an occupation for adults should allow of intellectual freedom, should give character as much chance as cleverness, and should be subject to the tonic of difficulty and the spice of danger.

> *Collected Papers,* "Emergency," Sect. 3

To the experimenter immersed in his research and to the clinician struggling with the load of experience and the needs of patients, it may seem unpractical to be concerned with the theory of medical knowledge. On the other hand, it is perhaps the lack of rational doctrine and a general interest in the problems of method that has made medicine the scene of so much disunited and contradictory effort, and helped to

put it down from its historical position as the mother and the nurse of science.
Ibid., "Observation and Experiment and Their Use in the Medical Sciences"

Léon Bernard [1875–   ]

Medicine should be practiced as a form of friendship.
Aphorism

Irvin Abell [1876–1949]

With the exception of the ministry it stands closer than any other calling to the secret of eternity and watches death ever busy with her shuttle as she weaves her somber threads into the woof and warp of the affairs of men. It seeks to mitigate human sufferings, to prolong human life.
Annals of Surgery 107:641, 1938

René Sand [1877–   ]

The place of medicine is in the stream of life, not on its banks.
The Advance to Social Medicine, Pt. 9

Lawrence J. Henderson [1878–1942]

Somewhere between 1910 and 1912 in this country, a random patient, with a random disease, consulting a doctor chosen at random had, for the first time in the history of mankind, a better than fifty-fifty chance of profiting from the encounter.[1]
Quoted in *New England Journal of Medicine* 270:449, 1964

Sir Henry Howarth Bashford ("Peter Harding") [1880–1961]

Here is an aspect of medicine worth consideration. To the seeing eye and the tender hand there is no easier door into the warm heart of humanity. There is no other profession that will lead you quite so close to reality. And

[1] Cf. Petrarch, p. 391b.

by this I don't mean realism in the modern sense, wherein, as it seems to me, the altogether ugly looms so disproportionately large. For after thirty years of tolerably wide opportunity I have still failed to find the altogether ugly. And though of course you will meet ugliness in plenty — a cancer that will find you shocked and, alas, largely impotent — yet, if you look long enough, and carefully enough, how often will you discover it to be but the shadow of some clearly shining spiritual beauty. No, you need not fear, I think, to tread behind the veil.
The Corner of Harley Street, Ch. 2

H. L. Mencken [1880–1956]

The aim of medicine is surely not to make men virtuous; it is to safeguard and rescue them from the consequences of their vices.
Prejudices, "Types of Men: The Physician"

Francis Weld Peabody [1881–1927]

There is no more contradiction between the science of medicine and the art of medicine than between the science of aeronautics and the art of flying.
The Care of the Patient

O. H. Perry Pepper [1884–1962]

It is often said that the master word of medicine is work. Of course this is true in one sense of the word *work.* But I don't like masters and I don't like work — in the other sense. The best that I can wish . . . is that you will find in medicine not a master, but a mistress: charming, intelligent, amusing; arousing love, passion, and a desire to serve. If this happens to you, your career will be happy and successful.
Address to Senior Class, University of Pennsylvania School of Medicine, Spring 1955

Victor Robinson [1886–1947]

The first cry of pain through the primitive jungle was the first call for a physician. . . . Medicine is a natural art, conceived in sympathy and born of necessity; from instinctive procedures developed the specialized science that is practiced today.
>*The Story of Medicine*

Sir F. M. R. Walshe [1888–   ]

Medicine has a changing and unchanging face, and it is as necessary to learn the meaning of the first as it is to recognize and to cherish the second.
>*Canadian Medical Association Journal* 67:395, 1952

Alan Gregg [1890–1957]

You are an artist if you pay homage through one medium to all that you feel from another. The scientific training permits of reliability and accuracy, not of adequacy. Thus, from these it follows that medicine may be both a science and an art.
>Aphorism (Quoted by Wilder Penfield in *The Difficult Art of Giving,* Appendix A)

What binds our profession together throughout the world is not so much the facts we agree upon or the knowledge we share, as the experiences we have all gone through, and the way we understand them and fit them to the pattern of our values.
>*Transactions of the Association of American Physicians* 67:47, 1954

Henry E. Sigerist [1891–1957]

Science progressed rapidly from the seventeenth century on; medicine became scientific, highly technical, highly specialized, and very costly.
>*Canadian Journal of Public Health* 35:253, 1944

Medical science has infinitely more to give than the people actually receive.
>*Civilization and Disease,* Ch. 12

Dana W. Atchley [1892–   ]

Like all great art, the art of medicine is the skillful and creative application of a scientific discipline to a human problem. The musician without harmony, the painter with no knowledge of pigment and perspective, the architect unaware of the essential elements of engineering — all are amateurs, as is the physician unversed in the science of medicine, its methods of thought, and its accumulated facts.
>*Journal of Medical Education* 34(October, Pt. II):17, 1959

Henry Jackson, Jr. [1892–   ]

Science of course is necessary; it has its justified place and each year it becomes more important to the proper practice of medicine. But neither tests nor science can fully replace the art of medicine and that is fast disappearing, though occasionally one sees shy, frightened bits peering cautiously out at the man who is ill through the maze of millimols and hydrogen ions and tests for histoplasmosis, which mean precisely nothing.
>*New England Journal of Medicine* 254:910, 1956

Ben Hecht [1894–1964]

Solving the mysteries of heaven has not given birth to as many abortive findings as has the quest into the mysteries of the human body. When you think of yourselves as scientists, I want you always to remember everything you learn from me will probably be regarded tomorrow as the naive confusions of a pack of medical aborigines. Despite all our toil and progress, the art of medicine still falls somewhere between trout casting and spook writing.
>*Miracle of the Fifteen Murderers*

George Merck [1894–1957]

Medicine is for the patient. Medicine is for the people. It is not for the profits.

Hermann L. Blumgart [1895–   ]

The profession of medicine is "a house of many mansions."
New England Journal of Medicine 271:238, 1964

Sir Robert Platt [1900–   ]

Medicine consists of science, wisdom, and technology. We teach the science; we ignore the study of human behavior from which wisdom could derive; and we profess to despise technology though we see it all around us.
British Medical Journal 2:551, 1965

Raymond Whitehead [1904–1965]

Medicine is not a field in which sheep may safely graze.
British Medical Journal 2:491, 1956

Wilfrid G. Oakley [1905–   ]

I suppose the term "armchair medicine" is one most often used in a disparaging way by those who act without thinking about those who think without acting.
Transactions of the Medical Society of London 78:2, 1962

William A. Sodeman [1906–   ]

Born in mystery and superstition, burdened by ignorance, beset by quackery, overcome in its abortive attempts to progress, at times by the engulfment of civilizations in which a start upward had been made, held in check by political and spiritual thought at times for centuries, medicine has emerged from this long and at times seemingly fruitless struggle to become the world's greatest boon to mankind.
Journal of the American Medical Association 193:592, 1965

William W. Engstrom [1915–   ]

The so-called art of medicine is a supplement, not a substitute, for science.
Marquette Medical Review 23:3, 1957–58

Louis Lasagna [1923–   ]

Some will say that . . . whereas medicine can legitimately deal with the prolongation of life, it cannot cope with its enrichment. But if the physician is to be a social animal, he must reject the tyrannical limitations imposed by such a dichotomy. Otherwise the picture is tragic indeed, for then science is relegated to the role of robot-maker, to the building of brightly polished automata with smoothly functioning gears which permit their owners to stare eternally with vacant eyes at a world they are unable to perceive or enjoy.
The Doctors' Dilemmas, Epilogue

American Proverb

There ain't much fun in physic, but there's a great deal of physic in fun.

Chinese Proverb

Medicine is one of the nine low trades.

MEETINGS

See also COMMITTEE MEETINGS

August Bier [1861–1949]

Nowadays [1926] everybody talks, wherever you look, especially in the parliaments, but worst of all at the International Congresses. There, the flowery speakers of all nations convene and infect one another.
Aphorism

Béla Schick [1877–1967]

The scientific sessions are of secondary importance — *meetings are for meeting people.*

> Quoted by I. J. Wolf in *Aphorisms and Facetiae of Béla Schick,* "Early Years"

Sir F. M. R. Walshe [1888–   ]

The symposium as an informal meeting for discussion has its obvious usefulness *for the symposiast,* but, as an excuse for multiple publication, quite another view may be taken of it. Also, if every symposiast were a Dr. Samuel Johnson, perhaps the intercalated discussions at a symposium might strike more fire and distil less mutual admiration. Symposia, like hard liquor, should be taken in reasonable measure, at appropriate intervals.

> *Perspectives in Biology and Medicine* 2:197, 1959

MELANCHOLY

See also SORROW

Miguel de Cervantes [1547–1616]

Melancholy was made, not for beasts, but for men; but if men give way to it overmuch they turn to beasts.

> *Don Quixote*

William Shakespeare [1564–1616]

For so your doctors hold it very meet,
Seeing too much sadness hath congeal'd your blood
And melancholy is the nurse of frenzy.
Therefore they thought it good you hear a play
And frame your mind to mirth and merriment,
Which bars a thousand harms and lengthens life.

> *The Taming of the Shrew,* Induction, ii, 133

This is in thee a nature but infected,
A poor unmanly melancholy sprung
From change of fortune.

> *Timon of Athens,* IV, iii, 202

He straight declin'd, droop'd, took it deeply,
Fasten'd and fix'd the shame on't in himself,
Threw off his spirit, his appetite, his sleep,
And downright languish'd.

> *The Winter's Tale,* II, iii, 14

Robert Burton [1577–1640]

If there be a hell upon earth, it is to be found in a melancholy man's heart.

> *The Anatomy of Melancholy*

When a sad and sick Patient was brought unto him [Epicurus] to be cured, he laid him on a down bed, crowned him with a garland of sweet-smelling flowers, in a fair perfumed closet delicately set out, and after a potion or two of good drink, which he administred, he brought in a beautifull yong wench that could play upon a Lute, sing and dance, etc. . . . most of our looser Physicians in some cases . . . allow of this, and all of them will have a melancholy, sad, and discontented person, make frequent use of honest sports, companies, and recreations.

> *Ibid.,* Pt. 2, Sect. 2, Memb. 6, Subsect. 4

John Ford [1586?–1640?]

> Melancholy
Is not, as you perceive, indisposition
Of body, but the mind's disease. So Ecstasy,
Fantastic Dotage, Madness, Frenzy, Rapture
Of mere imagination, differ partly
From Melancholy; which is briefly this,
A mere commotion of the mind, o'ercharged

With fear and sorrow; first begot i'
the brain,
The seat of reason, from thence de-
rived
As suddenly in the heart, the seat
Of our affection.
> *The Lover's Melancholy*, Act
> III, Sc. ii

Voltaire [1694–1778]

Wounds of the soul . . . [are] a disease wherein the patient must minister
to himself.
> Letter to a friend, 1728 (tr. by
> S. G. Tallentyre)

I look on solemnity as a disease: I
had rather a thousand times be as feeble and feverish as I am now than
think lugubriously.
> Letter to Frederick, Prince
> Royal of Russia, 1737

Samuel Johnson [1709–1784]

I inherited . . . a vile melancholy
from my father, which has made me
mad all my life, at least not sober.
> Quoted by James Boswell in
> *Tour to the Hebrides*, Septem-
> ber 16, 1773

Thomas Gray [1716–1771]

Melancholy mark'd him for her own.
> *Elegy Written in a Country
> Church-Yard*, "The Epitaph"

Tobias Smollett [1721–1771]

The approbation of the public, which
he had earned or might acquire, like
a cordial often repeated, began to lose
its effect upon his imagination; his
health suffered by the sedentary life
and austere application; his eyesight
failed, his appetite forsook him, his
spirits decayed; so that he became
melancholy, listless, and altogether incapable of prosecuting the only means
he had left for his subsistence.
> *The Adventures of Peregrine
> Pickle*, Ch. 100

Sydney Smith [1771–1845]

Never give way to melancholy; resist
it steadily, for the habit will encroach.
> Quoted by Lady Holland in *A
> Memoir of the Rev. Sydney
> Smith*, Ch. 10

H. H. Munro ("Saki") [1870–1916]

He's simply got the instinct for being
unhappy highly developed.
> *Chronicles of Clovis*, "The
> Match-Maker"

Richard Asher [1912–   ]

Despair is better treated with hope,
not dope.
> *Lancet* 1:954, 1958

METABOLISM

The Prasna Upanishad
[ca. 500 B.C.]

Food eaten is sundered in three. The
thickest stock thereof becometh excre-
ment, the middling flesh, and thinnest
mind. Water drunk is sundered in
three. The thickest stock thereof becometh the body's water, the middling
blood, and the thinnest breath. Heat
eaten is sundered in three. The thickest stock thereof becometh bone, the
middling marrow, the thinnest speech.

Claude Bernard [1813–1878]

We may, of course, strike a balance
between what a living organism takes
in as nourishment and what it gives
out in excretions. . . . This would be
like trying to tell what happens inside
a house by watching what goes in by
the door and what comes out by the
chimney.
> *An Introduction to the Study
> of Experimental Medicine*, Pt.
> II, Ch. 2, Sect. ix (tr. by H. C.
> Greene)

Sir Archibald E. Garrod
[1857–1936]

Actual derangements of the metabolic processes follow almost any deviations from the normal of health, but our interpretation of the urinary changes which result is, in many instances, greatly hampered by the scantiness of our knowledge of the intermediate steps of the paths of metabolism. Such knowledge as we have of these steps is derived from casual glimpses afforded when, as the outcome of one of Nature's experiments, some particular line is interfered with, and intermediate products are excreted incompletely burnt.

Inborn Errors of Metabolism, Ch. 1

It may well be that the intermediate products formed at the several stages [in metabolism] have only momentary existence as such, being subjected to further change almost as soon as they are formed; and that the course of metabolism along any particular path should be pictured as in continuous movement rather than as series of distinct steps. If any one step in the process fail the intermediate product in being at the point of arrest will escape further change, just as when the film of a biograph is brought to a standstill the moving figures are left foot in air.

Idem

Sir Frederick G. Hopkins
[1861–1947]

In the study of the intermediate processes of metabolism we have to deal, not with complex substances which elude ordinary chemical methods, but with simple substances undergoing comprehensible reactions.

British Medical Journal 2:713, 1913

MICROBES

See also ANTISEPSIS, INFECTION

Percy Bysshe Shelley [1792–1822]

I tell thee that those viewless beings,
Whose mansion is the smallest particle
Of the impassive atmosphere,
Think, feel and live like man.
Queen Mab, Sect. II

Jacob Henle [1805–1885]

I have shown, then, that the infective material must be independently alive, and thought to consist of organisms — either plant or animal — or of parts of animals which have achieved a limited independence.

One must assume that the infective material is alive or, at least, can survive on the outside. A healthy body is not a proper soil for it, and pre-existing tissue changes might be required to permit its growth and proliferation.[1]

Pathologische Untersuchungen (tr. by Max Samter)

William T. Helmuth [1833–1902]

Oh, powerful bacillus,
With wonder how you fill us,
Every day!
While medical detectives,
With powerful objectives,
Watch your play.
Ode to the Bacillus

Mark Twain (Samuel L. Clemens) [1835–1910]

I doubt if God has given us any refreshment which, taken in moderation, is unwholesome, except microbes.

Autobiography, Vol. I, "Chapters Begun in Vienna"

[1] Jacob Henle was Robert Koch's teacher, and his ideas on this subject must have influenced Koch strongly.

Robert Bridges [1844–1930]

Where she [Medicine] nam'd the disease she now separates the bacillus;
Sets the atoms of offence, those blind
and sickly bloodeaters,
'Neath lens and daylight, forcing their
foul propagations,
Which had ever prosper'd in dark impunity unguest,
Now to behave in sight, deliver their
poisonous extract
And their strange self-brew'd, self-
slaying juice to be handled,
Experimented upon, set aside and
stor'd to oppose them.
Now in Wintry Delights

Hilaire Belloc [1870–1953]

The Microbe is so very small
You cannot make him out at all,
But many sanguine people hope
To see him through a microscope.
His jointed tongue that lies beneath
A hundred curious rows of teeth;
His seven tufted tails with lots
Of lovely pink and purple spots,
On each of which a pattern stands,
Composed of forty separate bands;
His eyebrows of a tender green;
All these have never yet been seen —
But Scientists, who ought to know,
Assure us that they must be so. . . .
Oh! let us never, never doubt
What nobody is sure about!
Cautionary Verses, "The Mi-
crobe"

Roy Atwell [1878–   ]

Some little bug is going to find you
some day,
Some little bug will creep behind you
some day.
*Some Little Bug Is Going to
Find You Some Day*

Martin H. Fischer [1879–1962]

Bacteria keep us from heaven and put
us there.
Quoted by Howard Fabing and
Ray Marr in *Fischerisms*

Wallace Wilson [fl. 20th Cent.]

He prayeth best who loveth best
All things both great and small.
The Streptococcus is the test —
I love it least of all.
Letter to Dr. E. P. Scarlett

Anonymous

In the Nineteenth Century men lost
their fear of God and acquired a fear
of microbes.

MIDDLE AGE

See also AGE, MATURITY,
YOUTH

Confucius [551–478 B.C.]

If a man has reached forty or fifty
without being heard of, he, indeed, is
incapable of commanding respect!
Analects, Bk. IX, Ch. XXII
(tr. by William E. Soothill)

Mencius [372?–289? B.C.]

At forty I attained to an unperturbed
mind.
Discourses, II

Martin Luther [1483–1546]

One's thirty-eighth year is an evil and
dangerous year, bringing many heavy
and great sicknesses.
Table-Talk, No. 787, "Of
Death" (tr. by William Hazlitt)

Francis Beaumont [1584–1616]
and John Fletcher [1579–1625]

Fat old women, fat and five and fifty.
Women Pleased, Act III, Sc. ii

John Dryden [1631–1700]

I am resolved to grow fat, and look
young till forty, and then slip out of
the world with the first wrinckle and
the reputation of five and twenty.
Secret Love, Act III

Edward Young [1683–1765]

A fool at forty is a fool indeed.
Love of Fame, Satire II

At *thirty* man *suspects* himself a fool;
Knows it at *forty*, and reforms his
plan.
Night Thoughts, Night I

Lady Mary Wortley Montagu
[1689–1762]

At the age of forty, she is very far
from being cold and insensible; her
fire may be covered with ashes, but
it is not extinguished.
Letter to Lady ———, January
13, 1716 [1]

Sir Walter Scott [1771–1832]

Fair, fat and forty.
St. Ronan's Well, Ch. 7

Esaias Tegnér [1782–1846]

Today is my forty-third birthday. I
have thus long passed the peak of life
where the waters divide.
Letter to F. M. Franzén, November 13, 1825

George Gordon, Lord Byron
[1788–1824]

A lady of a 'certain age,' which
means
Certainly aged.
Don Juan, Canto VI, Stanza 68

Though her years were waning,
Her climacteric teased her like her
teens.
Ibid., Canto XII, Stanza 1

Of all the barbarous middle ages, that
Which is most barbarous is the mid-
dle age
Of man!
Ibid., Canto XII, Stanza 1

Too old for youth, — too young, at
thirty-five,

[1] This letter, regarded as spurious, is listed
only by title in collections of her letters.

To herd with boys, or hoard with
good threescore, —
I wonder people should be left alive;
But since they are, that epoch is a
bore.
Ibid., Stanza 2

Arthur Schopenhauer [1788–1860]

On passing his fortieth year, any man
of the slightest power of mind — any
man, that is, who has more than the
sorry share of intellect with which nature has endowed five-sixths of mankind — will hardly fail to show some
trace of misanthropy.
Counsels and Maxims, "The
Ages of Life" (tr. by T. B.
Saunders)

Ralph Waldo Emerson
[1803–1882]

Men over forty are no judges of a book
written in a new spirit.
Lectures, "The Man of Letters"

William Makepeace Thackeray
[1811–1863]

Forty times over let Michaelmas pass,
Grizzling hair the brain doth clear —
Then you know a boy is an ass,
Then you know the worth of a lass,
Once you have come to Forty Year.
The Age of Wisdom

George Bernard Shaw [1856–1950]

Every man over forty is a scoundrel.
Man and Superman, "Maxims
for Revolutionists"

Karin Michaëlis [1872–1950]

The Dangerous Age.
Title of a book

Hans Zinsser [1878–1940]

Our task, as we grow older in a rapidly
advancing science, is to retain the capacity of joy in discoveries which correct older ideas and theories and to
learn from our pupils as we teach
them. That is the only sound prophy-

laxis against the dodo-diseases of middle age.
> *As I Remember Him,* Ch. 9, Sect. 1

Robert Benchley [1889–1945]

Just think of all the things you can do after 40! Professor Webster was 57 when he cut up Dr. Parkman and threw him into the furnace of the Harvard Medical School, and Dr. Parkman was 70 himself! Nero was 52 when he set fire to Rome. Thomas Jukes was 54 when he married his own daughter to conceal the fact that he had killed her first husband. And I myself was 42 when I fell down a flight of steps and got water on the knee. Middle-age? Bosh!
> *From Bed to Worse,* "Life Begins at (fill in space)"

Alvan L. Barach [1895–   ]

Middle age has been said to be the time of a man's life when, if he has two choices for an evening, he takes the one that gets him home earlier.
> *Journal of the American Medical Association* 181:393, 1962

MIDWIFE

See also CHILDBIRTH

Charles Dickens [1812–1870]

Mrs. Gamp . . . in her highest walk of art, a monthly nurse, or, as her signboard boldly had it, "Midwife" . . . was a fat old woman . . . with a husky voice and a moist eye, which she had a remarkable power of turning up, and only showing the white of it. . . . She wore a very rusty black gown, rather the worse for snuff, and a shawl and bonnet to correspond. . . . The face of Mrs. Gamp — the nose in particular — was somewhat red and swollen, and it was difficult to enjoy her society without becoming conscious of a smell of spirits.
> *Martin Chuzzlewit,* Ch. 19

The Bible

God dealt well with the midwives: and the people multiplied, and waxed very mighty.
> *Exodus* 1:20

Proverb

Meddlesome midwifery is bad.

Persian Proverb

When there are two midwives, the baby's head is crooked.

MILITARY MEDICINE

Tobias Smollett [1721–1771]

This inhuman disregard [on hospital ships] was imputed to the scarcity of surgeons; though it is well known that every great ship in the fleet could have spared one at least for this duty; an expedient which would have been more than sufficient to remove this shocking inconvenience.
> *The Adventures of Roderick Random,* Ch. 33

Benjamin Rush [1745?–1813]

Soldiers bore operations of every kind immediately *after* a battle, with much more fortitude than they did at any time afterwards.
> *An Account of the Influence of the Military and Political Events of the American Revolution upon the Human Body*

Newton D. Baker [1871–1937]

The devotion and success of the American doctors in our war [World War I] experience makes a record about which those who are still to enter that noble

profession can safely and proudly build their ideals of public usefulness.
> Foreword to Franklin H. Martin's *The Joy of Living*, Vol. II

Hans Zinsser [1878–1940]

To the average professional officer, the military doctor is an unwillingly tolerated noncombatant who takes sick call, gives cathartic pills, makes transportation troubles, complicates tactical plans, and causes the water to smell bad.
> *Rats, Lice and History*, Ch. 8

MILK SICK

Daniel Drake [1785–1852]

It must be admitted that the plant on which Mr. Rowe experimented, possesses some active properties, as four animals under its use, died with what were pronounced to be symptoms of Trembles. Still, the mode of conducting the experiments, differed too widely from that in which the animal is likely to eat the poisonous plant, in the woods; and the decision that the animals killed by it, *had* the Trembles, is far from conclusive or binding. . . . A professional scrutiny only can be relied on in such cases. The testimony adduced by Mr. Rowe is, therefore, defective and inconclusive, even if nothing could be found to oppose it; but there are several facts which directly invalidate it.[1]
> *Western Journal of Medicine and Surgery* 3:161, 1841

Dennis Hanks [2] [1799–1892]

The Reson is this we war perplext By a Disese cald Milk Sick my Self Being the oldest I was Determed to Leve and hunt a Cuntry whare the milk was not I maried his oldest Step Daughter I Sold out and they concluded to gow with me. . . . My wifs mother could not think of parting with hir and we Riped up Stakes and Started to Illinois.
> Letter to William H. Herndon, March 7, 1866

Anna Pierce Hobbs Bixby [1808–1869]

Sheep and goats are careful in selecting their foods, and horses are what teachers call graminivorous; that is, grasseaters, while cattle are herbiverous and not careful in selecting. These things prove to us that it is not a grass, but an herb that is spreading sorrow and death among us.[1]
> *Diary*

Abraham Lincoln [1809–1865]

I said I would remove him [Gen. George McClellan] if he let Lee's army get away from him, and I must do so. He's got the "slows." [2]

MIND

See also BODY AND MIND, BRAIN, INSANITY, PSYCHIATRY, PSYCHOANALYSIS, PSYCHOLOGY, PSYCHOSOMATICS

Lucretius [96?–55 B.C.]

The mind like a sick body can be healed and changed by medicine.
> *On the Nature of Things*, III. 510 (tr. by W. H. D. Rouse)

---

[1] In 1839 John Rowe, a farmer, decided that white snakeroot caused milk sick; he fed the plant to calves and produced typical trembles. After a review of the evidence Dr. Drake drew this arrogant and incorrect conclusion.

[2] A cousin of Abraham Lincoln.

[1] Mrs. Bixby discovered that milk sick was caused by white snakeroot (*Eupatorium urticaefolium*).

[2] The lethargy that characterizes milk sick has helped give it the name of "the sloes" or "slows."

Ovid [43 B.C.–A.D. 17?]

All things can corrupt perverted minds.
> *Tristia*, II.301 (tr. by A. L. Wheeler)

Marcus Aurelius [121–180]

Tranquility is nothing else than the good ordering of the mind.
> *Meditations*, IV.3 (tr. by G. Long)

Sir Francis Bacon [1561–1626]

The cause and root of nearly all evils in the sciences is this — that while we falsely admire and extol the powers of the human mind we neglect to seek for its true helps.
> *Novum Organum*, "Aphorisms," IX

The human understanding is moved by those things most which strike and enter the mind simultaneously and suddenly, and so fill the imagination; and then it feigns and supposes all other things to be somehow, though it cannot see how, similar to those few things by which it is surrounded.
> *Ibid.*, XLVII

The human understanding is no dry light, but receives an infusion from the will and affections; whence proceed sciences which may be called "sciences as one would." For what a man had rather were true he more readily believes. Therefore he rejects difficult things from impatience of research; sober things, because they narrow hope; the deeper things of nature, from superstition; the light of experience, from arrogance and pride, lest his mind should seem to be occupied with things mean and transitory; things not commonly believed, out of deference to the opinion of the vulgar. Numberless in short are the ways, and sometimes imperceptible, in which the affections colour and infect the understanding.
> *Ibid.*, XLIX

David Hartley [1705–1757]

The white medullary Substance of the Brain is also the immediate Instrument, by which Ideas are presented to the Mind; or, in other Words, whatever Changes are made in this Substance, corresponding Changes are made in our Ideas; and *vice versâ*.
> *Observations on Man*, Ch. 1, Prop. 2

Samuel Johnson [1709–1784]

Depend upon it, Sir, when a man knows he is to be hanged in a fortnight, it concentrates his mind wonderfully.
> Quoted by James Boswell in *Life of Samuel Johnson*, September 19, 1777

The fountain of contentment must spring up in the mind; and he who has so little knowledge of human nature as to seek happiness by changing anything by his own disposition, will waste his life in fruitless efforts and multiply the griefs which he purposes to remove.

David Hume [1711–1776]

What we call a mind is nothing but a heap or collection of different perceptions, united together by certain relations, and suppos'd, tho' falsely, to be endow'd with a perfect simplicity and identity.
> *A Treatise of Human Nature*, Bk. I, Pt. IV, Sect. 2

Charles Churchill [1731–1764]

With curious Art the Brain too finely wrought,
Preys on herself, and is destroy'd by Thought.
> *Epistle to Hogarth*

James Currie [1756–1805]

But though we may never know *how* mind acts on matter, we may, by a careful attention, possibly discover the general principles of this action; which is all, indeed, that we are able to attain in regard to the action of matter on matter.

> Letter to Dr. George Bell, October 20, 1781

Charles Lamb [1775–1834]

It is the mind, . . . and not the limbs, that taints by long sitting.

> Letter to Bernard Barton, November 22, 1823

John Keats [1795–1821]

The only means of strengthening one's intellect is to make up ones mind about nothing — to let the mind be a thoroughfare for all thoughts. Not a select party.

> Letter to George and Georgiana Keats, September 17–27, 1819

Jean Martin Charcot [1825–1893]

It is the mind which is really alive and sees things, yet it hardly sees anything without preliminary instruction.

Samuel Butler [1835–1902]

The more a thing knows its own mind, the more living it becomes.

> *Note-Books*

Ambrose Bierce [1842–1914?]

MIND, n. A mysterious form of matter secreted by the brain. Its chief activity consists in the endeavor to ascertain its own nature, the futility of the attempt being due to the fact that it has nothing but itself to know itself with.

> *The Devil's Dictionary*

Gerard Manley Hopkins [1844–1889]

O the mind, mind has mountains; cliffs of fall
Frightful, sheer, no-man-fathomed. Hold them cheap
May who ne'er hung there. Nor does long our small
Durance deal with that steep or deep.

> *No Worst, There Is None*

James J. Putnam [1846–1918]

No argument is needed to show what transforming power the mind can exert. The energy set free by the magic agencies of hope, courage, desperation, fanaticism, or by the enthusiasm for a great cause, may reveal the possession of a force undreamed of, or so husband the resources of the body as to keep the flame of life burning for a time when the oil seems exhausted.

> *Boston Medical and Surgical Journal* 141:53, 1899

Santiago Ramón y Cajal [1852–1934]

We disdain and hate from lack of self-comprehension and we understand in proportion as we study ourselves.

> *Charlas de Café*

James Harvey Robinson [1863–1936]

There are four historical layers underlying the minds of civilized men — the animal mind, the child mind, the savage mind, and the traditional civilized mind.

> *The Mind in the Making,* Ch. III, Sect. 6

Wilfred Trotter [1872–1939]

Has the Intellect a Function?

> Title of lecture, June 20, 1939

Wilder Penfield [1891–   ]

It is fair to say that science provides no method of controlling the mind. Scientific work on the brain does not explain the mind — not yet. Neither the work of Pavlov on conditioned reflexes nor that of any other worker has proven the thesis of materialism. Surgeons can remove areas of brain, physicians can destroy or deaden it with drugs and produce unpredictable fantasies, but they cannot force it to do their bidding.

> Dartmouth Convocation on *The Great Issues of Conscience in Modern Medicine* (1960), Third Panel Discussion

René J. Dubos [1901–　　]

The mind can be a piercing searchlight which reveals many of the hidden mysteries of the world, but unfortunately, it often causes such a glare that it prevents the eyes from seeing the natural objects which should serve as guideposts in following the ways of nature.
Louis Pasteur, Free Lance of Science, Ch. V

The Bible

In his right mind.
Mark 5:15

Latin Proverb

Pain of mind is worse than pain of body.

MOUTH

Henry Gibbons, Sr. [1808–1884]

[Definition of a kiss:] The anatomical juxtaposition of two orbicularis oris muscles in a state of contraction.

Ambrose Bierce [1842–1914?]

MOUTH, n. In man, the gateway to the soul; in woman, the outlet of the heart.
The Devil's Dictionary

Japanese Proverb

Diseases enter by the mouth.

MURDER

William Shakespeare [1564–1616]

Murther most foul, as in the best it is;
But this most foul, strange, and unnatural.
Hamlet, I, v, 27

See how the blood is settled in his face. . . .
But see, his face is black and full of blood;

His eyeballs further out than when he liv'd,
Staring full ghastly, like a strangled man;
His hair uprear'd, his nostrils stretch'd with struggling;
His hands abroad display'd, as one that grasp'd
And tugg'd for life and was by strength subdu'd.
Look, on the sheets his hair, you see, is sticking; . . .
It cannot be but he was murd'red here.
Henry VI, Part II, III, ii, 160

R. H. Barham ("Thomas Ingoldsby") [1788–1845]

'Tis plain,
As anatomists tell us, that never again
Shall life revisit the foully slain,
When once they've been cut through the jugular vein.
The Ingoldsby Legends, "The Hand of Glory"

James Anthony Froude [1818–1894]

Wild animals never kill for sport. Man is the only one to whom the torture and death of his fellow-creatures is amusing in itself.
Oceana, Ch. 5

The Bible

Thou shalt not kill.
Exodus 20:13

MUSCLE

Leonardo da Vinci [1452–1519]

No muscle uses its power in pushing but always in drawing to itself the parts that are joined to it.
Dell' Anatomia, Fogli B (tr. by Edward MacCurdy in *The Notebooks of Leonardo da Vinci*, Vol. I, Ch. III)

The function of muscle is to pull and not to push except in the case of genitals and the tongue.
Idem

The muscles always begin and end in the bones that touch one another, and they never begin and end in the same bone, for it would not be able to move anything unless this was itself in a state of rarity or density.
Idem

NATURE

Hippocrates [460?–377? B.C.]

Natural forces are the healers of disease.
Epidemics, VI.V.1

Nature is sufficient in all for all.
Nutriment, XV (tr. by W. H. S. Jones)

Celsus [25 B.C.–A.D. 50]

Whatever the malady luck no less than the art can claim influence for itself; seeing that with nature in opposition the art of medicine avails nothing.
De Medicina, III.i.4 (tr. by W. G. Spencer)

Leonardo da Vinci [1452–1519]

Those who study only the authorities and not the works of nature are . . . the grandsons and not the sons of nature, which is the supreme guide of the good authorities.
Codice Atlantico, 141 (tr. by Edward MacCurdy in *The Notebooks of Leonardo da Vinci*, Vol. II, Ch. XXIX)

Necessity is the mistress and guardian of nature.
Necessity is the theme and artificer of nature — the bridle, the law, and the theme.
Forster Bequest MS. III, Victoria and Albert Museum (*ibid.*, Vol. I, Ch. II)

Although human subtlety makes a variety of inventions answering by differ-

ent means to the same end, it will never devise an invention more beautiful, more simple or more direct than does nature, because in her inventions nothing is lacking, and nothing is superfluous.
Quaderni d'Anatomia, Vol. IV (*ibid.*, Vol. I, Ch. III)

Paracelsus [1493?–1541]

The physician is only the servant of nature, not her master. Therefore it behooves medicine to follow the will of nature.
Three Books on the French Disease, Bk. III, Ch. XI (tr. by Norbert Guterman in *Selected Writings*)

He who would explore nature must tread her books with his feet. Holy Scripture is explored through its letters, but nature is explored from country to country; it has as many pages as there are countries. This is the code of nature, and thus must her leaves be turned.
Seven Defenses, Ch. 4

The art of healing comes from nature, not from the physician. Therefore the physician must start from nature, with an open mind.

Michel de Montaigne [1533–1592]

Let us let things take their course: the scheme of things that takes care of fleas and moles also takes care of men who have the same patience to let themselves be governed as fleas and moles. . . . Let us follow along, in God's name, let us follow! It leads those who follow; those who do not follow, it drags along, and their rage and their medicine too. Order a purge for your brain; it will be better employed there than on your stomach.
Essays, Bk. II, Ch. 37, "Of the Resemblance of Children to Fathers" (tr. by Donald M. Frame)

William Shakespeare [1564–1616]

In nature's infinite book of secrecy
A little I can read.
Antony and Cleopatra, I, ii, 9

Sir Thomas Browne [1605–1682]

All things are artificiall, for Nature is
the Art of God.
Religio Medici, Pt. I, Sect. 16

Thus there are two bookes from
whence I collect my Divinity; besides
that written one of God, another of
his servant Nature, that universall
and publik Manuscript, that lies ex-
pans'd unto the eyes of all; those that
never saw him in the one, have discovered him in the other.
Idem

There is therefore no deformity but
in monstrosity, wherein notwithstanding there is a kind of beauty, Nature
so ingeniously contriving those irregular parts, as they become sometimes
more remarkable than the principall
Fabrick.
Idem

Thomas Sydenham [1624–1689]

I watched what method Nature might
take, with intention of subduing the
symptom by treading in her footsteps.
Medical Observations, Sect. 5,
Ch. 2 (tr. by R. G. Latham in
Works, Vol. I)

John Locke [1632–1704]

Nature never makes excellent things,
for mean or no uses.
*Essay Concerning Human Un-
derstanding*, Bk. II, Ch. 1, Sect.
15

Sir Isaac Newton [1642–1727]

The changing of bodies into Light, and
Light into Bodies, is very conformable
to the Course of Nature, which seems
delighted with Transmutations.
Opticks

Stephen Hales [1677–1761]

The searching into the works of Nature, while it delights and inlarges
the mind, and strikes us with the
strongest assurance of the wisdom and
power of the divine Architect, in framing for us so beautiful and well regulated a world, it does at the same time
convince us of his constant benevolence
and goodness towards us.
Vegetable Staticks, Dedication

Edward Young [1683–1765]

The *Course* of *Nature* is the *Art* of
GOD.
Night Thoughts, Night IX

William Smellie [1697–1763]

I diligently attended to the course of
operations of Nature which occurred
in my practice, regulating and improving myself by that infallible standard.

Sir John Forbes [1787–1861]

In a large proportion of cases treated
by physicians, the disease is cured by
nature, not by them.

Thomas Carlyle [1795–1881]

Nature admits no lie.[1]
Latter-Day Pamphlets, No. 5

Elisha Bartlett [1804–1855]

Far, far beyond this visible boundary,
and hidden within unapproachable recesses, actions may be going on, between the ultimate constituents of
matter, not only utterly removed from
our knowledge, but as truly beyond
our powers of conception even, as
eternity and space are beyond our
powers of measurement, or estimate.
Philosophy of Medical Science,
Pt. I, Ch. 4

[1] Cf. Charles Darwin, p. 500a.

Oliver Wendell Holmes
[1809–1894]

Nature is a benevolent old hypocrite; she cheats the sick and the dying with illusions better than any anodynes.
> *Medical Essays,* "The Young Practitioner"

Sir William Withey Gull
[1816–1890]

Fixed as is the course of nature, it does not seem fixed by blind necessity, but ordered so that the intellect of man may learn it and dispose it for his good.
> *British Medical Journal* 2:425, 1874

That the course of nature may be varied we have assumed by our meeting here today. The whole object of the science of medicine is based on this assumption.
> *Idem*

Henry David Thoreau
[1817–1862]

If you would learn the secrets of Nature, you must practice more humanity than others.
> *Journal,* October 23, 1855

Samuel Haughton [1821–1897]

I will tell you what Nature wants; she wants to put the man in his coffin. [When told that the evacuations of cholera were an effort of Nature to cure the disease.]
> Quoted by Sir William Withey Gull in the President's Address to the Clinical Society, 1872

Abraham Jacobi [1830–1919]

Nature does not kill and does not heal. If there were consciousness in Nature, she would feel indifferent about what she is, *viz.,* mere evolution.

Haven Emerson [1874–1957]

Nature heals, under the auspices of the medical profession.
> Lecture

Albert Szent-Györgyi [1893–   ]

There is no real difference between the grass and he who mows it. The muscles which move the mower need the very same two substances for their motion as the grass needs for its growth, potassium and phosphate, the two substances we put on our lawn as fertilizers so as to have something to mow — a strikingly simple demonstration of the basic unity of living Nature.

Anonymous

If when the tide is falling you take out water with a twopenny pail, you and the moon can do a great deal.
> Quoted by W. I. B. Beveridge in *The Art of Scientific Investigation,* Ch. II

Nature builds up one side of a paired system when the other drags. As when you have a leg that is short by half an inch, the opposite member turns out to be longer by precisely the same measure.
> *Tufts Folia Medica* 9:73, 1963

Nature is the great experimenter.

Chinese Proverb

Nature is better than a middling doctor.

Latin Phrase

The healing power of nature.

NAUSEA

William Shakespeare [1564–1616]

Prithee do not turn me about. My stomach is not constant.
> *The Tempest,* II, ii, 118

NAVEL

Bishop Richard Cumberland [1631–1718]

All other men, being born of woman, have a navel, by reason of the umbilical vessels inserted into it, which from the placenta carry nourishment to children in the womb of their mothers; but it could not be so with our first parents. It cannot be believed that God gave them navels which would have been altogether useless.

James Bridie [1888–1951]

In anatomy, then, it is little better than a mere landmark. When we assume the spectacles of the embryologist, however, it takes on great importance. If one may be allowed a poetical image, it is all that remains of the stem that bound us to the parental stalk. It is a reminder that we have been plucked and must sooner or later die. It might be said that when the stem is severed, we cease to live in any true sense. We may be ornamental like roses or useful like cabbages, but only for a little. Our dissolution has begun.
Tedious and Brief, Pt. II, "The Umbilicus"

NERVES

Leonardo da Vinci [1452–1519]

The frog instantly dies when the spinal cord is pierced; and previous to this it lived without head, without heart or any bowels or intestines or skin; and here therefore it would seem lies the foundation of movement and life.
Quaderni d'Anatomia, Vol. V (tr. by Edward MacCurdy in *The Notebooks of Leonardo da Vinci*, Vol. I, Ch. V)

William Shakespeare [1564–1616]

Thy nerves are in their infancy again
And have no vigour in them.
The Tempest, I, ii, 484

William Heberden [1710–1801]

The power of moving in every part of the body by means of the muscles which obey the will, or by means of others the actions of which are involuntary; the various perceptions by the five external senses; and lastly those mental powers named memory, imagination, attention, and judgment, together with the passions of the mind; all these seem to be exercised by the ministry of the nerves; and are impaired, disturbed, or destroyed, in proportion to any injury done to the brain, the spinal marrow, and nerves, not only by their peculiar diseases, of which we know little, but by contusions, wounds, ulcers, and distortions, and by many poisons of the intoxicating kind.
Commentaries on the History and Cure of Diseases, Ch. 69

Mary Baker Eddy [1821–1910]

Nerves have no more sensation, apart from what belief bestows upon them, than the fibres of a plant.
Science and Health, Ch. XIV

Alfred Korzybski [1879–1950]

God may forgive you your sins, but your nervous system won't.

NEUROSIS

See also HYPOCHONDRIA, INSANITY, PSYCHIATRY, PSYCHOANALYSIS, PSYCHOLOGY, PSYCHOSOMATICS

Hippocrates [460?–377? B.C.]

I advise maidens who suffer from hysteria to marry as soon as possible.

For if they conceive, they will be cured.
About Maidens

William Heberden [1710–1801]

The hysteric globe in the throat is scarcely ever heard of among men, but is one of the most familiar symptoms with hysteric women.
Commentaries on the History and Cure of Diseases, Ch. 49

Thomas Jefferson [1743–1826]

Idleness begets ennui, ennui the hypochondriac, and that a diseased body. No laborious person was ever yet hysterical.
Letter to Martha Jefferson, March 28, 1787

Robert G. Ingersoll [1833–1899]

Many people think they have religion when they are troubled with dyspepsia.
Liberty of Man, Woman and Child, Sect. 3

Sigmund Freud [1856–1939]

The true believer is in a high degree protected against the danger of certain neurotic afflictions; by accepting the universal neurosis he is spared the task of forming a personal neurosis.
The Future of an Illusion, Ch. 8 (tr. by W. D. Robson-Scott)

The expectation that every neurotic phenomenon can be cured may, I suspect, be derived from the layman's belief that the neuroses are something quite unnecessary which have no right whatever to exist. Whereas in fact they are severe, constitutionally fixed illnesses, which rarely restrict themselves to only a few attacks but persist as a rule over long periods or throughout life. Our analytic experience that they can be extensively influenced . . . has led us to neglect the constitutional factor in our therapeutic practice and

in any case we can do nothing about it; but in theory we ought always to bear it in mind.
New Introductory Lectures on Psychoanalysis, Lect. XXXIV (tr. by J. Strachey)

Marcel Proust [1871–1922]

All the greatest things we know have come to us from neurotics. It is they and they only who have founded religions and created great works of art. Never will the world be conscious of how much it owes to them, nor above all of what they have suffered in order to bestow their gifts on it. We enjoy fine music, beautiful pictures, a thousand exquisite things, but we do not know what they cost those who wrought them in sleeplessness, tears, spasmodic laughter, rashes, asthma, epilepsy, a terror of death which is worse than any of these.
The Guermantes Way, Pt. I, "My Grandmother's Illness" (tr. by C. K. Scott-Moncrieff)

Neurosis has an absolute genius for malingering. There is no illness which it cannot counterfeit perfectly. It will produce life-like imitations of the dilatations of dyspepsia, the sickness of pregnancy, the broken rhythm of the cardiac, the feverishness of the consumptive. If it is capable of deceiving the doctor, how should it fail to deceive the patient?
Idem

Neurotic subjects are perhaps less addicted than any, despite the time-honoured phrase, to "listening to their insides": they can hear so many things going on inside themselves, by which they realise later that they did wrong to let themselves be alarmed, that they end by paying no attention to any of them. Their nervous systems have so often cried out to them for help, as though from some serious malady, when it was merely because snow was

coming, or because they had to change their rooms, that they have acquired the habit of paying no more heed to these warnings.
Within a Budding Grove, Pt. I (tr. by C. K. Scott-Moncrieff)

Lord Robert Webb-Johnstone [1879–]

A neurotic is the man who builds a castle in the air. A psychotic is the man who lives in it. And a psychiatrist is the man who collects the rent.
Collected Papers

David Seegal [1899–]

A little neurosis may be a valuable asset, even though a heavy one may be hard to take.
Journal of the American Medical Association 182:1031, 1962

The member of the neurotic population may console himself with the knowledge that his chronic disorder places him among the majority of the population; that his difficulties arise from a common wellspring of the human condition; and that the dynamism of the neurosis may contribute energy to his particular personality or genius.
Idem

Cyril Connolly [1903–]

A mistake which is commonly made about neurotics is to suppose that they are interesting. It is not interesting to be always unhappy, engrossed with oneself, malignant and ungrateful, and never quite in touch with reality.
The Unquiet Grave, Pt. II

NIGHT CALLS

Karl F. H. Marx [1796–1877]

Almost every one who goes to bed counts upon a full night's rest: Like a picket at the outposts, the doctor must be ever on call.
Quoted by F. H. Garrison in *Bulletin of the New York Academy of Medicine* 5:156, 1929

George Bernard Shaw [1856–1950]

He may be hungry, weary, sleepy, run down by several successive nights disturbed by that instrument of torture, the night bell; but who ever thinks of this in the face of sudden sickness or accident? We think no more of the condition of a doctor attending a case than the condition of a fireman at a fire.
The Doctor's Dilemma, "Preface on Doctors"

Reginald L. Hine [1883–]

"When I die," said dear and whimsical old Doctor Pycroft, "I shall have a bell hung on my head-stone, with an inscription asking the compassionate passer-by to ring it long and loud. *And I shan't get up.*"
Confessions of an Uncommon Attorney, Pt. II, Ch. 3

Paul B. Magnuson [1884–]

Ring the Night Bell.
Title of a book

NOSE

Epictetus [fl. ca. 90]

Sit down now and pray forsooth that the mucus in your nose may not run! Nay, rather wipe your nose and do not blame God!
Discourses, II.xvi.13 (tr. by W. A. Oldfather)

William Shakespeare [1564–1616]

My nose fell a-bleeding on Black Monday last.
The Merchant of Venice, II, v, 24

Francis Beaumont [1584–1616] **and John Fletcher** [1579–1625]

Nose, nose, jolly red nose,
And who gave thee this jolly red nose? . . .
Nutmegs and ginger, cinnamon and cloves;
And they gave me this jolly red nose.
The Knight of the Burning Pestle, Act I, Sc. iv

Charles Farrar Browne ("Artemus Ward") [1834–1867]

Their noses blossom as the Lobster.
Artemus Ward His Book, "Fourth of July Oration"

James Gibbons Huneker [1860–1921]

A venerable man [1] with a purple nose — a Cyrano de Cognac nose.
Old Fogy, Ch. IX

The Bible

The wringing of the nose bringeth forth blood.
Proverbs 30:33

NOSTRUMS

See also QUACKS

Oliver Goldsmith [1728–1774]

There is scarcely a disorder incident to humanity against which our advertising doctors are not possessed with a most infallible antidote.
On Quack Doctors

Thomas Carlyle [1795–1881]

Brothers, I am sorry I have got no Morrison's Pill for curing the maladies of Society.
Past and Present, Bk. I, Ch. 4

[1] Franz Liszt.

Oliver Wendell Holmes [1809–1894]

But the good bishop [Berkeley] got excited; he pleased himself with the thought that he had discovered a great panacea; and having once tasted the bewitching cup of self-quackery, like many before and since his time, he was so infatuated with the draught that he would insist on pouring it down the throats of his neighbors and all mankind.
Medical Essays, "Homoeopathy and Its Kindred Delusions"

Charles Evans Hughes [1862–1948]

Allowing the broadest range to the conflict of medical views, there still remains a field in which statements as to curative properties are downright falsehoods.

Samuel Hopkins Adams [1871–1958]

With a few honorable exceptions the press of the United States is at the beck and call of the patent medicines. Not only do the newspapers modify news possibly affecting these interests, but they sometimes become their active agents.[1]
Collier's Weekly, October 7, 1905

Ignorance and credulous hope make the market for most proprietary remedies.
Ibid., December 2, 1905

NURSES

Sushruta [5th Cent.? B.C.]

That person alone is fit to nurse or to attend the bedside of a patient, who

[1] From the first in a series of ten articles entitled "The Great American Fraud," which led to the passage of the Pure Food and Drug Act, signed by Theodore Roosevelt on January 1, 1907.

is cool-headed and pleasant in his demeanor, does not speak ill of any body, is strong and attentive to the requirements of the sick, and strictly and indefatigably follows the instructions of the physician.

> *Sushruta-Samhitá*, "Sutrasthánam," Ch. 34 (tr. by K. K. L. Bhishagratna)

Euripides [484–406 B.C.]

It's better to be sick than nurse the sick. Sickness is single trouble for the sufferer: but nursing means vexation of the mind, and hard work for the hands besides.

> *Hippolytus*, 186 (tr. by D. Grene)

Andrew Boorde [1490–1549]

It is necessary for hym that is sycke to have two or .iii. good kepers.

> *The Dyetary of Helth*, Ch. XL

William Cowper [1731–1800]

The nurse sleeps sweetly, hired to watch the sick,
Whom snoring she disturbs.

> *The Task*, Bk. I

Henry Wadsworth Longfellow [1807–1882]

A Lady with a Lamp [1] shall stand
In the great history of the land,
A noble type of good,
Heroic womanhood.

> *Santa Filomena*

Florence Nightingale [1820–1910]

My life now is as unlike my Hospital life when I was concerned with the souls and bodies of men as reading a cookery book is unlike a good dinner.

> Letter to Rev. Mother Bermondsey, 1864

It seems a commonly received idea among men and even among women themselves that it requires nothing but a disappointment in love, the want

[1] Florence Nightingale.

of an object, a general disgust, or incapacity for other things, to turn a woman into a good nurse.

> *Notes on Nursing: What It Is and What It Is Not*, Conclusion

I can always talk better to a medical man than to anyone else.

> Quoted by Zachary Cope in *Florence Nightingale and the Doctors*, Ch. 1

You cannot select the good from the inferior by any test or system of examination. . . . Most of all and first of all must the moral qualifications be made to stand preeminent in estimation.[1]

Theodor Billroth [1829–1894]

Taking care of such an unhappy patient, with so little prospect of any success, is one of the heaviest loads one can lay on a human being, which only women can carry for any length of time with never-ending patience.

> Letter to Johannes Brahms, January 7, 1874 (tr. by H. Barkan)

S. Weir Mitchell [1829–1914]

Do not think too much of the dignity of your profession or what it is beneath you to do. It is a moral disorder of young nurses and, I may add, of young doctors.

Ever since the Crimean war, nurses have been getting into novels.

While I can understand the patient falling in love with the nurse, I do not as easily comprehend the nurse falling in love with the sick patient.

William Ernest Henley [1849–1903]

A well-bred silence always at command.

> *In Hospital*, "Lady Probationer"

[1] Discussing the establishment of an examining board for registration of nurses.

Sir William Osler [1849–1919]

The trained nurse has become one of the great blessings of humanity, taking a place beside the physician and the priest, and not inferior to either in her mission.

> *Aequanimitas, with Other Addresses,* "Nurse and Patient"

Stephen Paget [1855–1926]

Talk of the patience of Job, said a Hospital nurse, *Job was never on night duty.*

> *Confessio Medici,* Ch. 6

Rudyard Kipling [1865–1936]

Let us now remember many honourable women,
    Such as bade us turn again when we
    were like to die.

> *Dirge of Dead Sisters*

Charles H. Mayo [1865–1939]

The trained nurse has given nursing the human, or shall we say, the divine touch, and made the hospital desirable for patients with serious ailments regardless of their home advantages.

> *Collected Papers of the Mayo Clinic and Mayo Foundation* 13:1242, 1921

Finley Peter Dunne ("Mr. Dooley") [1867–1936]

"I think," said Mr. Dooley, "that if th' Christyan Scientists had some science an' th' doctors more Christianity, it wudden't make anny diff'rence which ye called in — if ye had a good nurse."

> *Mr. Dooley's Opinions,* "Christian Science"

Frank H. Lahey [1880–1953]

We have strived here to avoid the sin which tends to beset all institutions, that is to become impersonal and mechanized. At the head of every department has been placed a mature and sympathetic nurse with the desire to appreciate that sick people are not numbered individuals and just cold medical problems, one with whom patients can become acquainted and to whom they can turn for information, direction and sympathy at the time of their visits.

> *Lahey Clinic Bulletin* 4:226, 1946

Otto Weininger [1880–1903]

It is very shortsighted of anyone to consider the nurse as a proof of the sympathy of women, because it really implies the opposite. For a man could never stand the sight of the sufferings of the sick; he would suffer so intensely that he would be completely upset and incapable of lengthy attendance on them. Any one who has watched nursing sisters is astounded at their equanimity and "sweetness" even in the presence of most terrible death throes; and it is well that it is so, for man, who cannot stand suffering and death, would make a very bad nurse.

> *Sex and Character,* Pt. II, Ch. 9

Christopher Morley [1890–1957]

As calmly detached as nurses in a hospital who smile at what the patients say under ether.

Catherine Black [1] [fl. 20th Cent.]

Every nurse learns that there are moments when it is better to leave a patient alone, because sympathy would only make matters worse.

> Quoted by Sir Harold Gillies and D. Ralph Millard, Jr., in *The Principles and Art of Plastic Surgery,* Vol. I, Ch. 1

Margaret Lee Runbeck [1905–   ]

The head nurse, a very broom of a presence, swept the place clean with a look.

> Quoted in *Archives of Internal Medicine* 117:152, 1966

[1] A nurse in an Army hospital during World War I.

Richard Asher [1912–   ]

Too often a sister puts all her patients back to bed as a housewife puts all her plates back in the plate-rack — to make a generally tidy appearance.

British Medical Journal 2:967, 1947

Anonymous

Behold, my daughter, I have parted from mine appendix, and my conscience is clear! Therefore do I fear but three things.

And the first of these is a mouse.

And the second is embonpoint.

But the third is a Trained Nurse!

For I have watched her at her work!

And, I charge thee, in the flutter of her eyelash there lurketh more danger than in the whole chorus of a comic opera. For a chorus girl practiseth her wiles upon strong men, but *she* seeketh him only that is stricken and at her mercy.

Yea, when he is down and out she getteth in her fine work.

Upon her head she weareth a cute cap, which glorifieth her as a halo in his sight. She walketh upon heels of velvet and cooeth unto him in a voice of silver.

Her smile runneth over and will not come off. She hath dove's eyes.

She batheth his brow with spikenard and myrrh, and anointeth him with alcohol. She arrangeth his pillows and comforteth his soul with words of cheer. *She taketh his pulse!*

He yearneth to be babied — and she babyeth him.

He pineth for sympathy — and she sympathizeth.

He seeketh comfort — and she maketh him comfortable.

And what chance hath a damsel at a pink tea beside a ministering angel such as one of these?

Go, thou simple one! What strength is there in a sick man that he shall flee before all the temptations of St. Anthony, in one?

Nay, though he be of stone and of adamant, though his heart be incased in barbed wire, yet shall he turn upon his pillow sighing:

"Alas, Miriam is all right, but a *wife* was never like this!"

Yet how guileless is human nature! For ye will keep your silver in a strong box and your jewels behind bars of iron; yet will ye trust your beloved in the hands of one of these.

Verily, verily, the Lorelei is passé and witches are no more.

But a little trained nurse is a *dangerous thing!*

The Little Trained Nurse; Being the Advice of Mrs. Solomon (700th Wife of King Solomon)

Practical Nurse — one who marries a rich patient.

Turkish Proverb

It is better to be sick than care for the sick.

NUTRITION

See also DIET, EATING, VITAMINS

Hippocrates [460?–377? B.C.]

Power of nutriment reaches to bone and to all the parts of bone, to sinew, to vein, to artery, to muscle, to membrane, to flesh, fat, blood, phlegm, marrow, brain, spinal marrow, the intestines and all their parts; it reaches also to heat, breath, and moisture.

Nutriment, VII (tr. by W. H. S. Jones)

Plutarch [46?–120?]

It is true I [the stomach] first receive all meats that nourish man's body; but afterward I send it again to the nourishment of other parts of the same.

Lives, "Coriolanus," VI

Don Herold [1889–   ]

The short skirts of today reveal the malnutrition of yesterday.

OATHS

Oath of the Hindu Physician [ca. 1500 B.C.]

You must be chaste and abstemious, speak the truth, not eat meat; care for the good of all living beings; devote yourself to the healing of the sick even if your life be lost by your work; do the sick no harm; not, even in thought, seek another's wife or goods; be simply clothed and drink no intoxicant; speak clearly, gently, truly, properly; consider time and place; always seek to grow in knowledge. Do not treat women except their men be present; never take a gift from a woman without her husband's consent. When the physician enters a house accompanied by a man suitable to introduce him there, he must pay attention to all the rules of behavior in dress, deportment, and attitude. Once with his patient, he must in word and thought attend to nothing but his patient's case and what concerns it. What happens in the house must not be mentioned outside, nor must he speak of possible death to his patient, if such speech is liable to injure him or anyone else. In face of gods and man, you can take upon yourself these vows; may all the gods aid you if you abide thereby; otherwise may all the gods and the sacra, before which we stand, be against you; and the pupil shall consent to this, saying, "So be it."

> Quoted by Charles L. Dana in *The Peaks of Medical History,* Introduction

Hippocrates [460?–377? B.C.]

I swear by Apollo the physician, and Aesculapius, and Health, and All-heal,[1] and all the gods and goddesses, that, according to my ability and judgment, I will keep this Oath and this stipulation — to reckon him who taught me this Art equally dear to me as my parents, to share my substance with him, and relieve his necessities if required; to look upon his offspring in the same footing as my own brothers, and to teach them this art, if they shall wish to learn it, without fee or stipulation; and that by precept, lecture, and every other mode of instruction, I will impart a knowledge of the Art to my own sons, and those of my teachers, and to disciples bound by a stipulation and oath according to the law of medicine, but to none others. I will follow that system of regimen which, according to my ability and judgment, I consider for the benefit of my patients, and abstain from whatever is deleterious and mischievous. I will give no deadly medicine to any one if asked, nor suggest any such counsel; and in like manner I will not give to a woman a pessary to produce abortion. With purity and with holiness I will pass my life and practise my Art. I will not cut persons labouring under the stone, but will leave this to be done by men who are practitioners of this work. Into whatever houses I enter, I will go into them for the benefit of the sick, and will abstain from every voluntary act of mischief and corruption; and further, from the seduction of females or males, of freemen and slaves. Whatever, in connexion with my professional practice, or not in connexion with it, I see or hear, in the life of men, which ought not to be spoken of abroad, I will not divulge, as reckoning that all such should be kept secret. While I continue to keep this Oath unviolated, may it be granted to me to enjoy life and the

[1] "Health" and "All-heal" refer to Hygeia and Panacea, daughters of Aesculapius; he was the patron-god of the Aesclepiadae, or priest-physicians, of which Hippocrates was a member.

practice of the art, respected by all men, in all times! But should I trespass and violate this Oath, may the reverse be my lot!
> *The Oath* (tr. by Francis Adams)

Asaph ben Berachiah and Jochanan ben Zabda [fl. 6th Cent.]

Take heed that you kill not any man with a root decoction; do not prepare any potion that may cause a woman who has conceived in adultery to miscarry; and do not lust after beautiful women to commit adultery with them; and do not divulge a man's secret that he has confided unto you; and do not be bribed to do injury and harm and do not harden your heart against the poor and the needy; rather have compassion upon them and heal them. Do not speak of good as evil nor of evil as good.
> First known formal pledge of medical ethics among the Jews (tr. by Fred Rosner and Sussman Muntner in *Annals of Internal Medicine* 63:317, 1965)

Anonymous

I swear and pronounce faithfully to teach in a long gown with wide sleeves, a doctoral cap upon my head, and a knot of scarlet ribbon on my shoulder.
> Gallic idea of the Hippocratic Oath, sworn by those entering the medical department of the University of Paris

OBESITY

See also BODY, LEANNESS

Hippocrates [460?–377? B.C.]

Persons who are naturally very fat are apt to die earlier than those who are slender.
> *Aphorisms*, II.44 (tr. by Francis Adams)

William Shakespeare [1564–1616]

A gross fat man.
> As fat as butter.
> *Henry IV, Part I*, II, iv, 559

Let me have men about me that are fat,
Sleek-headed men, and such as sleep a-nights.
> *Julius Caesar*, I, ii, 192

Fat paunches have lean pates, and dainty bits
Make rich the ribs but bankrout quite the wits.
> *Love's Labour's Lost*, I, i, 26

Francis Beaumont [1584–1616] and John Fletcher [1579–1625]

Fat old women, fat and five and fifty.
> *Women Pleased*, Act III, Sc. ii

John Dryden [1631–1700]

I am resolved to grow fat, and look young till forty, and then slip out of the world with the first wrinckle and the reputation of five and twenty.
> *Secret Love*, Act III

Sir Charles Sedley [1639?–1701]

I am as sound as a Bell — Fat, Plump and Juicy, and have drunk my gallon a day these seven Years.
> *Bellamira*, Act III, Sc. ii

John Cotgrave [fl. 1655]

As fat as a pig.
> *Wit's Interpreter*

Sir William S. Gilbert [1836–1911]

I see no objection to stoutness, in moderation.
> *Iolanthe*, Act I

Thomas B. Reed [1839–1902]

I'll own up to two hundred pounds,

but no gentleman ever weighs over two hundred.

> Comment to David B. Henderson in lobby of U.S. House of Representatives

Santiago Ramón y Cajal [1852–1934]

A mature fat man excites pity, like a ship well stocked for its last voyage.
> *Charlas de Café*

Excessive corpulence, the index of good nature and deliberation in the man, is commonly a guarantee of fidelity in the woman. Aside from the shameless artistic error involved in exhibiting a monstrous figure, the heart of the rotund matron has enough to do in irrigating some hundred-weights of adipose tissue.
> *Idem*

Arthur Guiterman [1871–1943]

Down where I feel there's a terrible lot
    o' me,
Down where some people are hippopotami,
In the department of laparotomy,
    That's where the vest begins.
> *Song and Laughter,* "Vulgar Lines for a Distinguished Surgeon"

Cyril Connolly [1903–   ]

Obesity is a mental state, a disease brought on by boredom and disappointment.
> *The Unquiet Grave,* Pt. I

Imprisoned in every fat man a thin one is wildly signalling to be let out.
> *Ibid.,* Pt. II

William Boniface [1927–   ]

Fat people overeat
To feed yesterday, and tomorrow.
At the end of the line, today
Never gets enough. They suffer

Not so much from gluttony
As starvation.
> *Slim Pickings*

American Proverbs

Everybody loves a fat man.

Nobody loves a fat man.

English Proverb

Often and little eating makes a man fat.

OBITER DICTA

Ambroise Paré [1517?–1590]

I have publisht this apology to the end that each man may know with what foot I have always marched and I think there is not any man so ticklish, which taketh not in good part what I have said, seeing my Discourse is true, and that the effect sheweth the thing to the eye, Reason being my warrant against all Calumnies.
> *The Voyage of Bayonne,* Bk. 29 (tr. by T. H. Johnson in *Works*)

CHARLES IX: I hope that you will care for the King better than for the poor.
PARÉ: No, Sire, that is impossible.
CHARLES IX: Why so?
PARÉ: Because I care for them as I do for kings.

William Clowes [1544–1604]

But it is truly said, Hannibal knew well how to subdue the Romans, yet he knew not how to entertain his victories. It is not enough for a man to have begun a good work, unless he still persevere and continue in the same.
> *Treatise on Struma* (ed. by F. N. L. Poynter in *Selected Writings,* Ch. 1)

Sir Thomas Browne [1605–1682]

He who must needs have Company, must needs have sometimes bad Company. Be able to be alone.
Christian Morals, Pt. III, Sect. 9

I could never divide my selfe from any man upon the difference of an opinion, or be angry with his judgement for not agreeing with mee in that, from which perhaps within a few days I should dissent my selfe.
Religio Medici, Pt. I, Sect. 6

I feele not in me those sordid, and unchristian desires of my profession, I doe not secretly implore and wish for Plagues, rejoyce at Famines. . . . I desire every thing in its proper season, that neither men nor the times bee out of temper.
Ibid., Pt. II, Sect. 9

Now for my life, it is a miracle of thirty yeares, which to relate, were not a History, but a peece of Poetry, and would sound to common eares like a fable; for the world, I count it not an Inne, but an Hospitall, and a place, not to live, but to die in. . . . whilst I study to finde how I am a Microcosme or little world, I finde my selfe something more than the great. There is surely a peece of Divinity in us, something that was before the Elements, and owes no homage unto the Sun.
Ibid., Sect. 11

William Withering [1741–1799]

Sir, I received your note; the purport of which if I am not mistaken, is a request that I would fix upon a time and place that you may have an opportunity to kill me. But it further implies that I may also have an opportunity of killing you; and this you call satisfaction. Permit me, however, to assure you that it would be no satisfaction to me to kill you, or any other man; therefore, until your ideas can be more properly adjusted, you must allow me to decline to meet you.[1]
Quoted in *Annals of Medical History* (New Series) 8:198, 1926

Antoine Lavoisier [1743–1794]

Public usefulness and the interests of humanity ennoble the most disgusting work.

Benjamin Rush [1745?–1813]

I know by experience as well as observation that an indiscreet zeal for truth, justice, or humanity has cost more to the persons who have exercised it, than the total want of zeal for any thing good, or even zeal in false and unjust pursuits.
Autobiography, "Travels Through Life," Ch. IV

Edward Jenner [1749–1823]

Shall I, who even in the morning of my days sought the lowly and sequestered paths of life, the valley and not the mountain; shall I now my evening is fast approaching, hold myself up as an object for fortune and fame? Admitting it as a certainty that I obtain both, what stock should I add to my little fund of happiness? My fortune, with what flows in from my profession, is sufficient to gratify my wishes; indeed, so limited is my ambition, . . . that were I precluded from further practice, I should be enabled to obtain all that I want. And as for fame, what is it? A gilded butt, forever pierced with the arrows of malignancy.
Letter to John Hunter

The joy I felt at the prospect before me of being the instrument destined to take away from the world one of its greatest calamities . . . was so excessive that . . . I have sometimes found myself in a kind of reverie.
Quoted by John Baron in *Life of Edward Jenner,* Vol. I, Ch. 4

[1] Withering's reply to a challenge to a duel.

Benjamin Waterhouse
[1754–1846]

All the seed which I myself have broad-cast has not all rotted in the ground. Some of my feeble efforts must have prospered, even at this late hour of my day. Some very useful things would probably never have existed or been postponed to a late and chilling distance of time, but for my exertions. I cut the claws and wings of small pox, and . . . uprooted if not destroyed several contagious disorders. . . . I am not, I hope, a boaster, but I have done my part.

> *Diary*, April 14, 1844

Johann Christian Reil [1759–1813]

Our time has been ruined by the ubiquity of its own conceit.

> Valedictory address, 1810 (tr. by Max Samter)

Sir Benjamin Collins Brodie
[1783–1862]

There is no greater happiness in life than that of surmounting difficulties and nothing will conduce more than this to improve your intellectual faculties, or to make you satisfied with the situation which you have attained in life, whatever it may be.

> *Clinical Lectures on Surgery*, Introductory Discourse

Peter Mere Latham [1789–1875]

Crowds keep one another in countenance where individuals feel sharply.

> *Collected Works*, Vol. II, "A Word or Two on Medical Education"

There is much indifferent taste and worse judgment in the world, which are apt to applaud in the wrong place, and so to injure many things really good by their undiscerning patronage of them.

> *Diseases of the Heart*, Lect. IV

It is easy to talk disparagingly of the best things.

> *Ibid.*, Lect. XXIX

Fortunate, indeed, is the man who takes exactly the right measure of himself, and holds a just balance between what he can acquire and what he can use, be it great or be it small!

> *Lectures on Clinical Medicine*, Lect. I

The great Lord Chatham, it is said, had such power of inspiring self-complacency into the minds of other men, that no one was ever a quarter of an hour in his company without believing that Lord Chatham was the first man in the world, and himself the second.

> *Ibid.*, Lect. III

John Keats [1795–1821]

I am certain of nothing but of the holiness of the Heart's affections and the truth of Imagination — What the imagination seizes as Beauty must be truth — whether it existed before or not.

> Letter to Benjamin Bailey, November 22, 1817

The setting sun will always set me to rights — or if a Sparrow come before my Window I take part in its existence and pick about the Gravel.

> *Idem*

At once it struck me, what quality went to form a Man of Achievement especially in Literature & which Shakespeare possessed so enormously — I mean *Negative Capability*, that is when man is capable of being in uncertainties, Mysteries, doubts, without any irritable reaching after fact & reason.

> Letter to George and Tom Keats, December 21, 1817

Baron Karl von Rokitansky
[1804–1878]

I am willing to state that we are on the

threshold of decadence, that the so-called modern individualism is about to turn the realistic, and just developing, concept of the individual into a cult which accepts the most ruthless egotism, accepts success without considering the ways and means by which it has been attained, which absolves the guilty of responsibility for the crime, and manipulates punishment and the conditions for which it may be applied. Would it be surprising if society, drunk from triumphant delusions of freedom, would find itself face to face with a reaction which, spurred on by moral indignation, would demand intervention by government, restriction and rigid authority?

> Valedictory address, 1857 (tr. by Max Samter)

Oliver Wendell Holmes [1809–1894]

I'll tell you, though, if you want to know it, what is the real offence of Boston. It drains a large water-shed of its intellect, and will not itself be drained.

> *The Autocrat of the Breakfast Table*, Sect. VI

A moment's insight is sometimes worth a life's experience.

> *The Professor at the Breakfast Table*, Sect. X

Rudolf Virchow [1821–1902]

I uphold my own rights and therefore I also recognize the rights of others.

> *Cellular Pathology*, Preface (tr. by Frank Chance)

Louis Pasteur [1822–1895]

Two contrary laws seem to be wrestling with each other nowadays: the one, a law of blood and of death, ever imagining new means of destruction and forcing nations to be constantly ready for the battlefield — the other,

a law of peace, work and health, ever evolving new means for delivering man from the scourges which beset him.

> Speech opening the Pasteur Institute, Paris, November 14, 1888 (tr. by René J. Dubos in *Pasteur and Modern Science*)

Sir Clifford Allbutt [1836–1925]

There are times in the lives of all of us when the flame of the Spirit burns low; when we are out of heart; we hardly know what to believe; the evil in the world dejects us, or, which is worst of all, we drift into indifference; the lamp drops from our hands; and, if we watch ourselves as we ought to do, we find we are losing the finer edge of our kindliness, our truthfulness, our purity. In these cold and arid seasons the message is, keep right on in a steady faithfulness, hoping all things.

> Address, London, 1922

John Shaw Billings [1838–1913]

Speaking to a body of scientific men, each of whom has, I hope, also certain unscientific beliefs, desires, hopes, and longings, I will only say: "Be strong and of good courage." As scientific men, let us try to increase and diffuse knowledge; as men and citizens, let us try to be useful; and, in each capacity, let us do the work that comes to us honestly and thoroughly and fear not the unknown future.

> Speech to the Philosophical Society of Washington, December 4, 1886

Sir William Osler [1849–1919]

The quest for righteousness is Oriental, the quest for knowledge, Occidental.

> Address to the Jewish Historical Society of England, April 27, 1914

Silence is always possible, than which we have no better weapon in our armoury against evil-speaking, lying, and slandering.

> *Aequanimitas, with Other Addresses,* "Chauvinism in Medicine"

What I inveigh against is a cursed spirit of intolerance, conceived in distrust and bred in ignorance, that makes the mental attitude perennially antagonistic, even bitterly antagonistic to everything foreign, that subordinates everywhere the race to the nation, forgetting the higher claims of human brotherhood.

> *Idem*

I have three personal ideals. One to do the day's work well and not to bother about to-morrow. . . .

The second ideal has been to act the Golden Rule, as far as in me lay, towards my professional brethren and towards the patients committed to my care.

And the third has been to cultivate such a measure of equanimity as would enable me to bear success with humility, the affection of my friends without pride and to be ready when the day of sorrow and grief came to meet it with the courage befitting a man.

> *Ibid.,* "L'Envoi"

Take away with you a profound conviction of the value of system in your work.

> *Ibid.,* "The Master-Word in Medicine"

Common sense in matters medical is rare, and is usually in inverse ratio to the degree of education.

> *Ibid.,* "Teaching and Thinking"

Advice is sought to confirm a position already taken.

> Quoted by William B. Bean in *Sir William Osler: Aphorisms,* Ch. 2

William H. Welch [1850–1934]

I plead for a little more of the cultural side in medicine.

Sigmund Freud [1856–1939]

There is something comic about the incongruity between one's own and other people's estimation of one's work.

> Letter to Dr. Wilhelm Fliess, May 21, 1894 (tr. by Eric Mosbacher and James Strachey)

John B. Murphy [1857–1916]

It is the purpose of every man's life to do something worthy of the recognition and appreciation of his fellow men. . . . By their superior intellectual qualifications, their fidelity to purpose and above all their indefatigable labor the few become leaders.

> *Journal of the American Medical Association* 57:1, 1911

Havelock Ellis [1859–1939]

The Promised Land always lies on the other side of a wilderness.

> *The Dance of Life,* Ch. 5

I wish that I might go from door to
door,
And lay my hand on every heart that's
sore;
And say sweet words, and comfort lids
that weep.

> *The Gospel of Consolation*

As this, I say, I know, and know as
well,
I never knew a heart I might not love.

> *In the Strand*

George David Stewart [1862–1933]

The Lord helps those who help themselves and the Lord help those who don't!

> Aphorism

J. Chalmers Da Costa [1863–1933]

Every now and then I see a judge on the bench who reminds me of a fly in amber. I know he is there, but I can't imagine how he got there.

The Trials and Triumphs of the Surgeon, Ch. 1

Sometimes cowardice, sometimes laziness, sometimes selfishness saves a man from being called irritable, combative, and cantankerous. What a man doesn't do is not always a sign of what he is and isn't. We must know why he doesn't do it in order to reach a conclusion.

Idem

The world is very small if we would avoid an enemy — huge if we would find a friend.

Idem

George Santayana [1863–1952]

Fanaticism consists in redoubling your effort when you have forgotten your aim.

The Life of Reason, Vol. I, Introduction

Harvey Cushing [1869–1939]

Who have made the greatest gifts to their fellow man? Those who have left an idea that has supplied, like the utterances of Christ, what minds have yearned for? Those who have added to his physical comforts and have found ways to lessen hunger and want? Those who have added to his conveniences and devised means to lighten his labor? Those who have, like Lincoln, freed him from bondage and like Lister released him from the horror of suppuration? One answer certainly can be made: that only when the gift requires self-denial and only if the giver be one that walketh uprightly, and worketh righteousness and speaketh the truth in his heart, will he, like Saint Francis, come to be canonized and forever blest.

Consecratio Medici, Ch. XIV

Wilfred Trotter [1872–1939]

In this respect I shall ask you to be indulgent to a weakness of seniority by which it tends to over-estimate the value of the elementary and the simple.

Collected Papers, "Emergency," Sect. 8

W. Somerset Maugham [1874–1965]

People ask you for criticism, but they only want praise.

Of Human Bondage, Ch. I

The normal's the one thing you practically never get. That's why it's called the normal.[1]

Ibid., Ch. LIV

By the time I was twenty-four I had constructed a complete system of philosophy. It rested on two principles: The Relativity of Things and The Circumferentiality of Man. I have learnt since that the first of these was not a very original discovery. It may be that the other was profound, but though I have racked my brains I cannot for the life of me remember what on earth it meant.

The Summing Up, Sect. lxvi

Albert Schweitzer [1875–1965]

The knowledge of life, therefore, which we grown-ups have to pass on to the younger generation will not be expressed thus: "Reality will soon give way before your ideals," but "Grow into your ideals, so that life can never rob you of them." If all of us could become what we were at fourteen, what a different place this world would be!

Memoirs of Childhood and Youth, Ch. 5 (tr. by C. T. Campion)

Oliver St. John Gogarty [1878–1957]

Three great inventions came from Ireland — the invention of soda water whereby whiskey outdoes champagne, the invention of the pneumatic tyre

---

[1] Discussing cadaver while dissecting.

whereby was made possible the evolution of an engine to scale the blue, and the invention of the system whereby disease is made to support patient, nurse and doctor, and horses to carry hospitals!

> *As I Was Going Down Sackville Street,* Ch. 3

In studying the external universe we have neglected the universe within ourselves.

> *I Follow Saint Patrick,* Ch. XV

Albert Einstein [1879–1955]

Perfection of means and confusion of goals seem — in my opinion — to characterize our age.

> *Out of My Later Years,* Ch. 15

Martin H. Fischer [1879–1962]

Any man who does not make himself proficient in at least two languages other than his own is a fool. Such men have the quaint habit of discovering things fifty years after all the world knows about them.

> Quoted by Howard Fabing and Ray Marr in *Fischerisms*

H. L. Mencken [1880–1956]

Life in America interests me, not as a moral phenomenon, but simply as a gaudy spectacle. I enjoy it most when it is most uproarious, preposterous, inordinate and melodramatic. I am perfectly willing to give a Roosevelt, a Wilson, a Fall, an Elder Hays, an Andy Mellon, or a Tom Heflin such small part of my revenues as he can gouge out of me in return for a show that he offers. Such gorgeous mountebanks take my mind off my gallstones, my war wounds, my public duties and my unfortunate love affairs, and so make existence agreeable. I had rather read the *Congressional Record* — or, failing that, any good tabloid — than go to see a bishop hanged.

> *Baltimore Evening Sun,* May 28, 1928

Charles Wilson, Lord Moran [1882–]

Courage is a moral quality; it is not a chance gift of nature like an aptitude for games. It is a cold choice between two alternatives, the fixed resolve not to quit; an act of renunciation which must be made not once but many times by the power of the will. Courage is will power.

> *The Anatomy of Courage,* Ch. V

William Carlos Williams [1883–1963]

Unless every age claims the world for its own and makes it so by its own efforts in its own day and unless the mark of this effort and success is left upon all the forms of that age including those formal expressions which we call art, no one can be said to have lived in any age or at any time.

> Letter to Whit Burnett, June 14, 1942

Alan Gregg [1890–1957]

Derogatory remarks are the barrow pits we dig to make an embankment of our own pride.

> Aphorism (Quoted by Wilder Penfield in *The Difficult Art of Giving,* Appendix A)

Good horse sense is the sense that horses have, never to bet on human beings.

> *For Future Doctors,* "Creativeness in Medicine"

In the effort to take the world as a real place and not evade its reality you may on occasion find wisdom in the art of timing, in taking advantage of the fact that life ebbs and flows, that the work of the world, like the work of the heart, goes on by means of diastole as well as systole, that children pass through phases, that enough is enough, that a sense of humor and proportion has its uses as well as being perfectly delightful.

Texas Reports on Biology and Medicine 11:440, 1953

Dana W. Atchley [1892–   ]

The joy of understanding is both the closest rival of the joy of service and its most effective partner.

Journal of Medical Education 34(October, Pt. II):17, 1959

Earle P. Scarlett [1896–   ]

A large number of people have, in the face of bewildering events and issues, adopted a struthionine practice; that is, burying their heads in the sand (the adjective *struthionine* which I have used has a certain polite and esoteric aura, deriving from the Latin *struthio* = an ostrich). But in medical matters this will just not do. Professional secrecy cannot be regarded as an idle matter, and, like some other medical customs, be disposed of as an ancient shibboleth that should be liquidated.

Archives of Internal Medicine 118:606, 1966

Thomas A. Dooley [1927–1961]

It is better to light a candle than to sit and drink beer in the darkness.

Aphorism in lectures

Have no qualms, my dear. I've been eating here for five years and all I've got is cancer. [To a newspaperwoman who asked if the food served in a Vientiane restaurant was safe.]

Told to Dr. William D. Snively, Jr.

OBSERVATION

See also SCIENTIFIC METHOD

Hippocrates [460?–377? B.C.]

We must turn to nature itself, to the observations of the body in health and disease to learn the truth.

Thomas Sydenham [1624–1689]

I am conscious of having omitted certain distinctive observations now inaccessible in the lumber-room of my memory. The fact that they are inaccessible only shows that I did not attend to them at the time or register them afterwards as carefully as I should. Nothing in medicine is so insignificant as to merit inattention.

Medical Observations (tr. by R. G. Latham in *Works*, Vol. I)

Sir Gilbert Blane [1749–1834]

The truth seems to be, that a higher order of intellect, a more rare and happy genius, a more correct and better tutored understanding, is required to elicit practical truths by observation, than to coin theories.

Elements of Medical Logic

Johann Wolfgang von Goethe [1749–1832]

The observation of nature requires a certain purity of mind, which cannot be disturbed or pre-occupied by anything.

Quoted by J. P. Eckermann in *Conversations with Goethe*, May 18, 1824 (tr. by J. Oxenford)

What is the hardest of all? That which you hold the most simple; seeing with your own eyes what is spread out before you.

Richard Bright [1789–1858]

It is quite impossible for any man to gain information respecting *acute* disease, unless he watch its progress. Day after day it must be seen; the lapse of eight-and-forty hours will so change the face of disease. . . . Acute disease must be seen at least once a-day by those who wish to learn; in many cases twice a-day will not be too often.

> *Address Delivered at the Commencement of a Course of Lectures on the Practice of Medicine*

Peter Mere Latham [1789–1875]

Observation runs sadly to waste when it is made upon cases piecemeal.

> *Diseases of the Heart,* Lect. XXVII

Armand Trousseau [1801–1867]

To know the natural progress of diseases is to know more than the half of medicine. . . . Observe the practice of many physicians; do not implicitly believe the mere assertion of your master; be something better than servile learners; go forth yourselves to see and to compare. . . . Knowing, henceforth, the physiognomy of the disease when allowed to run its own course, you can, without risk of error, estimate the value of the different medications which have been employed. You will discover which remedies have done no harm, and which have notably curtailed the duration of the disease; and thus for the future you will have a standard by which to measure the value of the medicines which you see employed to counteract the malady in question. What you have done in respect of one disease, you will be able to do in respect of many; and by proceeding in this way you will be able, on sure data, to pass judgment on the treatment pursued by your masters.

> *Clinical Medicine,* Vol. I, Introduction

Sir Dominic J. Corrigan [1802–1880]

The trouble with doctors is not that they don't know enough, but that they don't see enough.

Elisha Bartlett [1804–1855]

With certain unimportant qualifications, our knowledge of the causes of disease is the direct and exclusive result of observation and study of the causes themselves.

> *Philosophy of Medical Science,* Pt. II, Ch. 6

The art of observation is always a very difficult art; and nowhere is it more so, than in the science of medicine. It is one of the rarest accomplishments; and although the annals of medical science are crowded with the names of men, who were famous for their learning, or for their reasoning and speculative powers, they bear those of but few who were distinguished as observers.

> *Ibid.,* Ch. 12

Look at any single disease, even of the simplest and best settled character; and let us suppose that all its elements, as far as this is possible, in the nature of things, have been accurately ascertained. Before our therapeutical knowledge of this disease can be said, in literal strictness, to be complete, we must know the effects and influences, which all the substances and agencies in nature are capable of producing upon it; and we can know this only by direct observation of the effects themselves.

> *Ibid.,* Ch. 16

Jean Martin Charcot [1825–1893]

If the clinician, as observer, wishes to see things as they really are, he must make a *tabula rasa* of his mind and proceed without any preconceived notions whatever.

In the last analysis, we see only what we are ready to see, what we have been taught to see. We eliminate and ignore everything that is not a part of our prejudices.

Theodor Billroth [1829-1894]

Let what you observe penetrate your inmost soul, let it so warm and replenish you that your thoughts constantly refer to it, and then you will find true pleasure and delight in your intellectual labours.
> *Lectures on Surgical Pathology and Therapeutics*

Walter Pater [1839-1894]

The growth [of observation] consists in a continual analysis of facts of rough and general observation into groups of facts more precise and minute.
> *Appreciations*, "Coleridge"

Thomas McCrae [1870-1935]

More is missed by not looking than by not knowing.
> Aphorism

Alexis Carrel [1873-1944]

A few observations and much reasoning leads to error; many observations and a little reasoning to truth.

Russell John Howard [1875-1942]

The only competent observer is yourself.
> Quoted by F. G. St. Clair Strange in *The Hip*, Ch. 1

Sir Robert Platt [1900–   ]

Indeed a great deal of recent medical knowledge is based on observation rather than experiment. No kind of controlled human experiment was needed to unravel the clinical significance of the haemoglobinopathies, for instance.
> *Universities Quarterly* 17:327, 1963

Richard Schatzki [1901–   ]

The eyes must finish their work before the gray cells take over.
> *Clinical Aphorisms from the Harvard Medical School* (1957), "Medicine"

OCCUPATIONAL DISEASE

See also PUBLIC HEALTH

Bernardino Ramazzini [1633-1714]

"When you come to a patient's house, you should ask him what sort of pains he has, what caused them, how many days he has been ill, whether the bowels are working and what sort of food he eats." So says Hippocrates in his work *Affections*. I may venture to add one more question: what occupation does he follow?
> *Diseases of Workers*, Preface (tr. by W. C. Wright)

The mortality of those who dig minerals in mines is very great, and women who marry men of this sort marry again and again. According to Agricola, at the mines in the Carpathian mountains women have been known to marry seven times.
> *Ibid.*, Ch. 1

Charles T. Thackrah [1795-1833]

Evils are suffered to exist, even where the means of correction are known and easily applied. Thoughtlessness or apathy is the only obstacle to success.
> *The Effects of the Principal Arts, Trades and Professions . . . on Health and Longevity,* "Comparative Mortality"

Alice Hamilton [1869–   ]

It is a pity that I cannot recall any instance of help from the organized industrialists. . . . [they] [1] fought the passage of occupational disease compensation as they fought laws against child labor, laws establishing a minimum wage for women and a maximum working day. Yet members . . . are many of them humane and benevolent employers. But as an organiza-

[1] The National Association of Manufacturers.

tion they have shown themselves to be as devoid of a sense of responsibility to the public as the most self-seeking of the trade-unions.
> *Exploring the Dangerous Trades*

Henry E. Sigerist [1891–1957]

The development of industry has created many new sources of danger. Occupational diseases are socially different from other diseases, but not biologically.
> Quoted in *Journal of the History of Medicine and Allied Sciences* 13:214, 1958

OLD AGE

See also AGE, LONGEVITY, MATURITY, MIDDLE AGE, SENILITY, YOUTH

I. GENERAL

Sophocles [496?–406 B.C.]

No man loves life as he who's growing old.
> *Fragments,* II.66, from *Acrisius*

Pausanias [fl. 479 B.C.]

When the physician said to him, "You have lived to be an old man," he [Pausanias] said, "That is because I never employed you as my physician."
> Quoted by Plutarch in *Moralia,* "Sayings of Spartans," 231.A.6 (tr. by F. C. Babbitt)

Hippocrates [460?–377? B.C.]

Old people, on the whole, have fewer complaints than young; but those chronic diseases which do befall them generally never leave them.
> *Aphorisms,* II.39 (tr. by Francis Adams)

Statius [220–168 B.C.]

Let him draw out his old age to dotage drop by drop.
> *Hymnis,* Fragment (Quoted by Festus, tr. by E. H. Warmington)

Cicero [106–43 B.C.]

No one is so old as to think he cannot live one more year.
> *On Old Age,* VII.24 (tr. by W. A. Falconer)

Plutarch [46?–120?]

Tiberius Caesar once said that a man over sixty who holds out his hand [pulse] to a physician is ridiculous.[1]
> *Moralia,* "Advice About Keeping Well" (tr. by F. C. Babbitt)

Juvenal [60?–140?]

Old men all look alike.
> *Satires,* X.198 (tr. by G. G. Ramsay)

Wang Wei [699–759]

Day after day
In vain we labor —
And grow old.

So come,
Empty a cup of wine
With me.

Waste no pity
On the falling blossoms.
Year after year
They will come again
With Spring.
> *Nature and Man* (tr. by H. H. Hart)

Michel de Montaigne [1533–1592]

There is no man so decrepit that as long as he sees Methuselah ahead of him, he does not think he has another twenty years left in his body.
> *Essays,* Bk. I, Ch. 20, "That to Philosophize Is to Learn to Die" (tr. by Donald M. Frame)

[1] Cf. Tacitus, p. 390b.

Who ever saw old age not praising times past and blaming the present?
> *Ibid.*, Bk. II, Ch. 13, "Of Judging of the Death of Others"

Shall I, who in all matters have so worshiped that *golden mean* of the past, and have taken the moderate measure as the most perfect, aspire to an immoderate and prodigious old age?
> *Ibid.*, Bk. III, Ch. 13, "Of Experience"

Duc François de La Rochefoucauld [1613–1680]

Few people know how to be old.
> *Maxims*

Walter Pope [1630–1714]

I hope I shall have no occasion to send
For Priests, or Fysicians, till I am so
    near mine End
That I have eat all my bread, and
    drunk my last Glass,
Let them come then, and set their
    Seals to my Pass.
> *The Wish*, Sect. XVI

Book of Common Prayer [1662]

I have been young, and now am old.
> *Psalter* 37:25

Jonathan Swift [1667–1745]

Threescore, I think, is pretty high;
'Twas time in conscience he should
    die!
> *A Satirical Elegy on the Death of a Late Famous General*

Nicholas Rowe [1674–1718]

The Ev'ning of my Age.
> *The Fair Penitent*, Act IV, Sc. i

Thomas Parnell [1679–1718]

If Truth in spight of Manners must
    be told,
Why really Fifty Five is something old.
> *An Elegy, To an Old Beauty*

Philip Stanhope, Lord Chesterfield [1694–1773]

Tyrawley and I have been dead these two years; but we don't choose to have it known.
> Quoted by James Boswell in *Life of Samuel Johnson*, April 3, 1773

John Armstrong [1709–1779]

Cease, reverend Fathers! from those
    youthful Sports
Retire, before unfinish'd *Feats* betray
Your slacken'd Nerves.
> *The Economy of Love*

Samuel Johnson [1709–1784]

It is unjust to claim the privileges of age, and retain the playthings of childhood.
> *The Rambler*, No. 50 (September 8, 1750)

Percivall Pott [1714–1788]

My lamp is almost extinguished. I hope it has burned for the benefit of others.
> *Chirurgical Works*, Vol. I, Janus Earle's "A Short Account of the Life of Mr. Pott"

Hester Lynch Piozzi (Mrs. Henry Thrale) [1741–1821]

The tree of deepest root is found
Least willing still to quit the ground;
'Twas therefore said by ancient sages
That love of life increased with years,
So much that in our later stages,
When pains grow sharp, and sickness
    rages,
The greatest love of life appears.
> *The Three Warnings*

Johann Wolfgang von Goethe [1749–1832]

No skill or art is needed to grow old; the trick is to endure it.

Napoleon Bonaparte [1769–1821]

There ought [not] to be any Generals

over sixty years of age on active service.

> The St. Helena Journal, December 11, 1816 (tr. by Sydney Gillard)

I have made noise enough in the world already, perhaps too much, and am now getting old, and want retirement.

> Quoted by Barry O'Meara in *Napoleon in Exile*, October 1, 1816

Sydney Smith [1771–1845]

That sign of old age, extolling the past at the expense of the present.

> Quoted by Lady Holland in *A Memoir of the Rev. Sydney Smith*, Ch. 11

Charles Lamb [1775–1834]

The growing infirmities of age manifest themselves in nothing more strongly, than in an inveterate dislike of interruption.

> *The Last Essays of Elia*, "Popular Fallacies," XII

Daniel Drake [1785–1852]

As old age is ruminant, youth ought to prepare for it as many savory cuds as possible.

> *Pioneer Life in Kentucky*, Letter VII

Ralph Waldo Emerson [1803–1882]

We do not count a man's years, until he has nothing else to count.

> *Society and Solitude*, "Old Age"

Henry Wadsworth Longfellow [1807–1882]

To be seventy years old . . . is like climbing the Alps. You reach a snow-crowned summit, and see behind you the deep valley stretching miles and miles away, and before you other summits higher and whiter, which you may have strength to climb, or may not. Then you sit down and meditate and wonder which it will be.

> Letter to George W. Childs, March 13, 1877

Whatever poet, orator, or sage
May say of it, old age is still old age.

> *Morituri Salutamus*

Oliver Wendell Holmes [1809–1894]

A general flavor of mild decay,
But nothing local, as one may say.

> *The Deacon's Masterpiece*

Joseph Sheridan Le Fanu [1814–1873]

Old persons are sometimes as unwilling to die as tired-out children are to say good night and go to bed.

John Godfrey Saxe [1816–1887]

I'm growing fonder of my staff;
  I'm growing dimmer in the eyes;
I'm growing fainter in my laugh;
  I'm growing deeper in my sighs;
I'm growing careless of my dress;
  I'm growing frugal of my gold;
I'm growing wise; I'm growing, — yes, —
             I'm growing old!

> *I'm Growing Old*

Henri Amiel [1821–1881]

To know how to grow old is the master-work of wisdom, and one of the most difficult chapters in the great art of living.

> *Journal Intime*, September 21, 1874 (tr. by Mrs. Humphrey Ward)

Mortimer Collins [1827–1876]

The true way to render age vigorous is to prolong the youth of the mind.

> *The Village Comedy*, Pt. I

339

Sir James Crichton-Browne
[1840–1938]

Old age begins at the cradle, and youth still lingers in decrepitude.
The Prevention of Senility

Sir William Osler [1849–1919]

Who serves the gods dies young — Venus, Bacchus, and Vulcan send in no bills in the seventh decade.
Quoted by Harvey Cushing in *Life of Sir William Osler*, Ch. XXI

Santiago Ramón y Cajal
[1852–1934]

In youth we say: "I am immortal." In age we say: "I die without having lived." And it would be the same if we lived the three hundred years of the crocodile or the two hundred of the elephant.
Charlas de Café

It is notorious that the desire to live increases as life itself shortens.
Idem

Ed Howe [1853–1937]

After a man is fifty you can fool him by saying he is smart, but you can't fool him by saying he is pretty.
Country Town Sayings

James B. Herrick [1861–1954]

I never miss the death notes and weather report in the papers.[1]
Memories of Eighty Years, Ch. XV

Sir Humphry Davy Rolleston
[1862–1944]

[There is] more danger of the individual rusting out than wearing out.
Some Medical Aspects of Old Age

[1] Comment on his visual acuity at the age of 87.

Logan Pearsall Smith [1865–1946]

The denunciation of the young is a necessary part of the hygiene of older people, and greatly assists the circulation of their blood.
All Trivia, "Last Words"

Charles Judson Herrick
[1868–1960]

You don't grow old; when you cease to grow, you are old.

Constantin Brancusi
[1876–1957]

When we are no longer young, we are already dead.

Maude Royden [1876–1956]

If you want to be a dear old lady at seventy, you should start early, say about seventeen.

Maxwell Anderson [1888–1959]

But it's a long, long while from May
    to December
And the days grow short when you
    reach September,
And I've lost one tooth and I walk a
    little lame,
And I haven't got time for the waiting
    game,
For the days turn to gold as they
    grow few,
September, November,
And these few golden days I'd spend
    with you.
These golden days I'd spend with you.
Knickerbocker Holiday, Act I, "September Song"

Alan Gregg [1890–1957]

We don't drowse because we're old: we're old because we have gotten to the point of having so few relevant stimuli that we become inattentive, actionless and drowsy.
Aphorism (Quoted by Wilder Penfield in *The Difficult Art of Giving*, Appendix A)

John F. Kennedy [1917–1963]

A proud and resourceful nation can no longer ask its older people to live in constant fear of a serious illness for which adequate funds are not available. We owe them the right of dignity in sickness as well as in health.

> *Message to Congress on Problems of the Aged,* February 21, 1963

The Bible

They all shall wax old as a garment; the moth shall eat them up.

> *Isaiah* 50:9

Anonymous

Auld men will die, and bairns will soon forget.

> *Black-Letter Ballads*

Everyone faces at all times two fateful possibilities: one is to grow older, the other not.

Proverb

Old age, though despised, is coveted by all men.

French Proverb

Forty is the old age of youth; fifty is the youth of old age.

Greek Proverb

It is useless to physic the dead or to advise an old man.

Latin Proverb

Become old early if you would be old long.[1]

Polish Proverb

Do not ask the old, "How are you?" but "What ails you?"

---

[1] English Proverb: They who would be young when they are old must be old when they are young.

II. GOOD ASPECTS

Huang Ti (The Yellow Emperor) [2697–2597 B.C.]

Those who search beyond the natural limits will retain good hearing and clear vision, their bodies will remain light and strong, and although they grow old in years they will remain able-bodied and flourishing; and those who are able-bodied can govern to great advantage.

> *Nei Ching Su Wên,* Bk. 2, Sect. 5 (tr. by Ilza Veith in *The Yellow Emperor's Classic of Internal Medicine*)

Homer [ca. 850 B.C.]

A green old Age unconscious of Decays.

> *Iliad,* XXIII.791 (929 as tr. by Alexander Pope)

Euripides [484–406 B.C.]

It is meaningless, the way the old men pray for death and complain of age and the long time they have to live. Let death only come close, not one of them still wants to die. Their age is not a burden any more.

> *Alcestis,* 669 (tr. by R. Lattimore)

Cicero [106–43 B.C.]

It is not by muscle, speed, or physical dexterity that great things are achieved, but by reflection, force of character, and judgement; in these qualities old age is usually not only not poorer, but is even richer.

> *On Old Age,* VI.17 (tr. by W. A. Falconer)

For just as I approve of the young man in whom there is a touch of age, so I approve of the old man in whom there is some flavour of youth. He who strives thus to mingle youthfulness and age may grow old in body, but old in spirit he will never be.

> *Ibid.,* XI.38

William Shakespeare [1564–1616]

Though I look old, yet I am strong and
  lusty;
For in my youth I never did apply
Hot and rebellious liquors in my blood,
Nor did not with unbashful forehead
  woo
The means of weakness and debility;
Therefore my age is as a lusty winter,
Frosty, but kindly.
> *As You Like It,* II, iii, 47

Thomas Campion [1567–1620]

Good thoughts his onely friendes,
  His wealth a well-spent age,
The earth his sober Inne
  And quiet Pilgrimage.
> *A Booke of Ayres,* "The Man
> of Life Upright"

Though you are yoong and I am olde,
though your vaines hot and my bloud
  colde,
though youth is moist and age is drie,
yet embers live when flames doe die.
> *Ibid.,* "Though You Are
> Yoong"

Walter Pope [1630–1714]

If I live to be Old, for I find I go down,
Let this be my Fate. In a Country
  Town,
May I have a warm House, with a
  Stone at the Gate,
And a cleanly young Girl, to rub my
  bald Pate.
May I govern my Passions with an
  absolute Sway,
And grow Wiser, and Better as my
  Strength wears away,
Without Gout, or Stone, by a gentle
  decay.
> *The Wish,* Sect. I

Hermann Boerhaave [1668–1738]

What a hope that is, to have the philosophers' stone! To hold to an unfailing bodily health, a constant vigour
and tranquillity of mind, to preserve
these into a green and rugged old age,
until without a struggle or a sickness
body and soul part company. . . . nay
more, to regain. lost youth — the old
granddam to win back a merry supple-
ness, . . . the wrinkles of her brow
to fill and level, so that she straightens
and she shines, . . . even old moulted
fowls to feather and lay eggs again.
Yet alas for that fortunate hope: the
nearer they win to it, so much the more
does possession threaten present dangers to them that all but have it, and
how these may be avoided I do not
know.
> *Dissertatio academica de gaudiis
> alchemistarum*

Samuel Johnson [1709–1784]

But in the decline of life shame and
grief are of short duration; whether
it be that we bear easily what we have
born long, or that, finding ourselves in
age less regarded, we less regard
others; or, that we look with slight
regard upon afflictions, to which we
know that the hand of death is about
to put an end.
> *Rasselas,* Ch. IV

James Grainger [1723–1767]

But when old age has silver'd o'er thy
  head,
When memory fails, and all thy vigour's fled,
Then may'st thou seek the stillness of
  retreat,
Then hear aloof the human tempest
  beat,
Then will I greet thee to my woodland
  cave,
Allay the pangs of age, and smooth
  thy grave.
> *Solitude*

Thomas Jefferson [1743–1826]

Tranquillity is the old man's milk.
> Letter to Edward Rutledge,
> June 24, 1797

William Drennan [1754-1820]

Time has touched me gently in his
    race,
And left no odious furrows in my face.
    Tales of the Hall, Bk. XVII

Oliver Wendell Holmes
[1809-1894]

A man over ninety is a great comfort
to all his elderly neighbors: he is a
picket-guard at the extreme outpost;
and the young folks of sixty and seventy feel that the enemy must get by
him before he can come near their
camp.
    The Guardian Angel, Ch. 2

To be seventy years young is sometimes far more cheerful and hopeful
than to be forty years old.
    Letter to Julia Ward Howe on
    her 70th birthday, May 27,
    1889

Alfred, Lord Tennyson
[1809-1892]

           You and I are old;
Old age hath yet his honor and his
    toil;
Death closes all: but something ere
    the end,
Some work of noble note, may yet be
    done.
    Ulysses

Robert Browning [1812-1889]

Grow old along with me!
The best is yet to be,
The last of life, for which the first was
    made.
    Rabbi Ben Ezra

George Santayana [1863-1952]

Old Age, on tiptoe, lays her jewelled
    hand
Lightly in mine.
    *A Minuet on Reaching the Age
    of Fifty*

Wilder Penfield [1891-   ]

Toward the end, senescence with its
comforting drowsiness closes stealthily
one door after another. And so when
death does come at last, it may not be
unwelcome after all. Science has not
changed these things. The span of life,
for those who escape its early perils, is
about the same today as when David
played on his harp before King Saul.
    The Second Career, Ch. I

III. BAD ASPECTS

See also SENILITY

Euripides [484-406 B.C.]

Oftener than not the old are uncon-
    trollable;
Their tempers make them difficult to
    deal with.
    Andromache, 727 (tr. by J. F.
    Nims)

O harsh old age! How hateful is your
    reign!
    The Suppliant Women, 1108
    (tr. by F. Jones)

Antiphanes [408?-334? B.C.]

Old age is, so to speak, the sanctuary
of ills: they all take refuge in it.
    Fragment from *The Dipnoso-
    phists*

Terence [185-159 B.C.]

Old age is an illness in itself.
    Phormio, Act IV (tr. by J.
    Sargeaunt)

Horace [65-8 B.C.]

Many ills encompass an old man,
whether because he seeks gain, and
then miserably holds aloof from his
store and fears to use it, or because, in
all that he does, he lacks fire and courage, is dilatory and slow to form hopes,

is sluggish and greedy of a longer life, peevish, surly, given to praising the days he spent as a boy, and to reproving and condemning the young. Many blessings do the advancing years bring with them; many, as they retire, they take away.

> *The Art of Poetry,* 169 (tr. by H. R. Fairclough)

Seneca [4? B.C.–A.D. 65]

Old age is a disease which we cannot cure.

> *Moral Epistles to Lucilius,* CVIII.28 (tr. by Richard M. Gummere)

St. Augustine [354–430]

When men desire old age, what else do they desire but prolonged infirmity?

> *Of the Catechizing of the Unlearned,* XVI.24 (tr. by J. P. Christopher)

Gabriele Zerbi [1468–1505]

Old men suffer from difficulty of breathing, catarrh accompanied by coughing, strangury, painful micturition, pains in the joints, kidney disease, dizziness, apoplexy, cachexia, pruritus of the whole body, sleeplessness, watery discharge from the bowels, the eyes and the nostrils, dullness of sight, cataract and hardness of hearing.

> *Gerontocomia*

Sir Thomas More [1478–1535]

They judge it a great poynt of crueltie, that anye body in their moste nede of helpe and comforte, shoulde be caste of and forsaken, and that olde age, whych both bringeth sicknes with it, and is a syckenes it selfe, should unkindly and unfaythfullye be delte withall.

> *Utopia,* Bk. II, Ch. 7 (tr. by R. Robinson)

Thomas, Lord Vaux [1510–1556]

For Age, with stealing steps,
Hath clawed me with his clutch.

> *Poems,* "The Aged Lover Renounceth Love"

Michel de Montaigne [1533–1592]

Old age puts more wrinkles in our minds than on our faces.

> *Essays,* Bk. III, Ch. 2, "Of Repentance"

Our mind grows constipated and sluggish as it grows old.

> *Ibid.,* Bk. III, Ch. 12, "Of Physiognomy"

Sir Francis Bacon [1561–1626]

Discern of the coming on of years, and think not to do the same things still; for age will not be defied.

> *Essays,* "Of Regiment of Health"

Men of age object too much, consult too long, adventure too little, repent too soon, and seldom drive business home to the full period, but content themselves with a mediocrity of success.

> *Ibid.,* "Of Youth and Age"

William Shakespeare [1564–1616]

The sixth age shifts

Into the lean and slipper'd pantaloon,
With spectacles on nose and pouch on
  side;
His youthful hose, well sav'd, a world
  too wide
For his shrunk shank, and his big
  manly voice,
Turning again toward childish treble,
  pipes
And whistles in his sound. Last scene
  of all,
That ends this strange eventful history,
Is second childishness and mere oblivion,
Sans teeth, sans eye, sans taste, sans
  everything.

> *As You Like It,* II, vii, 157

The satirical rogue says here that old men have grey beards; that their faces are wrinkled; their eyes purging thick amber and plum-tree gum; and that they have a plentiful lack of wit, together with most weak hams.

Hamlet, II, ii, 198

Do you set down your name in the scroll of youth, that are written down old with all the characters of age? Have you not a moist eye, a dry hand, a yellow cheek, a white beard, a decreasing leg, an increasing belly? Is not your voice broken, your wind short, your chin double, your wit single, and every part about you blasted with antiquity? And will you yet call yourself young?

Henry IV, Part II, I, ii, 201

A good leg will fall, a straight back will stoop, a black beard will turn white, a curl'd pate will grow bald, a fair face will wither, a full eye will wax hollow.

Henry V, V, ii, 168

The aged man that coffers up his gold
Is plagu'd with cramps and gouts and painful fits.

The Rape of Lucrece, line 855

Were I hard-favour'd, foul, or wrinkled old,
Ill-nurtur'd, crooked, churlish, harsh in voice,
O'erworn, despised, rheumatic, and cold,
Thick-sighted, barren, lean and lacking juice,
   Then mightst thou pause, for then I were not for thee.

Venus and Adonis, line 133

Thomas Middleton [1570?–1627]

These old folks talk of nothing but defects,
Because they grow so full of 'em themselves.

Women Beware Women, Act I, Sc. i

Ben Jonson [1573?–1637]

Their limbs faint,
Their senses dull, their seeing, hearing, going,
All dead before them; yea, their very teeth,
Their instruments of eating, fayling them.

Volpone, Act I, Sc. iv

Duc François de La Rochefoucauld [1613–1680]

Age loves to give good precepts to console itself for being no longer able to give bad examples.

Maxims, No. 93

The blemishes of the mind, like those of the face, increase with age.

Ibid., No. 112

Old age is a tyrant who has decreed that indulgence in the pleasures of youth shall be a capital offence.

Ibid., No. 461 (tr. by Constantine FitzGibbon)

Jeremy Taylor [1613–1667]

Before a man comes to be wise, he is half dead with gouts and consumptions, with catarrhs and aches, with sore eyes and a worn-out body.

The Rule and Exercises of Holy Dying, Ch. I, Sect. III

Jean de La Bruyère [1645–1696]

We fear old age, which we are never sure of being able to reach.

Characters, Ch. VI

Susannah Centlivre [1667?–1723]

'Tis the defect of Age to rail at the Pleasure's of Youth.

The Basset Table, Act I

Voltaire [1694–1778]

Man can have only a certain number of teeth, hair and ideas; there comes a time when he necessarily loses his teeth, hair and ideas.

Philosophical Dictionary

Samuel Johnson [1709–1784]

My diseases are an asthma and a dropsy, and what is less curable, seventy-five.

> Letter to W. G. Hamilton, October 20, 1784

William Heberden [1710–1801]

The love of life, or fear of death, makes most men unwilling to allow that their constitution is breaking; and for this reason they are ready to impute to any other cause what in reality are the signs of approaching and unavoidable decay.

> *Commentaries on the History and Cure of Diseases,* Ch. 9

Horace Walpole [1717–1797]

The loss of youth is melancholy enough; but to enter into old age through the gate of infirmity, most disheartening.

> Letter to George Montagu, July 28, 1765

Nobody grows stronger at seventy-five.

> Letter to Hannah More, August 21, 1792

Charles Churchill [1731–1765]

OLD AGE, a *second Child,* by Nature curs'd
With more and greater evils than the first,
Weak, sickly, full of pains; in ev'ry breath
Railing at life, and yet afraid of death.
> *Gotham,* Bk. I

Thomas Jefferson [1743–1826]

But I am past service. The hand of age is upon me. The decay of bodily faculties apprises me that those of the mind cannot be unimpaired, had I not still better proofs. Every year counts by increased debility, and departing faculties keep the score. The last year it was the sight, this it is the hearing, the next something else will be going, until all is gone.

> Letter to William Duane, October 1, 1812

But our machines have now been running seventy or eighty years, and we must expect that, worn as they are, here a pivot, there a wheel, now a pinion, next a spring, will be giving way; and however we may tinker them up for a while, all will at length surcease motion.

> Letter to John Adams, July 5, 1814

Napoleon Bonaparte [1769–1821]

At fifty, one can no longer love.
> *The St. Helena Journal,* April 7, 1817 (tr. by Sydney Gillard)

Sir Walter Scott [1771–1832]

Thus aged men, full loath and slow,
The vanities of life forego,
And count their youthful follies o'er,
Till Memory lends her light no more.
> *Rokeby,* Canto V, Stanza 1

Sydney Smith [1771–1845]

One evil in old age is, that as your time is come, you think every little illness is the beginning of the end. When a man expects to be arrested, every knock at the door is an alarm.

> Letter to Sir Wilmot-Horton, February 8, 1836

It is a bore, I admit, to be past seventy, for you are left for execution and are daily expecting the death-warrant; but, as you say, it is not anything very capital we quit. We are, at the close of life, only hurried away from stomach-aches, pains in the joints, from sleepless nights and unamusing days, from weakness, ugliness, and nervous tremors; but we shall all meet again in another planet, cured of all our defects.

> Letter to Lady Holland, September 13, 1842

Old age is not so much a scene of illness as of *malaise*. I think every day how near I am to death.
> Letter to Mrs. Grote, January 31, 1844

Walter Savage Landor
[1775–1864]

I am nearly blind and totally deaf. My son Charles undresses me, and I do not give any trouble. I dine on soup.
> Letter to Robert Browning, August 18, 1864

Charles C. Colton [1780?–1832]

An old man, like a spider, can never make love, without beating his own death watch.
> *Lacon*, Vol. II, No. CCLIX

George Gordon, Lord Byron
[1788–1824]

> Years steal
> Fire from the mind as vigour from the limb;
> And life's enchanted cup but sparkles near the brim.
>> *Childe Harold's Pilgrimage*, Canto III, Stanza 8

Percy Bysshe Shelley [1792–1822]

Old men are testy and will have their way.
> *The Cenci*, Act I, Sc. ii

John Keats [1795–1821]

> The weariness, the fever, and the fret
> Here, where men sit and hear each other groan;
> Where palsy shakes a few, sad, last gray hairs,
> Where youth grows pale, and spectre-thin, and dies.
>> *Ode to a Nightingale*

George P. R. James [1799–1860]

Age is the most terrible misfortune that can happen to any man; other evils will mend, but this is every day getting worse.
> *Richelieu*, Ch. XIV

Ralph Waldo Emerson
[1803–1882]

Nature abhors the old, and old age seems the only disease; all others run into this one.
> *Essays* (First Series), "Circles"

The man and woman of seventy assume to know all, they have outlived their hope, they renounce aspiration, accept the actual for the necessary, and talk down to the young.
> *Idem*

Tobacco, coffee, alcohol, hashish, prussic acid, strychnine, are weak dilutions: the surest poison is time.
> *Society and Solitude*, "Old Age"

Adolf Kussmaul [1822–1902]

> It seems that happenings of yore
> Might have occurred the day before
> But what transpired yesterday
> Already wants to fade away.
>> Poem (tr. by Hans Waine)

S. Weir Mitchell [1829–1914]

The arctic loneliness of age.

Orpheus C. Kerr [1836–1901]

> As Age advances, ails and aches attend,
> Backs builded broadest burdensomely bend;
> Cuttingly cruel comes consuming Care,
> Dealing delusions, drivelry, despair.
>> *Versatilities*, "Age Bluntly Considered"

Ambrose Bierce [1842–1914?]

AGE, n. That period of life in which we compound for the vices that we still cherish by reviling those that we have no longer the enterprise to commit.
> *The Devil's Dictionary*

Gerard Manley Hopkins
[1844–1889]

> Nothing can be done
> To keep at bay

Age and age's evils, hoar hair,
Ruck and wrinkle, drooping, dying,
    death's worst, winding sheets,
    tombs and worms and tumbling to
    decay.
> *The Leaden Echo and the
> Golden Echo*

Elie Metchnikoff [1845–1916]

Old age is an infectious chronic disease, characterized by the degeneration or enfeebling of the noble elements and by the excessive activity of the phagocytes.

Sir William Osler [1849–1919]

The teacher's life should have three periods, study until twenty-five, investigation until forty, profession until sixty, at which age I would have him retired on a double allowance. Whether Anthony Trollope's suggestion of a college and chloroform should be carried out or not I have become a little dubious, as my own time is getting so short.[1]
> *Aequanimitas, with Other Ad-
> dresses,* "The Fixed Period"

I have two fixed ideas. . . . The first is the comparative uselessness of men above forty years of age. . . . My second fixed idea is the uselessness of men above sixty years of age, and the incalculable benefit it would be in commercial, political and in professional life if, as a matter of course, men stopped work at this age.
> *Idem*

As it can be maintained that all the great advances have come from men under forty, so the history of the world shows that a very large proportion of the evils may be traced to the sexagenarians — nearly all the great mistakes politically and socially, all of the worst poems, most of the bad pic-

[1] Although Osler spoke in jest, this speech fostered the misapprehension that he proposed to retire, or even chloroform, all men at 60.

tures, a majority of the bad novels, not a few of the bad sermons and speeches.
> *Idem*

To every man over sixty whose spirit I may have thus unwittingly bruised, I tender my heartfelt regrets. Let me add, however, that the discussion which followed my remarks has not changed, but has rather strengthened my belief that the real work of life is done before the fortieth year and that after the sixtieth year it would be best for the world and best for themselves if men rested from their labours.
> *Ibid.* (2nd ed.), Preface

Santiago Ramón y Cajal [1852–1934]

It is idle to dispute with old men. Their opinions, like their cranial sutures, are ossified.
> *Charlas de Café*

Alfred Worcester [1855–1951]

The aged, as we must never forget, are always lonesome. They have outlived the preceding and, very likely also their own generation; or, if any survive, only by extra good fortune can there be any more meetings. Their family separations too often have caused the additional loss of their old homes and former neighbors. To the ways and manners of the present they are not accustomed. They belong to the unforgiving past. They are as strangers in the land.
> *The Care of the Aged, the Dy-
> ing and the Dead,* Ch. 1

W. Somerset Maugham [1874–1965]

What makes old age hard to bear is not the failing of one's faculties, mental and physical, but the burden of one's memories.
> *Points of View,* Ch. 1

I am sick of this way of life. The weariness and sadness of old age make it intolerable. I have walked with death in hand, and death's own hand is warmer than my own. I don't wish to live any longer.

> Remarks to the press on his 90th birthday

T. S. Eliot [1888–1965]

Damp, jaggèd, like an old man's mouth drivelling, beyond repair.
> *Ash-Wednesday,* III

Alvan L. Barach [1895–   ]

Since the ego of the man past 65 is rarely satisfied by a new occupation, the sources of self-applause and praise from others tend to disappear.
> *Journal of the American Geriatric Society* 12:262, 1964

John F. Kennedy [1917–1963]

A medical revolution has extended the life of our elder citizens without providing the dignity and security those later years deserve.
> Acceptance speech, Democratic National Convention, Los Angeles, July 15, 1960

Prolonged and costly illness in later years robs too many of our elder citizens of pride, purpose and savings.
> *Message to Congress on the Nation's Health Needs,* February 27, 1962

Too many elderly people with small incomes skimp on food at a time when their health requires greater quantity, variety, and balance in their diets.
> *Message to Congress on Problems of the Aged,* February 21, 1963

Too many senior citizens are wasting away in obsolete mental institutions without adequate treatment or care.
> *Idem*

The Bible

The days of our years are threescore years and ten; and if by reason of strength they be fourscore years, yet is their strength labour and sorrow; for it is soon cut off, and we fly away.
> *Psalms* 90:10

Proverb

Age breeds aches.

English Proverb

An old man is a bed full of bones.

German Proverb

Old age is a hospital that takes in all diseases.

Latin Proverb

The sins of youth are paid for in old age.

IV. TREATMENT

Frank Kittredge Paddock [1841–1901]

Physicians who care much for the elderly may find their lives slowly shredded to pieces as their seniors pick at them with minor worries magnified by the rapidly diminishing sands. If the telephone should come into common use, this state of affairs would worsen.
> Aphorism

David Seegal [1899–   ]

The principle of minimal interference is paramount in the management of the elderly. The older a patient, the less his way of life should be disturbed. Destruction of an established pattern of life may result in confusion and tragedy. The young amorphous personality can usually be vigorously molded without danger. In contrast, the older, more rigid personality is like a crystal, easily shattered by unwise impacts.
> *Journal of Chronic Diseases* 3:101, 1956

Don't challenge and thus gamble with the vitality of the elderly patient by quickly subjecting him to more tests and treatments than he can tolerate with reasonable safety.

Ibid., 17:299, 1964

The nature of the medical profession fosters the doctor's role as an "orderer." He becomes accustomed to a mildly imperious manner. In dealing with the elderly he may become impatient when the oldster insists on taking his special laxative (a nightly act for 30 years) or changing nurses. In many such instances, the physician can gain much by foregoing his luxury, like that of the baseball umpire, of always winning the argument. In the long run, the young doctor, facing the egocentricities of the aged, will find it rewarding to heed symbolically the sign on the highway: "Yield Right of Way," unless a major problem of health is involved.

Idem

The proper study of geriatrics begins with pediatrics.

Journal of Pediatrics 63:685, 1963

OPERATIONS

See also SURGERY

Sydney Smith [1771–1845]

It requires a surgical operation to get a joke well into a Scotch understanding. Their only idea of wit . . . is laughing immoderately at stated intervals.[1]

Quoted by Lady Holland in *A Memoir of the Rev. Sydney Smith*, Ch. 2

George Bernard Shaw [1856–1950]

In surgery all operations are recorded as successful if the patient can be got

out of the hospital or nursing home alive, though the subsequent history of the case may be such as would make an honest surgeon vow never to recommend or perform the operation again.

The Doctor's Dilemma, "Preface on Doctors"

Now it cannot be too often repeated that when an operation is once performed, nobody can ever prove that it was unnecessary. If I refuse to allow my leg to be amputated, its mortification and my death may prove that I was wrong; but if I let the leg go, nobody can ever prove that it would not have mortified had I been obstinate. Operation is therefore the safe side for the surgeon as well as the lucrative side.

Idem

Remy de Gourmont [1858–1915]

Before undergoing a surgical operation arrange your temporal affairs — you may live.

August Bier [1861–1949]

I never say of an operation that it is without danger.

Irvin S. Cobb [1876–1944]

But after all, when all is said and done, the king of all topics is operations.

Speaking of Operations

E. B. White [1899–   ]

The operation wasn't bad. I quite enjoyed the trip up from my room to the operating parlors, as a closely confined person does enjoy any sort of outing. The morphine had loosened my tongue, and while we waited in the corridor for the surgeon to arrive, the orderly and I let down our hair and had a good chat about fishing tackle.

The Second Tree from the Corner, "A Weekend with the Angels"

[1] Cf. Anonymous Scotsman, p. 351a.

Henry, Lord Cohen of Birkenhead [1900–   ]

The feasibility of an operation is not the *best* indication for its performance.
Annals of the Royal College of Surgeons of England 6:3, 1950

Anonymous

Exploratory operation: a remunerative reconnaissance.

The operation was successful — but the patient died.

Attributed to an Anonymous Scotsman

They tell me it takes a surgical operation to get a joke into a Scotsman's head, but I don't see how you could get a joke into anyone's head by a surgical operation.[1]
Quoted by H. L. Mencken in *A New Dictionary of Quotations*

OPIUM

See also DRUGS

Molière [1622–1673]

Quia est in eo
Virtus dormitiva
Cujus est natura
Sensus tranquillizare.[2]

[There is in it
A dormitive virtue
The nature of which
Is to lull the senses.]
Le Malade Imaginaire, Finale

Tobias Smollett [1721–1771]

The opium which had been given to Jolter, together with the wine he had

drank, produced such a perturbation in his fancy, that he was visited with horrible dreams, and among other miserable situations, imagined himself in danger of perishing in the flames.
The Adventures of Peregrine Pickle, Ch. 38

Edmund Burke [1729–1797]

Opium is pleasing to Turks, on account of the agreeable delirium it produces.
On the Sublime and Beautiful, "On Taste"

Michel de Crèvecoeur ("J. Hector St. John") [1735–1813]

They [the Quaker women of Nantucket] have adopted these many years, the Asiatic custom of taking a dose of opium every morning; and so deeply rooted is it, that they would be at a loss how to live without this indulgence; they would rather be deprived of any necessary than forego their favourite luxury.
Letters from an American Farmer, Letter VIII

Samuel Taylor Coleridge [1772–1834]

Laudanum gave me repose, not sleep; but you, I believe, know how divine this repose is, what a spot of enchantment, a green spot of fountain and flowers and trees in the very heart of a waste of sands.

Thomas De Quincey [1785–1859]

Thou hast the keys of Paradise, oh, just, subtle, and mighty opium!
Confessions of an English Opium-Eater, Pt. II

Opium gives and takes away. It defeats the steady habit of exertion; but it creates spasms of irregular exertion! It ruins the natural power of life; but it develops preternatural paroxysms of intermitting power.

---

[1] Cf. Sydney Smith, p. 350a.
[2] This is Argan's Latin hodgepodge reply to a question on how opium produces sleep.

Peter Mere Latham [1789–1875]

Opium once given is gone beyond your power to recall.
General Remarks on the Practice of Medicine, Ch. XV

Oliver Wendell Holmes [1809–1894]

Opium . . . the Creator himself seems to prescribe, for we often see the scarlet poppy growing in the cornfields, as if it were foreseen that wherever there is hunger to be fed there must also be pain to be soothed.
Medical Essays, "Currents and Counter-Currents in Medical Science"

Charles Dickens [1812–1870]

There's nothin' so refreshin' as sleep, Sir, as the servant girl said afore she drank the egg-cup-full o' laudanum.
Pickwick Papers, Ch. 16

Christina Rossetti [1830–1894]

The poppy saith amid the corn:
'Let but my scarlet head appear
And I am held in scorn;
Yet juice of subtle virtue lies
Within my cup of curious dyes.'
Consider the Lilies of the Field

Sir Leslie Stephen [1832–1904]

To tell the story of Coleridge without the opium is to tell the story of Hamlet without mentioning the Ghost.
Hours in a Library, "Coleridge"

Mary A. Barr [1852– ?]

The Poppy hath a charm for pain and woe.
White Poppies

René and Jean Dubos [1901–] [1918–]

It is probable that every consumptive became, in some measure, an opium addict, and it may be wondered whether the drug did not contribute to the mental effervescence that expressed itself in poetry and artistic creation.
The White Plague, Ch. V

ORGANS

Edmund Burke [1729–1797]

The stomach, the lungs, the liver, as well as other parts, are incomparably well adapted to their purposes; yet they are far from having any beauty.
On the Sublime and Beautiful, Pt. III, Sect. VI

Thomas Mann [1875–1955]

This body, then, which hovered before him, this individual and living I, was a monstrous multiplicity of breathing and self-nourishing individuals, which, through organic conformation and adaptation to special ends, had parted to such an extent with their essential individuality, their freedom and living immediacy, had so much become anatomic elements that the functions of some had become limited to sensibility toward light, sound, contact, warmth; others only understood how to change their shape or produce digestive secretions through contraction; others, again, were developed and functional to no other end than protection, support, the conveyance of the body juices, or reproduction. There were modifications of this organic plurality united to form the higher ego: cases where the multitude of subordinate entities were only grouped in a loose and doubtful way to form a higher living unit.
The Magic Mountain, Ch. V, "Research" (tr. by H. T. Lowe-Porter)

W. I. B. Beveridge [1908–]

Vitalism, which postulated mysterious "vital" forces, and teleology, which postulated a supernatural directing agency, have long ago been abandoned by experimental biologists. However, teleology is admissible in a modified sense that an organ or function fulfils a purpose toward aiding the survival of the organism as a whole or survival of the species.

> *The Art of Scientific Investigation,* Ch. X

OVERHEARD IN A DOCTOR'S OFFICE

The doctor is away this month?

Let's have a look at it.

Bend over.

You just tell me when it hurts.

How long have you had this?

That's funny. I never knew it to do that before.

The x-ray doesn't show a thing.

Unfortunately, we still have a lot to learn about this.

If this doesn't work, we'll have to try something else.

If the druggist questions it, ask him to call me.

I'm going to send you to this man. He's a specialist.

We're going to put you in the hospital for a few days.

PAIN

See also PLEASURE AND PAIN, SUFFERING

Hippocrates [460?–377? B.C.]

When two pains occur together, but

not in the same place, the more violent obscures the other.

> *Aphorisms,* II.46 (tr. by W. H. S. Jones)

Democritus [5th–4th Cent. B.C.]

The pain which is intolerable carries us off; but that which lasts a long time is tolerable.

> Quoted by Marcus Aurelius in *Meditations,* VII.33 (tr. by G. Long)

Antiphanes [408?–334? B.C.]

All pain's one malady with many names.

> Fragment from *The Doctor* (tr. by J. M. Edmonds)

Seneca [4? B.C.–A.D. 65]

Remember that pain has this most excellent quality: if prolonged it cannot be severe, and if severe it cannot be prolonged.

> *Moral Epistles to Lucilius,* XCIV (tr. by Richard M. Gummere)

St. Augustine [354–430]

The greatest evil is physical pain.

> *Soliloquies,* I.21

Petrarch [1304–1374]

It is by poultices, not by words, that pain is ended, although pain is by words both eased and diminished.

> Letter to Guido Sette, 1359

William Shakespeare [1564–1616]

For let our finger ache, and it endues
Our other, healthful, members even to
    that sense
Of pain.

> *Othello,* III, iv, 146

John Milton [1608–1674]

But pain is perfect miserie, the worst
Of evils, and excessive, overturnes
All patience.

> *Paradise Lost,* Bk. VI

Marie, Marquise de Sévigné [1626–1696]

There is no real evil in life except great pain; all the others are in the imagination and depend on the way one thinks of things. All other evils find their remedy either in time, or in moderation, or in strength of mind; reflection, devotion, philosophy can soften them.
> Letter to Mme. de Grignan, May 4, 1672

Matthew Henry [1662–1714]

So great was the extremity of his pain and anguish, that he did not only sigh but roar.
> *An Exposition on the Old and New Testament, Job* 3:24

Samuel Johnson [1709–1784]

The mind is seldom quickened to very vigorous operations but by pain, or the dread of pain.
> *The Idler,* No. 18 (August 12, 1758)

Those who do not feel pain seldom think that it is felt.
> *The Rambler,* No. 48 (September 1, 1750)

Thomas Gray [1716–1771]

See the Wretch, that long has tost
  On the thorny bed of Pain,
At length repair his vigour lost,
  And breathe and walk again.
> *Ode on the Pleasure Arising from Vicissitude*

Adam Smith [1723–1790]

A man may sympathize with a woman in childbed, though it is impossible that he should conceive himself as suffering her pains in his own proper person and character.
> *The Theory of Moral Sentiments,* Pt. VII, Sect. 3, Ch. 1

Thomas Jefferson [1743–1826]

The art of life is the art of avoiding pain.
> Letter to Maria Cosway, October 12, 1786

Jeremy Bentham [1748–1832]

Pain is in itself an evil; and, indeed, without exception, the only evil.
> *Principles of Morals and Legislation,* Ch. X

Johann Wolfgang von Goethe [1749–1832]

A toast to Allah? Yes, I shall propose it:
For giving pain, but not the knowledge why.
A patient might as well despair and die,
Knew he disease as the physician knows it.
> *West-Eastern Divan,* Sect. VI, No. 40 (tr. by Max Samter)

Friedrich von Schiller [1759–1805]

The transformation of pain to aversion is a fundamental law of the soul.
> *Prosäische Schriften* (Erste Periode), "Ueber den Zusammenhang der thierischen Natur des Menschen mit seiner geistigen," Sect. 9 (tr. by Hans Waine)

John Abernethy [1764–1831]

"Mr. Abernethy," said a patient, "I have something the matter, Sir, with this arm. There, oh! (making a particular motion with the limb), that, Sir, gives me great pain." "Well, what a fool you must be to do it, then," said Abernethy.
> Quoted by George Macilwain in *Memoirs of John Abernethy,* Ch. XXIII

Samuel Taylor Coleridge [1772–1834]

Real pain can alone cure us of imag-

inary ills. We feel a thousand miseries till we are lucky enough to feel misery.
Notebooks

Sir Charles Bell [1774–1842]

Pain is the necessary contrast to pleasure; it ushers us into existence or consciousness: it alone is capable of exciting the organs into activity: it is the compassion and the guardian of human life.
The Hand, Its Mechanism and Vital Endowments as Evincing Design, Ch. 7

Charles Lamb [1775–1834]

Pain is life — the sharper, the more evidence of life.
Letter to Bernard Barton, January 9, 1824

I am sitting opposite a person who is making strange distortions with the gout, which is not unpleasant — to me at least. What is the reason we do not sympathise with pain, short of some terrible Surgical operation?
Ibid., Spring 1824

Peter Mere Latham [1789–1875]

Not only degrees of Pain, but its existence, in any degree, must be taken upon the testimony of the patient.
Diseases of the Heart, Lect. XI

It would be a great thing to understand Pain in all its meanings.
General Remarks on the Practice of Medicine, Ch. XIV

No man, wise or foolish, ever suffered Pain, who did not invest it with a *quasi* materialism.
Idem

Percy Bysshe Shelley [1792–1822]

Pain, whose unheeded and familiar speech
Is howling, and keen shrieks, day after day.
Prometheus Unbound, Act II, Sc. iv

Alfred, Lord Tennyson [1809–1892]

He loves to make parade of pain.
In Memoriam, Sect. XXI

Robert Browning [1812–1889]

When pain ends, gain ends too.
A Death in the Desert

George Eliot (Marian Evans Cross) [1819–1880]

A man deep-wounded may feel too much pain
To feel much anger.
Spanish Gypsy, Bk. I

Charles Kingsley [1819–1875]

Pain is no evil
Unless it conquers us.
St. Maura. A.D. 304

Margaret Junkin Preston [1820–1897]

Pain is no longer pain when it is past.
Old Songs and New, "Nature's Lesson"

Herbert Spencer [1820–1903]

Pain is the correlative of some species of wrong — some kind of divergence from that course of action which perfectly fills all requirements.
The Data of Ethics, Ch. XV, Sect. 101

S. Weir Mitchell [1829–1914]

The birth of pain! . . .
What mighty forces pledged the dust to life!
What awful will decreed its silent strife!
Till through vast ages rose on hill and plain,
Life's saddest voice, the birthright wail of pain. . . .
Yet still, forever, he who strove to gain
By swift despatch a shorter lease for pain
Saw the grim theatre, and 'neath his knife

Felt the keen torture, in the quivering
life.
The Birth and Death of Pain

As to pain, I am almost ready to say
that the physician who has not felt it
is imperfectly educated.

Santiago Ramón y Cajal
[1852–1934]

Physical pain is easily forgotten, but
a moral chagrin lasts indefinitely.
Charlas de Café

Sir William Watson [1858–1935]

Pain with the thousand teeth.
The Dream of Man (1899)

Francis Thompson [1859–1907]

Nothing begins, and nothing ends,
    That is not paid with moan;
For we are born in other's pain,
    And perish in our own.
    Daisy

Georg Groddeck [1866–1934]

To insure oneself from hurt is to insure oneself from growth.
The Book of the It

Marcel Proust [1871–1922]

Illness is the doctor to whom we pay
most heed: to kindness, to knowledge
we make promises only; pain we obey.
Cities of the Plain, Pt. I, Ch. 1,
"My Social Life" (tr. by C. K.
Scott-Moncrieff)

Paul Valéry [1871–1945]

At certain moments my body is illuminated. . . . It is very curious. Suddenly I see into myself. . . . I can
make out the depth of the layers of my
flesh; and I feel zones of pain, rings,
poles, plumes of pain. Do you see these
living figures, this geometry of my
suffering? Some of these flashes are
exactly like ideas. They make me understand — from here, to there. . . .
And yet they leave me *uncertain*.
Monsieur Teste, Ch. 1 (tr. by
J. Mathews)

W. Somerset Maugham
[1874–1965]

The new-born child does not realise
that his body is more a part of himself than surrounding objects, . . . and
it is only by degrees, through pain,
that he understands the fact of the
body.
Of Human Bondage, Ch. XIII

Albert Schweitzer [1875–1965]

We must all die. But that I can save
him from days of torture, that is what
I feel as my great and ever new priv-
ilege. Pain is a more terrible lord of
mankind than even death himself.
*On the Edge of the Primeval
Forest*, Ch. 5 (tr. by C. T.
Campion)

The Fellowship of those who bear the
Mark of Pain. Who are the members
of this Fellowship? Those who have
learnt by experience what physical
pain and bodily anguish mean, belong
together all the world over; they are
united by a secret bond.
Ibid., Ch. 11

René Leriche [1879–   ]

Physical pain is not a simple affair of
an impulse, travelling at a fixed rate
along a nerve. It is the resultant of a
conflict between a stimulus and the
whole individual.
Surgery of Pain

Wade Oliver [1890–   ]

I too, have gone down
The long, lone night of pain;
Therefore I know, now,
The longing of the rain.
Sky-Rider, "Kinship"

Charles F. W. Illingworth
[1899–   ]

Every sentient being knows what is meant by pain but the true significance of pain eludes the most sapient. For philosophers, pain is a problem of metaphysics, and exercise for stoics; for mystics it is an ecstasy, for the religious, a travail meekly to be borne, for clinicians a symptom to be understood and an ill to be relieved.
Peptic Ulcer

David Seegal [1899–   ]

Pain, messenger of harm
Nature's poignant alarm
Often man's wily friend
To signal means to mend.
The Pharos of Alpha Omega Alpha 28:126, 1965, "Pain as Friend"

Peter Fleming [1907–   ]

If you come to think about it, physical pain has many singularities. Of all human experiences it is, as long as it lasts, the most absorbing; and it is the only human experience which, when it comes to an end, automatically confers a real if not perhaps a very high kind of happiness. It is also the only experience this side of death which is by its nature solitary. But the oddest thing about it is that despite its intensity, despite its unequaled power over mind and body, when it is over you cannot really remember it at all.
My Aunt's Rhinoceros and Other Reflections, "On Pain"

Anonymous

Man endures pain as an undeserved punishment; woman accepts it as a natural heritage.

Proverbs

Great pains quickly find ease.

He preaches patience that never knew pain.

Dutch Proverb

Where a man feels pain he lays his hand.

PALSY

William Shakespeare [1564–1616]

DICK: Why dost thou quiver, man?
SAY: It is the palsy, and not fear, provokes me.
Henry VI, Part II, IV, vii, 97

O, then how quickly should this arm
    of mine,
Now prisoner to the palsy, chastise thee.
Richard II, II, iii, 103

                    The faint defects of age
Must be the scene of mirth: to cough
    and spit,
And, with a palsy fumbling on his
    gorget,
Shake in and out the rivet.
Troilus and Cressida, I, iii, 172

PARASITES

Jonathan Swift [1667–1745]

So, Nat'ralists observe, a Flea
Has smaller Fleas that on him prey,
And these have smaller Fleas to bite
    'em,
And so proceed *ad infinitum.*
On Poetry: A Rhapsody

Siegfried J. Thannhauser
[1885–1962]

Patients may have both fleas and lice.[1]
    Comment during ward rounds,
    New England Center Hospital

Japanese Proverb

Every man carries a parasite some-where.

[1] Emphasizing that a patient may be afflicted with two distinctly unrelated diseases.

West African Proverb

Put the meat away and you'll get rid of the flies.

PARENTS

See also MATERNITY

Homer [ca. 850 B.C.]

It is a wise child that knows his own father.
> *Odyssey,* I.216

William Shakespeare [1564–1616]

It is a wise father that knows his own child.
> *The Merchant of Venice,* II, ii, 80

H. Gideon Wells [1875–1943]

Maternity is a matter of fact—paternity is a matter of speculation.
> Aphorism

The Bible

Honour thy father and thy mother.
> *Exodus* 20:12

Anonymous

The mother of what is called her child is no real parent of it but the nurse only of the young life that is sown in her: the real parent is the male.
> Greek saying, ca. 400 B.C.

An observant parent's evidence may be disproved but should never be ignored.
> Quoted in *Lancet* 1:688, 1951

PATHOLOGY

Plutarch [46?–120?]

Medicine, to produce health, has to examine disease.
> *Lives,* "Demetrius," I.3 (tr. by John Dryden, rev. by A. H. Clough)

Elisha Bartlett [1804–1855]

Pathology is not founded upon physiology. . . . Our knowledge of the morbid processes and susceptibilities of the several organs and tissues of the body cannot be inferred or deduced from our knowledge of their healthy processes.
> *Philosophy of Medical Science,* Pt. II, Ch. 6

Rudolf Virchow [1821–1902]

Pathology also has its place in the science of biology, certainly a very honorable one, for to pathology we owe the realization that the contrast between health and disease is not to be sought in a fundamental difference of two kinds of life, nor in an alteration of essence, but only in an alteration of conditions.
> *Disease, Life, and Man,* "The Place of Pathology Among the Biological Sciences" (tr. by L. J. Rather)

Pathology has been released from the anomalous and isolated position which it has occupied for thousands of years. Through the application of its doctrines not only to diseases of man, but also to those of even the smallest and lowest of animals, and to those of plants, it helps to deepen biological knowledge, and to light up still further that region of the unknown which still envelops the intimate structure of living matter. It is no longer merely applied physiology — it has become physiology itself.
> *Idem*

Austin O'Malley [1858–1932]

Ugliness is a point of view: an ulcer is wonderful to a pathologist.

Edward Martin [1859–1938]

Pathology is the accomplished tragedy; physiology the basis on which our treatment rests.

Gordon Holmes [1876–   ]

The pathologist (in the United States one would say the laboratory) is useful when kept to heel.
Quoted in *Archives of Internal Medicine* 116:164, 1965

H. L. Mencken [1880–1956]

Pathology would remain a lovely science, even if there were no therapeutics, just as seismology is a lovely science, though no one knows how to stop earthquakes.
A Mencken Chrestomathy, Ch. XXX

Simeon Burt Wolbach [1880–1954]

It is often difficult to ascertain the nature of the edifice that has burnt down from a study of the ashes.
Aphorism

Anonymous

Hic est locus ubi mors gaudet succurrere vitae.
[This is the place where death rejoices to come to the aid of life.]
Motto of the Pathological Institute of McGill University

This is like staging the play *Hamlet* without the Prince of Denmark! [1]

PATIENCE

John Florio [1553?–1625]

Pacience is the best medicine that is, for a sicke man, the most precious plaister that is, for any wounde.
First Frutes, Folio 44

Robert Burton [1577–1640]

Hope and Patience are two soveraigne remedies for all, the surest reposals,

[1] Comment after a clinicopathological conference when the pathologist failed to show sections of the kidneys of a patient who had died of renal failure.

the softest cushions to lean on in adversity.
The Anatomy of Melancholy, Pt. II, Sect. iii, Memb. 3

Henry Vaughan [1622–1695]

Patience then is the best medicine of Evills; it is the cure of the Incurable, the last Physitian, the Ease in death, the mollifying Oyle, the gentle purge, the pleasant Potion, and that I may recover its right to another Title which death usurped from the pen of *Boethius, It is a sanctuary that lies alwaies open to the distressed.*
Flores Solitudinis

Charles Churchill [1731–1764]

Patience is sorrow's salve.
The Prophecy of Famine

Proverb

Patience is a plaster for all sores.

PATIENT–PHYSICIAN RELATIONSHIP

See also BEDSIDE MANNER, PATIENTS, TRUTH

I. GENERAL

Judah ha-Levi [1085?–1140?]

Every ill man fears death and hopes that he may be cured; and when told that the physician is coming he feels happy and he longs to wait for the utterances of his mouth. For this reason any fool and inexperienced man finds it possible to be a physician.
Liber Cosri

John Owen [1560?–1622]

Physicians take Gold, but seldom give:
They Physick give, take none; yet healthy live.
A Diet They prescribe; the Sick must for 't

Give Gold; Each other Thus supply-support.
> *Latine Epigrams* (1612), Bk. I, No. 53 (tr. by Thomas Harvey)

John Donne [1573–1631]

I observe the *Phisician,* with the same diligence, as hee the *disease.*
> *Devotions Upon Emergent Occasions,* VI

Whilst my Physitians by their love are growne
Cosmographers, and I their Mapp, who lie
Flat on this bed.
> *Hymne to God my God, in My Sicknesse*

Paul Laymann [1574–1635]

A doctor, on being consulted, may give an advice, not only probable according to his own opinion, but contrary to his opinion, provided this judgment happens to be more favorable or more agreeable to the person that consults him. Nay, I go further, and say, that there would be nothing unreasonable in his giving those who consult him a judgment held to be probable by some learned person, even though he should be satisfied in his own mind that it is absolutely false.
> *Theologia moralis*

Jean de La Bruyère [1645–1696]

Those who are well get sick; they need people whose business it is to assure them they won't die: as long as men go on dying, and love living, the doctor will be made game of and well-paid.
> *Characters,* Ch. XIV

Laurence Sterne [1713–1768]

I'll tell it, cried Smelfungus,[1] to the world. You had better tell it, said I, to your physician.
> *A Sentimental Journey,* Bk. I?, Ch. 18

---

[1] Smelfungus is Sterne's caricature of Tobias Smollett, whose complaints about his health and comfort in *Travels Through France and Italy* annoyed Sterne.

Karl F. H. Marx [1796–1877]

In nature, those who cry out with pain and those who prescribe remedies therefor are different persons: in politics, they are one and the same.
> Quoted by F. H. Garrison in *Bulletin of the New York Academy of Medicine* 4:1001, 1928

Sir William Jenner [1815–1898]

Never believe what a patient tells you his doctor has said.

George Eliot (Marian Evans Cross) [1819–1880]

It's no trifle at her time of life to part with a doctor who knows her constitution.
> *Janet's Repentance,* Ch. 3

John Shaw Billings [1838–1913]

He who aspires to be his brother's keeper must know how his brother lives.
> *Medical News* 60:230, 1892

Frank Kittredge Paddock [1841–1901]

It is always amusing when a patient states that he is "ordered" into the hospital. The last time I did that, the patient departed in his horse and buggy and never consulted me again. It thus appears that the "ordering" occurred only in retrospect and relieves the patient of personal responsibility for the outcome.
> Aphorism

Thanks to the wide distribution of and belief in medical folklore, it comes as a constant surprise to my patients that sometimes I appear to know almost as much medicine as they do.
> Aphorism

The personal responsibility of the physician for his patient is magnified in a rural community and diminished in a metropolis. This is caused by the greater speed and area of communication — of gossip — in the small region. Everyone knows if the rural physician has made an erroneous diagnosis whereas the city physician's errors are lost to all but a handful of the patient's immediate family or friends. The resultant difference in attitude might be called "The Great Metropolitan Fallacy."

Aphorism

Robert Tuttle Morris [1857–1945]

Gratitude commonly belongs chemically among the lighter hydrocarbons, and follows their laws of diffusion.
Doctors Versus Folks, Ch. 3

James G. Mumford [1863–1914]

Probably to no other [than the physician] are the strengths and weakness of humanity so completely laid bare.

Harvey Cushing [1869–1939]

A physician is obligated to consider more than a diseased organ, more even than the whole man — he must view the man in his world.
Quoted by René J. Dubos in *Man Adapting,* Ch. XII

Burton J. Hendrick [1870–1949]

The consultant's first obligation is to the patient, not to his brother physician.

Marcel Proust [1871–1922]

Inasmuch as a great part of what doctors know is taught them by the sick, they are easily led to believe that this knowledge which patients exhibit is common to them all, and they pride themselves on taking the patient of the moment by surprise with some remarks picked up at a previous bedside.
The Guermantes Way, Pt. I, "My Grandmother's Illness" (tr. by C. K. Scott-Moncrieff)

Wilfred Trotter [1872–1939]

The ordinary patient goes to his doc-

tor because he is in pain or some other discomfort and wants to be comfortable again; he is not in pursuit of the ideal of health in any direct sense. The doctor on the other hand wants to discover the pathological condition and control it if he can. The two are thus to some degree at cross purposes from the first, and unless the affair is brought to an early and happy conclusion this divergence of aims is likely to become more and more serious as the case goes on. The good doctor therefore has to learn to serve two objects at the same time — the diagnosis and treatment of the patient's ailment on one hand, and to keep him comfortable on the other.
Collected Papers, "Art and Science in Medicine," Sect. 6

W. Somerset Maugham [1874–1965]

I do not know a better training for a writer than to spend some years in the medical profession. . . . the doctor . . . sees [human nature] bare. Reticences can generally be undermined; very often there are none. Fear for the most part will shatter every defence; even vanity is unnerved by it.
The Summing Up, Sect. xix

Albert Schweitzer [1875–1965]

It is our duty to remember at all times and anew that medicine is not only a science, but also the art of letting our own individuality interact with the individuality of the patient.

Martin H. Fischer [1879–1962]

Medicine is the one place where all the show is stripped off the human drama. You, as doctors, will be in a position to see the human race stark naked — not only physically, but mentally and morally as well.
Quoted by Wherry, Holmes, and Baehr in *Fischerisms*

Dorothy Parker [1893–1967]

The doctors were very brave about it.[1]
Quoted in *Journal of the American Medical Association* 194:211, 1965

Graham Greene [1904–   ]

The secrets of the consulting-room, my dear boy, are one-sided. . . . The patient, though not the doctor, is at liberty to tell everything.
The New Statesman, October 8, 1965, "Dr. Crombie"

Marguerite H. Wolf [1914–   ]

I have never looked a gift horse in the mouth: not that I lack curiosity, but none of my husband's patients ever happened to give him a horse.
Tufts Folia Medica 8:115, 1962

Anonymous Latin Poem

Three shapes a doctor wears. At first we hail
   The angel; then the god, if he prevail.
Last, when, the cure complete, he asks his fee,
   A hideous demon he appears to be.
Doctor and Patient (tr. by W. F. H. King in *Classical Foreign Quotations*)

Medieval Maxim

In the presence of the patient, Latin is the language.

II. GOOD

Sushruta [5th Cent.? B.C.]

The patient, who may mistrust his own parents, sons and relations, should repose an implicit faith in his own physician, and put his own life into his hands without the least apprehension of danger; hence a physician should

[1] An observation made after a bout with a serious illness.

protect his patient as his own begotten child.
Sushruta-Samhitá, "Sutrasthánam," Ch. 25 (tr. by K. K. L. Bhishagratna)

Hippocrates [460?–377? B.C.]

Some patients, though conscious that their condition is perilous, recover their health simply through their contentment with the goodness of the physician.
Precepts, VI (tr. by W. H. S. Jones)

Plato [427?–347 B.C.]

No physician, in so far as he is a physician, considers his own good in what he prescribes, but the good of his patient; for the true physician is also a ruler having the human body as a subject, and is not a mere moneymaker.
Republic, I.342.D (tr. by Benjamin Jowett)

Celsus [25 B.C.–A.D. 50]

Presuming their state to be equal, it is more useful to have in the practitioner a friend rather than a stranger.
De Medicina, Prooemium (tr. by W. G. Spencer)

Epictetus [60?–120?]

And yet what harm have I done you? None at all, unless the mirror also does harm to the ugly man by showing him what he looks like; unless the physician insults the patient, when he says to him, 'Man, you think there is nothing the matter with you; but you have a fever; fast today and drink only water'; and no one says, 'What dreadful insolence!'
Discourses, II.xiv.21 (tr. by W. A. Oldfather)

Paracelsus [1493?–1541]

But pay heed further how I justify myself in this accusation that I give a rough answer. The other physicians

know little of the arts; they resort to friendly, pleasing, charming words; they advise people with breeding and fine words; they set forth all things at length, delightfully, with distinct differentiations, and say: Come again soon, my dear sir; my dear wife, go and accompany the gentleman, etc. I say thus: What wilt thou? I have no time now; it is not so urgent. Now I have upset the applecart! They have made such fools of the patients that they are completely of the belief that a friendly, affectionate manner, ceremony, ingratiating ways, much ado, constitute art and medicine. They call him "young sir" who only comes from the shopkeeper's; they call another "Sir, wise Sir" who is a cobbler and a dullard, where I say "Thou"; but with this I throw away my resources. My intention is to gain nothing with my tongue, but only with works. As they, however, are not of this opinion, they can well say in their way that I am a strange, queer-headed fellow, that I give little good advice. I do not believe in feeding myself on friendly caresses, wherefore I cannot use what befits me not, nor what I have not learned.
> *Seven Defensiones,* "The Sixth Defense" (tr. by C. Lilian Temkin in *Four Treatises*)

John Caius [1510–1573]

Therefor seke ye out a good Phisicien, and knowen to have skille, and at the leaste be so good to your bodies as you are to your hosen and shoes.

Sir Francis Bacon [1561–1626]

Physicians are some of them so pleasing and conformable to the humour of the patient, as they press not the true cure of the disease; and some other are so regular in proceeding according to art for the disease, as they respect not sufficiently the condition of the patient. Take one of a middle temper; or if it may not be found in one man, combine two of either sort; and forget not to call as well the best acquainted with your body, as the best reputed of for his faculty.
> *Essays,* "Of Regiment of Health"

Izaak Walton [1593–1683]

The Tench is the Physician of fishes, for the Pike especially. . . . the Pike, being either sick or hurt, is cured by the touch of the Tench. And it is observed, that the tyrant Pike will not be a wolf to his physician, but forbears to devour him though he be never so hungry.
> *The Compleat Angler,* Pt. I, Ch. XI

Sir Thomas Browne [1605–1682]

Let mee be sicke my selfe, if often times the malady of my patient be not a disease unto me. I desire rather to cure his infirmities than my owne necessities. Where I do him no good me thinkes it is scarce honest gaine, though I confess 'tis but the worthy salary of our well intended endeavours. I am not onely ashamed, but heartily sorry that besides death, there are diseases incurable; yet not for my own sake, or that they be beyond my art, but for the general cause & sake of humanity, whose common cause I apprehend as my own.
> *Religio Medici,* Pt. II, Sect. 9

John Coakley Lettsom [1744–1815]

I think a humane physician, who evinces by his conduct a tender interest in the recovery of his patient, never loses reputation by an event which no human means could prevent; on the contrary, oftentimes nearer attachments are acquired; for the sympathy of the physician makes him appear almost as one of the family, and mutual anxiety begets mutual endearment.
> Letter to a friend, September 6, 1791

Hannah More [1745–1833]

I used to wonder why people should be so fond of the company of their physician, till I recollected that he is the only person with whom one dares to talk continually of oneself, without interruption, contradiction or censure; I suppose that delightful immunity doubles their fees.

> Letter to Horace Walpole, July 27, 1789

Benjamin Rush [1745?–1813]

Do not condemn, or oppose unnecessarily, the simple prescriptions of your patients. Yield to them in matters of little consequence, but maintain an inflexible authority over them in matters that are essential to life.

> Lecture, University of Pennsylvania, February 7, 1789

Make it a rule never to be angry at anything a sick man says or does to you. Sickness often adds to the natural irritability of the temper. We, therefore, bear the reproaches of our patients with meekness and silence.

> *Idem*

Never resent an affront offered to you by a *sick* man. . . .
Never make light (to a patient) of *any* case.
Never appear in a hurry in a sickroom, nor talk of indifferent matters till you have examined and prescribed for your patient.

> Letter to Dr. William Claypoole, July 29, 1782

Thomas Gisborne [1758–1846]

It is frequently of much importance, not to the comfort only, but to the recovery of the patient, that he should be enabled to look upon his Physician as his friend.

> *The Duties of Physicians*

Christoph Wilhelm Hufeland [1762–1836]

The physician must generalize the disease, and individualize the patient.

> Quoted by Oliver Wendell Holmes in *Medical Essays,* "Scholastic and Bedside Teaching"

Sir Henry Halford [1766–1844]

And here you will forgive me, perhaps, if I presume to state what appears to me to be the conduct proper to be observed by a physician in withholding, or making his patient acquainted with, his opinion of the probable issue of a malady manifesting mortal symptoms. I own I think it my first duty to protract his life by all practicable means, and to interpose myself between him and everything which may possibly aggravate his danger. And unless I shall have found him averse from doing what was necessary in aid of my remedies, from a want of a proper sense of his perilous situation, I forbear to step out of the bounds of my province in order to offer any advice which is not necessary to promote his cure. At the same time, I think it indispensable to let his friends know the danger of his case, the instant I discover it. An arrangement of his worldly affairs, in which the comfort or unhappiness of those who are to come after him is involved, may be necessary. . . . If friends can do these good offices at a proper time, and under the suggestions of the physician, it is far better that they should undertake them than the medical adviser. They do so without destroying his hopes, for the patient will still believe that he has an appeal to his physician beyond their fears; whereas if the physician lay open his danger to him, however delicately he may do this, he runs a risk of appearing to pronounce a sentence of condemnation to death, against which there is no appeal—no hope.

> *Essays and Orations*

William Beaumont [1785–1853]

Physicians, when tending upon patients, should make their health their first object. So gentle and sympathizing should be their dispositions and manner in the apartment of the sick that pain and distress should seem suspended in their presence. So exhilarating ought their visits to be that hope should follow their footsteps, so salutary their prescriptions that death should drop his commission in combat with their skill.

> *Notebook* (ed. by J. S. Myers in *Life and Letters*, Ch. 3)

James Syme [1799–1870]

As in the case of thriving plants, it is of more consequence that the roots of your character should strike deep in public confidence than that there should be a premature production of flower, or fruit.

> *Edinburgh Medical Journal* 13:197, 1867

Oliver Wendell Holmes [1809–1894]

Let me recommend you, as far as possible, to keep your doubts to yourself, and give the patient the benefit of your decision.

> *Medical Essays,* "The Young Practitioner"

Once in a while you will have a patient of sense, born with the gift of observation, from whom you may learn something.

> *Idem*

What I call a good patient is one who, having found a good physician, sticks to him till he dies.

> *Idem*

Your patient has no more right to all the truth you know than he has to all the medicine in your saddle-bags, if you carry that kind of cartridge-box

for the ammunition that slays disease.

> *Idem*

And last, not least, in each perplexing case,
Learn the sweet magic of a *cheerful face;*
Not always smiling, but at least serene,
When grief and anguish cloud the anxious scene.
Each look, each movement, every word and tone,
Should tell your patient you are all his own;
Not the mere artist, purchased to attend,
But the warm, ready, self-forgetting friend,
Whose genial visit in itself combines
The best of cordials, tonics, anodynes.

> *The Morning Visit*

If you are making choice of a physician, be sure you get one, if possible, with a cheerful and serene countenance.

> *The Professor at the Breakfast Table,* Sect. VI

Truth is the breath of life to human society. It is the food of the immortal spirit. Yet a single word of it may kill a man as suddenly as a drop of prussic acid.

> Valedictory address, Harvard Commencement, March 10, 1858

William Makepeace Thackeray [1811–1863]

It is not only for the sick man, it is for the sick man's friends that the Doctor comes. His presence is often as good for them as for the patient, and they long for him yet more eagerly.

> *The History of Pendennis,* Ch. LII

Theodor Billroth [1829–1894]

A person may have learned a very great deal and still be an exceedingly unskillful physician, who awakens little confidence in his powers. . . . The manner of dealing with patients, of winning their confidence, the art of listening to them (the patient is always more anxious to talk than to listen), of soothing and consoling them, or of drawing their attention to serious matters, — all this cannot be learned from books. The student can learn these things only from immediate contact with the teacher, whom he will unconsciously imitate. . . . The patient longs for the doctor's daily visit; it is the event upon which all his thoughts and emotions turn. The physician can do all he has to do with speed and precision, but he must never appear to be in a hurry, and never absent-minded.

The Medical Sciences in the German Universities, Pt. III

Samuel Butler [1835–1902]

We in England never shrink from telling our doctor what is the matter with us merely through the fear that he will hurt us. We let him do his worst upon us, and stand it without a murmur, because we are not scouted for being ill, and because we know that the doctor is doing his best to cure us, and that he can judge of our case better than we can; but we should conceal all illness if we were treated as the Erewhonians are when they have anything the matter with them; we should do the same as with moral and intellectual diseases, — we should feign health with the most consummate art, till we were found out.

Erewhon, Ch. X

Harriet E. Hamilton King [1840–1920]

What restless forms to-day are lying, bound
On sick-beds, waiting till the hour comes round
That brings thy foot upon the chamber stair,
Impatient, fevered, faint, till thou art there,

Then one short smile of sunshine to make light
The long remembrance of another night.

Frank Kittredge Paddock [1841–1901]

The patient is content with a doctor not because of his medical ability or knowledge but rather because he is sufficiently near him in intellectual capacity and social background. Too great a separation of these levels leads to failure of communication and unhappiness for both.

Aphorism

James J. Putnam [1846–1918]

We cannot really know the man whom we are called upon to treat without going far beyond his outward relations and penetrating in imagination deep into his mental life. "The man" is, above all else, the mind of the man, and not only the mind as an organ of conscious thought but the mind as an organ of bodily nutrition, and the mind as a vast theatre for the interplay of contending forces that do not always recognize the personal consciousness as their ruler. This is the man that the doctor should learn to know and treat.

Boston Medical and Surgical Journal 141:53, 1899

Edward Hickling Bradford [1848–1926]

Neither the precision of science nor the efficiency of business methods will suffice, for above all else the practitioner must preserve and exercise the kindly indulgence of a considerate friend.

Harvard Graduate Magazine 35:70, 1926

Robert Tuttle Morris [1857–1945]

It is the human touch after all that counts for most in our relation with our patients.

Doctors Versus Folks, Ch. 3

J. Chalmers Da Costa [1863–1933]

Tact is a valuable attribute in gaining practice. It consists in telling a squint-eyed man that he has a fine, firm chin.
The Trials and Triumphs of the Surgeon, Ch. 1

C. Jeff Miller [1874–1936]

Body and soul cannot be separated for purposes of treatment, for they are one and indivisible. Sick minds must be healed as well as sick bodies. Whether he will or no, the doctor's office is very often a confessional of spiritual as well as of physical disability. Mankind's eternal cry is for release, and the physician must answer it with something more than a test tube, something beyond faultless technique. The cure — which really means the care — of the sick, the relief of suffering, the salvation of life, these are the high aims of the medical profession, as they were the high aims of the priesthood from which it sprung, and scientific knowledge and medical skill will not of themselves bring them to pass.
Surgery, Gynecology & Obstetrics 52:488, 1931

Warfield T. Longcope [1877–1953]

The relationship between doctor and patient partakes of a peculiar intimacy. It presupposes on the part of the physician not only knowledge of his fellow men, but sympathy. . . . This aspect of the practice of medicine has been designated as the art; yet I wonder whether it should not, most properly, be called the essence.
Bulletin of the Johns Hopkins Hospital 50:4, 1932

Each patient ought to feel somewhat the better after the physician's visit, irrespective of the nature of the illness.
Quoted by David Seegal in *The Pharos of Alpha Omega Alpha* 26:7, 1963

Martin H. Fischer [1879–1962]

Let your entrance into the sick room decrease, not increase, the irritability of your patient.
Quoted by Howard Fabing and Ray Marr in *Fischerisms*

Sir Alfred Webb-Johnson [1880–1958]

The well-equipped clinician must possess the qualities of the artist, the man of science, and the humanist, but he must exercise them only in so far as they subserve the getting well of the individual patient. He must feel directly responsible *to* his patient, not *for* him — to someone else.
Medical Press 216:312, 1946

Francis Weld Peabody [1881–1927]

One of the essential qualities of the clinician is interest in humanity, for the secret of the care of the patient is in caring for the patient.
The Care of the Patient

The treatment of a disease may be entirely impersonal; the care of a patient must be completely personal.
Idem

Sir John Parkinson [1885–   ]

The common duty required of a physician lies in the recognition and treatment of disease. If he enlarges his study to cover life as affected by disease, and masters the psychology of the individual sick in body, he will widen his usefulness and reach a fuller life himself as a physician. He will dare to enter into the mind of his patient with imaginative sympathy, proving himself a friend in need. To professional skill he will join human warmth and understanding. By so doing, and only by so doing, will he accept the whole burden and fulfill his destiny. If anyone seeks happiness, here it may prove to be. It is the second mile enjoined in the text, "And whosoever shall compel thee to go a mile, go with him twain." The good physician will accompany his patient on the second mile — and to the end of the road.

Annals of Internal Medicine 35:307, 1951

Frederick A. Coller [1887–   ]

Medicine never has been followed wholly in the scientific spirit. Science serving mankind needs and has had another expression that can be called humanism. It implies an understanding of the mental state of the patient and a sympathy for him as a purposeful being. It is this that distinguishes the physician from the barber-leech. . . . [When] a physician could not be found to minister to their pains at two o'clock in the morning, they forget about the scourges that have disappeared and wonder "Where is the doctor?" Availability in times of fear and suffering ranks higher as a popular asset than does the ability to prevent the disease.

Bulletin of the American College of Surgery 36:29, 1951

Sir James Calvert Spence [1892–1954]

The doctor needs to know the individual with basic, expert, and specialized understanding if he is to work with success. He sees men of all ages from childhood to senility. He is present at birth and at death. He observes man in his confidence of full health and in his fear of sickness. He observes him near the noon of day when courage is at its height, and in the small hours of morning when it so often ebbs away. Not only must he understand the individual but he must understand him in many of these variations from the norm.

The Purpose and Practice of Medicine, Ch. 18

The real work of a doctor . . . is not an affair of health centres, or public clinics, or operating theatres, or laboratories, or hospital beds. These techniques have their place in medicine, but they are not medicine. The essential unit of medical practice is the occasion when, in the intimacy of the consulting room or sick room, a person who is ill, or believes himself to be ill, seeks the advice of a doctor whom he trusts. This is a consultation and all else in the practice of medicine derives from it.

Idem

Robert F. Loeb [1895–   ]

The patient should be managed the way the doctor or a member of his family would wish to be treated if he were that patient in that bed at that time.

Quoted by David Seegal in *Journal of the American Medical Association* 177:641, 1961

Gentlemen, the thing that I am doing is greeting another human being. [When asked whether it was to determine the temperature, moisture, or strength of the arm that he shook hands with a patient on rounds at Bellevue Hospital in 1962.]

Dickinson W. Richards [1895–   ]

If you would know about suffering, study your patient, as he lies there, as he looks at you, his eyes, his voice, how he moves, what he says, how he says it. Then from here you build up the whole structure of your care, a broad structure, as broad as the measure of his distress. Surely this is no denial of medical science, but its fulfillment.

Transactions of the Association of American Physicians 75:1, 1962

Sir Hugh Cairns [1896–1952]

How does one learn to devote oneself unsparingly to one's patients? You cannot get this from books or from formal clinical instruction. It is something which is passed on from one generation of doctors to the next, and the easiest way to acquire it is to work with a doctor who already has it in his blood. Lister, for example, was a good doctor: he used to visit his patients in King's every day, including Sundays, and his eminence and his preoccupation with research did not prevent him from showing great understanding and consideration of their feelings.
Lancet 2:665, 1949

Your patients . . . do not come to you to be cured; they come to be relieved of their pains and other symptoms and to be comforted. Forced to choose, they would usually prefer a kind doctor to an efficient one. Never forget that the patient and his relations are usually frightened and anxious — upset in their normal life to such an extent that they are prepared to call *you* into their lives and to tell you the most intimate facts about themselves, though you may be unknown to them except as a member of an honourable profession.
Idem

William Faulkner [1897–1962]

He had surrendered all reality, all dread and fear, to the doctor beside him, as people do.
Light in August, Ch. 17

Sir George W. Pickering [1904–　　]

Unless the doctor is utterly devoted to his patients and prepared to take immense trouble to understand their problems he is inferior to a machine. It is only by virtue of that rather intangible and neglected quality, his at-

titude of mind as expressed by devotion to his patient, the real ethos of medicine, that he becomes superior.
British Medical Journal 2:133, 1963

Maurice B. Strauss [1904–　　]

The fact that to-day a physician may be trained in and work in molecular biology no more destroys his capacity to "care for the patient" if he "cares for the patient" than did the training in investigative fields of Peabody's day.[1]
Medicine 43:619, 1964

Robert H. Ebert [1914–　　]

I have never been convinced that the physician concerned with the science of medicine was any less concerned for his patient than his less scientifically oriented counterpart of a generation ago. . . . There are probably as many "kindly old specialists" as there are "kindly old family physicians."
Address to the National Tuberculosis Association, May 30, 1965

Anonymous

In illness the physician is a father; in convalescence, a friend; when health is restored, he is a guardian.
Brahmanic saying

Hebrew Proverb

Honour a physician before thou hast need of him.

III. BAD

Aristotle [384–322 B.C.]

It is no part of a physician's . . . business to use either persuasion or compulsion upon the patients.
Politics, VII.ii (tr. by H. Rackham)

---

[1] Cf. Francis Weld Peabody, p. 367b.

Oxyrhynchus Logia (Agrapha) [1] [2nd Cent.]

A prophet is not acceptable in his own homeland, nor does a physician work cures on those who know him.
> Eleventh Logion (tr. by Grenfell and Hunt) [*Gospel of Thomas*, Saying 31]

Bachya ben Joseph ibn Paauda [fl. 11th Cent.]

A sick person who lies to his physician cheats only himself, wastes the physician's efforts and aggravates his sickness.
> *Duties of the Heart*, Third Treatise, Ch. 5 (tr. by Moses Hyamson)

Euricius Cordus [1486–1535]

God and the Doctor we alike adore
When on the brink of danger, not before;
The danger past, both are alike requited.
God is forgotten and the Doctor slighted.

Michel de Montaigne [1533–1592]

Why do the doctors work on the credulity of their patient beforehand with so many false promises of a cure, if not so that the effect of the imagination may make up for the imposture of their decoction?
> *Essays*, Bk. I, Ch. 21, "Of the Power of the Imagination" (tr. by Donald M. Frame)

John Owen [1560?–1622]

God and the Doctor we alike adore,
But only when in danger, not before;
The danger o'er, both are alike requited,
God is forgotten, and the doctor slighted.
> Epigram

[1] This Greek manuscript is a scrap of the *Gospel of Thomas*, a document containing sayings of Jesus found in 1945 at Nag Hamadi in Egypt.

Sir Francis Bacon [1561–1626]

Even as if you would call a physician that is thought good for the cure of the disease you complain of, but is unacquainted with your body; and therefore may put you in way for a present cure, but overthroweth your health in some other kind; and so cure the disease and kill the patient.
> *Essays*, "Of Friendship"

William Shakespeare [1564–1616]

The patient dies while the physician sleeps.
> *The Rape of Lucrece*, line 904

Jonathan Swift [1667–1745]

No man values the best medicine if administered by a physician whose person he hates or despises.

Voltaire [1694–1778]

Who are the greatest deceivers? The doctors? And the greatest fools? The patients?

Samuel Johnson [1709–1784]

I deny the lawfulness of telling a lie to a sick man for fear of alarming him. You have no business with consequences; you are to tell the truth. Besides, you are not sure what effect your telling him that he is in danger may have. It may bring his distemper to a crisis, and that may cure him. Of all lying, I have the greatest abhorrence of this, because I believe it has been frequently practised on myself.
> Quoted by James Boswell in *Life of Samuel Johnson*, June 13, 1784

John Bard [1716–1799]

The physician who confines his attention to the body knows not the extent of his art. If he knows not how to soothe the irritation of a troubled and enfeebled mind, to calm the fretfulness of impatience, to rouse the courage of the timid, and even to quiet the compunctions of an over-tender conscience, it will very much confine the efficacy of his prescriptions; and these he cannot do, without he gain the confidence, esteem and even the love of his patients.

Tobias Smollett [1721–1771]

Mr. Morgan being nettled at this treatment, told him, his indignation ought to be directed to Cot [1] Almighty, who visited his people with distempers, and not to him, who contributed all in his power towards their cure.
> *The Adventures of Roderick Random,* Ch. 27

Yet I cannot help thinking I have some right to discharge the overflowing of my spleen upon you, whose province it is to remove those disorders that occasioned it.
> *The Expedition of Humphry Clinker,* Letter 14

Johann Peter Frank [1745–1821]

When I was young, patients were afraid of me; now that I am old, I am afraid of patients.
> Quoted by F. H. Garrison in *Bulletin of the New York Academy of Medicine* 5:157, 1929

George Gordon, Lord Byron [1788–1824]

This is the way physicians mend or end us,
  Secundum artem: but although we sneer
In health — when ill, we call them to attend us,
Without the least propensity to jeer.
> *Don Juan,* Canto X, Stanza 42

Eugene Field [1850–1895]

When one's all right, he's prone to spite

The doctor's peaceful mission;
But when he's sick, it's loud and quick
He bawls for a physician.
> *Doctors*

James Howard Means [1885–1967]

The custom of giving patients appointments weeks in advance, during which time their illness may become seriously aggravated, seems to me to fall short of the ideal doctor-patient relationship.
> *Daedalus* 92:701, 1963

John Steinbeck [1902–   ]

The medical profession is unconsciously irritated by lay knowledge.
> *East of Eden,* Ch. 54

Marguerite Yourcenar [1905–   ]

I have ceased to quarrel with physicians; their foolish remedies have killed me, but their presumption and hypocritical pedantry are work of our making; if we were not so afraid of pain they would tell fewer lies.
> *Memoirs of Hadrian,* Ch. 6 (tr. by Grace Frick)

Proverb

He's a fool that makes the doctor his heir.[1]

Bantu (Chuana) Proverb

If you despise the doctor, despise the sickness also.

Italian Proverb

While the doctor is reflecting the patient dies.[2]

Latin Proverb

The intemperate patient makes the doctor cruel.

---

[1] Latin Proverb: A sick man does ill for himself who makes the doctor his heir.
  Romanian Proverb: If you wish to die soon, make your physician your heir.
[2] Cf. Proverb, p. 67a.

[1] "Cot" instead of "God" is a peculiarity of Mr. Morgan's pronunciation.

371

PATIENTS

See also INVALID, PATIENT–
PHYSICIAN RELATIONSHIP,
SICKNESS

I. GENERAL

Sushruta [5th Cent.? B.C.]

The patient, who believes in a kind and
all-merciful Providence, and possesses
an unshakable fortitude and strong
vital energy, and who is laid up with a
curable form of disease, and is not
greedy, and who further commands all
the necessary articles at his disposal,
and firmly adheres to the advice of his
physician, is a patient of the proper or
commendable type.

> *Sushruta-Samhitá,* "Sutrasthá-
> nam," Ch. 34 (tr. by K. K. L.
> Bhishagratna)

Ovid [43 B.C–A.D. 17?]

Strong things have powers of their own,
and need no Machaon; [1] the sick man
in his danger has recourse to the art
of healing.

> *Pontic Epistles,* III.iv.7 (tr. by
> A. L. Wheeler)

St. Benedict of Nursia [480?–543?]

Before all things and above all things
care is to be had of the sick. . . . And
let the sick themselves remember that
they are served for the honour of God,
and not grieve the brethren who serve
them by unnecessary demands. Yet
must they be patiently borne with, because from such as these is gained a
more abundant reward. Let it be therefore the Abbot's greatest care that they
suffer no neglect. And let a cell be set
apart by itself for the sick brethren,
and one who is God-fearing, diligent,
and careful, be appointed to serve
them. Let the use of baths be allowed

[1] A physician, son of Aesculapius, mentioned in Homer's *Iliad.*

to the sick as often as may be expedient; but to those who are well, and
especially to the young, let it be
granted more seldom. Let the use of
flesh meat also be permitted to the sick
and to those who are very weakly, for
their recovery; but when they are restored to health, let all abstain from
meat in the accustomed manner.

> *The Rule of St. Benedict,* Ch.
> XXXVI (tr. by Oswald Hunter-
> Blair)

Rhazes [850–923]

When the disease is stronger than the
patient, the physician will not be able
to help him at all, and if the strength
of the patient is greater than the
strength of the disease, he does not
need a physician at all. But when both
are equal, then one needs a physician
who will support the patient's strength
and help him against the disease.

> Quoted by Moses ben Maimon
> in *The Preservation of Youth*
> (tr. by Fi Tadbir as-Sihha)

The patient who consults a great many
physicians is likely to have a very confused state of mind.

Moses ben Maimon (Maimonides)
[1135–1204]

One who is ill has not only the right
but also the duty to seek medical aid.

Martin Luther [1483–1546]

Medicine makes sick patients, for doctors imagine diseases, as mathematics
makes hypochondriacs and theology
sinners.

Paracelsus [1493?–1541]

Every physician must be rich in knowledge, and not only of that which is
written in books; his patients should
be his book, they will never mislead
him.

> *The Book of Tartaric Diseases,*
> Ch. 13 (tr. by Norbert Guter-
> man in *Selected Writings*)

Robert Burton [1577–1640]

Many things are necessarily to be observed and continued on the patient's behalf: First that he be not too niggardly miserable of his purse, or think it too much he bestows upon himself, and to save charges endanger his health. . . . 'Tis a part of his cure to wish his own health; and not to defer it too long. . . . A third thing to be required in a patient, is confidence, to be of good cheer, and have sure hope that his physician can help him.
> *The Anatomy of Melancholy,* Pt. 2, Sect. 1, Memb. 4, Subsect. II

Giorgio Baglivi [1669–1707?]

Let the young know they will never find a more interesting, more instructive book than the patient himself.

Samuel Johnson [1709–1784]

What can a sick man say, but that he is sick?
> Letter to William Windham, August 1784

A sick man wishes to be where he is not.
> *Ibid.,* October 2, 1784

William Cowper [1731–1800]

Some men employ their health, an ugly trick,
In making known how oft they have been sick.
> *Conversation*

Nicholas de Belleville [1753–1831]

If you have patients of good sense, and they need no medicine, only advice, explain the matter to them, but if you are treating damned fools, give them bread pills.
> Quoted by Fred B. Rogers in *Help-Bringers,* "Belleville"

George Washington Custis [1781–1857]

His [George Washington's] illnesses were of rare occurrence, but were particularly severe. His aversion to the use of medicine was extreme; and, even when in great suffering, it was only by the entreaties of his lady, and the respectful, yet beseeching look of his oldest friend and companion in arms (Dr. James Craik), that he could be prevailed upon to take the slightest preparation of medicine.
> *Recollections of Washington,* Ch. II

Boston Dispensary [1796]

First, the sick without being pained by a Separation from their Families may be attended and relieved in their own Houses. Secondly, The Sick can in this way be Assisted at a less expense to the public than at a Hospital. Thirdly, Those who have seen better Days may be comforted without being humiliated: and all the Poor receive the Benefits of a Charity the more refined as it is the more secret.[1]

Oliver Wendell Holmes [1809–1894]

The insurance companies do not commonly charge a different percentage on the lives of the patients of this or that physician.
> *Medical Essays,* "Border Lines of Knowledge in Some Provinces of Medical Science"

There are many very good people who are not what I call good patients. I was once requested to call on a lady suffering from nervous and other symptoms. It came out in the preliminary conversational skirmish, half medical, half social, that I was the *twenty-sixth* member of the faculty into whose arms, professionally speaking, she had successively thrown herself. Not being a believer in such a rapid rotation of scientific crops, I gently deposited the burden, commending it to the care of

[1] The first charter in the United States providing for domiciliary care.

number twenty-seven, and, him, whoever he might be, to the care of Heaven.
> *Ibid.*, "The Young Practitioner"

Some old lady told the story o'er
Whose endless stream of tribulation flows
For gastric griefs and peristaltic woes.
> *Rip Van Winkle, M.D.*, Canto I

The sick man's faltered blessing reaches heaven through the battered roof of his hovel before the Te Deum that reverberates in vast cathedrals.
> Valedictory address, Harvard Commencement, March 10, 1858

John Brown [1810–1882]

It is not a case we are treating; it is a living, palpitating, alas, too often suffering fellow creature.
> Quoted in *Lancet* 1:464, 1904

Frank Kittredge Paddock [1841–1901]

The very rich and the very poor, the highly intelligent and the dull witted present the greatest problems in patient care. The latter can grasp no concept greater than the administration of a pill while the former will deny the most logical of diagnoses in favor of the advice of their cook.
> Aphorism

Joel Chandler Harris [1848–1908]

I'm sickly but sassy.
> *Nights with Uncle Remus*, Ch. 50

Robert Tuttle Morris [1857–1945]

It is difficult indeed for a layman in the city to find the right physician if he has been so unfortunate as to have had good health until some emergency arises.
> *Doctors Versus Folks*, Ch. 3

William J. Mayo [1861–1939]

It is worth-while to secure the happiness of the patient as well as to prolong his life.

Rudyard Kipling [1865–1936]

There are only two classes of mankind in the world—doctors and patients.
> *A Doctor's Work*, address to medical students at London's Middlesex Hospital, October 1, 1908

Stephen B. Leacock [1869–1944]

Whatever is wrong with the patient, the doctor insists on snipping off parts and pieces and extracts of him and sending them mysteriously away to be analysed. He cuts off a lock of the patient's hair, marks it, "Mr. Smith's Hair, October, 1910." . . . Then he looks the patient up and down, with the scissors in his hand, and if he sees any likely part of him he clips it off and wraps it up. Now this, oddly enough, is the very thing that fills the patient up with that sense of personal importance which is worth paying for. "Yes," says the bandaged patient, later in the day to a group of friends much impressed, "the doctor thinks there may be a slight anaesthesia of the prognosis, but he's sent my ear to New York and my appendix to Baltimore and a lock of my hair to the editors of all the medical journals, and meantime I am to keep very quiet and not exert myself beyond drinking a hot Scotch with lemon and nutmeg every half-hour." With that he sinks back faintly on his cushions, luxuriously happy.
> *Literary Lapses*, "How to Be a Doctor"

Béla Schick [1877–1967]

First, the patient, second the patient, third the patient, fourth the patient, fifth the patient, and then maybe comes science. We first do everything for the patient; science can wait, research can wait.
> Quoted by I. J. Wolf in *Aphorisms and Facetiae of Béla Schick*

Salvador de Madariaga y Rojo [1886–   ]

There are no diseases, there are only patients.
> *Essays with a Purpose,* "On Medicine"

T. S. Eliot [1888–1965]

Or, take a surgical operation.
In consultation with the doctor and
  the surgeon,
In going to bed in the nursing home,
In talking to the matron you are still
  the subject,
The centre of reality. But, stretched on
  the table,
You are a piece of furniture in a repair
  shop
For those who surround you, the
  masked actors;
All there is of you is your body
And the 'you' is withdrawn.
> *The Cocktail Party,* Act I, Sc. i

Isaac Starr [1895–   ]

Perhaps one half of all patients or more
have nothing wrong with them in terms
of prospective death. But can we say
that there is nothing wrong with them
in terms of prospective life?
> Quoted by S. W. Bloom in *The Doctor and His Patient,* Ch. 6

Robert J. Needles [1903–   ]

Follow the doctor, but don't run over
him.
> *Your Heart & Common Sense,* Sect. 4

Maurice B. Strauss [1904–1974]

Medicine can never abdicate the obligation to care for the patient and to
teach patient care.
> *Medicine* 43:19, 1964

The Talmud

If the patient says, I need [food],
whilst the physician says: He does not
need it, we hearken to the patient.
> *Yoma,* VIII.83a (tr. by L. Jung)

Anonymous

A bore is one who, when you ask him
"How are you?" tells you.

All honour to those who have the courage of their convictions. I include in
their number the patients who have
gone out of hospital against my advice.
I have seen them pioneer the modern
treatment of . . . many diseases. I
would pay special tribute to the casualties; but the funny thing is that I can't
remember any.
> *Lancet* 1:760, 1964

The best patient is a millionaire with a
positive Wassermann.[1]

Hindu Proverb

Ask the patient, not the doctor, where
the pain is.

Indian Proverbs

Physicians live by rich patients, officials by unlucky princes, princes by
litigants, and clever men by fools.

Soldiers long for war, physicians for
patients, clay for water, Brahmins for
land, and beggar-monks for the fat of
the land.

Swahili Proverb

The sick man is the garden of the physicians.

II. VISITORS TO

Francis Hawkins [1628–1681]

Visiting any sick body do not play suddenly the Doctor of Phisicks part, if
thou therein understand nothing.
> *Youth's Behavior,* Pt. I, Ch. 2

Benjamin Franklin [1706–1790]

A cheerful face is nearly as good for an
invalid as healthy weather.

[1] A comment from the pre-penicillin era.

375

Samuel Johnson [1709–1784]

Visitors are no proper companions in the chamber of sickness. They come when I could sleep or read, they stay till I am weary, they force me to attend when my mind calls for relaxation, and to speak when my powers will hardly actuate my tongue. The amusements and consolations of languor and depression are conferred by familiar and domestic companions, which can be visited or called at will, and can occasionally be quitted or dismissed, who do not obstruct accomodation by ceremony, or destroy indolence by awakening effort.

> Letter to Mrs. Henry Thrale, December 27, 1783

The Bible

I was sick, and ye visited me.
> *Matthew* 25:36

The Bible: Apocrypha

Be not slow to visit the sick: for that shall make thee to be beloved.
> *Ecclesiasticus* 7:35

Bantu (Chuana) Proverb

Visitors' footfalls are like medicine; they heal the sick.

PHILOSOPHY

Aristippus [435?–356? B.C.]

Those that study particular sciences and neglect philosophy are like Penelope's wooers, that made love to the waiting-women.
> Quoted by Sir Francis Bacon in *Apothegms*, No. 189

Celsus [25 B.C–A.D. 50]

At first the science of healing was held to be part of philosophy, so that the curing of diseases and the contemplation of the nature of things came in through the same authorities; clearly because it was needed especially by those whose bodily strength had become weakened by quiet thinking and watching by night.
> *De Medicina,* Prooemium (tr. by W. G. Spencer)

Epictetus [60?–120?]

Men, the lecture-room of the philosopher is a hospital; you ought not to walk out of it in pleasure, but in pain. For you are not well when you come; one man has a dislocated shoulder, another an abscess, another a fistula, another a headache. And then am I to sit down and recite to you dainty little notions and clever little mottoes, so that you will go out with words of praise on your lips, one man carrying away his shoulder just as it was when he came in, another his head in the same state, another his fistula, another his abscess?
> *Discourses,* III.xxiii.30 (tr. by W. A. Oldfather)

Marcus Aurelius [121–180]

Just as physicians always keep their lancets and instruments ready to their hands for emergency operations, so also do thou keep thine axioms ready for the diagnosis of things human and divine, and for the performing of every act, even the pettiest, with the fullest consciousness of the mutual ties between these two.
> *Meditations,* III.13 (tr. by C.R. Haines)

Thomas Hewitt Key [1799–1875]

What is Matter? — Never mind.
What is Mind? — No matter.
> *Punch,* July 14, 1855, "A Short Cut to Metaphysics"

Alfred North Whitehead [1861–1947]

The very purpose of philosophy is to delve below the apparent clarity of common speech.
> *Adventures of Ideas,* Ch. 15

PHYSICIANS

See also CLINICIAN, GEN-
ERAL PRACTITIONER, SUR-
GEON

I. GENERAL

Hippocrates [460?–377? B.C.]

Physicians are many in title but very
few in reality.
> *The Law,* I (tr. by Francis
> Adams)

Plautus [254?–184 B.C.]

When sickness comes call for the physician.
> *Amphitruo,* Fragment 12

Celsus [25 B.C.–A.D. 50]

We should not impute the faults of the
physician to his art.

Petronius [fl. 1st Cent.]

After all, a doctor is just to put your
mind at rest.
> *Satyricon,* 42 (tr. by J. Sulli-
> van)

Pliny the Elder [23–79]

But for these Physitians, who are the
judges themselves to determine of our
lives, and who many times are not long
about it, but give us a quick dispatch
and send us to heaven or hell; what
regard is there had, what inquiry and
examination is made of their quality
and worthiness?
> *Natural History,* XXIX.i (tr.
> by Philemon Holland)

The medical profession is the only one
in which anybody professing to be a
physician is at once trusted, although

nowhere else is an untruth more dangerous.
> *Ibid.,* XXIX.viii.17 (tr. by
> W. H. S. Jones)

Epictetus [60?–120?]

As physicians are the preservers of the
sick, so are the laws of the injured.
> *Fragments,* CXVIII (tr. by E.
> Carter)

Galen [fl. 2nd Cent.]

The physician is Nature's assistant.
> *Commentary on Hippocrates'*
> De Humoribus, Bk. I, Prooem-
> ium

Isaac Israeli [830?–932?]

Suffer not thy mouth to condemn when
something happens to a physician, for
everyone has his evil day.
> *Aphorisms,* 29 (tr. by Harry
> Friedenwald in *The Jews and
> Medicine,* Vol. I)

Rhazes [850–923]

When the disease is stronger than the
patient, the physician will not be able
to help him at all, and if the strength
of the patient is greater than the
strength of the disease, he does not
need a physician at all. But when both
are equal, then one needs a physician
who will support the patient's strength
and help him against the disease.
> Quoted by Moses ben Maimon
> in *The Preservation of Youth*
> (tr. by Fi Tadbir as-Sihha)

John of Salisbury [d. 1180]

Theoretical physicians do indeed perform their function, and (perchance in
view of their regard for you they will
draw more generously upon their resources) you will learn from them the
cause and nature of each and every
thing.
> *Policraticus,* Bk. II, Ch. 29 (tr.
> by J. Pike)

Michael Servetus (Villanovanus)
[1511–1553]

You who are going to concoct the crude humors and restore health to the human body. Observe the teachings of this book.

> *Syruporum,* title page (tr. by C. D. O'Malley)

Christopher Marlowe [1564–1593]

> *Galen* come:
> Seeing, *ubi desinit philosophus, ibi incipit medicus,*[1]
> Be a physitian, *Faustus,* heape up golde,
> And be eternizd for some wondrous cure.
> *Summum bonum medicinae sanitas,*[1]
> The end of physicke is our bodies health:
> Why *Faustus,* hast thou not attaind that end?
> Is not thy common talke sound Aphorismes?
> Are not thy billes hung up as monuments,
> Wherby whole Citties have escapt the plague,
> And thousand desprate maladies been easde,
> Yet art thou still but *Faustus,* and a man.
> Wouldst thou make men to live eternally?
> Or being dead, raise them to life againe?
> Then this profession were to be esteemd.
> > *The Tragicall History of Doctor Faustus,* line 40

William Shakespeare [1564–1616]

> How long is't, count,
> Since the physician at your father's died? . . .
> If he were living, I would try him yet.
> . . . The rest have worn me out
> With several applications. Nature and sickness

---

[1] The two Latin quotations are from Aristotle.

Debate it at their leisure.
> *All's Well That Ends Well,* I, ii, 69

Shall I lose my doctor? No! he gives me the potions and the motions.
> *The Merry Wives of Windsor,* III, i, 104

Ben Jonson [1573?–1637]

Many funerals discredit a physician.

John Ford [1586?–1640?]

Physicians are the cobblers, rather the botchers, of men's bodies; as the one patches our tattered clothes, so the other solders our diseased flesh.
> *The Lover's Melancholy,* Act I, Sc. ii

Francis Quarles [1592–1644]

Physitians of all men are most happy; what good successe soever they have, the world proclaimes, and what faults they commit, the earth covers.
> *Hieroglyphickes of the Life of Man,* Hierogliph IV

Johann Oberndoerffer
[fl. 1600–1621]

The Physitian is a great Commaunder, hath as subordinate to him the Cookes for diet, the Surgions for manuall operation, the Apothecaries for confecting and preparing Medicines.
> *The Anatomye of the True Physitian* (tr. by F. Herring)

Samuel Butler [1612–1680]

There's but the twinkling of a *Star*
Between a Man of *Peace* and *War* . . .
A formal *Preacher* and a *Player,*
A learn'd *Physitian* and *Man-slayer.*
> *Hudibras,* Pt. II, Canto III

Jean de La Fontaine [1621–1695]

Doctor So-Much-the-Worse . . . and Doctor All-the-Better.
> *Fables,* Bk. V, Fable 12

Gideon Harvey [1640?–1700?]

In which curative particular the Thinking Physician has the advantage, though the Prating Physician by his pretended Anatomy ingrosses the opinion of mankind.

> *The Art of Curing Disease by Expectation*, Ch. 22

Voltaire [1694–1778]

I know of nothing more laughable than a doctor who does not die of old age.

> Letter to Charles Augustin Feriol, comte d'Argental, November 6, 1767

Samuel Johnson [1709–1784]

A physician in a great city seems to be the mere plaything of fortune; his degree of reputation is, for the most part, totally casual; they that employ him know not his excellence; they that reject him know not his deficience.

> *Lives of the Poets*, "Life of Mark Akenside"

Arthur Young [1741–1820]

Who is it that says there is a great difference between a good physician and a bad one; yet very little between a good one and none at all?

> *Travels in France*, September 9, 1787

Thomas Jefferson [1743–1826]

The office of surgeon has been considered as on a footing with that of chaplain, and the administering of medicine to be as inoffensive as giving religious instruction to those with whom we are contending.

> Letter to Philip Turpin, July 29, 1783

Benjamin Rush [1745?–1813]

The circumstances that influence opinion and choice and of course the fate of a physician are too numerous and many of them too trifling to be mentioned. . . . medical skill has but little share in them.

> *Autobiography*, "Travels Through Life," Ch. IV

Sir Gilbert Blane [1749–1834]

It has been sarcastically said, that there is a wide difference between a good physician and a bad one, but a small difference between a good physician and no physician at all; by which it is meant to insinuate, that the mischievous officiousness of art does commonly more than counterbalance any benefit derivable from it.

> *Elements of Medical Logic*

Nicholas de Belleville [1753–1831]

If you get one *good* doctor, you get one *good* thing, but if you get one *bad* doctor, you get one *bad* thing. If you have a lawsuit, you get one bad lawyer, you lose your suit — you can appeal; but if you have one bad doctor, and he kills you, then there can be no appeal.

> Quoted by Stephen Wickes in *History of Medicine in New Jersey*, Pt. 2

George Crabbe [1754–1832]

Next, to a graver tribe we turn our view,
And yield the praise to worth and science due;
But this with serious words and sober style,
For these are friends with whom we seldom smile:
Helpers of men they're call'd, and we confess
Theirs the deep study, theirs the lucky guess.

> *The Borough*, Letter VII

Sir Walter Scott [1771–1832]

A slight touch of the cynic in manner and habits, gives the physician, to the common eye, an air of authority which greatly tends to enlarge his reputation.

> *The Surgeon's Daughter*, Ch. 1

379

Sir Charles Bell [1774–1842]

Nor is the public aware of the Temptations which men of our profession withstand. Credit for great abilities, gratitude for services performed, and high emoluments are ready to be bestowed for a little deception, and that obliquity of conduct, which does not amount to actual crime.

> *Illustrations of the Great Operations in Surgery,* Preface

James Jackson [1777–1867]

I have often remarked that, though a physician is sometimes blamed very unjustly, it is quite as common for him to get more credit than he is fairly entitled to; so that he has not, on the whole, any right to complain.

> *Letters to a Young Physician,* 1855

William Prout [1785–1850]

That the physician of another age will be as familiar with the operations of the animal economy as he is at present with its anatomy, I have not the least doubt and — I will venture to predict that what the knowledge of anatomy at present is to the surgeon, in conducting his operations, so will chemistry be to the physician in directing him generally, what to do and what to shun; and, in short, enabling him to wield his remedies with a certainty and precision.

Karl F. H. Marx [1796–1877]

The individualized physician is, in the truest sense, a man of the world.

> Quoted by F. H. Garrison in *Bulletin of the New York Academy of Medicine* 4:1001, 1928

Honoré de Balzac [1799–1850]

The physician strives for the good as the artist strives for the beautiful, each pushed on by that admirable feeling we call virtue.

Samuel Warren [1807–1877]

There are no members of society whose pursuits lead them to listen more frequently to what has been exquisitely termed

> The still sad music of humanity.
> *Diary of a Late Physician* (1864), Introduction

John Greenleaf Whittier [1807–1892]

The paths of pain are thine. Go forth With healing and with hope.

> *To a Young Physician*

Oliver Wendell Holmes [1809–1894]

But the practising physician's office is to draw the healing waters, and while he gives his time to this labor he can hardly be expected to explore all the sources that spread themselves over the wide domain of science. The traveller who would not drink of the Nile until he had tracked it to its parent lakes, would be like to die of thirst; and the medical practitioner who would not use the results of many laborers in other departments without sharing their special toils, would find life far too short and art immeasurably too long.

> *Medical Essays,* "Scholastic and Bedside Teaching"

Doctors are oxydable products, and the schools must keep furnishing new ones as the old ones turn into oxyds; some of first-rate quality that burn with a great light, — some of a lower grade of brilliancy, some honestly, unmistakably, by the grace of God, of moderate gifts, or in simpler phrase, dull.

> *Idem*

Prince Otto von Bismarck [1815–1898]

Physicians still retain something of their priestly origin: they would gladly do what they forbid.

Florence Nightingale [1820–1910]

We were lucky in our Medical Heads. Two of them are brutes and four are angels — for this is a work which makes angels or devils of men.
> Letter to Dr. Bowman, November 14, 1854

Gustave Flaubert [1821–1880]

DOCTOR: Always preceded by "the good." Among men, in familiar conversation, "Oh! balls, doctor!" Is a wizard when he enjoys your confidence, a jackass when you're no longer on terms. All are materialists: "You can't probe for faith with a scalpel."
> *Dictionary of Accepted Ideas*
> (tr. by Jacques Barzun)

Rudolf Virchow [1821–1902]

Only those who regard healing as the ultimate goal of their efforts can, therefore, be designated as physicians.
> *Disease, Life, and Man*, "Standpoints in Scientific Medicine" (tr. by Jacques Barzun)

Jakob Laurenz Sonderegger [1826–1896]

Medicine must be (and everything depends on this) your religion and your politics, your fortune and misfortune. Therefore do not advise anyone to become a physician. If he still wants to become one, warn him against it, repeatedly and earnestly; if none the less he persists, then give him your blessing; if it is worth anything, he will have need of it.
> Letter

Count Leo Tolstoy [1828–1910]

This is where the strength of the physician lies, be he a quack, a homoeopath or an allopath. He supplies the perennial demand for comfort, the craving for sympathy that every human sufferer feels.
> *War and Peace*, Pt. 9, Ch. 16

Robert, Marquis of Salisbury [1830–1903]

Doctors are a social cement.

Ambrose Bierce [1842–1914?]

PHYSICIAN, n. One upon whom we set our hopes when ill and our dogs when well.
> *The Devil's Dictionary*

William Ernest Henley [1849–1903]

Bland as a Jesuit, sober as a hymn.
> *In Hospital*, Sect. xvi, "House-Surgeon"

Sir William Osler [1849–1919]

Permanence of residence, good undoubtedly for the pocket, is not always best for wide mental vision in the physician.
> *Aequanimitas, with Other Addresses*, "The Army Surgeon"

Perhaps no sin so easily besets us as a sense of self-satisfied superiority to others.
> *Ibid.*, "Chauvinism in Medicine"

There are only two sorts of doctors: those who practise with their brains, and those who practise with their tongues.
> *Ibid.*, "Teaching and Thinking"

John Watson ("Ian Maclaren") [1850–1907]

A've often thocht oor doctor's little better than the Gude Samaritan.

Stephen Paget [1855–1926]

Every year, young men enter the medical profession who neither are born doctors, nor have any great love of science, nor are helped by name or influence. Without a welcome, without money, without prospects, they fight their way into practice, and in practice; they find it hard work, ill-thanked, ill-paid: there are times when they say, *What call had I to be a doctor? I should have done better for myself and my wife and the children in some other calling.* But they stick to it, and that not only from necessity, but from pride, honor, conviction: and Heaven, sooner or later, lets them know what it thinks of them. The information comes quite as a surprise to them, being the first received, from any source, that they were indeed called to be doctors; and they hesitate to give the name of divine vocation to work paid by the job, and shamefully underpaid at that. Calls, they imagine, should master men, beating down on them: surely, a diploma, obtained by hard examination and hard cash, and signed and sealed by earthly examiners, cannot be a summons from Heaven. But it may be. For, if a doctor's life may not be a divine vocation, then no life is a vocation, and nothing is divine.

Confessio Medici, Ch. 1

It is certain, that some men are indeed called to be doctors: and so are some women. They are, as we say, born doctors: they were shapen in Medicine. So apt are they to their work, and it to them, that they almost persuade me to hold opinion with Pythagoras, and to believe that in some previous existence they were in general practice. Or their ability may be the result of inheritance: but we know next to nothing about inheritance, neither is it imaginable by what physical processes the babe unborn is predisposed for one profession. Still, there are men and women, but not a great number, created for the service of Medicine: who were called to be doctors when they were not yet called to be babies.

Idem

George Bernard Shaw [1856–1950]

But the true doctor is inspired by a hatred of ill-health, and a divine impatience of any waste of vital forces.

Unless a man is led to medicine or surgery through a very exceptional technical aptitude, or because doctoring is a family tradition, or because he regards it unintelligently as a lucrative and gentlemanly profession, his motives in choosing the career of a healer are clearly generous.

The Doctor's Dilemma, "Preface on Doctors"

Even the fact that doctors themselves die of the very diseases they profess to cure passes unnoticed. We do not shoot out our lips and shake our heads, saying, "They save others: themselves they cannot save": their reputation stands, like an African king's palace, on a foundation of dead bodies.

Idem

Make it compulsory for a doctor using a brass plate to have inscribed on it, in addition to the letters indicating his qualifications, the words "Remember that I too am mortal."

Idem

When men die of disease they are said to die from natural causes. When they recover (and they mostly do) the doctor gets the credit of curing them.

Idem

Did you ever see a boy cultivating a moustache? Well, a middle-aged doctor cultivating a grey head is much the same sort of spectacle.

Ibid., Act I

William J. Mayo [1861–1939]

As he [William J. Mayo] approached the place where a meeting of doctors was being held, he saw some elegant limousines and remarked, "The surgeons have arrived." Then he saw some cheaper cars and said, "The physicians are here, too." A few scattered model-T Fords led him to infer that there were pathologists present. And when he saw a row of overshoes inside,

under the hat rack, he is reported to have remarked, "Ah, I see there are laboratory men here."
> Quoted by Walter B. Cannon in *The Way of an Investigator*, Ch. 19

Rudyard Kipling [1865–1936]

There are only two classes of mankind in the world — doctors and patients.
> *A Doctor's Work*, address to medical students at London's Middlesex Hospital, October 1, 1908

You [doctors] have been, and always will be, exposed to the contempt of the gifted amateur — the gentleman who knows by intuition everything that it has taken you years to learn.
> *Idem*

Charles H. Mayo [1865–1939]

All who are benefited by community life, especially the physician, owe something to the community.
> *Medical Life* 34:165, 1927

Abraham Flexner [1866–1959]

The sick man's progress is nature's comment and criticism. The professional competency of the physician is in proportion to his ability to heed the response which nature thus makes to his ministrations.
> *Medical Education, A Comparative Study*

Marcel Proust [1871–1922]

In this man, so insignificant, so common, there was, in these brief moments in which he deliberated, in which the relative dangers of one and another course of treatment presented themselves alternately to his mind until he arrived at a decision, the same sort of greatness as in a general who, vulgar in all the rest of his life, decides upon what is from the military point of view the wisest course, and gives the order: "Advance eastwards."
> *The Guermantes Way*, Pt. II, "My Grandmother's Illness" (tr. by C. K. Scott-Moncrieff)

Thomas Mann [1875–1955]

A true doctor devoted to science and to the pursuit of medicine for its own sake is easiest of all to deceive.
> *Confessions of Felix Krull, Confidence Man*, Bk. I, Ch. 6

Warfield T. Longcope [1877–1953]

In rare instances, however, the practising physician becomes the creative scientist. His imagination conceives of an hypothesis, based on frequent, accurate, well controlled observation.
> *Bulletin of the Johns Hopkins Hospital* 50:4, 1932

Sir Auckland Geddes [1879–1954]

So many come to the sickroom thinking of themselves as men of science fighting disease and not as healers with a little knowledge helping nature to get a sick man well.
> Quoted by Sir Robert Hutchison in *The Practitioner*

Walton H. Hamilton [1881–1958]

I suspect that, aside from the alleviation of suffering, the strongest impulse which moves the physician is the professional motive of winning the esteem of his fellows. And I am inclined to believe that the ordinary physician is an artist who esteems, far more highly than the dubious chance at wealth, a regular and an adequate income, the feeling of security and freedom to devote himself in an uncompromising way to his calling.
> *Dissenting Opinion on the Report of the Committee on American Medicine*, 1932

James Howard Means [1885–1967]

The most conspicuous change in the behavior of the doctor is that nowadays he is usually in such a hurry that he is less accessible and less communicative.

Daedalus 92:701, 1963

James Bridie [1888–1951]

There is a temptation for any creature who seems obviously to be doing the work of the Almighty to imagine himself a god. This is particularly so in medicine, and an almost unavoidable error in the hospital physician or surgeon. He is surrounded by respectful and even adoring acolytes, and he holds the power of life and death over helpless persons. It is small wonder if he becomes, like the superintendent's dog, an orgulous animal. If he is to avoid madness, he must stand aside from the business from time to time and deride himself and his colleagues.

Tedious and Brief, Pt. II, "The Umbilicus"

John A. Ryle [1889–1950]

Whereas the hope and interest of the theologians and their pupils are for personal survival, [the physician's] interest, not greatly regarding self, is in the survival of matter, of the atoms which were his share of the universe and will return to earth and space when he is dead; in the survival within his offspring, if he have them, and in the collaterals of the race of those germs of inheritance which he drew, let us hope with pride and gratitude, from his sires; and in the survival of such influence for happiness, for wisdom and for good as his personality may have imparted to those around him while he walked with them on earth.

Fears May Be Liars, Ch. 3

Vannevar Bush [1890–   ]

Originally . . . the profession had its quota of men of character, more of a quota than the other professions undoubtedly because of the heavy direct and personal responsibilities involved, devoted and intelligent men who took the oath of Hippocrates seriously. . . . All this has now changed.

Modern Arms and Free Men, Ch. XVI

Wilder Penfield [1891–   ]

'Work today and be happy tomorrow' — that's the physician's rule of life.

The Torch, Ch. 10

Henry E. Sigerist [1891–1957]

When we look back into the past, we see an endless train of doctors on the march. Their dress, their language, their social position varies; their outlooks and their methods change from age to age. Some have a urine-glass in their hands, others a stethoscope. Yet one and all, from the shamans of primitive tribes down to the scientific physicians of our own day, are inspired by the same will. They seek the same goal and are guided by the same idea. Many of them have been veritably great.

The Great Doctors, Preface (tr. by Eden and Cedar Paul)

The physician is by no means the only medical worker. . . . In a country like the United States more than a million people are actively engaged in health work. . . . The physician, however, is the key medical expert of society.

Medicine and Human Welfare, Ch. 3

Ben Hecht [1894–1964]

The talent for secrecy is highly developed among doctors who, even with nothing to conceal, are often as close mouthed as old-fashioned bomb throwers on their way to a rendezvous.

Miracle of the Fifteen Murderers

Temple Fay [1895–1963]

Your books and teachings
You will find of value

Experience and skill are slow to be
acquired
But your success will oft depend
Upon the message that your hands
themselves
Bear to your patient when you first
grasp his
When quest for help brings him to your
door
Or when you count the pulse
Of those who face the ebbing tide of
life.
These Hands of Ours

Fuller Albright [1900–   ]

As with eggs, there is no such thing
as a poor doctor, doctors are either
good or bad.

> *Textbook of Medicine* (9th ed.
> by Russell L. Cecil and Robert
> F. Loeb), "Diseases of the
> Ductless Glands," Introduction

Lindsay E. Beaton [1911–   ]

In medicine the scientist-educator and
the practitioner have each his own
faith. The faith of the physician em-
braces both.

> *Journal of the American Med-
> ical Association* 189:40, 1964

As yet among the vocal segment of the
medical profession there is little inclination to adapt. Rather the effort is
to stem the tide, and in his own defense, borrowing from psychiatry,
which Sinclair Lewis in *Arrowsmith*
called a plot against medicine, the
private practitioner at last falls back
to the barricade of the free choice of
physician. It matters not that the sacred efficacy of this has yet to be demonstrated by any scientific study. It
is an item of faith and, as such, un-
challengeable.

> *Journal of Medical Education*
> 40:35, 1965

I am a practicing private physician;
I want most desperately to be also a
practicing member of the medical college community. For myself and my

brothers, currently adrift on a restless
sea, I ask for a mooring place. We
have been taught a great deal; we use
it for our patients the best we can.
We think that we have perceived how
to live with the sick. We need more.
The fact that men are decent human beings at last makes them compassionate; only learning makes them
physicians. And only continuing and
never-ending basic knowledge and fundamental learning will make them
good physicians. Where is the vision
that will give us this future? For it is
written that without vision the people
perish.

> *Ibid.*, 40:278, 1965

Budd Schulberg [1914–   ]

Today we are sending you out to
battle. Only you are not armed with
poison gas and bayonets, but with antiseptic, chloroform and healing hands.
For you march not in the path
of Alexander and Napoleon, but of
Semmelweis, Lister and Pasteur. Fight
your war with courage and honesty,
young men, for yours is a war against
death.

> *The Writer's Radio Theater
> 1941* (ed. by N. S. Weiser),
> "Hollywood Doctor"

John L. McClenahan [1915–   ]

It is because we have begun to act
like merchants, and in many instances
to observe the same hours, that the
public expects us to be regulated by
the same restraints.

> *X-ray Technician* 32:498, 1961

Charles Brook [fl. 1945]

It can be reasonably supposed that
the average person, if asked to define
the difference between a physician and
a surgeon, would reply "a surgeon
uses the knife while the physician
prescribes medicines," but the real distinction is that the physician and the
surgeon belong to entirely different
schools of medical thought. The good

physician is a disciple of Paracelsus, who was a sceptic, while the good surgeon is a disciple of Galen, who was a good dogmatist.

Battling Surgeon, Ch. 1

The Bible

Is there no balm in Gilead; is there no physician there?

Jeremiah 8:22

The Bible: Apocrypha

And He gave men discernment,
  That they might glory in His mighty works.
By means of them the physician assuageth pain
  And likewise the apothecary prepareth a confection
That His work may not cease,
  Nor health from the face of His earth.

Ecclesiasticus 38:6

He that sinneth before his Maker, let him fall into the hand of the physician.

Ecclesiasticus 38:15

Anonymous

[Two women discussing a new doctor in their district:] Is he a pooh-pooh-er or a wind-up-er?

Punch

A doctor is the only man who can suffer from good health.

Anonymous Arabian Poet

What ails the physician that he dies of the disease which in times gone by he claimed to cure?

Quoted by Victor Robinson in *The Story of Medicine*

Anonymous Indian Saying
[ca. 1000–1500]

The Physician who understands the healing powers of roots and herbs is a man; he who understands the waters and fire, a demon; he who understands the efficacy of prayer, a prophet; he who understands the virtues of quicksilver, a god.

Proverbs

Nature, time, and patience are the three great physicians.

The best Physicians are Dr. Diet, Dr. Quiet, and Dr. Merryman.[1]

Arabic Proverb

When fate arrives the physician becomes a fool.

Bechuanaland Proverb

When the clever doctor fails, try one less clever.

Chinese Proverbs

The superior doctor prevents sickness;
The mediocre doctor attends to impending sickness;
The inferior doctor treats actual sickness.

The unlucky doctor treats the head of a disease; the lucky doctor its tail.

French Proverb

Happy is the physician who is called in at the end of the illness.

Indian (Tamil) Proverb

A loquacious doctor is successful.

Polish Proverb

Every Czech is a musician; every Italian, a doctor; every German, a merchant; every Pole, a nobleman.

Scottish Proverbs

If the doctor cures, the sun sees it; but if he kills, the earth hides it.

Old wives and bairns make fools of physicians.

[1] Adapted from the School of Salerno's *Regimen Sanitatis Salernitanum.* Cf. p. 487a.

II. FOR

Homer [ca. 850 B.C.]

A leech is of the worth of many other men for the cutting out of arrows and the spreading of soothing simples.

> *Iliad*, XI.514 (tr. by A. T. Murray)

John of Salisbury [d. 1180]

What am I to say of the practicing physicians? Far be it from me to say anything detrimental to them; I have too frequently fallen into their hands as atonement for my sins. Their resentment is not to be aroused by words; rather are they to be soothed by compliance. I do not wish them to deal harshly with me nor yet do I dare entertain the views that all proclaim. I shall therefore say with the holy man Solomon that medicine is from the Lord God and no wise man will despise it. There is indeed no one more indispensable than the doctor, provided he be a man of faith and wisdom. Who may sound the praises of him who as builder of salvation and protector of life imitates the Lord and performs his function in that he as agent and servant regulates and dispenses the salvation which He effects and as Lord and Prince grants?

> *Policraticus*, Bk. II, Ch. 29 (tr. by J. Pike)

Desiderius Erasmus [1466?–1536]

[The doctor] does not merely cure the body, which is man's baser part, but he cures the whole man, even though the theologian begins with the Soul and the doctor with the body. . . . Who is so persistent a preacher of abstinence, sobriety, restraining anger, fleeing care, avoiding gluttony, rejecting love, moderating sex, as the Doctor?

> *Declamatio in laudem artis medicae*

We owe gratitude to those who drive off the enemy who flies at our throats; are we not more indebted to the doctor who fights daily for our safety against so many deadly enemies to life?

> *Idem*

Paolo Giovio [1483–1552]

At the end of an unhappy reign, he [Pope Adrian VI] died of drinking too much beer — whereupon the house of his physician was hung with garlands by midnight revellers, and adorned with the inscription, "Liberatori Patriae S. P. Q. R."

> *Biography of Adrian VI* (Paraphrased by Jakob Burckhardt in *The Civilization of the Renaissance in Italy*, tr. by S. G. C. Middlemore)

Michel de Montaigne [1533–1592]

I honor doctors, not, according to the precept, out of necessity — . . . but for love of themselves, having known many honest and lovable men among them.

> *Essays*, Bk. II, Ch. 37, "Of the Resemblance of Children to Fathers" (tr. by Donald M. Frame)

Thomas Dekker [1572?–1632?]

Make much of thy Physitian: let not an Emperick or Mounti-bancking Quacksalver peepe in at thy window, but set thy Gates wide open to entertaine thy learned Physitian: Honour him, make much of him. Such a Physitian is Gods second, and in a duell or single fight (of this nature) will stand bravely to thee. A good Physitian, comes to thee in the shape of an *Angell*, and therefore let him boldly take thee by the hand, for he has been in Gods garden, gathering herbes: and soveraine rootes to cure thee; A good Physitian deales in simples, and will be simply honest with thee in thy preservatiõ.

> *London Looke Backe*

Ben Jonson [1573?–1637]

Life and *Health,* which are both inestimable, we have of the *Physician.*
> *Discoveries,* "Valor rerum"

Samuel Butler [1612–1680]

A skilful Leech is better far
Than half a hundred Men of War.
> *Hudibras,* Pt. I, Canto II

Jeremy Taylor [1613–1667]

To preserve a man alive in the midst of so many chances and hostilities, is as great a miracle as to create him.
> *The Rule and Exercises of Holy Dying,* Ch. I, Sect. I

Richard Steele [1672–1729]

There is not a more useful Man in the Commonwealth than a good Physician; and by Consequence no worthier a Person than he that uses his Skill with Generosity, even to Persons of Condition, and Compassion to those in Want.
> *The Tatler,* Vol. II, No. 78 (October 6–8, 1709)

Alexander Pope [1688–1744]

They [physicians] are in general the most amiable companions and the best friends, as well as the most learned men I know.
> Letter to Ralph Allen, September 13, 1743

Voltaire [1694–1778]

Men who are occupied in the restoration of health to other men, by the joint exertion of skill and humanity, are above all the great of the earth. They even partake of divinity, since to preserve and renew is almost as noble as to create.
> *A Philosophical Dictionary,* "Physicians"

Samuel Johnson [1709–1784]

Every man has found in physicians great liberality and dignity of sentiment, very prompt effusion of beneficence, and willingness to exert a lucrative art where there is no hope of lucre.
> *Lives of the Poets,* "Life of Samuel Garth"

They [doctors] do more good to mankind without a prospect of reward than any profession of men whatever.

Felix Vicq-d'Azyr [1748–1794]

If a doctor's offices are admirable, it is in fact less in palaces and in the midst of grandeur, where the motives of self-interest, whether apparent or real, leave no room for those of humanity, than in the cramped, unhealthy dwelling of the poor. . . . It is there that one may do good, that man may help man, without stir and even without witnesses; it is there that generosity, true beneficence, tender pity thrive; it is there that one will surely find tears to dry, unfortunates to comfort. To the praise of doctors let us say: what other group of citizens discharges these august duties with so much zeal and courage?
> *Éloges Historiques,* "Éloge de Fothergill"

Johann Wolfgang von Goethe [1749–1832]

Certainly physicians cannot prolong our lives by a single day: we live as long as God wills; but it makes a great difference whether we live miserably, like poor dogs, or keep well and fresh, and here a wise physician can do much for us.

John, Lord Russell [1792–1878]

I admire the habits of a physician; he sees the weakness of our nature; he is generally just and conscientious; though somewhat selfish from the contempt which his profession must give him of mankind, his mind is rather accurate than exalted.

George Eliot (Marian Evans Cross) [1819–1880]

Many of us looking back through life would say that the kindest man we have ever known has been a medical man, or perhaps that surgeon whose fine tact, directed by deeply-informed perception, has come to us in our need with a more sublime beneficence than that of miracle-workers.
> *Middlemarch,* Ch. 66

Walt Whitman [1819–1892]

I love doctors and hate their medicine.

Sir William Osler [1849–1919]

In the records of no other profession is there to be found so large a number of men who have combined intellectual pre-eminence with nobility of character.
> *Aequanimitas, with Other Addresses,* "Books and Men"

A well-trained, sensible doctor is one of the most valuable assets of a community, worth to-day, as in Homer's time, many another man.
> *Ibid.,* "Chauvinism in Medicine"

Robert Louis Stevenson [1850–1894]

You doctors have a serious responsibility. You call a man from the gates of death, you give health and strength once more to use or abuse. But for your kindness and skill, this would have been my last book, and now I am in hopes that it will be neither my last nor my best.
> Inscription in a copy of *Travels with a Donkey* sent to his physician, Dr. William Bambord, 1879

There are men and classes of men that stand above the common herd: the soldier, the sailor, and the shepherd not unfrequently; the artist rarely; rarelier still, the clergyman; the physician almost as a rule. He is the flower (such as it is) of our civilization. . . . Generosity he has, such as is possible to those who practise an art, never to those who drive a trade; discretion, tested by a hundred secrets; tact, tried in a thousand embarrassments; and what are more important, Heraclean cheerfulness and courage.
> *Underwoods,* Dedication

Stephen Paget [1855–1926]

If Medicine is a trade, why should the doctor so often work for nothing? If it is an art, what works of art does he produce? None, says Claude Bernard, *Le Médecin Artiste ne crée rien:* but surely he is wrong. The doctor, so far from creating nothing, creates life: for he who saves or prolongs life, creates more life. If Miss X is seventy, and the doctor, by an operation, enables her to live till she is seventy-five, he has not prolonged the seventy years, for they were ended before he came; but he has created five brand-new years. If he had not been there, they would not be here: that is creation. He has not lengthened her past, nobody could; he has called into existence her present and her future: and they are she, therefore he has called into existence her. Not that he thinks much of that tremendous act.
> *Confessio Medici,* Ch. 5

William Ralph Inge [1860–1954]

On the whole the doctors I have known have been amongst the finest men of my acquaintance. . . . their generosity far surpasses what I have found in any other profession.
> Address to students of the London Hospital, 1933

Ben Hecht [1894–1964]

Doctors have a sense for things unseen and complications unstated.
> *Miracle of the Fifteen Murderers*

Nigel Dennis [1912–   ]

If there is one good thing to be said of the medical profession it is that their promiscuousness makes class-distinction impossible.

Cards of Identity, Pt. I

The Bible: Apocrypha

Honour a physician with the honour due unto him for the uses which ye may have of him: for the Lord hath created him.

For of the most High cometh healing, and he shall receive honour of the King.

The skill of the physician shall lift up his head; and in the sight of great men he shall be in admiration.

Ecclesiasticus 38:1

Then give place to the physician, for the Lord hath created him: let him not go from thee, for thou hast need of him. There is a time when in their hands there is good success.

Ecclesiasticus 38:12

Chinese Proverb

A skillful physician can revive the springtime of life.

German Proverb

A half doctor near is better than a whole one far away.

III. AGAINST

Philemon [361?–263? B.C.]

There is not a doctor who desires the health of his friends; not a soldier who desires the peace of his country.

Fabulae Incertae, Fragment 46 (Quoted by Stobaeus in *Florilegium*, CII.5)

Lucilius [2nd Cent. B.C.]

Diophantus saw Hermogenes the doctor in his sleep and never woke up again, although he was wearing an amulet.

Quoted in *The Greek Anthology*, XI.257 (tr. by W. R. Paton)

Martial [fl. 1st Cent.]

Diaulus has been a doctor, he is now an undertaker. He begins to put his patients to bed in his old effective way.

Epigrams, I.30 (tr. by W. C. A. Ker)

Lately was Diaulus a doctor, now he is an undertaker. What the undertaker now does the doctor too did before.

Ibid., I.47

I was sickening; but you at once attended me, Symmachus, with a train of a hundred apprentices. A hundred hands frosted by the North wind have pawed me; I had no fever before, Symmachus; now I have.

Ibid., V.9

Nicarchus [fl. 1st Cent.]

The physician Marcus laid his hand yesterday on the stone Zeus, and though he is of stone and Zeus he is to be buried to-day.

The Greek Anthology, XI.113 (tr. by W. R. Paton)

Pliny the Elder [23–79]

Physicians acquire their knowledge from our dangers, making experiments at the cost of our lives. Only a physician can commit homicide with impunity.

Natural History, XXIX.viii.18 (tr. by W. H. S. Jones)

Tacitus [55?–after 117]

[Tiberius] was wont to jest at the arts of the physician and at all who, after the age of thirty, require another man's advice to distinguish between what is beneficial or hurtful to their constitutions.[1]

> *Annals*, VI.46 (tr. by Church and Brodribb)

Valens [328?–378]

Keep the physician from your door as long as you can.

John of Salisbury [d. 1180]

The common people say, that physicians are the class of people who kill other men in the most polite and courteous manner.

> *Policraticus*, Bk. II, Ch. 29

Joseph ben Meir ibn Sabara [ca. 1150–1200]

You may kill a man for to plunder him,
Society will leave you at large;
You've a better thing than the Reaper grim:
He can't charge.

> *The Book of Delights*, Ch. X (tr. by Moses Hadas)

Roger Bacon [1214?–1294]

The typical medical man is ignorant of his own simple medicine and puts himself in the hands of unlearned apothecaries.

> *De Erroribus Medicorum*

Medical men don't know the drugs they use, nor their prices.

> *Idem*

Petrarch [1304–1374]

If a hundred or a thousand people, all of the same age, of the same constitution and habits, were suddenly seized by the same illness, and one half of them were to place themselves under the care of doctors, such as they are in our time, whilst the other half intrusted themselves to Nature and to their own discretion, I have not the slightest doubt that there would be

more cases of death amongst the former, and more cases of recovery among the latter.[1]

> *Invectives*, Preface, Letter to Pope Clement VI

Life in itself is short enough, but the physicians with their art, know to their amusement, how to make it still shorter.

> *Idem*

My friend, if a doctor did himself what he advises others to do or bade them do the same as he does, he would either suffer in health or in estate.

> *Idem*

Neither is there any doubt, as Pliny gracefully says, that they are always hunting after renown for some novelty and so traffic in our lives . . . that anyone who holds himself out as a physician is at once accepted as such; but although in no form of fraud is there greater danger, yet we do not regard it, so great is the attraction of a man's own particular delusion.

> *Idem*

Michel de Montaigne [1533–1592]

No doctor takes pleasure in the health even of his friends.

> *Essays*, Bk. I, Ch. 22, "One Man's Profit Is Another Man's Harm" (tr. by Donald M. Frame)

The doctors are not content with having control over the sickness; they make health itself sick, in order to prevent people from being able at any time to escape their authority.

> *Ibid.*, Bk. II, Ch. 37, "Of the Resemblance of Children to Fathers"

Barnabe Rich [1540?–1617]

They say it is an argument of a licentious commonwealth, where Phisitians

---

[1] Cf. Plutarch, p. 337b.

[1] Cf. Lawrence J. Henderson, p. 302a.

and Lawyers have too great comminges in, but it is the surfeits of peace that bringeth in the Phisitians gain, yet in him there is some dispatch of businesse, for if he cannot speedily cure you, he will yet quickly kill you.
> *The Honestie of This Age*

François Rabelais [1494?–1553]

[Pantagruel] thought of studying medicine here but decided the profession was too troublesome and morbid. Besides, physicians smelled hellishly of enemas.
> *Gargantua and Pantagruel*, Bk. II, Ch. 5 (tr. by Jacques Le Clercq)

Maximilianus Urientius [1559–1613]

I tell you, the one by his drugs and pills,
By his knife the other, the churchyard fills:
The diff'rence only from the Hangman's seen,
Their work's clumsy and slow, his quick and clean.
> *The Physician, Surgeon, and Hangman* (tr. by H. P. Dodd)

William Shakespeare [1564–1616]

He hath abandon'd his physicians, madam; under whose practices he hath persecuted time with hope, and finds no other advantage in the process but only the losing of hope by time.
> *All's Well That Ends Well*, I, i, 15

Will you cast away your child on a fool and a physician?
> *The Merry Wives of Windsor*, III, iv, 100

Trust not the physician;
His antidotes are poison, and he slays More than you rob.
> *Timon of Athens*, IV, iii, 434

Thomas Dekker [1572?–1632?]

He might have met with three Fencers in this time, and have received lesse hurt than by meeting one Doctor of Phisicke.
> *The Honest Whore*, Pt. I, Act IV, Sc. iv

Francis Beaumont [1584–1616] and John Fletcher [1579–1625]

The doctors are our friends; wish them no ill,
For though they kill but slow, they're certain.
> *The Spanish Curate*, Act II, Sc. i

James Howell [1594?–1666]

As *Adrian* VI said, he is very necessary to a populous country, for *were it not for the Physician, Men would live so long and grow so thick, that one could not live for the other; and he makes the Earth cover all his faults*. But what . . . Pope Adrian [said] of the physician was spoken, I conceive, in merriment.
> *Familiar Letters*, Vol. III, Letter 8

Samuel Butler [1612–1680]

Whence men are brought to Desprater distresses,
By catching Physique rather than Diseases:
Whence 'tis observed they frequently Recover
As soon as Doctors do but give them over.
> *Physique*

Molière [1622–1673]

Let us maintain agreement in the presence of our patients. Thus we may take to ourselves the credit when their maladies end happily, and put the blame on nature when they don't.
> *L'Amour Médecin*, Act III, Sc. i (tr. by John Wood)

I find [medicine]. . . one of the greatest follies of mankind; and if I look at it from a philosophical point of view,

I've never seen a sillier lot of humbuggery. I don't think there is anything more ridiculous than that one man should undertake to cure another. . . . [Doctors] have had a very good education, they know how to talk very good Latin, and how to name all the diseases in Greek, and define them and classify them; but as for curing them, that's what they don't know at all.
> *Le Malade Imaginaire*, Act III, Sc. iii (tr. by Morris Bishop)

I reckon I shall stick to Medicine for good. I find it's the best of all trades because whether you do any good or not you still get your money. We never get blamed for bad workmanship. . . . If we blunder it isn't our look out: it's always the fault of the fellow who's dead and the best part of it is that there's a sort of decency among the dead, a remarkable discretion: you never find them making any complaint against the doctor who killed them!
> *Le Médecin Malgré Lui*, Act III, Sc. i (tr. by John Wood)

He's not one of those doctors that make a market of their patients: he's a man that's expeditious, expeditious, who loves to dispatch his patients: and when they are to die, 'tis done with him the quickest in the world.
> *Monsieur de Pourceaugnac*, Act I, Sc. v

Blaise Pascal [1623–1662]

If the physicians had not their cassocks and their mules, if the doctors had not their square caps and their robes four times too wide, they would never have duped the world, which cannot resist so original an appearance.
> *Pensées*, Sect. II, No. 82 (tr. by W. F. Trotter)

John Dryden [1631–1700]

The first Physicians by Debauch were made:

Excess began, and Sloth sustains the Trade.
> *Fables Ancient and Modern*, "To John Driden of Chesterton"

Baron Gottfried Wilhelm von Leibnitz [1646–1716]

I often say a great doctor kills more people than a great general.

Sir Samuel Garth [1661–1719]

The Patient's Ears remorseless he assails,
Murthers with Jargon where his Med'cine fails.
> *The Dispensary*, Canto II

Oxford and all her passing Bells can tell,
By this Right Arm, what mighty Numbers fell.
Whilst others meanly ask'd whole Months to slay,
I oft dispatch'd the Patient in a Day:
With Pen in Hand I push'd to that degree,
I scarce had left a Wretch to give a Fee.
Some fell by *Laudanum*, and some by *Steel*,
And Death in Ambush lay in ev'ry Pill.
For save or slay, this Privilege we claim,
Tho' Credit suffers, the Reward's the same.
> *Ibid.*, Canto IV

Matthew Prior [1664–1721]

But, when the wit began to wheeze,
  And wine had warm'd the politician,
Cur'd yesterday of my disease,
  I died last night of my physician.
> *The Remedy Worse than the Disease*

Edward (Ned) Ward [1667–1731]

Physicians kill more than ever they can cure.
> *The World Bewitched*

Joseph Addison [1672–1719]

If . . . we look into the Profession of Physick, we shall find a most formidable Body of Men: The Sight of them is enough to make a Man serious, for we may lay it down as a Maxim, that when a Nation abounds in Physicians it grows thin of People.
The Spectator, Vol. I, No. 21 (March 24, 1711)

William Broome [1689–1745]

Though patients die the doctor's paid:
Licens'd to kill, he gains a palace
For what another mounts the gallows.
Poverty and Poetry

John Taylor [1694–1761]

A doctor is a man who writes prescriptions till the patient either dies or is cured by nature.

Voltaire [1694–1778]

Doctors are men who prescribe medicine of which they know little to cure diseases of which they know less in human beings of which they know nothing.

Benjamin Franklin [1706–1790]

To be hurried about perpetually from one sick chamber to another is not living. Do you please yourself with the fancy that you are doing good? Half the lives you save are not worth saving, as being useless, and almost all the other half ought not to be saved, as being mischievous. Does your conscience never hint to you the impiety of being in constant warfare against the plans of Providence?
Letter to Dr. John Fothergill, March 14, 1764

John Armstrong [1709–1779]

Many more Englishmen die by the lancet at home, than by the sword abroad.

Jean Jacques Rousseau [1712–1778]

A feeble body makes a feeble mind. Hence the influence of physic, an art which does more harm to man than all the evils it professes to cure. I do not know what the doctors cure us of, but I know this: they infect us with very deadly diseases, cowardice, timidity, credulity, the fear of death. What matter if they make the dead walk, we have no need of corpses; they fail to give us men, and it is men we need.
Émile, Bk. I (tr. by Barbara Foxley)

If you live according to Nature, are patient, and dismiss your doctors, you will not escape death, but you will feel it only once; whereas they bring it daily before your troubled imagination, and their lying art, instead of prolonging your life, only takes away your power of enjoying it.
Ibid., Bk. II

Denis Diderot [1713–1784]

The best doctor is the one you run for and can't find.

Horace Walpole [1717–1797]

I abhor physicians.
Letter to Sir Horace Mann, December 20, 1762

In physicians I believe no more than in divines.
Letter

Physicians, though they commit more deaths than soldiers, never are tried.
Letter

Tobias Smollett [1721–1771]

A young man, in whose air and countenance appeared all the uncouth gravity and supercilious self-conceit of a physician piping hot from his studies.
The Adventures of Peregrine Pickle, Ch. 42

José Julian Lopez de Castro [1723–1762]

But the King gains one great thing
If he dies of this. . . .
Freedom from doctors and prescriptions,
Which are the most rapid couriers
To the other world.
> *Mas vale tarde que nunca,* Act
> II

For where a doctor enters,
Immediately a dead man leaves.
> *Idem*

Oliver Goldsmith [1728–1774]

The people here judge as they do in the east; where it is thought absolutely requisite that a man should be an ideot before he pretend to be either a conjuror or a doctor.
> *The Citizen of the World,* Letter XXIV

Thomas Jefferson [1743–1826]

I believe we may safely affirm, that the inexperienced & presumptuous band of medical tyros let loose upon the world, destroys more of human life in one year, than all the Robinhoods, Cartouches, & MacHeaths do in a century.
> Letter to Dr. Caspar Wistar,
> June 21, 1807

It is not the physic that I object to so much as to physicians.

Johann Wolfgang von Goethe [1749–1832]

It is so hard that one cannot really have confidence in doctors and yet cannot do without them.

Joseph Jekyll [1754–1837]

The parson shows the way to heaven,
And then with tender care
The doctor consummates the work
And sends the patient there.

Gaspar Zavala y Zamora [d. 1813]

The doctor says there is no hope, and as he does the killing he ought to know.
> *El triunfo del Amor y de la Amistad,* Act II, Sc. viii

John Abernethy [1764–1831]

Abernethy, leaving his house, kicked his foot against a paving stone where the road was under repair. He shouted to a workman (who was Irish) to take it out of the way. "And where shall I take it?" asked the Irishman. "Take it to H–ll for all I care." "May be," said the Irishman, "if I take it to Heaven it will be more out of your Honor's way."
> Quoted by Howard Marsh in
> *St. Bartholomew's Hospital Journal* 2:82, 1904

Napoleon Bonaparte [1769–1821]

You medical people will have more lives to answer for in the other world than even we generals.
> Quoted by Barry O'Meara in
> *Napoleon in Exile,* September
> 29, 1817

William Wordsworth [1770–1850]

Physician art thou? — one, all eyes,
Philosopher! — a fingering slave,
One that would peep and botanize
Upon his mother's grave?
> *A Poet's Epitaph*

Sydney Smith [1771–1845]

The sixth commandment is suspended by one medical diploma from the North of England to the South.

Jean Baptiste Biot [1774–1862]

I do not see that the quality of their science becomes the more obvious for their lack of literary culture.
> Quoted by René J. Dubos in
> *Louis Pasteur, Free Lance of Science*

William Lamb, Lord Melbourne [1779–1848]

English physicians kill you, the French let you die.
> Quoted by Elizabeth Longford in *Queen Victoria*, Ch. V

William Tully [1785–1859]

"The lancet is a minute instrument of mighty mischief"—a weapon which annually slays more than the sword. . . . The King of Great Britain, without doubt, loses every year more subjects, by these means [depleting remedies], than the battle and campaign of Waterloo cost him, with all their glories.
> *Essays on Fever*, Pt. II, Essay 4

John Wilson ("Christopher North") [1785–1854]

Doctors are generally dull dogs.

Thomas Hood [1799–1845]

In fact he did not find M.D.'s
Worth one D——M.
> *Jack Hall*

Thomas Huxley [1825–1895]

Nothing is too good for the patient, provided it doesn't involve any extra effort on my part.

William Snowden Battles [1827–1895?]

For many hold 'twould be so hard
Through Heaven's gate to wheedle
A doctor as to drive a camel through
A hypodermic needle.
> *The Doctor's Dream*

Baroness Marie von Ebner-Eschenbach [1830–1916]

Physicians are hated either from conviction or from economy.
> *Aphorisms* (tr. by Mrs. Annis L. Wister)

Robert Louis Stevenson [1850–1894]

Doctors is all swabs.
> *Treasure Island*, Ch. 3

Charles L. Dana [1852–1935]

All the real, solid, elemental jests against doctors were uttered some one or two thousand years ago.

David Lloyd George [1863–1945]

The doctors are always changing their opinions. They always have some new fad.[1]
> Quoted by Lord Riddell in *War Diary*, Ch. XXXVI

Thomas Mann [1875–1955]

Indeed, the medical profession is not different from any other: its members are, for the most part, ordinary empty-headed dolts, ready to see what is not there and to deny the obvious.
> *Confessions of Felix Krull, Confidence Man*, Bk. I, Ch. VI

Franz Kafka [1883–1924]

Certainly doctors are stupid, or rather they are not more stupid than other people but their pretensions are ridiculous, nevertheless one has to count with the fact that they become more and more stupid the moment one is in their hands and what the doctor demands for the moment is neither very stupid nor impossible.
> *Letters to Milena* (tr. by Tania and James Stern)

Humbert Wolfe [1885–1940]

The doctors are a frightful race.
I can't see how they have the face
to go on practising their base
profession; but in any case
I mean to put them in their place.
> *Cursory Rhymes*, "Poems Against Doctors," I

---

[1] Comment to Lord Riddell, who had told him that an eminent surgeon suggested that people should sleep on their stomachs.

The doctor lives by chicken pox,
  by measles, and by mumps.
He keeps a microbe in a box
  and cheers him when he jumps

at unsuspecting children, who
  have two important nurses;
but if it bounds where less than two
  are kept, he simply curses.

His greed is such that though you ache
  in every limb, be sure
if there is nothing else to take,
  he'll take your temperature.

And if at first he can't succeed,
  he has another try,
and takes your pulse. Some people
  plead
  "The man must live!" But why?
    Ibid., II

Salvador de Madariaga y Rojo [1886–   ]

There is no medicine; there are only
medicine-men.
    Essays with a Purpose, "On
    Medicine"

T. S. Eliot [1888–1965]

Well I *hope* we shan't have to call a
  doctor
Doris just hates having a doctor.
    *Sweeney Agonistes, Fragment of
    a Prologue*

The Bible

And a certain woman . . . had suffered many things of many physicians,
and had spent all that she had, and was
nothing bettered, but rather grew
worse.
    Mark 5:25

The Talmud

The best of doctors will go to hell.
    Kiddushin, IV. 82a

Anonymous

First of the pedant you borrow the air,
And with a long wig cover up all of
  your hair:

Then trick out your habit with fur and
  with satin,
And constantly babble in Greek and in
  Latin.
In this combination, you'll readily see,
You've most all that's needed to be an
  M.D.
    17th-century poem

One physician cures you of the colic;
two physicians cure you of the medicine.
    Quoted by Vincent J. Derbes in
    *Journal of the American Medi-
    cal Association* 190:765, 1964

The physician walks along and the Angel of Death walks behind him with
sleeves turned up for work.

What is a doctor?
A licensed executioner.
    Mazarinade

From food twice cooked
From an ignorant doctor
From an enemy reconciled
From an evil woman
From all evil
Liberate us, Lord!
    Latin prayer

Proverb

One doctor makes work for another.

Czech Proverb

Where the sun never comes, the doctor
comes often.[1]

French Proverbs

The doctor is often more to be feared
than the disease.

Young doctors make humpy cemeteries.

German Proverb

When you call the physician, call the
judge to make your will.

[1] Chinese Proverb: When you shut out the
sun from coming through the window, the
doctor comes in at the door.

Hebrew Proverb

Do not dwell in a city whose governor is a physician.

Indian (Kashmiri) Proverb

Until a physician has killed one or two he is not a physician.[1]

Italian Proverb

He who doesn't know a trade becomes a doctor.

Medieval Latin Proverb

All idiots, priests, Jews, actors, monks, barbers and old women think they are physicians.

Portuguese Proverbs

If you have a friend who is a physician, send him to the house of your enemy.

The more doctors, the more diseases.

Spanish Proverb

Fond of lawyer, little wealth; fond of doctor, little health.

Swedish Proverb

With a young lawyer you lose your inheritance; with a young doctor your health.

IV. GOOD PHYSICIANS

Sushruta [5th Cent.? B.C.]

A physician well versed in the principles of surgery, and experienced in the practice of medicine, is alone capable of curing distempers, just as only a

two-wheeled cart can be of service in a field of battle.

> *Sushruta-Samhitá,* "Sutrasthá-nam," Ch. 3 (tr. by K. K. L. Bhishagratna)

A physician having thoroughly studied the Science of medicine, and fully pondered on and verified the truths he has assimilated, both by observation and practice, and having attained to that stage of (lucid) knowledge, which would enable him to make a clear exposition of the science (whenever necessary), should open his medical career (commence practising) with the permission of the king of his country. He should be cleanly in his habits and well shaved, and should not allow his nails to grow. He should wear white garments, put on a pair of shoes, carry a stick and an umbrella in his hands, and walk about with a mild and benignant look as a friend of all created beings, ready to help all, and frank and friendly in his talk and demeanour, and never allowing the full control of his reason or intellectual powers to be in any way disturbed or interfered with.

> *Ibid.,* Ch. 10

A physician should abjure the company of women, nor should he speak in private to them or joke with them. A physician is forbidden to take anything but cooked rice from the hands of a woman.

> *Idem*

A physician, who is well versed in the science of medicine and has attended to the demonstrations of surgery and medicine, and who himself practices the healing art, and is clean, courageous, light-handed, fully equipped with supplies of medicine, surgical instruments and appliances, and who is intelligent, well read, and is a man of ready resources, and one who commands a decent practice, and is further endowed with all moral virtues, is alone fit to be called a physician.

> *Ibid.,* Ch. 34

---

[1] Polish Proverb: Before a doctor can cure one he will kill ten.

Indian (Tamil) Proverb: He who kills a thousand people is half a doctor.

Indian (Bengali) Proverb: The destruction of a bushel of eyes makes an oculist; the destruction of one hundred patients makes a doctor; the destruction of a thousand a physician.

Hippocrates [460?–377? B.C.]

A physician who is a lover of wisdom is the equal of a god.
> *Decorum*, V (tr. by W. H. S. Jones)

The physician must have at his command a certain ready wit, as dourness is repulsive both to the healthy and to the sick.
> *Ibid.*, VII

The dignity of a physician requires that he should look healthy, and as plump as nature intended him to be; for the common crowd consider those who are not of this excellent bodily condition to be unable to take care of others. Then he must be clean in person, well dressed, and anointed with sweet-smelling unguents that are not in any way suspicious.
> *The Physician*, I (tr. by W. H. S. Jones)

Plato [427?–347 B.C.]

The best physicians are those who both know their art and have had the greatest experience of disease. They would better not be themselves too robust in health.
> *Republic*, III.408.D (tr. by Benjamin Jowett)

Herophilus [fl. 300 B.C.]

[When asked who was the most perfect physician:] He who can discriminate between what is possible and what is impossible.
> Quoted by Stobaeus in *Florilegium*, "De Medicis"

Celsus [25 B.C.–A.D. 50]

A man of few words who learns by practice to discern well, would make an altogether better practitioner than he who, unpractised, overcultivates his tongue.
> *De Medicina*, Prooemium (tr. by W. G. Spencer)

St. Isidore of Seville [560?–636]

The physician ought to know literature, to be able to understand or to explain what he reads. Likewise also rhetoric, that he may delineate in true arguments the things which he discusses; dialectic also so that he may study the causes and cures of infirmities in the light of reason. Similarly also arithmetic, in view of the temporal relationships involved in the paroxysms of diseases and in diurnal cycles.
> *Etymologiae*, IV (tr. by W. D. Sharpe)

Avicenna [980–1037]

Galen's art heals only the body,
But Abou Amram's the body and soul.
With his wisdom he could heal the sickness of ignorance.
> Quoted by Ibn Abi Usaibi'a in his biographical sketch of Maimonides

John Lydgate [1370?–1451?]

Good leche is he that himself can recure.
> *The Daunce of Machabree*

Savonarola [1452–1498]

The physician that bringeth love and charity to the sick, if he be good and kind and learned and skilful, none can be better than he. Love teacheth him everything, and will be the measure and rule of all the measures and rules of medicine.

Antonio de Guevara [1480?–1545?]

Medicine is to be praised when it is in the hands of a Phisition that is learned, grave, wise, stayed and of experience.
> *Familiar Epistles*, "Of Seven Notable Benefits Proceeding from the Good Physition" (tr. by Edward Hellows)

Paracelsus [1493?–1541]

If you wish to be a true physician you must be able to do your own thinking, and not merely employ the thoughts of others.

Sir Francis Bacon [1561–1626]

They are the best physicians, who being great in learning most incline to the traditions of experience, or being distinguished in practice do not reject the methods and generalities of art.

The Advancement of Learning, Bk. IV, Ch. II

Thomas Fuller [1608–1661]

He [the good physician] hansells not his new experiments on the bodies of his patients: letting loose mad receipts into the sick man's body. . . . To poore people he prescribes cheap but wholesome medicines: not removing the consumption out of their bodies into their purses; nor sending them to the East Indies for drugs, when they can reach better out of their gardens.

The Holy State, Ch. XVII

Voltaire [1694–1778]

Nothing is more estimable than a physician who, having studied nature from his youth, knows the properties of the human body, the diseases which assail it, the remedies that will benefit it, exercises his art with caution, and pays equal attention to the rich and the poor.

Philosophical Dictionary, "Physicians" (tr. by J. K. Hoyt)

The efficient physician is the man who successfully amuses his patients while Nature effects a cure.

John Bard [1716–1799]

A neat and simple manner of prescribing is a great proof of a physician's skill and greatly conducive to the patient's safety. . . . In your taste of clothes preserve a plain and manly fashion, as well as in your manners.

Letter to his son Samuel, February 19, 1765

Johann Wolfgang von Goethe [1749–1832]

The physician himself must be productive, if he really intends to heal; if he is not so, he will only succeed now and then, as if by chance; but, on the whole, he will be only a bungler.

Quoted by J. P. Eckermann in *Conversations with Goethe,* March 11, 1828 (tr. by J. Oxenford)

Sir Benjamin Collins Brodie [1783–1862]

You must feel and act as a gentleman. . . . But let there be no misunderstanding as to who is to be regarded as a gentleman. It is not he who is fashionable in his dress, expensive in his habits, fond of fine equipages, pushing himself into the society of those who are above himself in their worldly station, that is entitled to that appelation. It is he who sympathizes with others, and is careful not to hurt their feelings even on trifling occasions; who, in little things as well as in great, . . . assumes nothing which does not belong to him, and yet respects himself; this is the kind of gentleman which a medical practitioner should wish to be. Never pretend to know what cannot be known; make no promises which it is not probable that you will be able to fulfil; you will not satisfy every one at the moment, for many require of our art that which our art can not bestow.

Clinical Lectures on Surgery, Introductory Discourse

Integrity and generosity of character; the disposition to sympathize with others; the power of commanding your own temper, of resisting your selfish instincts; and that self respect, so important in every profession, but especially so in our own profession, which would prevent you from doing in secret what you would not do before all the world; these things are rarely acquired, except by those who have been careful to scrutinize and regulate their own conduct in the very outset of their career.

Idem

Nathaniel Hawthorne [1804–1864]

If the [physician] possess native sagacity, and a nameless something more, — let us call it intuition; if he show no intrusive egotism, nor disagreeably prominent characteristics of his own; if he have the power, which must be born in him, to bring his mind into such affinity with his patient's, . . . then, at some inevitable moment, will the soul of the sufferer be dissolved, and flow forth in a dark, but transparent stream, bringing all its mysteries into the daylight.

The Scarlet Letter, Ch. 9

Oliver Wendell Holmes [1809–1894]

The face of a physician, like that of a diplomatist, should be impenetrable.

Medical Essays, "The Young Practitioner"

John Brown [1810–1882]

Sagacity, manual dexterity, quiet reserve, a kind heart, and a conscience — these, if there at all, are always at hand, always inestimable; and if wanting, . . . I can profit my patient and myself nothing.

Horae Subsecivae

It is the lot of the successful medical practitioner, who is more occupied with discerning diseases and curing them, than with discoursing about their essence, and arranging them into systems, who observes and reflects in order to act rather than to speak, — it is the lot of such men to be invaluable when alive, and to be forgotten soon after they are dead; and this not altogether or chiefly from any special ingratitude or injustice on the part of mankind, but from the very nature of the case.

Ibid., Series I, "Locke and Sydenham"

The prime qualifications of a physician may be summed up in the words *Capax, Perspicax, Sagax, Efficax. Capax* — there must be room to receive, and arrange and keep knowledge; *Perspicax* — senses and perceptions keen, accurate, and immediate, to bring in materials from all sensible things; *Sagax* — a central power of knowing what is what and what is worth, of choosing and rejecting, of judging; and finally, *Efficax* — the will and the way — the power to turn all the other three — capacity, perspicacity, sagacity, to account, in the performance of the thing in hand, and thus rendering back to the outer world, in a new and useful form, what you have received from it.

Ibid., Series II, "With Brains, Sir"

John Ruskin [1819–1900]

They, on the whole, desire to cure the sick; and, — if they are good doctors, and the choice were fairly put to them, — would rather cure their patient and lose their fee, than kill him, and get it.

The Crown of Wild Olive

Henri Amiel [1821–1881]

To me the ideal doctor would be a man endowed with profound knowledge of life and of the soul, intuitively divining any suffering or disorder of whatever kind, and restoring peace by his mere presence.

Journal Intime, August 22, 1873 (tr. by Mrs. Humphrey Ward)

Joseph, Lord Lister [1827–1912]

I trust I may be enabled in the treatment of patients always to act with a single eye to their good, and therefore to the glory of our Heavenly Father. If a man is able to act in this spirit, and is favoured to feel something of the sustaining love of God in his work, truly the practice of surgery is a glorious occupation.

Letter to his sister Jane, March 3, 1857

Theodor Billroth [1829–1894]

He who combines the knowledge of physiology and surgery, in addition to the artistic side of his subject, reaches the highest ideal in medicine.

Quoted in *Surgery* 50:697, 1961

S. Weir Mitchell [1829–1914]

Do not think too much of the dignity of your profession or what it is beneath you to do. It is a moral disorder of young nurses and, I may add, of young doctors.

Abraham Jacobi [1830–1919]

The magnetic needle of professional rectitude should, in spite of occasional deviations, always point in the direction of pity and humanity.

James Little [1836–1885]

The first qualification for a physician is hopefulness.

Edward L. Trudeau [1848–1915]

The practicing physician and surgeon must have optimism if he is to develop a full degree of efficiency.

The Value of Optimism in Medicine

Sir William Osler [1849–1919]

Now a certain measure of insensibility is not only an advantage, but a positive necessity in the exercise of a calm judgment, and in carrying out delicate operations. Keen sensibility is doubtless a virtue of high order, when it does not interfere with steadiness of hand or coolness of nerve; but for the practitioner in his working-day world, a callousness which thinks only of the good to be effected, and goes ahead regardless of smaller considerations, is the preferable quality.

Aequanimitas, with Other Addresses, "Aequanimitas"

Acquire early the *Art of Detachment,* by which I mean the faculty of isolating yourselves from the pursuits and pleasures incident to youth.

Ibid., "Teacher and Student"

Stephen Paget [1855–1926]

Pray to the Gods, also, for a fair measure of the love of science, a good memory, a quiet manner, the accurate use of your hands and your senses, and the necessity of making money. Pray even for opposites; for humility and pride, for plodding business-ways and for the wings of ambition, for a will both stubborn and flexible: and, above all, for that one gift which has been the making of the best men in our profession, the grace of simplicity of purpose.

Confessio Medici, Ch. 7

Alfred North Whitehead [1861–1947]

One of the most advanced types of human being on earth today is the *good* American doctor. . . . he is sceptical toward the data of his own profession, welcomes discoveries which upset his previous hypotheses, and is still animated by humane sympathy and understanding.

Dialogues, Dialogue XXI (June 28, 1941)

John M. T. Finney [1863–1942]

Integrity, intelligence and industry — these three are fundamental to success in medicine, as well as in any other walk of life. Add to these certain characteristics of greater or less importance, such as a pleasing personality, tact, patience, love of his fellow man, and one's success in his chosen profession is assured.

The Physician, Ch. 5

Sir Alfred Fripp [1865–1930]

If we cannot be clever, we can always be kind.
> Quoted by C. Allan Birch in *Emergencies in Medical Practice*

Martin H. Fischer [1879–1962]

Observation, Reason, Human understanding, Courage; these make the physician.
> Quoted by Howard Fabing and Ray Marr in *Fischerisms*

Robert Haven Schauffler [1879–   ]

The ideal doctor is a judicial observer.
> Aphorism

The ideal doctor is patient.
> Aphorism

Murray H. Bass [1882–1962]

The ideal physician should be a combination of three persons — a clergyman, a fireman and a scientist. He must know how to handle and console the patient and his family. . . . he must be ready to answer an "alarm" day and night; he must know the science of medicine . . . using its present potentialities to the utmost of his ability.
> *Clinical Pediatrics* 3:50, 1964 [1]

Paul B. Magnuson [1884–   ]

Just what is a good doctor? . . . I should say the first attribute is a burning and unquenchable desire to make sick people well. That desire will surmount all sorts of difficulties. It will sacrifice comfort and convenience. Time and effort mean nothing.
> *Quarterly Bulletin of the Northwestern University Medical School* 19:7, 1945

[1] "Notes on Fifty Years of Pediatric Practice," Bass's unfinished autobiography.

William Doolin [1887–   ]

Forty years of teaching have taught me this: that it is relatively easy to become a competent specialist, but it is much more difficult to become a good doctor — and it takes much longer.
> *Lancet* 2:1364, 1958

Kenneth M. Lynch [1887–   ]

Keep always bright by using the desire to serve that all of you expressed when you sought admission to the study of medicine.

A. Benson Cannon [1889–1950]

It is a good thing for a physician to have prematurely grey hair and itching piles. The first makes him appear to know more than he does, and the second gives him an expression of concern which the patient interprets as being on his behalf.

Alan Gregg [1890–1957]

What this country needs is not a good 5-cent cigar but more medical men patterned after the ideal prototype. And what are the characteristics of that prototype? Among other things: an open mind, a burning desire to learn, and — above all — a truly creative imagination.

Dana W. Atchley [1892–   ]

[A true physician is] a scientific scholar of human biology who practices his profession as a perceptive humanist.

Sir Hugh Cairns [1896–1952]

How does one become a good doctor? When one doctor says of another, "He is a good doctor," the words have a particular meaning. You will hear the expression used not only about some general practitioners, but also about some specialists. As I understand it a good doctor is one who is shrewd in diagnosis and wise treatment; but,

more than that, he is a person who never spares himself in the interest of his patients; and in addition he is a man who studies the patient not only as a case but also as an individual. . . . The good doctor, whether general practitioner or specialist, is also a man who studies the patient's personality as well as his disease.
> *Lancet* 2:665, 1949

Paul Reznikoff [1896–   ]

A physician is judged by the three A's, Ability, Availability and Affability.
> Aphorism

Sir Theodore Fox [1899–   ]

The patient may well be safer with a physician who is naturally wise than with one who is artificially learned.
> *Lancet* 2:801, 1965

William A. R. Thomson [1906–   ]

The doctor is not primarily a scientist. He (or she) is a person who has been trained to think, to observe critically, and to realize that a human being is not a conglomeration of integrated complex systems, but an individual with a personality of his own.
> *Institute of Public Health and Hygiene* 23:290, 1960

W. H. Auden [1907–   ]

Give me a doctor partridge-plump,
Short in the leg and broad in the rump,
An endomorph with gentle hands
Who'll never make absurd demands
That I abandon all my vices
Nor pull a long face in a crisis,
But with a twinkle in his eye
Will tell me that I have to die.
> *Nones,* "Footnotes to Dr. Sheldon"

William B. Bean [1909–   ]

The one mark of maturity, especially in a physician, and perhaps it is even rarer in a scientist, is the capacity to deal with uncertainty.
> *Archives of Internal Medicine* 112:2, 1963

George A. Perera [1911–   ]

Curiosity is the hallmark of scholarship and science, but it is also the hallmark of service. Curiosity is not confined to the research laboratory; it is obligatory at the bedside as well. To act in the role of scientific advisor, to restore confidence and a measure of health to one's patient, these require an honest appraisal utilizing every available bit of evidence. Only by being curious as to basic mechanisms, with a genuine regard for who is ill, how did he become so, and why this disorder or that sign or symptom, can one become and remain a competent physician.
> *Journal of Medical Education* 38:44, 1963

Anonymous

Fifty years ago the successful doctor was said to need three things; a top hat to give him Authority, a paunch to give him Dignity, and piles to give him an Anxious Expression.
> *Lancet* 1:169, 1951

Chinese Proverb

A doctor's character should be square, his knowledge round, his gallbladder large, and his heart small.[1]

German Proverb

A lucky physician is better than a learned one.

V. BAD PHYSICIANS

Sushruta [5th Cent? B.C.]

The endeavours of a man who has studied the entire Ayurveda [medical

---

[1] A large gallbladder signifies bravery, and a small heart indicates carefulness.

scriptures] but fails to make a clear exposition of the same, are vain like the efforts of an ass that carries a load of sandal-wood (without ever being able to enjoy its pleasing scent).

> *Sushruta-Samhitá,* "Sutrasthá-nam," Ch. 4 (tr. by K. K. L. Bhishagratna)

A physician (surgeon) making a wrong operation on the body of his patient either through mistake, or through the want of necessary skill or knowledge, or out of greed, fear, nervousness or haste, or in consequence of being spurned or abused, should be condemned as the direct cause of many new and unforeseen maladies. A patient, with any instinct of self-preservation, would do well to keep aloof from such a physician, or from one who makes a wrong or injudicious application of the cautery, and should shun his presence just as he would shun a conflagration or a cup of fatal poison.

> *Ibid.,* Ch. 25

Hippocrates [460?–377? B.C.]

It is disgraceful in any art, and especially in medicine, to make parade of much trouble, display, and talk, and then do no good.

> *On Joints,* 44 (tr. by E. T. Withington)

You must also avoid adopting, in order to gain a patient, luxurious headgear and elaborate perfume. For excess of strangeness will win you ill repute, but a little will be considered in good taste.

> *Precepts,* X (tr. by W. H. S. Jones)

Seneca [4? B.C.–A.D. 65]

Only a poor physician gives up.
> *De Clementia,* I.xvii.2

Callicter

Alexis the physician purged by a clyster five patients at one time and five others by drugs; he visited five, and again he rubbed five with ointment. And for all there was one night, one medicine, one coffin-maker, one tomb, one Hades, one lamentation.

> *Greek Anthology,* IX.122 (tr. by W. R. Paton)

Galen [fl. 2nd Cent.)

That physician will hardly be thought very careful of the health of others who neglects his own.
> *Of Protecting the Health,* Bk. V

The observation that most athletes would like to win in Olympic Games, but are unwilling to undertake anything by which they might bring it about, applies equally to many physicians. They praise Hippocrates and consider him the chief of all things. They would like to emulate him, but they act in all things contrary to this. Hippocrates, for example, says that astronomy as well as that geometry which of necessity precedes it contribute significantly to medicine. Yet, physicians do not merely avoid both, but actually criticize those who devote time to these disciplines. Hippocrates emphasizes the necessity for a thorough knowledge of the nature of the body, which he establishes as the foundation of all medicine. But most physicians have studied in such a manner that they are ignorant not only of the size, structure, and relationships of the parts of the body, but indeed of where they are situated. Consequently, since the classification of diseases by types and species is unknown to them, they will therefore mistake the aims of treatment — as Hippocrates observes when he exhorts us to systematic study. To-day's physicians, however, are so averse to this course that they say that those who spend time upon it are attempting useless things.

> *Quod Optimus Medicus Sit Quoque Philosophus,* I

Avicenna [980–1037]

An ignorant doctor is the aide-de-camp of death.

Petrarch [1304–1374]

Shun the physician who is eminent not for his knowledge, but solely for his powers of speech, as you would a lurking assassin or a poisoner.
> *Invectives,* Preface, Letter to Pope Clement VI

Moreover, when the sick are dying, though the end be unfortunate, they give themselves airs by tangling up Hippocratic problems in a web of Ciceronian oratory.
> *Idem*

Sir Thomas More [1478–1535]

He is a folyshe phisition, that cannot cure his patientes disease, unless he caste him in an other syckenes.
> *Utopia,* Bk. I (tr. by R. Robinson)

Paracelsus [1493?–1541]

So great is the ill-will among physicians that each denies honour and praise to the other; they would rather harm a patient and even kill him than grant a colleague his meed of praise. From this, everyone can judge why a man has become a physician: not out of love for the patient, which should be the physician's first virtue, but for the sake of money. Where money is the goal, envy and hatred, pride and conceit, are sure to appear — and may God protect and preserve us all from such temptations!
> *Die grosse Wundarznei,* Bk. II, Conclusion (tr. by Norbert Guterman in *Selected Writings*)

There are two kinds of physician — those who work for love, and those who work for their own profit. They are both known by their works; the true and just physician is known by his love and by his unfailing love for his neighbour. The unjust physicians are known by their transgressions against the commandment; for they reap, although they have not sown, and they are like ravening wolves; they reap because they want to reap, in order to increase their profit, and they are heedless of the commandment of love.
> *Seven Defenses,* Ch. 5 (*idem*)

Michel de Montaigne [1533–1592]

They know Galen well, but the patient not at all.
> *Essays,* Bk. I, Ch. 25, "Of Pedantry" (tr. by Donald M. Frame)

William Shakespeare [1564–1616]

He brings his physic After his patient's death.
> *Henry VIII,* III, ii, 40

Izaak Walton [1593–1683]

There are too many foolish meddlers in physick and divinity that think themselves fit to meddle with hidden secrets, and so bring destruction to their followers. But I'll not meddle with them, any farther than to wish them wiser.
> *The Compleat Angler,* Pt. I, Ch. XI

Sir Thomas Browne [1605–1682]

No one should approach the temple of science with the soul of a money changer.

Thomas Jefferson [1743–1826]

When a boy, I knew a Doctor Seymour . . . who imagined he could cure the diseases of his tobacco plants; he bled some, administered lotions to others, sprinkled powders on a third class, and so on — they only withered and perished the faster.
> Letter to Dr. Benjamin Rush, March 6, 1813

Laurence Balzac [1802–1825]

This Monsieur Nacquart, with his long words, his loud laughter, his grand airs and grand pretentions, his small talent and great show of devotion, seems to me a doctor like any other. He cares precious little about his patient, and when he has run out of talk he sends you into the country or orders you back to your native air or tells you to go on a journey, it amounts to the same thing.
> Letter, 1821

Oliver Wendell Holmes [1809–1894]

A physician who talks about *ceremony* and *gratitude,* and *services rendered,* and the *treatment he got,* surely forgets himself.
> *Medical Essays,* "The Contagiousness of Puerperal Fever"

The life of a physician becomes ignoble when he suffers himself to feed on petty jealousies and sours his temper in perpetual quarrels.
> *Ibid.,* "The Young Practitioner"

George Eliot (Marian Evans Cross) [1819–1880]

Ignorance is not so damnable as humbug, but when it prescribes pills it may happen to do more harm.
> *Felix Holt,* Ch. 5

James Russell Lowell [1819–1891]

He could gauge the old books by the old set of rules,
And his very old nothings pleased very old fools;
But give him a new book, fresh out of the heart,
And you put him at sea without compass or chart.
> *A Fable for Critics*

Friedrich Nietzsche [1844–1900]

The most dangerous physicians are those who can act in perfect mimicry of the born physician.
> *Human, All Too Human,* Pt. II (tr. by Hans Waine)

Charles Warrington Earle [1845–1893]

He isn't competent and he doesn't ring true. It is well known among West Side doctors that, when this man sees that a patient is going to die, he has a sudden call out of town or is himself taken ill, or he is so busy that he can't come. So he suggests that the family get someone else. But people are on to him. When things look serious, they drop him. Perhaps you don't realize it . . . but the best doctors sign the most death certificates.
> Quoted by James B. Herrick in *Memories of Eighty Years,* Ch. 6

Sir Robert Hutchison [1871–1960]

It is unnecessary — perhaps dangerous — in medicine to be too clever.
> *Lancet* 2:61, 1938

Adam Hall [1920–   ]

We're like doctors. We can't do the job if we let pity into it.
> *The Quiller Memorandum,* Ch. 14

Anonymous

Despite all of Dr. ———'s faults, he is still an extremely difficult person to get along with.

He has steadily deteriorated for the past twenty years, and he really wasn't much in 1940.
> Overheard at a medical convention, 1960

Of all others, perhaps, the most provoking is the talkative doctor.
> Quoted by Frederick Saunders in *Salad for the Social,* "The Mysteries of Medicine"

Hebrew (Aramaic) Proverb

A doctor from a distance is like a blind eye.

Welsh Proverb

Heaven defend me from a busy doctor.

VI. DUTIES

Celsus [25 B.C.–A.D. 50]

Asclepiades said that it is the office of the practitioner to treat safely, speedily, and pleasantly.

> *De Medicina,* III.iv.1 (tr. by W. G. Spencer)

Paracelsus [1493?–1541]

This is my vow: To perfect my medical art and never to swerve from it so long as God grants me my office, and to oppose all false medicine and teachings. Then, to love the sick, each and all of them, more than if my own body were at stake. Not to judge anything superficially, but by symptoms, not to administer any medicine without understanding, nor to collect any money without earning it. Not to trust any apothecary, nor to do violence to any child. Not to guess, but to know.

> *Sketches, Notes, and Revisions,* "Jus jurandum" (tr. by Norbert Guterman in *Selected Writings*)

William Shakespeare [1564–1616]

Give physic to the sick, ease to the pained?
The poor, lame, blind, halt, creep, cry out for thee.

> *The Rape of Lucrece,* line 901

John Gregory [1725–1773]

It is as much of the business of a physician to alleviate pain, and to smooth the avenues of death, when unavoidable, as to cure diseases.

> *Lectures on the Duties and Qualifications of a Physician,* Lect. II

Benjamin Rush [1745?–1813]

While I thus wish to direct attention to everything that can improve the gentleman, the philosopher, and the man of the world so as to qualify you to mix with all those classes of people who are to be your patients to advantage, always recollect that your first duties will be to the sick, and that the physician and surgeon should predominate over all other human attainments in your character.

> Letter to his son James, June 8, 1810

Peter Mere Latham [1789–1875]

But Nature, in all her powers and operations, allows herself to be led, directed, and controlled. And to lead, direct, or control for purposes of good, this is the business of the physician.

> *Diseases of the Heart,* Lect. X

My business is to attend the sick and to aid the studies of those who seek the knowledge of disease at the bedside of the patient.

Karl F. H. Marx [1796–1877]

To support and help others on occasion is every one's whim. It is the chief end of the doctor's existence.

> Quoted by F. H. Garrison in *Bulletin of the New York Academy of Medicine* 5:156, 1929

Armand Trousseau [1801–1867]

Get that patient well.

> Quoted by F. H. Garrison in *Bulletin of the New York Academy of Medicine* 5:157, 1929

Oliver Wendell Holmes [1809–1894]

A physician's business is to avert disease, to heal the sick, to prolong life, and to diminish suffering.

> *Medical Essays,* "Scholastic and Bedside Teaching"

Thomas Laycock [1812–1876]

You have to collect evidence where no oath binds the speaker; to penetrate disguises; to sift conflicting statements; to reconcile improbabilities. Without the power to experimentalize — that is, to vary at will the circumstances, so as to disentangle the essential from the non-essential, or without even the power to cross-examine, you must come to a conclusion; often with but a moment for deliberation, you must act. And when you have determined what is to be done under the circumstances, still you will usually have no power to compel to the necessary course of conduct, except through those motives to action which are consonant with the hopes, the fears, the prejudices of your patient. To investigate a case rightly, and to secure that the necessary measures be executed promptly and fully, you must be able to judge quickly as to these motives. This judgment can only be founded on a thorough knowledge of human nature, and this knowledge and the use of it, therefore, constitute important elements of professional skill and tact.
> *Lectures on the Principles and Methods of Medical Observation and Research,* Introduction

Sir James Paget [1814–1899]

Your responsibilities are as various as are the ills that flesh is heir to; they are as deep as the earnestness with which men long to be delivered from suffering, or from the grasp of death. Why, we sometimes see the beam of life and death so nearly balanced, that it turns this way or that, according to the more or less skill that may be cast into the scale of life.
> *Memoirs and Letters,* "On the Motives to Industry in the Study of Medicine"

Sir William Osler [1849–1919]

To prevent disease, to relieve suffering and to heal the sick — this is our work.
> *Aequanimitas, with Other Addresses,* "Chauvinism in Medicine"

Our mission is of the highest and of the noblest kind, not alone in curing disease but in educating the people in the laws of health, and in preventing the spread of plagues and pestilences.
> *Ibid.,* "Teaching and Thinking"

J. Chalmers Da Costa [1863–1933]

The days of waiting for practice are very hard and very dangerous. Those days may make a man or mar him. The same wind which blows out the penny dip urges the flames of the forest fire. Those days go far in determining what sort of man he is and is to be. During them he should study ceaselessly, learn to work, to observe, to think, and to teach himself. He should ponder deeply and often on the responsibilities and the duties of his calling. Thus he should become a real man, an individual, a man with genuine ideas, definite beliefs, established principles, and high ideals.
> *New York Medical Journal* 101:709, 1915

Richard Clarke Cabot [1868–1939]

The job of the physician as a physician and teacher is not just to tell but to convince.
> Quoted by David Seegal in *Journal of Medical Education* 39:1030, 1964

Martin H. Fischer [1879–1962]

A doctor must work eighteen hours a day and seven days a week. If you cannot console yourself to this, get out of the profession.
> Quoted by Howard Fabing and Ray Marr in *Fischerisms*

Robert de Vernéjoul [1890–]

The first duty of the doctor is in all cases and all circumstances to respect

the personality of the patient who places himself in his hands.
> *Medical Tribune,* August 31, 1964

Anonymous

These are the duties of a physician: First . . . to heal his mind and to give help to himself before giving it to anyone else.
> Epitaph of an Athenian Doctor, A.D. 2 (Quoted in the *Journal of the American Medical Association* 189:989, 1964)

To cure sometimes, to relieve often, to comfort always.[1]

VII. REWARDS AND SORROWS

Sushruta [5th Cent.? B.C.]

By doing good to humanity with his professional skill, a physician achieves glory, and acquires the plaudits of the good and the wise in this life, and shall live in Paradise in the next.
> *Sushruta-Samhitá,* "Sutrasthánam," Ch. 25 (tr. by K. K. L. Bhishagratna)

Hippocrates [460?–377? B.C.]

The medical man sees terrible sights, touches unpleasant things, and the misfortunes of others bring a harvest of sorrows that are peculiarly his.
> *Breaths,* I (tr. by W. H. S. Jones)

Laurence Sterne [1713–1768]

There are worse occupations in this world *than feeling a woman's pulse.*
> *A Sentimental Journey,* Bk. I, Ch. 33

William Hunter [1718–1783]

The little good I have done is that which has cost me the greatest trouble and has encountered the most numerous obstacles.

Thomas Jefferson [1743–1826]

The physician is happy in the attachment of the families in which he practises. All think he has saved some one of them, and he finds himself everywhere a welcome guest, a home in every house. If, to the consciousness of having saved some lives, he can add that of having at no time, from want of caution, destroyed the boon he was called on to save, he will enjoy, in age, the happy reflection of not having lived in vain.
> Letter to Judge David Campbell, January 28, 1810

Samuel Bartlett Parris [1806-1827]

A richer pleasure, earth cannot afford
Than when it is your lot, a friend to save
From sinking down to his untimely grave.
> *Anticipations and Recollections,* Pt. I

Sir James Young Simpson [1811–1870]

If you follow these the noble objects of your profession in a proper spirit of love and kindness to your race, the pure light of benevolence will shed around the path of your toils and labours a brightness and beauty, that will faithfully cheer you onwards, and keep your steps from being weary in well doing — while, if you practice the art that you profess with a cold-hearted view to its results merely as a matter of lucre and trade, your course will be as dark and miserable, as that low and groveling love that dictates it.
> *Physicians and Physic,* Ch. 1

---

[1] Guerir quelquefois, soulager souvent, consoler toujours.
This folk saying, dating to the fifteenth century or earlier, is inscribed on Gutzon Borglum's statue of Dr. Edward Livingston Trudeau at Saranac Lake, N.Y.

I prefer to have my reward in the gratitude of my patients.

Rudolf Virchow [1821–1902]

You can soon become so engrossed in study, then professional cares, in getting and spending, you may so lay waste your powers that you find too late with hearts given away that there is no place in your habit-stricken souls for those gentler influences that make life worth living.

William Snowden Battles
[1827–1895?]

I dreamed of all the ups and downs
  Of thirty years of practice,
That brought with many a scented
    rose,
Its compensating cactus. . . .

About the doctors and their bills,
  The good and bad we did,
The lives our skill so often saved,
  Mistakes the earth had hid.
    The Doctor's Dream

Joseph, Lord Lister [1827–1912]

If we had nothing but pecuniary rewards and worldly honours to look to, our profession would not be one to be desired. But in its practice you will find it to be attended with peculiar privileges; second to none in intense interest and pure pleasures. It is our proud office to tend the fleshly tabernacle of the immortal spirit, and our path, if rightly followed, will be guided by unfettered truth and love unfeigned.
    Graduation address, 1876

I must confess that highly, and very highly, as I esteem the honours which have been conferred upon me, I regard that all worldly distinctions are as nothing in comparison with the hope that I may have been the means of reducing in some degree the sum of human misery.
    Address at Edinburgh, June 1898

Theodor Billroth [1829–1894]

The pleasure of a physician is little, the gratitude of patients is rare, and even rarer is material reward, but these things will never deter the student who feels the call within him.

Jacob M. Da Costa [1833–1900]

An aspiration of every true physician is that the time may come when he shall have no incurable cases; when old age alone shall baffle him. Do not think that, especially in encountering acute disease, you will ever see the day when you can feel other than distress at what you know must prove, with the means of resistance which we possess, an unequal and futile struggle. The youngest of us who to-day holds his newly-won diploma will have in his first unsuccessful case no deeper sense of misery than he who has had the experience of half a century. I declare I have known men of wide learning and of great and tried skill who could neither eat nor sleep when contending with a dangerous malady. I have seen those who never flinched for a moment while anything was to be done, depressed and worn by the knowledge of the inevitable result. . . . Can the time come when you will see without emotion a child suffocating with croup and be aware that not even an operation offers more than the faintest chance? Can you watch placidly the horrible struggles of lockjaw? Can you witness without distress the gasping for breath in an organic disease of the heart? If you can, you had better leave the profession: cast your diploma into the fire; you are not worthy to hold it.
    College and Clinical Record
    12:103, 1891

Sir Clifford Allbutt [1836–1925]

In all honest work there is ultimate good, but in Medicine the rewards of devotion, of forgetting self in helping the sick and sorrowful, are more immediate; the harvest is gathered on the field.

William Henry Drummond
[1854–1907]

Ole Docteur Fiset of Saint Anicet,
  Sapré tonnerre! he was leev long
  tam!
I'm sure he's got ninety year or so,
Beat all on de Parish 'cept Pierre
  Courteau,
  An' day affer day he work all de
  sam'.

But Docteur Fiset, not moche fonne
  he get,
  Drivin' all over de whole contree,
If de road she's bad, if de road she's
  good,
W'en ev'ryt'ing's drown on de Spring-
  tam flood,
  An' workin' for not'ing half tam'
  mebbe!
      The Habitant and Other Poems,
      "Ole Docteur Fiset"

Stephen Paget [1855–1926]

The natural dignity of our work, its unembarrassed kindness, its insight into life, its hold on science — for these privileges, and for all that they bring with them, up and up, high over the top of the tree, the very heavens open, preaching thankfulness.
      Confessio Medici, Epilogue

J. Chalmers Da Costa [1863–1933]

Objectionable people are numerous. They have one trait in common, that is, a most unfortunate tendency to longevity. Few die and none resign. They haunt physicians' offices. Among them I would mention: That breathing outrage, the fierce female who glares petrifaction on all who enter the private office ahead of her.

The human disaster who constantly borrows trouble and pays some of it off to you whenever he calls.

That unescapable calamity, the doc-

tor who has a row on his hands and wants to get you into it.

The lawyer whose client has traumatic neurasthenia and wants to sue a street car company. . . .

The life insurance agent. . . .

The religious beggar who has a mission and a peculiar hat. . . .

The patient who is always late and catches you just as you are ready to leave. . . .

The sexual hypochondriac who desires to describe it all. The drug agent loaded down with specimens. The patient who does not know when to leave. . . . The book agent. . . . The man who wants to sell mining stock.
      Selected Papers and Speeches,
      "Behind the Office Doors"

Rudyard Kipling [1865–1936]

The world . . . has long ago decided that you have no working hours that anybody is bound to respect, and nothing except extreme bodily illness will excuse you in its eyes from refusing to help a man who thinks he may need your help at any hour of the day or night. Nobody will care whether you are in your bed or in your bath, on your holiday or at the theatre.
      A Doctor's Work, address to
      students at London's Middlesex
      Hospital, October 1, 1908

Carl Augustus Hamann
[1868–1930]

The people in this world put on a tremendous show, and doctors have a front row seat.
      Aphorism

John McCrae [1872–1918]

It will be in your power every day to store up for yourselves treasures that will come back to you in the consciousness of duty well done, of kind acts performed, things that having given away freely you yet possess. It has often seemed to me that when in the Judgment those surprised faces look up and say, Lord, when saw we Thee ahungered and fed Thee; or thirsty and gave Thee drink; a stranger and took Thee in; naked and clothed Thee; and there meets them that warrant-royal of all charity, Inasmuch as ye did it unto one of the least of these, ye have done it unto Me, there will be amongst those awed ones many a practitioner of medicine.

> Address at McGill University (Quoted by Sir Andrew Mac-Phail in "An Essay in Character" in *In Flanders Field and Other Poems*)

Wilfred Trotter [1872–1939]

The good doctor . . . will find that the world gives him little attention except to impose restrictions and to exact responsibilities, and he will find his patients but little able to co-operate with him, uneasy and subject to strange moods. But he will not be without consolations: first, the knowledge that its difficulties make his task one fit for grown men in a real world; and secondly, in co-operation with his single steady friend — the natural power of the body to resist injury and disease. It is in work with this inimitable ally that he will earn his least corruptible reward.

> *Collected Papers*, "Emergency," Sect. viii

Hans Carossa [1878–1956]

"Who would become a physician if he could foresee the hardships which are in store for him?" However justified, this question — asked by the aging Goethe — has surely not kept anyone from studying medicine. As to the hardships, they are likely to be spread out over long stretches of life, and they are rarely disastrous. Guilt and grief caused by lack of concern or lack of concentration are far worse than hardships.

> *Der Tag des jungen Artzes* (tr. by Max Samter)

Martin H. Fischer [1879–1962]

In my experience no good doctor was ever asked to stay hungry, cold, or unliquored for long.

> Quoted by Howard Fabing and Ray Marr in *Fischerisms*

Life is a ticket to the greatest show on earth. As a doctor you'll have a front seat.

> *Idem*

The most self-satisfying thought left the physician is that he does not have to rush with any crowd.

> *Idem*

Carlton K. Matson [1890–1948]

But a doctor who has gone into lonely and discouraged homes, where there was fear for the sick, and no one else at hand to administer remedy, and give hope, can really say, "I amount to something. I'm worth while."

> *The Cleveland Press*

W. Russell, Lord Brain [1895–1966]

The doctor occupies a seat in the front row of the stalls of the human drama, and is constantly watching, and even intervening in, the tragedies, comedies and tragi-comedies which form the raw material of the literary art.

> Foreword to R. Coope's *The Quiet Art: A Doctor's Anthology*

David Seegal [1899–]

Although many members of the medical profession might agree that their chosen discipline often leads to periods of weariness, frustration, or anxiety, the great majority of individuals in active practice would find it difficult to single out a dull day in their way of life.

> *Yale Scientific Magazine* 36:31, 1962

Merrill Moore [1903–1957]

If the average man is a harp on whom Nature occasionally plays, the physician is an instrument on whom the emotions are played continuously during his waking hours and that is not too good for any man.

>Epilogue to Mary Lou Mc-Donough's *Poet Physicians*

Charles L. Hudson [1904–   ]

I am at my desk, having just returned from seeing a patient . . . who is alive and at the moment well because of the miracle of medical progress. In recalling her happiness and the look of fondness and gratitude she gave me, I cannot help reaching out in appreciation to those persons, some known to me and many unknown, whose efforts have permitted me this, the supreme reward to the physician.

>*Journal of Medical Education* 40 (Pt. 2): 11, 1965

Lindsay E. Beaton [1911–   ]

We are physicians. It is a proud title. It carries prerogatives; it carries privileges. Most of all it carries accountability, not only for the future of a great profession but for the very lives of our fellow sufferers from the human condition. We would not fail these responsibilities for any personal advantage. If we do fail, we fail the sick. If we fail, we fail the well. If we fail, we fail ourselves. If we fail, we fail mankind. But if we succeed in taking a step toward our own grail, we shall illumine the brightest page in medical history. The brightest, for such must be our faith, until the next is turned.

>*Journal of Medical Education* 40:35, 1965

Italian Proverb

If the patient dies, it is the doctor who has killed him, and if he gets well, it is the saints who have cured him.

VIII. PHYSICIANS AS PATIENTS

Aeschylus [525–456 B.C.]

Thou art forsaken of thy wits and art gone astray; and like an unskilled leech, fallen ill, thou losest heart and canst not discover what remedies to minister to thine own disease.

>*Prometheus Bound,* 471 (tr. by H. W. Smyth)

Philemon [361?–263? B.C.]

Doctors order for their patients a strict regime; when they themselves are ill in bed they do everything that they have forbidden to others.

>Fragment (Quoted by Stobaeus in *Florilegium,* CII.4)

Huai-nan Tzu (Liu An) [d. 122 B.C.]

Doctors cannot cure their own complaints.

Sulpicius [d. 43 B.C.]

Do not imitate bad physicians who, in treating the diseases of others, profess to have mastered the whole art of healing, but themselves they cannot cure.

>Letter to Cicero collected in Cicero's *Epistulae ad familiares,* IV.v.5 (tr. by W. Glynn Williams)

François Rabelais [1494?–1553]

We entrust . . . our bodies to physicians, who, to a man, loathe medicine and refuse to take physics.

>*Pantagruel,* Bk. III, Ch. XXIX (tr. by Jacques Le Clercq)

William Shakespeare [1564–1616]

He will be the physician that should be the patient.

>*Troilus and Cressida,* II, iii, 223

Ivan Turgenev [1818–1883]

As to how I am, well, a respectable doctor is never sick. If ever anything

happens to him, he dies at once, and that is all.
> *A Month in the Country*, Act I

Stephen Paget [1855–1926]

You cannot be a perfect doctor, till you have been a patient.
> *Confessio Medici*, Ch. 7

George Bernard Shaw [1856–1950]

The most tragic thing in the world is a sick doctor.
> *The Doctor's Dilemma*, Act I

Thomas Mann [1875–1955]

He had settled down as one of the physicians who are companions in suffering to the patients in their care; who do not stand above disease, fighting her in the armour of personal security, but who themselves bear her mark — an odd, but by no means isolated case, and one which has its good as well as its bad side.
> *The Magic Mountain*, Ch. IV, "Doubts and Considerations" (tr. by H. T. Lowe-Porter)

Sympathy between doctor and patient is surely desirable, and a case might be made out for the view that only he who suffers can be the guide and healer of the suffering. And yet — can true spiritual mastery over a power be won by him who is counted among her slaves? Can he free others who himself is not free? The ailing physician remains a paradox to the average mind, a questionable phenomenon. May not his scientific knowledge tend to be clouded and confused by his own participation, rather than enriched and morally reinforced? He cannot face disease in clear-eyed hostility to her; he is a prejudiced party, his position is equivocal. With all due reserve it must be asked whether a man who himself belongs among the ailing can give himself to the cure or care of others as can a man who is himself entirely sound.
> *Idem*

The Bible

Physician, heal thyself.
> *Luke* 4:23

Proverb

Doctors make the very worst patients.

Chinese Proverb

No man is a good doctor who has never been sick himself.[1]

Italian Proverb

No good doctor ever takes physic.

IX. YOUNG AND OLD

Thomas Percival [1740–1804]

A Physician who is advancing in years, yet unconscious of any decay in his faculties, may occasionally experience some change in the wonted confidence of his friends. Patients, who before trusted solely to his care and skill, may now request that he will join in consultation, perhaps with a younger coadjutor. It behooves him to admit this change without dissatisfaction or fastidiousness, regarding it as no mark of disrespect, but as the exercise of a just and reasonable privilege in those by whom he is employed.
> *Medical Ethics*, Ch. 2

James Gregory [1753–1821]

Young men kill their patients; old men let them die.
> Quoted by John Brown in *Horae Subsecivae*, Series I, "Locke and Sydenham"

Daniel Drake [1785–1852]

The first acts of a graduate are apt to be his precedents through coming years, for there is no era in his life in which his self-complacency is so exalted, as the time which passes between

---

[1] Cf. Stephen Paget, p. 588a; Proverb, p. 592b.

receiving his diploma with its blue ribbon, and receiving crape and gloves, to wear at the funeral of his first patient.
Western Journal of Medicine and Surgery 2:354, 1844

Oliver Wendell Holmes
[1809–1894]

The old age of a physician is one of the happiest periods of his life. He is loved and cherished for what he has been, and even in the decline of his faculties there are occasions when his experience is still appealed to, and his trembling hands are looked to with renewing hope and trust.
Medical Essays, "The Young Practitioner"

The young man knows the rules, but the old man knows the exceptions. . . . The young man feels uneasy if he is not continually doing something to stir up his patient's internal arrangements. The old man takes things more quietly, and is much more willing to let well enough alone.
Idem

He had, in fact, an ancient, mildewed air,
A long gray beard, a plenteous lack of hair, —
The musty look that always recommends
Your good old Doctor to his ailing friends.
Talk of your science! after all is said
There's nothing like a bare and shiny head;
Age lends the graces that are sure to please;
Folks want their doctors mouldy, like their cheese.
Rip Van Winkle, M.D., Canto II

Sir William Osler [1849–1919]

The killing vice of the young doctor is intellectual laziness.
Aequanimitas, with Other Addresses, "On the Educational Value of the Medical Society"

G. K. Chesterton [1874–1936]

That combination of *savoir-faire* with a sort of well-groomed coarseness which is not uncommon in young doctors.
The Man Who Was Thursday, Ch. V

Alan Gregg [1890–1957]

Know you what it is to be sixty?
It is to believe in love, to believe
in loveliness, to believe in belief —
all as never before: it is to be so
old that young men can reach
to whisper in your ear; it is to turn
RF [1] funds into coaches and mice into men
and timidity into self-confidence,
ambition into unselfishness and dreams into realities;
for every old doctor has a fairy godmother in his own soul;
it is to live in an office and count
yourself the link between youth and knowledge
and immeasurable compassion.[2]
Quoted by Wilder Penfield in *The Difficult Art of Giving,* Ch. 21

Ben Hecht [1894–1964]

There is nothing as pleasing to a graying medicine man as the opportunity of slapping a dunce-cap on the young of science.
Miracle of the Fifteen Murderers

Thornton Wilder [1897–   ]

Doctors are mostly impostors. The older a doctor is and the more venerated he is, the more he must pretend to know everything. Of course, they grow worse with time. Always look for a doctor who is hated by the best doctors. Always seek out a bright young doctor before he comes down with nonsense.

[1] Rockefeller Foundation, of which Gregg was Director of the Division of Medical Sciences.
[2] Gregg wrote this poem, which he labeled "After Francis Thompson on Shelley," a week after his sixtieth birthday.

David Seegal [1899–   ]

Emeritus
Quit making fuss;
You've had your say.
Hand others clay
To shape *their* way.
Banish dismay.
Write sonnets gay.[1]
New England Journal of Medicine 272:487, 1965

Paul Kimmelstiel [1900–   ]

[When asked why he was not wearing his name badge at the Third International Congress of Nephrology, September 27, 1966:] I'm so tired of having people read it and then say, "I thought you were dead!" [2]

Proverb

Beware of the young doctor and the old barber.

French Proverb

If youth only knew! If age only could!

French and Italian Proverb

A surgeon should be young, a physician old.

X. FICTIONAL

Geoffrey Chaucer [1340?–1400]

With us ther was a Doctour of Phisik; [3]
In al this world ne was ther noon hym
  lik,
To speke of phisik and of surgerye,
For he was grounded in astronomye.
He kepte his pacient a ful greet deel
In houres by his magyk natureel.
Wel koude he fortunen the ascendent

Of his ymages for his pacient.
He knew the cause of everich maladye,
Were it of hoot, or coold, or moyste, or
  drye,
And where they engendred, and of what
  humour.
He was a verray, parfit praktisour.
The Canterbury Tales, Prologue

William Shakespeare [1564–1616]

This young gentlewoman had a father [Dr. Gerard de Narbon] . . . whose skill was almost as great as his honesty; had it stretch'd so far, would have made nature immortal, and death should have play for lack of work. Would for the King's sake he were living! I think it would be the death of the King's disease. . . . He was famous, sir, in his profession, and it was his great right to be so. . . . He was skilful enough to have liv'd still, if knowledge could set up against mortality.
All's Well That Ends Well, I, i, 19

Hundreds call themselves
Your creatures, who by you have been
  restor'd;
And not your knowledge, your personal
  pain, but even
Your purse, still open, hath built Lord
  Cerimon
Such strong renown as time shall never
  raze.
Pericles, III, ii, 44

Alain René Lesage [1668–1747]

Sir, said I, one evening, to Doctor Sangrado, I call Heaven to witness on the spot that I have never strayed from your infallible method; and yet I have never saved a patient: one would think they died out of spite. . . . My good lad, replied he, my experience nearly comes to the same point. It is but seldom I have the pleasure of curing my kind and partial friends. If I had less confidence in my principles, I should think my prescriptions had set their faces against the work they were

---

[1] Lines written shortly after the author became emeritus.
[2] The "Kimmelstiel-Wilson" lesion was described in 1936.
[3] John of Gaddesden, Fellow of Merton College at Oxford, is supposedly the original of Chaucer's "Doctour of Phisik."

intended to perform. If you will take a hint, sir, replied I, we had better vary our system. Let us give, by way of experiment, chemical preparations to our patients: the worst they can do is to tread in the steps of our pure dilutions and phlebotomizing evacuations. I would willingly give it a trial, rejoined he, if it were a matter of indifference, but I have published on the practice of bleeding and the use of drenches: would you have me cut the throat of my own fame as an author! O, you are in the right, resumed I; our enemies must not gain this triumph over us; they would say that you are out of conceit with your own systems, and would ruin your reputation for inconsistency. Perish the people, perish rather our nobility and clergy! But let us go in the old path. . . .

We went on working double tides, and did so much execution, that in less than six weeks we made as many widows and orphans as the siege of Troy.

> *The Adventures of Gil Blas de Santillana,* Bk. II, Ch. 5 (tr. by Tobias Smollett)

Laurence Sterne [1713–1768]

Imagine to yourself a little, squat, uncourtly figure of a Doctor Slop, of about four feet and a half perpendicular height, with a breadth of back and a sesquipedality of belly, which might have done honour to a serjeant in the horse-guards.

> *Tristram Shandy,* Vol. II, Ch. 9

Oliver Goldsmith [1728–1774]

A man he was, to all the country dear,
And passing rich with forty pounds a
    year.

> *The Deserted Village*

Henry Wadsworth Longfellow [1807–1882]

Forth then issued Hiawatha,
Wandered eastward, wandered west-
    ward,
Teaching men the use of simples

And the antidotes for poisons,
And the cure of all diseases.

> *The Song of Hiawatha,* Pt. XV

Charles Dickens [1812–1870]

Mr. Bayham Badger, who had a good practice at Chelsea, and attended a large public Institution besides . . . was a pink, fresh-faced, crisp-looking gentleman, with a weak voice, white teeth, light hair, and surprised eyes: some years younger, I should say, than Mrs. Bayham Badger. He admired her exceedingly, but principally, and to begin with, on the curious ground (as it seemed to us) of her having had three husbands.

> *Bleak House,* Ch. 13

He [Mr. Chillip, the doctor] was the meekest of his sex, the mildest of little men. He sidled in and out of a room, to take up the less space. He walked as softly as the Ghost in Hamlet, and more slowly. He carried his head on one side, partly in modest depreciation of himself, partly in modest propitiation of everybody else.

> *David Copperfield,* Ch. 1

Doctor Parker Peps, one of the Court Physicians, and a man of immense reputation for assisting at the increase of great families, was walking up and down the drawing-room with his hands behind him, to the unspeakable admiration of the family Surgeon.

> *Dombey and Son,* Ch. 1

John Jobling, Esquire, M.R.C.S., [Medical Officer of the Anglo-Bengalee Disinterested Loan and Life Assurance Company] . . . had a portentously sagacious chin, and a pompous voice, with a rich huskiness in some of its tones that went directly to the heart, like a ray of light shining through the ruddy medium of choice old burgundy.

> *Martin Chuzzlewit,* Ch. 27

With which parting injunction, slowly and portentously delivered, the doctor departed, leaving the whole house in admiration of that wisdom which tallied so closely with their own. Everybody said he was a shrewd doctor indeed, and knew perfectly what people's constitutions were; which there appears some reason to suppose he did.

The Old Curiosity Shop, Ch. 46

Mr. Losberne, a surgeon in the neighbourhood, known through a circuit of ten miles round as "the doctor," had grown fat: more from good-humour than from good living: and was as kind and hearty, and withal as eccentric an old bachelor, as will be found in five times that space, by any explorer alive.

Oliver Twist, Ch. 29

George Eliot (Marian Evans Cross) [1819–1880]

The moment of vocation had come. . . . the world was made new to him. . . . From that hour Lydgate felt the growth of an intellectual passion.[1]

Middlemarch, Ch. 15

Lydgate's hair never became white. He died when he was only fifty, leaving his wife and children provided for by a heavy insurance on his life. He had gained an excellent practice, alternating, according to the season, between London and a Continental bathing-place; having written a treatise on Gout, a disease which has a good deal of wealth on its side. His skill was relied on by many paying patients, but he always regarded himself as a failure: he had not done what he once meant to do.

Ibid., Ch. 86

Sir Arthur Conan Doyle [1859–1930]

Good old Watson! You are the one fixed point in a changing age.

His Last Bow, Ch. VIII

[1] Reading for the first time of the wonders of the heart valves.

"Excellent!" I cried.
"Elementary," he said.

Memoirs of Sherlock Holmes, "The Crooked Man"

Richard Austin Freeman [1862–1943]

Thorndyke [of King's Bench Walk, Inner Temple, London] is a unique figure in the legal world. He is a barrister and a doctor of medicine. In the one capacity he is probably the greatest criminal lawyer of our time. In the other he is, among other things, the leading authority on poisons and on crimes connected with them; and so far as I know, he has never made a mistake.

As a Thief in the Night, Ch. IX

Stephen Vincent Benét [1898–1943]

[Doc Mellhorn, when asked by the reception clerk what he would like to do first:] "I think I'd like to sit down."

Doc Mellhorn and the Pearly Gates

XI. NAMED PHYSICIANS AND SCIENTISTS [1]

Jonathan Swift [1667–1745]

Removed from kind Arbuthnot's [2] aid,
Who knows his art, but not the trade,
Preferring his regard for me
Before his credit, or his fee.

In Sickness

Bliss Carman [1861–1929]

Arnoldus Villanova,[3]
Though earth is growing old,
As long as life has longing

[1] This subcategory is arranged alphabetically by the subjects' names rather than chronologically.
[2] Dr. John Arbuthnot [1667–1735], friend of Swift and Alexander Pope.
[3] Arnold of Villanova [1235?–1312?], a distinguished physician of the School of Montpellier, wrote an influential commentary on the School of Salerno's *Regimen Sanitatis Salernitanum.*

Your guess at truth will hold.
Still works the hidden power
After a thousand springs, —
The medicine for heartache
That lurks in lovely things.
          The Green Oasis, "Peony"

Sir Arthur Conan Doyle [1859–1930]

The most notable of the characters I met was one Joseph Bell,[1] surgeon at the Edinburgh Infirmary. . . . He was a very skillful surgeon, but his strong point was diagnosis, not only of disease, but of occupation and character. . . . In one of his best cases he said to a civilian patient: "Well, my man, you've served in the Army?" "Aye, sir."

"Not long discharged?" "No, sir."
"A Highland regiment?" "Aye, sir."
"A non-com. officer." "Aye, sir."
"Stationed at Barbados?" "Aye, sir."

"You see, Gentlemen," he would explain, "the man was respectful but did not remove his hat. They do not in the army, but he would have learned civilian ways had he been long discharged. He has an air of authority and he is obviously Scottish. As to Barbados, his complaint is elephantiasis, which is West Indian and not British."
          Memories and Adventures, Ch. 3

Martin H. Fischer [1879–1962]

Claude Bernard holds first rank among my gods.
          Quoted by Howard Fabing and
          Ray Marr in *Fischerisms*

René J. Dubos [1901–   ]

Claude Bernard, although trained in the Paris School of Medicine during its period of greatest clinical glory, shared Pasteur's irritation at his medical colleagues. Have you noticed, he would say, how physicians, when walking into a room, always carry about themselves

---

an air that seems to imply "Look at me, I have just saved another life"? . . . Today Pasteur and Bernard might find material for their scorn in the scientist who, unmindful of the long history of the world prior to his efforts, entertains the illusion that his last experiment will open a new era in thought.
          *Louis Pasteur, Free Lance of
          Science*, Ch. III

S. Weir Mitchell [1829–1914]

He [John Shaw Billings] was asked how many degrees he had received, and when they began to count the LL.D.'s and B.C.L.'s, he laughed and said, "Yes, that is my principal title to be considered a man of letters."
          British Medical Journal 2:686,
          1913

Sir Andrew MacPhail [1864–1938]

[Hermann] Boerhaave lectured five hours a day; his hospital contained only twelve beds, but by Sydenham's method he made of it the medical centre of Europe.
          British Medical Journal 1:445,
          1933

Frederick Irving [1883–1957]

When in 1738 the great Dutch physician Boerhaave died he left an elaborately bound book which was said to contain all the secrets of medicine. Upon opening the volume all the pages were found blank but one, and on that was written, "Keep the head cool, the feet warm, and the bowels open."
          Safe Deliverance, Pt. 2, Ch. 2

Izaak Walton [1593–1683]

We may say of angling, as Dr. Boteler[1] said of strawberries, "Doubtless God could have made a better berry, but doubtless God never did;" and so, (if I

---

[1] Dr. Bell, one of Doyle's professors, was the model for Sherlock Holmes.

[1] Dr. Boteler is William Butler [1535–1618], referred to by Thomas Fuller in *Worthies of England* as the "Aesculapius of our age."

might be judge) "God never did make a more calm, quiet, innocent recreation than angling."
> *The Compleat Angler* (5th ed.), Ch. V

George Gordon, Lord Byron [1788–1824]

Though nature's sternest painter, yet the best.[1]
> *English Bards and Scotch Reviewers*

John Tyndall [1820–1893]

Mr. Charles Darwin, the Abraham of scientific men, a searcher as obedient to the command of truth as was the patriarch to the command of God.
> *Fragments of Science for Unscientific People* (1892), "Science and Man"

Anonymous

He would have been known to the world as a Patriot, had he not been known as something greater — a Physician.
> Inscription on the statue of Dr. W. E. B. Davis, Birmingham, Alabama, unveiled in 1904

John Shaw Billings [1838–1913]

Dr. [Daniel] Drake was a great organizer, and a great disorganizer, a founder and a founderer.
> *Cincinnati Lancet-Clinic* 20: 297, 1888

Jean Martin Charcot [1825–1893]

How is it that, one fine morning, Duchenne discovered a disease [2] which probably existed in the time of Hippocrates?

Jerome Meyers [1883–]

Thy spirit ne'er shall bear the badge of death,

[1] George Crabbe [1754–1832].
[2] Pseudohypertrophic muscular paralysis.

For thou hast saved, and not destroyed in strife,
And thou hast conquered death, and given life.
> *Sonnet on the Death of Paul Ehrlich*

John Tyndall [1820–1893]

When an experimental result was obtained by [Michael] Faraday it was instantly enlarged by his imagination. I am acquainted with no mind whose power and suddenness of expansion at the touch of new physical truth could be ranked with his. Sometimes I have compared the action of his experiments on his mind to that of highly combustible matter thrown into a furnace; every fresh entry of fact was accompanied by the immediate development of light and heat. The light, which was intellectual, enabled him to see far beyond the boundaries of the fact itself, and the heat, which was emotional, urged him to the conquest of this newly-revealed domain.
> *Faraday as a Discoverer*, "Magnetism of Flame and Gases"

W. I. B. Beveridge [1908–]

When I asked Sir Alexander Fleming about his views on research his reply was that he was not doing research when he discovered penicillin, he was just playing.
> *The Art of Scientific Investigation*, Ch. XI

Sophie Kerr [1880–1965]

Freud and his three slaves, Inhibition, Complex and Libido.
> *The Saturday Evening Post*, April 9, 1932, "If Only He Wouldn't"

Henri de Mondeville [1260–1320]

God did not exhaust all his creative power in making Galen.

Thomas Hobbes [1588–1679]

[William Harvey] is the only man, I

know that, conquering envy, hath established a new Doctrine in his lifetime.
> *Elements of Philosophy*, "Concerning Body," Dedication (tr. by W. Molesworth)

Sir Robert Platt [1900–   ]

Even the lessons of Harvey had little impact on the practice of medicine for more than 200 years.
> *Universities Quarterly* 17:327, 1963

Aristotle [384–322 B.C.]

One would pronounce Hippocrates to be greater, not as a human being but as a physician, than somebody who surpassed him in bodily size.
> *Politics*, VII.iv (tr. by H. Rackham)

Galen [fl. 2nd Cent.]

Hippocrates . . . was the first known to us of all those who have been both physicians and philosophers inasmuch as he was the first to recognize what Nature effects.
> *On the Natural Faculties*, I.viii (tr. by Arthur J. Brock)

Marcus Aurelius [121–180]

Hippocrates, after curing many diseases, himself fell sick and died.
> *Meditations*, III.3 (tr. by G. Long)

Gustave Flaubert [1821–1880]

HIPPOCRATES: Always to be cited in Latin because he wrote in Greek, except in the maxim: "Hippocrates says Yes, but Galen says No."
> *Dictionary of Accepted Ideas* (tr. by Jacques Barzun)

Wilder Penfield [1891–   ]

Hippocrates . . . swept away religious superstition and the unprovable assumptions of philosophy, to record what he could see and hear and feel. He based his reasoning on observed fact and learned to assist the body in its vital struggle against disease.
> *The Second Career*, "Aegean Cradle of Medicine"

Oliver Wendell Holmes [1809–1894]

For faithful life-long study of science you will find no better example than John Hunter, never satisfied until he had the pericardium of Nature open and her heart throbbing naked in his hand.
> Valedictory address, Harvard Commencement, March 10, 1858

Sir William Macewen [1848–1924]

John Hunter has been placed in the same rank as Aristotle, Bichat, and Harvey, yet during his life he stood alone — as possibly all such men must. He never had more than 20 students at his lectures, and at the beginning, when a solitary student presented himself, he had to ask the attendant to bring in the skeleton, so that he might address them as "Gentlemen."
> Address to the British Medical Association, 1923

Sir James Learmonth [1895–1967]

All surgical roads lead to John Hunter. In the search for those first principles which have guided great men their successors should probe the workings of their minds rather than their technical successes.
> *The Life History of Inflammation*, Sir John Marnoch Lecture

Thomas Addison [1793–1860]

Were I to affirm that Laënnec contributed more towards the advancement of the medical art than any other single individual, either of ancient or of modern times, I should probably be advancing a proposition which, in the estimation of many, is neither extravagant nor unjust.

> *Collection of Published Writings,* "Diseases of the Chest"

Samuel Johnson [1709–1784]

In Misery's darkest cavern known,
His useful care was ever nigh,
Where hopeless Anguish pour'd his groan,
And lonely Want retir'd to die.

No summons mock'd by chill delay,
No petty gain disdain'd by pride;
The modest wants of ev'ry day
The toil of ev'ry day supplied.

> *On the Death of Mr. Robert Levet, a Practiser in Physic*

René J. Dubos [1901–   ]

This great man [Justus von Liebig], whose vision, learning and energy had founded the science of biochemistry, presents with particular acuity the tragic spectacle of a brilliant mind become slave of preconceived ideas and blinded by them.

> *Louis Pasteur, Free Lance of Science,* Ch. V

Sir Clifford Allbutt [1836–1925]

Lister saw the vast importance of the discoveries of Pasteur. He saw it because he was watching on the heights, and he was watching there alone.

William Ernest Henley [1849–1903]

His brow spreads large and placid, and his eye
Is deep and bright, with steady looks that still,
Soft lines of tranquil thought his face fulfil—
His face at once benign and proud and shy.
If envy scout, if ignorance deny,
His faultless patience, his unyielding will,
Beautiful gentleness and splendid skill,
Innumerable gratitudes reply.

His wise, rare smile is sweet with certainties,
And seems in all his patients to compel
Such love and faith as failure cannot quell.
We hold him for another Herakles,
Battling with custom, prejudice, disease,
As once the son of Zeus with Death and Hell.

> *In Hospital,* Sect. xv, "The Chief" [1]

Sir James M. Barrie [1860–1937]

Are we not all conscious, fitfully, of a white light that hovers for a moment before our lives? It comes back to us from time to time to the very gasp of our days. Comes back for us — to take us where? So quickly fades, as if unequal to its undertaking, like an escaped part of ourselves. . . . The inaccessible star. If any one of ours has reached his star, it was our Lister.

> *The Entrancing Life*

Sir Berkeley Moynihan [1865–1936]

On the roll of honour which, in letters of gold, bears the names of the saviours of mankind, no man is more worthy of remembrance than Lister. His living and enduring memorial is a great, and ever greater multitude of men, women, children, of every nation, of every race, of every creed, through his mercy and by the skill of his most gentle hand relieved from infirmity and suffering and sorrow, and made for a time triumphant over death itself.

> *Addresses on Surgical Subjects,* "Lister as a Surgeon"

Wilder Penfield [1891–   ]

He [Lord Lister] was a scientist by virtue of his habit of thought. . . . he did not accept the pronouncements and the explanations of the surgeons and physicians about him, or who had gone before him, without critical considera-

[1] Joseph, Lord Lister [1827–1912].

tion of the evidence. . . . He depended on those things that could be proven. Thus his thinking about clinical problems was scientific rather than authoritarian.
> *The Second Career,* "Surgery and Science"

The Bible

Luke, the beloved physician.
> *Colossians* 4:14

John Watson ("Ian Maclaren") [1850–1907]

[Dr. "Weelum" MacLure:] A tall, gaunt, loosely made man, without an ounce of superfluous flesh on his body, his face burned a dark brick color by constant exposure to the weather, red hair and beard turning grey, honest blue eyes that looked you ever in the face, huge hands with wrist bones like the shank of a ham, and a voice that hurled his salutations across two fields, he suggested the moor rather than the drawing room. . . . He was "ill pitten thegither" to begin with, but many of his physical defects were the penalties of his work, and endeared him to the Glen.
> *Beside the Bonnie Brier Bush,* Pt. VII, Ch. 1

Alfred Newton Richards [1876–1966]

I am glad that at last Marshall has found an animal that fits in with his theory.[1]
> Remark at a Woods Hole Seminar, 1930

Samuel Johnson [1709–1784]

Dr. Mead[2] lived more in the broad sunshine of life than almost any man.
> Quoted by James Boswell in *Life of Samuel Johnson,* 1778

---

[1] Referring to a paper delivered by Eli K. Marshall, Jr., on the formation of urine in the aglomerular fish.
[2] Richard Mead [1673–1754].

William B. Castle [1897–   ]

He [George R. Minot] was, as usual, at once interested in a new idea, irrespective of its source.
> Letter, April 27, 1964 (Quoted in *Medicine* 43:619, 1964)

Wilder Penfield [1891–   ]

[Ambroise] Paré . . . was guided by fearless compassion for the suffering of his patients, and by practical experiment. Thus it was that he established better methods of treatment and forbade gratuitous interference.
> *The Second Career,* "Surgery and Science"

Robert Bridges [1844–1930]

Grant us an hundred years, and man
  shall hold in abeyance
These foul distempers, and with this
  world's benefactors
Shall PASTEUR obtain the reward of
  saintly devotion,
His crown heroic, who fought not destiny in vain.
> *Now in Wintry Delights*

René J. Dubos [1901–   ]

He [Pasteur] was a symbol of the great creators who, despite poverty and at the cost of sacrifices and suffering, establish the foundations of science that less gifted men may continue to add slowly to the great structure arising from the struggles of genius.
> *Louis Pasteur, Free Lance of Science,* Ch. III

For him, doctrines and techniques were tools to be used only as long as they lent themselves to the formulation and performance of meaningful experiments. . . . In his hands, the experimental method was not a set of recipes, but a living philosophy adaptable to the ever-changing circumstances of natural phenomena.
> *Ibid.,* Ch. IX

C. D. Darlington [1903–]

Pasteur, like Darwin, was impelled through fifty years of active inquiry by an unfailing appetite for discovery. But the contrast between the affluent but dyspeptic English country gentleman and vigorous French peasant-artisan was as deep as it could be in every other respect.

Genetics and Man, Ch. 7

Paul H. Lavietes [1907–]

It is true that he [John Punnett Peters] did not bother to distinguish between good causes and lost ones, but he never mistook a figure of speech for a fact, and although he had many and high ideals, he had few illusions. To call him naïve was to confuse naïveté with courage.

Eulogy

Henry, Lord Cohen of Birkenhead [1900–]

He [Sir Charles Sherrington] had intended . . . to spend some time with [Eduard F. W.] Pflüger of Bonn, but found him somewhat superficial. He records that on arrival, Pflüger took him by the arm and said "und nun wir wollen einer Entdeckung machen,"[1] so they entered the laboratory and proceeded to discover a nerve in the gallbladder.

The Sherrington Lectures, IV, Sect. I

Thomas Jefferson [1743–1826]

In his theory of bleeding and mercury, I was ever opposed to my friend [Benjamin] Rush, whom I greatly loved; but who had done much harm, in the sincerest persuasion that he was preserving life and happiness to all around him.

Letter to Dr. Thomas Cooper, October 7, 1814

[1] "And now we will make a discovery."

Elisha Bartlett [1804–1855]

It may be safely said, I think, that in the whole vast compass of medical literature, there cannot be found an equal number of pages, containing a greater amount and variety of utter nonsense and unqualified absurdity, — a more heterogeneous and ill-adjusted an assemblage, not merely of unsupported, but of unintelligible and preposterous assertions, than are embodied in his exposition of this theory.[1]

Philosophy of Medical Science, Pt. II, Ch. 13

His speculative doctrines in regard to the nature of disease indisposed him to a careful and discriminating study of its phenomena and relationships, and in a great degree disqualified him for such study. They obscured his perceptions, and clouded his judgment. Worse than this, his false philosophy of disease was suffered to influence his practice, rendering this, also, more exclusive and faulty, than it would otherwise have been.

Idem

William B. Bean [1909–]

The heroic aspects of Benjamin Rush, his many ideas about mental health, his signing of the Declaration of Independence, have made us forget the harm he did. His willingness to follow the guttering candle of ignorance, his dogmatic conviction that he was right, his consummate ability to fool himself consistently helped to kill an unmeasured plenty of his patients in Philadelphia. That his motives were pure and serene constitutes another example of the unlimited capacity of man to fool himself. Only the genius or unsung hero can make an intellectual judgment when his feelings, emotions and beliefs are engaged.

Archives of Internal Medicine 117:1, 1966

[1] Comment on Benjamin Rush's *Theory of Fever.*

Charles R. Stockard [1879–1939]

He [Theobald Smith] built temples to nature and communed in them by whispering questions to her. And nature answered back to this favored son — and he understood.

Science 80:579, 1934

W. J. Kerr [1889–   ] and William B. Bean [1909–   ]

With such qualities and character he [1] brings to mind the grace and skill, élan and many-sidedness of the Elizabethan gentleman. Beyond anyone's thought he was impatient of delay and drove himself relentlessly but without bitterness to reach his goal. With so much of the path traversed he was suddenly overwhelmed, a martyr to his own idealism.

Transactions of the Association of American Physicians 63:15, 1950

Thomas Jefferson [1743–1826]

In Italy, the works of [Lazzaro] Spallanzani on Digestion and generation, are valuable. Though, perhaps, too minute, and therefore tedious, he has developed some useful truths, and his book is well worth attention.

Letter to Dr. Joseph Willard, March 24, 1789

Peter Mere Latham [1789–1875]

Perhaps, the very structure of his [Thomas Sydenham's] mind was such, that it was really incapable of gaining anything second-hand which it could gather fresh from the reality.

Lectures on Clinical Medical, Lect. I

Anonymous

He [Dr. James Syme] never wastes a word, a drop of ink, or a drop of blood.

Quoted by John Brown in *Horae Subsecivae,* Series I, Preface

[1] Mayo Hamilton Soley [1907–1949].

Antoine Perrenot, Cardinal de Granvelle [1517–1586]

Monsieur de Lalaing . . . is better, as I have heard, and does not much fear Vesalius' verdicts on his patients, because he always declares them about to die, so that if they do die, he is not at fault, and if they live, he has performed a miracle.

Letter, October 20, 1558

Sir William Osler [1849–1919]

In addition to a three-story intellect, [William H.] Welch has an attic on top.

Anonymous

Nobody knows what "Popsey" eats,
Nobody knows where "Popsey" sleeps,
Nobody knows the women he keeps,
Excepting God and "Popsey"! [1]

John Enders [1897–   ]

His [Hans Zinsser's] gallant and imaginative spirit saw in scientific research high adventure.

Harvard Medical Alumni Bulletin 15 (Supplement):1, 1940, "Tribute to Dr. Hans Zinsser"

PHYSIOLOGY

See also ANATOMY, BASIC SCIENCE

John Morgan [1735–1789]

As every disease we labour under is a disorder of the vital, animal, or natural functions; a thorough acquaintance with these in their sound state is implied before we can pretend to understand their morbid affections, or how to remedy them.

A Discourse upon the Institution of Medical Schools in America

[1] William H. Welch [1850–1934], one of the founders of the Johns Hopkins Hospital and Medical School and a lifelong bachelor, was familiarly referred to as "Popsey."

Claude Bernard [1813–1878]

The constancy of the internal environment is the condition of free and independent existence.
Leçons sur les phénomènes de la vie communs aux animaux et aux végétaux, Vol. I, Lesson 2, Pt. 3

Samuel Butler [1835–1902]

A physician's physiology has much the same relation to his power of healing as a cleric's divinity has to his power of influencing conduct.
Note-Books, Ch. XIV

Sir Michael Foster [1836–1907]

All the deeper problems of physiology turn on the mutual action of the tissues and the blood, as the stream of the latter sweeps among the elements of the former. Harvey showed that the blood did sweep through the tissues, Malpighi showed what the tissues were and how the blood swept through them. And thus the way was opened for those inquiries into the ways in which the blood acts on the tissue and the tissue acts on the blood, inquiries the results of which are the pride of modern times and the hope of times to come.
History of Physiology, Lect. 4

Edward Martin [1859–1938]

Pathology is the accomplished tragedy; physiology the basis on which our treatment rests.

Walter B. Cannon [1871–1945]

These changes — the more rapid pulse, the deeper breathing, the increase of sugar in the blood, the secretion from the adrenal glands — were very diverse and seemed unrelated. Then, one wakeful night, after a considerable collection of these changes had been disclosed, the idea flashed through my mind, that they could be nicely integrated if conceived as bodily preparations for supreme effort in flight or in fighting.
The Way of an Investigator, "The Role of Hunches"

There are still among us benighted persons who would sympathize with the member of the House of Commons who, commenting on the extravagance of the London School Board, declared: "Physiology, besides being costly and useless, is an immodest subject. When the Author of the Universe hid the liver of man out of sight He did not want frail human creatures to see how He had done it." Indeed, when my academic title was advanced to that of a full professorship, a sensitive Cambridge lady, who had learned somehow that I was working on the activities of the digestive tract, was heard to remark, "I do hope that now he will give up his disgusting researches on the stomach."
Ibid., "Making Science Understandable"

Martin H. Fischer [1879–1962]

Physiology is the stepchild of medicine. That is why Cinderella often turns out the queen.
Quoted by Howard Fabing and Ray Marr in *Fischerisms*

John Punnett Peters [1887–1955]

The disorders encountered in disease may be regarded as normal physiologic responses to unusual conditions produced by pathologic processes.
New England Journal of Medicine 239:353, 1948

PILES

See also BOWELS

Martial [fl. 1st Cent.]

Accept this saddle for thy hunting-nag,

For riding bare-back causes nasty piles.
> *Epigrams*, XIV.86

William Heberden [1710-1801]

Women during the state of pregnancy, and just after the menses have finally left them, are peculiarly subject to the piles.
> *Commentaries on the History and Cure of Diseases*, Ch. 44

Chinese Proverb

Nine out of every ten men have piles.

PLACEBO

Thomas Jefferson [1743-1826]

One of the most successful physicians I have ever known, has assured me, that he used more bread pills, drops of colored water, & powders of hickory ashes, than of all other medicines put together. It was certainly a pious fraud.
> Letter to Dr. Caspar Wistar, June 21, 1807

Waitstill R. Ranney [1792-1854]

It is better to let your patients die with the "powerful operation" of *bread pills* and colored drops from the "north side of the well," than to suffer medication misapplied.
> Letter to his son

Richard Clarke Cabot [1869-1939]

In my experience the educated physician who knows that only a few of his patients can be much benefited by drugs, gives out just as many prescriptions as the ignorant physician who believes all that the Pharmacopeia and the nostrum vendor tell him. The only difference is that the educated physician gives his drugs as placebos. In my opinion, the placebo habit does more harm than the habit of giving drugs to every patient with full faith in their pharmacologic action. . . . They weaken the confidence of the patient in the physician, because every placebo is a lie, and in the long run the lie is found out. We give a placebo with one meaning; the patient receives it with quite another. We mean him to suppose that the drug acts directly on his body, not through his mind by means of expectant attention. If the patient finds out what we are doing, he laughs at it or is rightly angry with us. I have seen both the laughter and the anger — at our expense. Placebo giving is quackery. It also fosters the nostrum evil.
> *Journal of the American Medical Association* 47:982, 1906

John L. McClenahan [1915-   ]

It requires a great deal of faith for a man to be cured by his own placebos.
> Aphorism

PLAGUE

See also EPIDEMICS

William Shakespeare [1564-1616]

ENOBARBUS: How appears the fight?
SCARUS: On our side like the token'd pestilence
Where death is sure.
> *Antony and Cleopatra*, III, x, 8

Biles and plagues
Plaster you o'er, that you may be abhorr'd
Farther than seen and one infect another
Against the wind a mile!
> *Coriolanus*, I, iv, 31

Now the red pestilence strike all trades in Rome,
And occupations perish!
> *Ibid.*, IV, i, 13

Thou art a boil,
A plague sore, an embossed carbuncle
In my corrupted blood.
King Lear, II, iv, 226

Write 'Lord have mercy on us' on those
three.
They are infected, in their hearts it
lies;
They have the plague, and caught it
of your eyes.
Love's Labour's Lost, V, ii, 419

The searchers of the town,
Suspecting that we both were in a
house
Where the infectious pestilence did
reign,
Seal'd up the doors, and would not let
us forth.
Romeo and Juliet, V, ii, 8

He is so plaguy proud, that the death
tokens of it
Cry 'No recovery.'
Troilus and Cressida, II, iii, 187

Samuel Pepys [1633–1703]

This day, much against my will, I did
in Drury Lane see two or three houses
marked with a red cross upon the
doors, and "Lord have mercy upon us"
writ there; which was a sad sight to
me, being the first of the kind that, to
my remembrance, I ever saw. It put
me into an ill conception of myself
and my smell, so that I was forced to
buy some roll-tobacco to smell to and
chaw, which took away the apprehension.
Diary, June 7, 1665

Lord! how sad a sight it is to see the
streets empty of people, and very few
upon the 'Change. Jealous of every
door that one sees shut up, lest it
should be the plague; and about us
two shops in three, if not more, generally shut up.
Ibid., August 16, 1665

Daniel Defoe [1659?–1731]

They had dug several pits in another
ground, when the distemper began to
spread in our parish, and especially
when the dead-carts began to go about,
which was not, in our parish, till the
beginning of August. Into these pits
they had put perhaps fifty or sixty
bodies each; then they made larger
holes, wherein they buried all that the
cart brought in a week, which, by the
middle to the end of August, came to
from 200 to 400 a week; and they
could not well dig them larger, because
of the order of the magistrates confining them to leave no bodies within
six feet of the surface.
A Journal of the Plague Year

Cotton Mather [1663–1728]

'Tis the *Destroyer*, or *the Devil*, that
scatters *Plagues* about the World. . . .
'Tis no uneasy thing for the Devil to
impregnate the Air with such Malignant *Salts* as, meeting with *the Salt*
of our *Microcosm*, shall immediately
cast us into that Fermentation and
Putrefaction, which will utterly dissolve all the Vital tyes within us.
*The Wonders of the Invisible
World*, "A Hortatory and Necessary Address," Prop. IV

John Armstrong [1709–1779]

Nothing but lamentable sounds was
heard,
Nor aught was seen but ghastly views
of death.
Infectious horror ran from face to face,
And pale despair.
The Art of Preserving Health,
Bk. III

Percy Bysshe Shelley [1792–1822]

O Wild West Wind, thou breath of
Autumn's being,
Thou, from whose unseen presence the
leaves dead
Are driven, like ghosts from an enchanter fleeing,

Yellow, and black, and pale, and hectic
red,
Pestilence-stricken multitudes.
    Ode to the West Wind, Sect. I

Albert Camus [1913–1960]

Dr. Rieux resolved to compile this
chronicle . . . to state quite simply
what we learn in a time of pestilence:
that there are more things to admire in
men than to despise.
    The Plague, Pt. V (tr. by Stuart
    Gilbert)

French Proverb

A Sunday's child never dies of the
plague.

PLASTIC SURGERY

John Marston [1575?–1634]

Do you know Doctor Plaster-face? by
this curd, he is the most exquisite in
forging of veins, sprightening of eyes,
dying of hair, sleeking of skins, blushing of cheeks, surphling [1] of breasts,
blanching and bleaching of teeth, that
ever made an old lady gracious by
torchlight.
    The Malcontent, Act II, Sc. iii

Sir Harold Gillies [1882–1960] **and
D. Ralph Millard, Jr.** [1919–   ]

The great ignominy to the plastic surgeon is his inability to remove a scar
without leaving another one. . . . the
best we can do is occasionally improve
on another surgeon's scar while indeed
he may be improving on several of ours.
    *The Principles and Art of Plas-
    tic Surgery,* Vol. I, Ch. 4

It is easy to agree to do a beauty
operation, but not always quite so easy
to be certain it is justified. A frightful-
looking old girl comes in for a face
lift; a deep swallow is taken before
the surgery is begun, for it is obvious

[1] surphling = washing with cosmetics.

even after the most wonderful lift she
will still look like the North Pole.
That is, only to us, not to her. She
is tickled with any improvement.
    Ibid., Vol. II, Ch. 20

If the world never suspects the face
has been lifted, that is the true test
of your handicraft.
    Idem

Jerome Pierce Webster
[1888–   ]

Is not . . . plastic surgery an art and
the plastic surgeon an artist? The plastic surgeon works with living flesh as
his clay, and his work of art is the
attempted achievement of normalcy in
appearance and function.
    Foreword to Sir Harold Gillies
    and D. Ralph Millard, Jr.'s *The
    Principles and Art of Plastic
    Surgery*

Living parts have a superabundance of
vitality, but if too great a burden is
put upon them, they cannot survive or
be used.
    Idem

Eugenia Sheppard [20th Cent.]

Anybody who is anybody seems to be
getting a lift — by plastic surgery —
these days. It's the new world wide
craze that combines the satisfactions
of psychoanalysis, massage, and a trip
to the beauty salon.
    New York Herald-Tribune,
    February 24, 1958

PLEASURE AND PAIN

See also PAIN, SUFFERING

Metrodorus [4th Cent. B.C.]

There is a certain pleasure which is
akin to pain.
    Quoted by Seneca in *Moral
    Epistles,* XCIX.25

Epicurus [342?–270 B.C.]

The magnitude of pleasure reaches its limit in the removal of all pain.
> *Sovran Maxims*, 3 (Quoted by Diogenes Laertes in *Lives of Eminent Philosophers*, X.139)

Ovid [43 B.C.–A.D. 17?]

Every man serves his own pleasure,
Sweeter perhaps, when it comes out of
   another man's pain.
> *The Art of Love*, I.747 (tr. by R. Humphries)

Samuel Butler [1612–1680]

Our *Pains* are real Things, and all
Our *Pleasures* but fantastical.
> *Satyr upon the Weakness and Misery of Man*

Benjamin Franklin [1706–1790]

Pain wastes the Body, Pleasures the Understanding.
> *Poor Richard's Almanack*, 1735

Edmund Burke [1729–1797]

The torments which we may be made to suffer are much greater in their effect on the body and mind, than any pleasures which the most learned voluptuary could suggest, or than the liveliest imagination, and the most sound and exquisitely sensible body, could enjoy.
> *On the Sublime and Beautiful*, Pt. I, Sect. VII

Jeremy Bentham [1748–1832]

Nature has placed mankind under the governance of two sovereign masters, *pain* and *pleasure*.
> *Introduction to the Principles of Morals and Legislation*, Ch. I

Arthur Schopenhauer [1788–1860]

The pleasure in this world, it has been said, outweighs the pain; or, at any rate, there is an even balance between the two. If the reader wishes to see shortly whether this statement is true, let him compare the respective feelings of two animals, one of which is engaged in eating the other.
> *Parerga und Paralipomena*, "On the Sufferings of the World" (tr. by T. B. Saunders)

John Keats [1795–1821]

Pleasure is oft a visitant; but pain
Clings cruelly to us.
> *Endymion*, Bk. I

Edward Bulwer-Lytton ("Owen Meredith") [1831–1891]

There is a pleasure which is born of pain.
> *The Wanderer*, Prologue, Pt. I

George Bernard Shaw [1856–1950]

The most intolerable pain is produced by prolonging the keenest pleasure.
> *Man and Superman*, "Maxims for Revolutionists"

The Bible

I take pleasure in infirmities, in reproaches, in necessities, in persecutions, in distresses for Christ's sake.
> *II Corinthians* 12:10

Proverb

An hour of pain is as long as a day of pleasure.

PLEURISY

William Shakespeare [1564–1616]

For goodness, growing to a plurisy,
Dies in his own too-much.
> *Hamlet*, IV, vii, 118

Elisha Bartlett [1804–1855]

No two cases of pleurisy are ever precisely identical. Still, the differences between them are not unlimited and indefinite; they are always confined within certain degrees.

Philosophy of Medical Science,
Pt. II, Ch. 11

Edith O. Somerville [1861–1949] and Martin Ross [1862–1915]

I couldn't give ye any patthern of it indeed, but it's like in me side as a pairson'd be polishin' a boot, and he with a brush in his hand.[1]

Irish Memories, Ch. XVII

PNEUMONIA

Sir William Osler [1849–1919]

In the mortality bills, pneumonia is an easy second, to tuberculosis; indeed, in many cities the death-rate is now higher and it has become, to use the phrase of Bunyan, "the Captain of the men of death."[2]

Aequanimitas, with Other Addresses, "Medicine in the Nineteenth Century"

POET PHYSICIANS

See also OBITER DICTA

Thomas Lodge [1558–1625]

Pluck the fruit and taste the pleasure,
   Youthful lordlings of delight;
Whilst occasion gives you seizure,
   Feed your fancies and your sight:
After death, when you are gone,
   Joy and pleasure is there none.
History of Robert, Second Duke of Normandy

Thomas Campion [1567–1620]

When thou must home to shades of underground,
And there arriv'd, a newe admired guest,

The beauteous spirits do ongirt thee round,
White Iope, blithe Hellen, and the rest,
To heare the stories of thy finisht love,
From that smoothe toongue whose musicke hell can move;

Then wilt thou speake of banqueting delights,
Of masks and revels which sweete youth did make,
Of Tournies and great challenges of knights,
And all these triumphes for thy beauties sake:
When thou hast told these honours done to thee,
Then tell, O tell, how thou didst murther me!
A Booke of Ayres, XX

There is a garden in her face
Where roses and white lilies grow;
A heavenly paradise is that place,
Wherein all pleasant fruits do flow.
There cherries grow which none may buy
Till "Cherry-ripe" themselves do cry.
Fourth Booke of Ayres

Never weatherbeaten Saile more willing bent to shore,
Never tyred Pilgrim's limbs affected slumber more,
Then my wearyd spright now longs to flye out of my troubled brest.
O come quickly, sweetest Lord, and take my soule to rest!

Ever blooming are the joyes of Heav'n's high paradice,
Cold age deafes not there our eares, nor vapour dims our eyes:
Glory there the sun outshines; whose beames the blessed onely see.
O come quickly, glorious Lord, and raise my spright to thee!
Two Bookes of Ayres, Bk. I, XI

John Byrom [1692–1763]

Christians awake, salute the happy morn,

---

[1] An old Irish woman describing an attack of pleurisy.
[2] Cf. John Bunyan, p. 642a.

Whereon the Saviour of the world was
born.
Hymn for Christmas Day

God bless the King — I mean the
faith's defender,
God bless — no harm in blessing — the
Pretender!
But who pretender is, or who is king, —
God bless us all! — that's quite an-
other thing.
Miscellaneous Poems, "To an
Officer of the Army, extempore"

Oliver Goldsmith [1728–1774]

O memory, thou fond deceiver,
Still importunate and vain,
To former joys recurring ever,
And turning all the past to pain. . . .

Thou, like the world, th' opprest op-
pressing,
Thy smiles increase the wretch's
woe;
And he who wants each other blessing,
In thee must ever find a foe.
*Song from The Captivity: An
Oratorio*

Ill fares the land, to hastening ills a
prey,
Where wealth accumulates, and men
decay.
The Deserted Village

I love everything that's old: old friends,
old times, old manners, old books, old
wine.
She Stoops to Conquer, Act I

Ask me no questions, and I'll tell you
no fibs.
Ibid., Act III

And learn the luxury of doing good.
The Traveller

You may all go to pot.
*Verses in Reply to an Invitation
to Dinner at Dr. Baker's*

When lovely woman stoops to folly,
And finds too late that men betray,

What charm can sooth her melancholy?
What art can wash her guilt away?

The only art her guilt to cover,
To hide her shame from every eye,
To give repentance to her lover,
And wring his bosom, is — to die.
The Vicar of Wakefield, Ch. 24

John Keats [1795–1821]

O, what can ail thee, knight-at-arms,
Alone and palely loitering?
The sedge has wither'd from the lake,
And no birds sing.
La Belle Dame Sans Merci

There is not a fiercer hell than the failure in a great object.
Endymion, Preface

A thing of beauty is a joy for ever:
Its loveliness increases; it will never
Pass into nothingness; but still will
keep
A bower quiet for us, and a sleep
Full of sweet dreams, and health, and
quiet breathing.
Ibid., Bk. I

Deep in the shady sadness of a vale
Far sunken from the healthy breath of
morn,
Far from the fiery noon, and eve's one
star,
Sat gray-hair'd Saturn, quiet as a
stone,
Still as the silence round about his lair.
Hyperion, Bk. I

I think Poetry should surprise by a fine
excess and not by Singularity — it
should strike the Reader as a wording
of his own highest thoughts, and appear almost a Remembrance — . . .
but it is easier to think what Poetry
should be than to write it — and this
leads me to another axiom. That if
Poetry comes not as naturally as the
Leaves to a tree it had better not come
at all.
*Letter to John Taylor, Febru-
ary 27, 1818*

'Beauty is truth, truth beauty' — that
  is all
Ye know on earth, and all ye need to
  know.
      Ode on a Grecian Urn

My heart aches, and a drowsy numb-
  ness pains
  My sense, as though of hemlock I
    had drunk,
Or emptied some dull opiate to the
  drains
  One minute past, and Lethe-wards
    had sunk.
      Ode to a Nightingale

Charm'd magic casements, opening on
  the foam
Of perilous seas, in faery lands forlorn.
      Idem

Much have I travell'd in the realms of
  gold,
And many goodly states and kingdoms
  seen.
      *On First Looking into Chap-
      man's Homer*

When I have fears that I may cease to
  be
Before my pen has glean'd my teeming
  brain.
      Sonnet from *Literary Remains*

Oliver Wendell Holmes
[1809–1894]

And as for all the "patronage" of all
  the clowns and boors
That squint their little narrow eyes at
  any freak of yours,
Do leave them to your prosier friends
  — such fellows ought to die
When rhubarb is so very scarce and
  ipecac so high!
      Nux Postcoenatica

Thomas Dunn English
[1819–1902]

Don't you remember sweet Alice, Ben
  Bolt —
  Sweet Alice whose hair was so brown,

Who wept with delight when you gave
  her a smile,
  And trembled with fear at your
    frown?
      Ben Bolt

Josiah Gilbert Holland
[1819–1881]

God give us men! A time like this de-
  mands
Strong minds, great hearts, true faith,
  and ready hands;
Men whom the lust of office does not
  kill;
  Men whom the spoils of office cannot
    buy;
Men who possess opinions and a will;
  Men who have honor, — men who
    will not lie;
Men who can stand before a dema-
  gogue,
  And damn his treacherous flatteries
    without winking!
Tall men, sun-crowned, who live above
  the fog
  In public duty, and in private think-
    ing:
For while the rabble, with their thumb-
  worn creeds,
Their large professions and their little
  deeds, —
Mingle in selfish strife, lo! Freedom
  weeps,
Wrong rules the land, and waiting Jus-
  tice sleeps!
      Wanted

S. Weir Mitchell [1829–1914]

I know the night is near at hand.
The mists lie low on hill and bay,
The autumn sheaves are dewless, dry;
But I have had the day.

Yes, I have had, dear Lord, the day;
When at Thy call I have the night,
Brief be the twilight as I pass
From light to dark, from dark to light.
      Vesperal

Robert Bridges [1844–1930]

I welcome fatigue
While frenzy and care

Like thin summer clouds
Go melting in air.

To dream as I may
And awake when I will
With the song of the birds
And the sun on the hill.

Or death — were it death —
To what should I wake
Who loved in my home
All life for its sake?

What good have I wrought?
I laugh to have learned
That joy cannot come
Unless it be earned.
Fortunatus Nimium

I will be what God made me, nor
protest
Against the bent of genius in my time,
That science of my friends robs all the
best,
While I love beauty, and was born to
rhyme.
Be they our mighty men, and let me
dwell
In shadow among the mighty shades of
old,
With love's forsaken palace for my
cell;
Whence I look forth and all the world
behold,

And say, These better days, in best
things worse,
This bastardy of time's magnificence,
Will mend in fashion and throw off the
curse,
To crown new love with higher excel-
lence.
Curs'd tho' I be to live my life alone,
My toil is for man's joy, his joy my
own.[1]
The Growth of Love, 62

When men were all asleep the snow
came flying,
In large white flakes falling on the city
brown,

[1] Written when he abandoned medicine for
poetry.

Stealthily and perpetually settling and
loosely lying,
Hushing the latest traffic of the
drowsy town.
London Snow

For when his [Hippocrates'] doctrine,
which Rome had wisely adopted,
Sank lost with the treasures of her
deep-foundering empire,
No art or science grew so contemptible,
order'd
So by mere folly, windy caprice, superstition and chance,
As boastful MEDICINE, with humours
fit for a madhouse,
Save when some Sydenham, like Samson among the Philistines,
Strode bond-bursting along with a
smile of genial instinct.
Now in Wintry Delights

Hast thou then thought that all this
ravishing music,
that stirreth so thy heart, making thee
dream of things
illimitable unsearchable and of heavenly import,
is but a light disturbance of the atoms
of air,
whose jostling ripples, gather'd within
the ear, are tuned
to resonant scale, and thence by the en-
thron'd mind received
on the spiral stairway of her audience
chamber
as heralds of high spiritual significance?
The Testament of Beauty, Bk.
I, Introduction

Our stability is but balance, and wisdom lies
in masterful administration of the unforeseen.
Idem

Spencer Michael Free [1856–1938]
'Tis the human touch in this world that
counts,
The touch of your hand and mine,
Which means far more to the fainting
heart

Than shelter and bread and wine.
For shelter is gone when the night is
   o'er
And bread lasts only a day,
But the touch of the hand and the
   sound of the voice
Sing on in the soul alway.
The Human Touch

George David Stewart [1862–1933]

When I, having finished with things be-
   low,
Lie out 'neath the sod alone,
Raise no cold monument to me
Of brass or bronze or stone;

But plant me beneath a big oak tree,
With its roots firmly fixed in the sod,
And its branches pointing everywhere
To the throne of the living God.
A Tired Doctor's Prayer

John McCrae [1872–1918]

In Flanders fields the poppies blow
   Between the crosses, row on row,
   That mark our place; and in the sky
   The larks, still bravely singing, fly
Scarce heard amid the guns below.

We are the Dead. Short days ago
We lived, felt dawn, saw sunset glow,
   Loved and were loved, and now we
   lie,
               In Flanders fields.

Take up our quarrell with the foe:
To you from failing hands we throw
   The torch; be yours to hold it high.
   If ye break faith with us who die
We shall not sleep, though poppies
   grow
               In Flanders fields.
In Flanders Fields

Oliver St. John Gogarty [1878–1957]

Our friends go with us as we go
   Down the long path where Beauty
   wends,
Where all we love forgathers, so
   Why should we fear to join our
   friends?

Who would survive them to outlast
   His children; to outwear his fame —
Left when the Triumph has gone
   past —
   To win from Age, not Time, a name?

Then do not shudder at the knife
That Death's indifferent hand drives
   home,
But with the Strivers leave the Strife
Nor, after Caesar, skulk in Rome.
An Offering of Swans, "Non
Dolet"

Hans Zinsser [1878–1940]

Now is death merciful. He calls me
   hence
Gently, with friendly soothing of my
   fears
Of ugly age and feeble impotence
And cruel disintegration of slow years.
Nor does he leap upon me unaware
Like some wild beast that hungers for
   its prey,
But gives me kindly warning to pre-
   pare:
Before I go, to kiss your tears away.
How sweet the summer! And the
   autumn shone
Late warmth within our hearts as in
   the sky,
Ripening rich harvests that our love
   had sown.
How good that 'ere the winter comes, I
   die!
Then, ageless, in your heart I'll come
   to rest
Serene and proud, as when you loved
   me best.
As I Remember Him, Ch. 26

William Carlos Williams [1883–1963]

They call me and I go.
It is a frozen road
past midnight, a dust
of snow caught
in the rigid wheeltracks.
The door opens.
I smile, enter and
shake off the cold.
Here is a great woman

on her side in the bed.
She is sick,
perhaps vomiting,
perhaps laboring
to give birth to
a tenth child. Joy! Joy!
Night is a room
darkened for lovers,
through the jalousies the sun
has sent one gold needle!
I pick the hair from her eyes
and watch her misery
with compassion.
    Complaint

Oh I suppose I should
wash the walls of my office
polish the rust from
my instruments and keep them
definitely in order
build shelves in the laboratory
empty out the old stains
clean the bottles
and refill them, buy
another lens, put
my journals on edge instead of
letting them lie flat
in heaps — then begin
ten years back and
gradually read them to date
cataloguing important
articles for ready reference.
I suppose I should
read the new books. . . .
Who can tell? I might be
a credit to my lady Happiness
and never think anything
but a white thought!
    Le Médecin Malgré Lui

Merrill Moore [1903–1957]

The noise that Time makes in passing
    by
Is very slight but even you can hear it,
Having not necessarily to be near it,
Needing only the slightest will to try!

Hold the receiver of a telephone
To your ear when no one is talking on
    the line
And what may at first sound to you
    like the whine

Of wind over distant wires is Time's
    own
Garments brushing against a windy
    cloud.

That same noise again but not so well
Can be heard by taking a small cockle
    shell
From the sand and holding it against
    your head;

Then you can hear Time's footsteps as
    they pass
Over the earth brushing the eternal
    grass.
    Sonnets from the Fugitive, "The
    Noise That Time Makes"

The Unconscious is incredibly wise.
It sees the world without aid of eyes,
It hears the world without aid of ears
And never mentions what it sees or
    hears.

It sits in silence, always listening.
It never misses, — takes in every word.
By the eyes' expression, glistening,
One can be aware that it has heard,

That it has taken in and utilized
What, in consciousness, might be de-
    spised.

It is the silent and unspoken part,
The under region, deeper than the
    heart.
It is the ancient and unuttered one,
As primitive and ageless as the sun.
    The Unconscious

Harvey Graham [1912–   ]

Venus found herself a goddess
In a world controlled by gods,
So she opened up her bodice
And evened up the odds.
    A Doctor's London, Ch. 7

POISON

Nicander [fl. 2nd Cent. B.C.]

The mouth it [lead] inflames and
    makes cold from within,

The gums dry and wrinkled are
parch'd like the skin,
The rough tongue feels harsher, the
neck muscles grip,
He soon cannot swallow, foam runs
from his lip,
A feeble cough tries it in vain to expel,
He belches so much, and his belly does
swell. . . .
Meanwhile there comes a stuporous
chill,
His feeble limbs droop and all motion
is still.[1]
Alexipharmaca, 74

Lucretius [96?–55 B.C.]

What is one man's meat is another
man's rank poison.
On the Nature of Things,
IV.637 (tr. by W. H. D. Rouse)

Paracelsus [1493?–1541]

Is not a mystery of nature concealed
even in poison? . . . What has God
created that He did not bless with some
great gift for the benefit of man? Why
then should poison be rejected and despised, if we consider not the poison
but its curative virtue?
Seven Defenses (tr. by Norbert
Guterman in *Selected Writings*)

William Shakespeare [1564–1616]

If they had swallow'd poison, 'twould
appear
By external swelling; but she looks
like sleep.
Antony and Cleopatra, V, ii, 348

I beseech your Grace, without of-
fence
(My conscience bids me ask), where-
fore you have
Commanded of me these most poison-
ous compounds,
Which are the movers of a languishing
death,
But though slow, deadly?
Cymbeline, I, v, 6

[1] A description of the effects of lead poisoning.

She doth think she has
Strange ling'ring poisons. I do know
her spirit
And will not trust one of her malice
with
A drug of such damn'd nature. Those
she has
Will stupefy and dull the sense awhile;
Which first, perchance, she'll prove on
cats and dogs,
Then afterward up higher; but there is
No danger in what show of death it
makes,
More than the locking up the spirits a
time,
To be more fresh, reviving.
Ibid., I, v, 33

She did confess she had
For you a mortal mineral, which, being
took,
Should by the minute feed on life, and
ling'ring,
By inches waste you.
Ibid., V, v, 49

Upon my secure hour thy uncle stole,
With juice of cursed hebona in a vial,
And in the porches of my ears did pour
The leperous distilment; whose effect
Holds such an enmity with blood of
man
That swift as quicksilver it courses
through
The natural gates and alleys of the
body,
And with a sudden vigour it doth
posset
And curd, like eager droppings into
milk,
The thin and wholesome blood. So did
it mine;
And a most instant tetter bark'd about,
Most lazar-like, with vile and loath-
some crust
All my smooth body.
Hamlet, I, v, 61

I bought an unction of a mountebank,
So mortal that, but dip a knife in it,
Where it draws blood no cataplasm so
rare,

Collected from all simples that have
virtue
Under the moon, can save the thing
from death
This is but scratch'd withal.
Ibid., IV, vii, 142

In poison there is physic, and these
news,
Having been well, that would have
made me sick,
Being sick, have in some measure made
me well.
Henry IV, Part II, I, i, 137

I had as live they would put ratsbane
in my mouth as offer to stop it with
security.
Ibid., I, ii, 47

I would the milk
Thy mother gave thee when thou
suck'dst her breast
Had been a little ratsbane for thy
sake!
Henry VI, Part I, V, iv, 27

Bid the apothecary
Bring the strong poison that I bought
of him.
Henry VI, Part II, III, iii, 17

Within me is a hell, and there the
poison
Is, as a fiend, confin'd to tyrannize
On unreprievable condemned blood.
King John, V, vii, 46

If you have poison for me, I will drink
it.
King Lear, IV, vii, 72

Or have we eaten on the insane root
That takes the reason prisoner?
Macbeth, I, iii, 84

The thought . . .
Doth, like a poisonous mineral, gnaw
my inwards.
Othello, II, i, 305

Within the infant rind of this small
flower

Poison hath residence, and medicine
power;
For this, being smelt, with that part
cheers each part;
Being tasted, slays all senses with the
heart.
Romeo and Juliet, II, iii, 23

I do remember an apothecary
And hereabouts 'a dwells, which late I
noted
In tatt'red weeds, with overwhelming
brows,
Culling of simples. . . .
Noting this penury, to myself I said,
'An if a man did need a poison now
Whose sale is present death in Mantua,
Here lives a caitiff wretch would sell it
him.'
Ibid., V, i, 37

Let me have
A dram of poison, such soon-speeding
gear
As will disperse itself through all the
veins
That the life-weary taker may fall
dead,
And that the trunk may be discharg'd
of breath
As violently as hasty powder fir'd
Doth hurry from the fatal cannon's
womb.
Ibid., V, i, 59

O true apothecary!
Thy drugs are quick.
Ibid., V, iii, 119

Like poison given to work a great time
after,
Now gins to bite the spirits.
The Tempest, III, iii, 105

Phineas Fletcher [1582–1650]

The coward's weapon, poyson.
Sicelides, Act V, Sc. iii

Francis Beaumont [1584–1616]
and John Fletcher [1579–1625]

What's one man's poison, Signior,
Is another's meat or drink.
Love's Cure, Act III, Sc. ii

Peter Mere Latham [1789–1875]

Poisons and medicine are oftentimes the same substance given with different intents.
General Remarks on the Practice of Medicine, Ch. IV

Ralph Waldo Emerson
[1803–1882]

The poisons are our principal medicines, which kill the disease and save the life.
The Conduct of Life, Ch. VII

Lewis Carroll (Charles L. Dodgson) [1832–1898]

She had never forgotten that, if you drink much from a bottle marked "poison," it is almost certain to disagree with you, sooner or later.
Alice's Adventures in Wonderland, Ch. I

Friedrich Nietzsche [1844–1900]

A little poison now and then: that maketh pleasant dreams. And much poison at last for pleasant death.
Thus Spake Zarathustra, "Zarathustra's Prologue," Sect. 5

Sir Max Beerbohm [1872–1956]

I maintain that though you would often in the fifteenth century have heard the snobbish Roman say, in a would-be off-hand tone, 'I am dining with the Borgias to-night,' no Roman ever was able to say, 'I dined last night with the Borgias.'
And Even Now, "Hosts and Guests"

Edna St. Vincent Millay
[1892–1950]

I know some poison I could drink;
  I've often thought I'd taste it;
But Mother bought it for the sink,
  And drinking it would waste it.
The Cheerful Abstainer

Joseph Kesselring [1902–1967]

Arsenic and Old Lace.
Title of a play

Henry Harrison [1903–   ]

Wan Lo has made an amazing discovery.
"I have found," he cries,
"That what is one man's poison
Is another man's poison."
Wan Lo Tanka

Bantu Proverb

Poison should be tried out on a frog.

Hindu Proverb

Even nectar is poison if taken to excess.

POLITICS

James C. Wilson [1847–1934]

Based upon political lines, it [the A.M.A.] is swayed and frequently controlled by political methods rather than by those of science.
Transactions of the Association of American Physicians 17:1, 1902

Charles V. Chapin [1856–1941]

Medical politics and medical bossism may be as pernicious as state politics.
A Report on State Public Health Work

James B. Herrick [1861–1954]

A study of past American history should cause the medical profession of today to fear the politicians even though they offer gifts.
Memories of Eighty Years, Ch. 8

J. Chalmers Da Costa [1863–1933]

Sometimes when a doctor gets too lazy to work he becomes a politician.
The Trials and Triumphs of the Surgeon, Ch. I

Everett C. Hughes [1897–   ]

The queen of the professions, medicine, is the avowed enemy of bureaucracy, at least of bureaucracy in medicine when others than physicians have a hand in it.

Daedalus 92:655, 1963

POPULATION

See also BIRTH CONTROL

Erasmus Darwin [1731–1802]

So human progenies, if unrestrain'd,
By climate friended, and by food sustain'd,
O'er seas and soils, prolific hordes! would spread
Ere long, and deluge their terraqueous bed;
But war and pestilence, disease, and dearth,
Sweep the superfluous myriads from the earth.
Thus while new forms reviving tribes acquire
Each passing moment, as the old expire;
Like insects swarming in the noontide bower,
Rise into being, and exist an hour;
The births and deaths content with equal strife,
And every pore of Nature teems with Life;
Which buds or breathes from Indus to the Poles,
And Earth's vast surface kindles as it rolls!

> *The Temple of Nature; or, The The Origin of Society,* Canto IV

Thomas Malthus [1766–1834]

Population, when unchecked, increases in a geometrical ratio. Subsistence increases only in an arithmetical ratio.

> *An Essay on the Principle of Population* (1798), Ch. 1

This perpetual struggle for room and food.

> *Ibid.,* Ch. 3

The vices of mankind are active and able ministers of depopulation. . . . But should they fail in this war of extermination, sickly seasons, epidemics, pestilence, and plague, advance in terrific array, and sweep off their thousands and ten thousands. Should success be still incomplete; gigantic inevitable famine stalks in the rear, and with one mighty blow, levels the population with the food of the world.

> *Ibid.,* Ch. 7

Charles Darwin [1809–1882]

Man tends to increase at a greater rate than his means of subsistence; consequently he is occasionally subjected to a severe struggle for existence.

> *The Descent of Man,* Ch. 21

Frank L. Lucas [1894–   ]

To man's future there are today perhaps two main dangers. . . . The first threat, of course, is nuclear war; the second is world overpopulation — a new Deluge, of a new kind, which *might* drown humanity in a Flood, not of water, but of themselves. . . .

At times, I have a vision of a crowd of villagers so anxiously intent on the heavings and rumblings of the mountain above them — will it erupt? — that they never notice how in smooth and sinister silence, from the far horizon behind them, there advances steadily and relentlessly the crest of a tidal wave.

> *The Greatest Problem and Other Essays,* "The Greatest Problem of To-Day"

René J. Dubos [1901–   ]

If men allow themselves to continue breeding like rabbits, their fate will inevitably be to live like rabbits, a precarious and limited existence.

> *Man Adapting,* Ch. XI

PRACTICE

See also GENERAL PRACTI-
TIONER, MEDICINE, PA-
TIENT–PHYSICIAN RELA-
TIONSHIP, PHYSICIANS,
THEORY AND PRACTICE

Antiphon [480?–411 B.C.]

We by skill gain mastery over things in
which we are conquered by nature.
> Quoted by Aristotle in *Mecha-
> nica*, I

Alexander of Tralles [525–605]

The physician should look upon the patient as a besieged city and try to rescue him with every means that art and
science place at his command.

Moses ben Maimon (Maimonides)
[1135–1204]

Medical practice is not knitting and
weaving and the labor of the hands, but
it must be inspired with soul and be
filled with understanding and equipped
with the gift of keen observation;
these together with accurate scientific
knowledge are the indispensable requisites for proficient medical practice.
> Quoted in *Bulletin of the Insti-
> tute of the History of Medicine*
> 3:555, 1935

William Douglass [1691–1752]

You complain of the Practice of Physick being undervalued in your parts
and with reason; we are not much
better in that respect in this place; we
abound with Practi[ti]oners tho no
other graduate than my self, we have
14 Apothecary shops in Boston, all our
Practi[ti]oners dispense their own
medicines, my self excepted being the
first who hath lived here by Practice
without the advantage of advance on
Medicines.
> Letter to Dr. Cadwallader Col-
> den, February 20, 1721

**Hendrick Van Beuren ("Dr.
Hendrick")** [1725–1797]

The daily and innumerable abuses that
are committed on the bodies of our
Fellow Creatures, in the practice of
Physic and Surgery by the unskilful
practitioners to both: and the deplorable instances of Havock and Devasta-
tion occasioned by such Intestine Enemies (destructive to any State as a raging pestilence) is obvious to all men
of Judgment and Observation.

How solicitous ought every Mon-
archy and Commonwealth to be about
the Health and Preservation of every
Individual. . . . A proper regulation
in this respect, so necessary in this
province, will be likely never to take
place without the Attention and Con-
currence of the Legislature. . . .
> Letter in the *New York Gazette,
> or Weekly Post Boy*, May 20,
> 1754

Joseph Black [1728–1799]

I have now studied the Theory of medicine & have likewise been taught every
thing upon the Practice which can be
learned in a College. I have also seen
some real Practice & have even practised a little myself. But all this is not
enough. I should be thoroughly acquainted with the real Practice & this
is a thing very different from what can
be learned in a College; thus for instance we are taught by our Professors
that if a sick person breathes with great
difficulty, one thing must be done; if
his respiration is yet more laborious,
another. But how shall we judge of the
nice degrees of laborious breathing unless from a dayly & familiar acquaintance with, & study of, the appearances
and looks of Patients &c. Most young
Physicians neglect this essential point
of their art in their education & very
often acquire it when they come to
Practice at the expense of their patients' safety.
> Letter to his father, June 1,
> 1754

Sir Gilbert Blane [1749–1834]

There is nothing in which a young practitioner should be more on his guard, than being misled by the sweeping dogmas of schools, and the indiscriminate practices of sects, or of favourite practitioners.

Elements of Medical Logick

John Warren [1753–1815]

The People here [Salem, Mass.] are accustomed to being dealt so very easily with by their Physician, Doctor Holyoke [1] having reduced the Fees to a very low Rate and never having troubled them with Accounts except they troubled him for them. A Physician who should change any thing nearly sufficient barely to support the Dignity of the Profession or should attempt to make any Innovations upon the ancient Usage of the Town would at once throw himself out of Practice.

Quoted in *Archives of Internal Medicine* 116:611, 1965

New York General Assembly [1760]

No person whatsoever shall practise as Physician or surgeon in the . . . City of New York before he shall have been examined in Physick or Surgery . . . by one of His Majesty's Council, the Judges of the Supreme Court, the King's Attorney General, and the Mayor of the City of New York.

Act to Regulate the Practice of Physick and Surgery in the City of New York, June 10, 1760

Peter Mere Latham [1789–1875]

Faith and knowledge lean largely upon each other in the practice of medicine.

General Remarks on the Practice of Medicine, Ch. VII

Physiology, pathology, and practice, often part company just where an in-

---

[1] Edward Holyoke [1728–1829], against whose practice Dr. Warren was attempting to set up as a rival.

telligent looker-on would make sure of their becoming sociable and co-operative. The practice of medicine is a perpetual compromise between what we know and what we can do, between our knowledge and our power.

Ibid., Ch. XI

Oliver Wendell Holmes [1809–1894]

How could a people which has a revolution once in four years, which has contrived the Bowie-knife and the revolver, which has chewed the juice out of all the superlatives in the language in Fourth of July orations, and so used up its epithets in the rhetoric of abuse that it takes two great quarto dictionaries to supply the demand; which insists on sending out yachts and horses and boys to out-sail, out-run, out-fight, and checkmate all the rest of creation; how could such a people be content with any but "heroic" practice?

Medical Essays, "Currents and Counter-Currents in Medical Science"

The best a physician can give is never too good for the patient.

Ibid., "Scholastic and Bedside Teaching"

'Tis a small matter in your neighbor's case,
To charge your fee for showing him your face;
You skip up-stairs, inquire, inspect, and touch,
Prescribe, take leave, and off to twenty such.

The Morning Visit

John Brown [1810–1882]

It is in medicine as in the piloting of a ship — rules may be laid down, principles expounded, charts exhibited; but when a man has made himself master of all these, he will often find his ship among breakers and quicksands, and must at last have recourse to his own craft and courage.

> *Horae Subsecivae*, Series I, "Locke and Sydenham"

Philip A. Austin [1819?– ?]

A preparation begun in pure science may end in correct practice, and the early habits of student life may follow the professional man throughout his career; but a preparation begun in practice will end there. The routine of professional duties often tempts the scholar to sink into a mere practicioner; it is rare indeed that one reverses the order of nature and sets aside the claims and emoluments of practice, to acquire slowly those habits of study so easily learned in youth.

> *The Principles and Practice of Dentistry*

Sir William Osler [1849–1919]

Even in populous districts the practice of medicine is a lonely road which winds up-hill all the way and a man may easily go astray and never reach the Delectable Mountains unless he early finds those shepherd guides of whom Bunyan tells, *Knowledge, Experience, Watchful* and *Sincere.*

> *Aequanimitas, with Other Addresses*, "Chauvinism in Medicine"

It must be confessed that the practice of medicine among our fellow creatures is often a testy and choleric business.

> *Idem*

The practice of medicine is an art, not a trade; a calling, not a business; a calling in which your heart will be exercised equally with your head. Often the best part of your work will have nothing to do with potions and powders, but with the exercise of an influence of the strong upon the weak, of the righteous upon the wicked, of the wise upon the foolish.

> *Ibid.*, "The Master-Word in Medicine"

As one watches a man handle a patient it is easy to tell whether or not he has had a proper training, and for this purpose fifteen minutes at the bedside are worth three hours at the desk.

> *British Medical Journal* 2:946, 1913

Samuel J. Meltzer [1851–1921]

The constitution does not keep you down exclusively to science, but let me tell you: beware of practice. It is a bewitching graveyard in which many a brain has been buried alive with no other compensation than a gilded tombstone.

> *Journal of the American Medical Association* 53:508, 1909

Sir James Mackenzie [1853–1925]

When I see the modern cardiologist getting his assistant to take an X-ray photograph of the heart and an electrocardiogram, and even a blood pressure reading, and then behold him sitting down to study these reports, I am truly amazed. I never could have realized that the practice of medicine could have become so futile and ineffective.

> Quoted by R. McNair Wilson in *The Beloved Physician*, Ch. 12

Stephen Paget [1855–1926]

As Matthew Arnold said of religion, that it is morality touched with emotion, so practice is science touched with emotion.

> *Confessio Medici*, Ch. 1

Sir Arthur Conan Doyle [1859–1930]

I have nothing to do to-day. My practice is never very absorbing.

> *The Adventures of Sherlock Holmes*, "The Red-Headed League"

Samuel Hopkins Adams [1871–1958]

To dogmatize on questions of medical

practice is to invite controversy and tempt disaster.

> *The Health Master,* Introductory Note

Warfield T. Longcope [1877–1953]

If you find that you resent having to look after the patients on your wards and want to get back to the laboratory, it probably means you'll be happier there. If on the contrary you find you are concerned all the time you are in the laboratory with what is going on in your patients, then that may indicate that you will be better off dealing with people.

> Comment to Dr. Lawrence A. Kohn

Béla Schick [1877–1967]

It is very difficult to slow down. The practice of medicine is like heart muscle contraction — it's *all or none.*

> Quoted by I. J. Wolf in *Aphorisms and Facetiae of Béla Schick,* "Early Years"

Martin H. Fischer [1879–1962]

Here's good advice for practice: go into partnership with nature; she does more than half the work and asks none of the fee.

> Quoted by Howard Fabing and Ray Marr in *Fischerisms*

It takes fifty years from the discovery of a principle in medicine to its adoption in practice.

> *Idem*

William Carlos Williams [1883–1963]

It's the humdrum, day-in, day-out, everyday work that is the real satisfaction of the practice of medicine; the million and a half patients a man has seen on his daily visits over a forty-year period of weekdays and Sundays that make up his life. . . .

I knew it was an elementary world that I was facing, but I have always been amazed at the authenticity with which the simple-minded often face the world when compared with the tawdriness of the public viewpoint exhibited in reports from the world at large.

> *Autobiography,* Ch. 54

Henry E. Sigerist [1891–1957]

Group medicine is a superior form of service. The best way to make full use of the present technology of medicine is to organize medical groups, teams that will practise in health centers. These must be close to the people, in industrial center, residential neighborhood, or farm.

> Quoted in *Journal of the History of Medicine and Allied Sciences* 13:214, 1958

Dana W. Atchley [1892–   ]

The principles of medical management are essentially the same for individuals of all ages, albeit the same problem is handled *differently* in *different* patients.

> Quoted by David Seegal in *Journal of Chronic Diseases* 17:299, 1964

Ben Hecht [1894–1964]

"There are two handicaps to the practice of medicine," Tick had repeated tenaciously through forty years of teaching. "The first is the eternal charlatanism of the patient who is full of fake diseases and phantom agonies. The second is the basic incompetence of the human mind, medical or otherwise, to observe without prejudice, acquire information without becoming too smug to use it intelligently, and most of all, to apply its wisdom without vanity."

> *Miracle of the Fifteen Murderers*

Walsh McDermott [1909–   ]

The revolution in medical science especially in the past ten years, has set an exceedingly fast pace for our medical centers but it has also had the effect of individualizing *the disease as well as the patient.* It is the failure to perceive this, that misleads lay magazines to perpetuate the folk myth that as medicine has become more scientific it has become less personal. In actuality, the whole effect of the scientific boom has been just the opposite, for it compels the physician to individualize the problems presented by each patient. And, it is the stimulation of the student to teach himself this ability to individualize, that represents our major teaching effort. Not just individualization of the science, but individualization of the human warmth and perceptivity with which the science is applied.

> *Journal of Chronic Diseases*
> 16:105, 1963

PRAYERS

See also RELIGION

Moses ben Maimon (Maimonides)
[1135–1204]

Thou has endowed man with the wisdom to relieve the suffering of his brother, to recognize his disorders, to extract the healing substances, to discover their powers and to prepare and to apply them to suit every ill.

Imbue my soul with gentleness and calmness when older colleagues, proud of their age, wish to displace me or to scorn me or disdainfully to teach me. May even this be of advantage to me, for they know many things of which I am ignorant.

Grant me an opportunity to improve and extend my training, since there is no limit to knowledge. Help me to correct and supplement my educational defects as the scope of science and its horizon widen day by day. Give me the courage to realize my daily mistakes so that tomorrow I shall be able to see and understand in a better light what I could not comprehend in the dim light of yesterday. Bless me with a spirit of devotion and self-sacrifice so that I can treat and heal thy suffering servants and prevent disease and preserve health to the best of my ability and knowledge.

Let me see in the sufferer the man alone. . . . Let me be intent upon one thing, O Father of Mercy, to be always merciful to Thy suffering children.

Grant that my patients have confidence in me and my art and follow my directions and counsel.

And now I turn unto my calling;
Ah, stand by me, my God, in this truly important task!
Grant me success! For —
Without Thy loving counsel and support,
Man can avail but naught.
Inspire me with true love for this my art
And for Thy creatures.
Oh, grant —
That neither greed for gain, nor thirst for fame, nor vain ambition,
May interfere with my activity.
For these, I know, are enemies of Truth and Love of men,
And might beguile one in profession
From furthering the welfare of Thy creatures.
Oh, strengthen me!
Grant energy unto both body and the soul,
That I may e'er unhindered ready be
To mitigate the woes,
Sustain and help,
The rich and poor, the good and bad, the enemy and friend,

Oh, let me e'er behold in the afflicted
　and the suffering,
Only the human being!
> Quoted in *Bulletin of the Insti-*
> *tute of the History of Medicine*
> 3:585, 1935

John Wheelock [1754–1817]

O Lord, we thank Thee for the Oxygen
Gas; we thank Thee for the Hydrogen
Gas; and for all gases. We thank Thee
for the Cerebrum; we thank Thee for
the Cerebellum; and for the Medulla
Oblongata. Amen!
> Prayer delivered at a Dart-
> mouth College session, 1798

Sir Robert Hutchison [1871–1960]

From inability to let well alone; from
too much zeal for the new and contempt for what is old; from putting
knowledge before wisdom, science before art, and cleverness before common
sense, from treating patients as cases,
and from making the cure of the disease more grievous than the endurance
of the same, Good Lord, deliver us.
> *British Medical Journal* 1:671,
> 1953

Anonymous

Dear Saint Luke, friend and advisor
to Saint Paul, guide my hand and eye
for the sake of my patient. Steady my
nerves and my scalpel; watch the
microbes and the nurses; make muscles, veins, arteries and nerves behave
according to the book; keep an eye on
the anesthetist. Save us all from lapses
of memory, fraying of tempers, confusion of bottles and instruments, mis-
counting of swabs, and blunders of
diagnosis. If it is "kill or cure," please
cure; if it is "kill or maim," please
maim, but save my patient. . . . And
as there is no more time for praying,
I say Amen.
> *The Linacre Quarterly*, August
> 1954, "A Prayer for Surgeons"

PREGNANCY

See also CHILDBIRTH, CON-
CEPTION, FETUS, ILLEGITI-
MACY, PREMATURITY

Scevola de Sainte-Marthé [1526–1623]

But teeming women, when desire grows
　strong,
Are apt for ev'rything they see to long.
Sand, chalk, and dirt, their appetite
　provoke,
The hearth's black ashes, and the
　chimney's smoke.
> *The Art of Bringing Up Chil-*
> *dren*

William Shakespeare [1564–1616]

He knows himself my bed he hath
　defil'd,
And at that time he got his wife with
　child.
Dead though she be, she feels her
　young one kick.
So there's my riddle: One that's dead
　is quick.
> *All's Well That Ends Well*, V,
> iii, 301

I am with child, ye bloody homicides.
Murther not then the fruit within my
　womb,
Although ye hale me to a violent death.
> *Henry VI, Part I*, V, iv, 62

For love of Edward's offspring in my
　womb.
This is it that makes me bridle passion
And bear with mildness my misfor-
　tune's cross.
Ay, ay, for this I draw in many a tear
And stop the rising of bloodsucking
　sighs,
Lest with my sighs or tears I blast or
　drown
King Edward's fruit, true heir to th'
　English crown.
> *Henry VI, Part III*, IV, iv, 18

She is two months on her way. . . .
She's quick; the child brags in her belly already.
> *Love's Labour's Lost,* V, ii, 679

This Mistress Elbow, being (as I say) with child, and being great-bellied, and longing (as I said) for prunes.
> *Measure for Measure,* II, i, 101

The Queen your mother rounds apace. We shall
Present our services to a fine new prince
One of these days. . . .
    She is spread of late
Into a goodly bulk.
> *The Winter's Tale,* II, i, 16

William Harvey [1578–1657]

Unquestionably the ordinary term of utero-gestation is that which we believe was kept in the womb of his mother by our Savior Christ, of men the most perfect; counting, viz. from the festival of the Annunciation, in the month of March, to the day of the blessed Nativity, which we celebrate in December [275 days]. Prudent matrons, calculating after this rule, as long as they note the day of the month in which the catamenia usually appear, are rarely out of their reckoning; but after ten lunar months have elapsed, fall in labour, and reap the fruit of their womb the very day on which the catamenia would have appeared, had impregnation not taken place.
> *On Parturition* (tr. by Robert Willis)

Benjamin Franklin [1706–1790]

A Ship under sail and a big-bellied Woman,
Are the handsomest two things that can be seen common.
> *Poor Richard's Almanack,* 1735

Rutherford Morison [1853–1939]

In men nine out of ten abdominal tumours are malignant; in women nine out of ten abdominal swellings are the pregnant uterus.
> Quoted in *The Practitioner,* October 1965

Anonymous

The building up of the placenta by the mother and the due performance of function of that wonderful organ require certain favouring conditions . . . and these conditions are certainly not to be found in factory labour.
> *Encyclopaedia Britannica,* 1884

Arabic (Syrian) Proverb

Love and pregnancy and riding upon a camel cannot be hid.

PREMATURITY

See also CHILDBIRTH, PREGNANCY

William Shakespeare [1564–1616]

This, my mother's son, was none of his;
And if it were, he came into the world
Full fourteen weeks before the course of time.
> *King John,* I, i, 111

If ever he have child, abortive be it,
Prodigious, and untimely brought to light,
Whose ugly and unnatural aspect
May fright the hopeful mother at the view.
> *Richard III,* I, ii, 21

Macduff was from his mother's womb
Untimely ripp'd.
> *Macbeth,* V, viii, 15

        On her frights and griefs
(Which never tender lady hath borne greater)
She is, something before her time, deliver'd.

. . . A daughter, and a goodly babe,
Lusty, and like to live.
The Winter's Tale, II, ii, 23

Dorothy C. Stetson [20th Cent.]

At times a premature baby will be
born to a couple who have been married less than nine months; have no
fear for the safety of the baby other
than that for a term baby. These premature babies are generally large and
vigorous. Prematurity in the first baby
in these cases does not indicate an
hereditary tendency toward prematurity; following issue are almost always
full-term gestations.[1]

PRESCRIPTION

Miguel de Cervantes [1547–1616]

Other Doctors kill their Patients, and
are paid for it too and yet they are at
ńo farther Trouble than scrawling two
or three cramp Words for some physical Slip-slop, which the 'Pothecaries
are at all Pains to make up.
Don Quixote, Pt. II, Ch. LXXI
(tr. by Peter Motteux)

Matthew Prior [1664–1721]

You tell your doctor, that ye're ill;
And what does he, but write a bill,
Of which you need not read one letter:
The worse the scrawl, the dose the
better.
For if you knew but what you take,
Tho' you recover he must break.
Alma, Canto III

Finley Peter Dunne ("Mr. Dooley") [1867–1936]

I wondher why ye can always read a
doctor's bill an' ye niver can read his
purscription.
Mr. Dooley Says, "Drugs"

[1] Pragmatic "medical wisdom" passed on
to Dr. John B. Stetson by his mother.

Burton J. Hendrick [1870–1949]

The most ridiculous lingering trace of
monkish superstition is the writing of
prescriptions in Latin.

PREVENTIVE MEDICINE

See also FITNESS, HYGIENE,
PUBLIC HEALTH, REGIMEN,
SOCIAL MEDICINE

Huang Ti (The Yellow Emperor)
[2697–2597 B.C.]

Hence the sages did not treat those
who were already ill; they instructed
those who were not yet ill. . . . To
administer medicines to diseases which
have already developed and to suppress
revolts which have already developed
is comparable to the behavior of those
persons who begin to dig a well after
they have become thirsty, and of those
who begin to cast weapons after they
have already engaged in battle.
Nei Ching Su Wên, Bk. 1, Sect.
2 (tr. by Ilza Veith in *The
Yellow Emperor's Classic of
Internal Medicine*)

The superior physician helps before
the early budding of the disease. . . .
The inferior physician begins to help
when (the disease) has already developed; he helps when destruction has
already set in. And since his help
comes when the disease has already
developed it is said of him that he is
ignorant.
Ibid., Bk. 8, Sect. 26

Ch'in Yueh-jen [ca. 225 B.C.]

The skilful doctor treats those who are
well but the inferior doctor treats those
who are ill.

Huai-nan Tzu (Liu An)
[d. 122 B.C.]

The good doctor pays constant attention to keeping people well so that there will be no sickness.

Liu Kung Cho

The able doctor acts before sickness comes.

Shao Tze

It is better to avert a malady with care than to use physic after it has appeared.

Sir Thomas More [1478–1535]

It is a wise mans part, rather to avoid sicknes, than to wishe for medicines.
> *Utopia*, Bk. II, Ch. 6 (tr. by R. Robinson)

Thomas Randolph [1605–1635]

One that is able to undoe the Company of Barbersurgeons, and Colledge of Physitians, by making all diseases fly the Country.
> *Aristippus*

Thomas Adams [fl. 1612–1653]

Hee is a better Physician that keepes diseases off us, than he that cures them being on us. Prevention is so much better than healing, because it saves the labour of being sick.
> *Works*, "The Happinesse of the Church"

Samuel Pepys [1633–1703]

Myself in good health, but mightily apt to take cold, so that this hot weather I am fain to wear a cloth before my belly.
> *Diary*, June 30, 1661

Now I am at a loss to know whether it be my hare's foot which is my preservation; for I never had a fit of the collique since I wore it, or whether it be my taking of a pill of turpentine every morning.
> *Ibid.*, March 26, 1665

Lemuel Shattuck [1793–1859]

We are not a theorist — a experimentalist. We have no sympathy with the opinions of some modern reformers, who seem to be governed by theories founded on uncertain, partial data, or vague conjecture. We are a statist — a dealer in facts. We wish to ascertain the laws of human life, developed by the natural constitution of our bodies, as they actually exist under the influences that surround them, and to learn how far they may be favorably modified and improved. This can only be done by an accurate knowledge of the facts that are daily occurring among us. These matters are important to the physician to aid him in curing the sick, but far more important to the people to aid them in *learning how to live without being sick*.
> Letter to the Secretary of State, Commonwealth of Massachusetts, 1845

William Farr [1807–1883]

The great source of misery of mankind is not their numbers, but their imperfections, and the want of control over the conditions in which they live. . . . there is a definite task before us — to determine from observation, the sources of Health, and the direct causes of death in the two sexes at different ages and under the different conditions. The exact determination of evils is the first step towards their remedies.
> *Vital Statistics*, Pt. 4

Oliver Wendell Holmes [1809–1894]

And lo! the starry folds reveal
The blazoned truth we hold so dear:
To guard is better than to heal, —
The shield is nobler than the spear!
> *Songs in Many Keys*, "For the Meeting of the National Sanitary Association," 1860

Sir William Withey Gull [1816–1890]

The diseases of the young are in large part preventable diseases. Epidemics carry off in great proportion the healthy members of a community.

> *Published Writings,* "Medicine in Modern Times"

Louis Pasteur [1822–1895]

When meditating over a disease, I never think of finding a remedy for it, but, instead, a means of preventing it.

> Address to the Fraternal Association of Former Students of the École Centrale des Arts et Manufactures, Paris, May 15, 1884

William H. Welch [1850–1934]

It is evident that efforts to preserve health will be most intelligently and effectually applied when they are based upon an accurate and full knowledge of the agencies which cause disease. Public and private hygiene, however, cannot and fortunately has not waited for the full light of that day, whose dawn has only begun to appear, when we shall have a clear insight into the causation of preventable diseases. Cleanliness and comfort demand that means shall be taken to render pure the ground on which we live, the air which we breathe, and the water and food with which we are supplied, and we must meet these needs without waiting to learn just what relation infectious agents bear to the earth, air, water and food.

> *Maryland Medical Journal* 21: 201, 1889

William J. Mayo [1861–1939]

The aim of medicine is to prevent disease and prolong life, the ideal of medicine is to eliminate the need of a physician.

> *National Education Association: Proceedings and Addresses* 66:163, 1928

Charles H. Mayo [1865–1939]

The prevention of disease today is one of the most important factors in the line of human endeavor.

> *Collected Papers of the Mayo Clinic and Mayo Foundation* 5:17, 1913

Harvey Cushing [1869–1939]

A rose by any other name is just as sweet, and there has been in common English usage for the past four hundred years what the doctor has known as prophylactic (to keep guard before), meaning precautionary, medicine. And it would be a slur on the students' intelligence for a surgeon, let us say, to point out, as he has been urged to do, that he wears rubber gloves to "prevent" infecting the patient, gives the anesthetic to "prevent" pain, removes the appendix to "prevent" peritonitis, and so on, *ad infinitum.* For his own part, he sits down and has a cup of tea to "prevent" fatigue, and then to "prevent" irritation keeps away from the faculty meeting where the great importance of preventive medicine will again be pointed out to him. Like many another catchword, — "reconstruction," for example, which was on everyone's lips after the War, — "prevention" can be very much overworked. There is only one ultimate and effectual preventive for the maladies to which flesh is heir, and that is death.

> *The Medical Career and Other Papers,* "Medicine at the Crossroads"

Three fifths of the practice of medicine depends on common sense, a knowledge of people and of human reactions. More than half of the remainder is technological and mechanical, the work of those medically trained artisans we call surgeons. What remains may be termed preventive; and this in bulk very properly and inevitably comes to be taken over by the state, though people, being what they are, find ways of evading a disagreeable statute as in the case of compulsory vaccination — intended for others but not them-

selves. Not everybody obeys the traffic light, and every regulation breeds its jaywalkers and its racketeers.
Idem

Fielding H. Garrison [1870–1935]

The ancient Hebrews were, in fact, the founders of prophylaxis, and the high priests were true medical police.
An Introduction to the History of Medicine, Ch. 3

Thomas, Lord Horder [1871–1955]

Inevitably, the doctor's work in the future will be more and more educational, and less and less curative. More and more will he deal with the physiology and psychology of his patient, less and less with his pathology. He will spend his time keeping the fit fit, rather than trying to make the unfit fit.

Haven Emerson [1874–1957]

The social cost of sickness is incalculable.
The prevention of disease is for the most part a matter of education, the cost is moderate, the results certain and easily demonstrated.
The Social Cost of Sickness

DeForest Clinton Jarvis
[1881–   ]

It is a lot harder to keep people well than it is to just get them over a sickness.
Folk Medicine, Foreword

Henry E. Sigerist [1891–1957]

Every child knows that prevention is not only better than cure, but also cheaper.
Atlantic Monthly, June 1939

Nicotinic acid cures pellagra, but a beefsteak prevents it.
Idem

Would it not be better business to spend more money to prevent the in-cidence of illness rather than to spend many times that amount to cure it?
Idem

Prevention of disease must become the goal of every physician.
Medicine and Human Welfare, Ch. 3

The barriers between preventive and curative medicine must be broken down.
Idem

The task of medicine has always been the same: to promote health by preventing illness and curing it.
Quoted in *Journal of the History of Medicine and Allied Sciences* 13:214, 1958

The Bible: Apocrypha

Learn before thou speak, and use physick or ever thou be sick.
Ecclesiasticus 18:19

Proverb

Prevention is better than cure.

Czech Proverb

He who eats apples every day takes the doctor's bread away.

English Proverb

An apple a day keeps the doctor away.

PROFESSIONAL RELATIONSHIPS

See also CONSULTATION, ETHICS

Plutarch [46?–120?]

Internists are seldom jealous of surgeons; nay, they back up and recommend one another.

John of Salisbury [d. 1180]

I am perfectly amazed and greatly disturbed by the fact that they [physicians] engage in such heated arguments and as a result are divided into factions. Of one thing I am convinced, that contraries can not at the same time be true.

> *Policraticus*, Bk. II, Ch. 29 (tr. by J. Pike)

Petrarch [1304–1374]

I know that your sick bed is continually besieged by physicians, a fact which is my chief cause of terror, for they disagree of set purpose, and even he who can bring forth nothing new is ashamed to follow in the footsteps of another.

> *Invectives*, Preface, Letter to Pope Clement VI

Michel de Montaigne [1533–1592]

Who ever saw a doctor use the prescription of his colleagues without cutting out or adding something?

> *Essays*, Bk. II, Ch. 37, "Of the Resemblance of Children to Fathers" (tr. by Donald M. Frame)

William Harvey [1578–1657]

To return evil speaking with evil speaking, however, I hold to be unworthy in a philosopher and searcher after the truth.

> *On the Circulation of the Blood*, "Second Essay to Jean Riolan" (tr. by Robert Willis)

For the honour of the Profession to continue in mutuall love and affeccion among themselves without which neither the dignity of the Colledge can bee preserved nor yet perticuler men receave that benefitt by their admission into the Colledge which els they might expect, Ever remembering that

Concordia res parvae crescunt, Discordia magnae dilabuntur.[1]

> Trust Deed to the Royal College of Physicians, June 21, 1656

William Wycherley [1640?–1716]

Well, Doctors differ.

> *Plain-Dealer*, Act I, Sc. i

Alexander Pope [1688–1744]

Who shall decide, when Doctors disagree,
And soundest Casuists doubt, like you and me?

> *Moral Essays*, Epistle III

Benjamin Rush [1745?–1813]

General Lee[2] once said: "Oh! that I were a dog, that I might not call man a brother!" With how much more reason might I say, "Oh! that I were a member of any other profession than that of medicine, that I might not call physicians my brethren!"

> Letter to Dr. David Hosack, August 15, 1810

Let us show the world that a difference of opinion upon medical subjects is not incompatible with medical friendships; and in so doing, let us throw the whole odium of the hostility of physicians to each other upon their competition for business and money.

> *Ibid.*, June 20, 1812

Daniel Drake [1785–1852]

The obligations of official duty might compel me to associate with such a man; but nature would defend me against his friendship.

> *A Second Appeal to the Justice of the Intelligent and Respectable People of Lexington*

[1] A slightly reworded quotation from Sallust's *War with Jugurtha*, X.6 (tr. by J. C. Rolfe): Harmony makes small nations great, while discord undermines the mightiest empires.

[2] Henry (Light-Horse Harry) Lee, father of Robert E. Lee.

Ralph Waldo Emerson
[1803–1882]

Don't *say* things. What you *are* stands over you the while, and thunders so that I cannot hear what you say to the contrary.
Letters and Social Aims, Ch. 2

Oliver Wendell Holmes
[1809–1894]

Doctors are the best-natured people in the world, except when they get fighting each other.

Claude Bernard [1813–1878]

The truly scientific spirit, then, should make us modest and kindly. We really know very little, and we are all fallible when facing the immense difficulties presented by investigation of natural phenomena. The best thing, then, for us to do is to unite our efforts, instead of dividing them and nullifying them by personal disputes.
An Introduction to the Study of Experimental Medicine, Pt. I, Ch. 2, Sect. 3 (tr. by H. C. Greene)

Rudolf Virchow [1821–1902]

Has not science the noble privilege of carrying on its controversies without personal quarrels?
Quoted by F. H. Garrison in *Bulletin of the New York Academy of Medicine* 4:995, 1928

Sir William Osler [1849–1919]

Worse still is the "lock and key" laboratory in which suspicion and distrust reign, and everyone is jealous and fearful lest the other should know of or find out about his work.
Aequanimitas, with Other Addresses, "Chauvinism in Medicine"

No sin will so easily beset you as uncharitableness toward your brother practitioner.
Ibid., "The Master-Word in Medicine"

If a man makes it a rule never under any circumstances to believe a story told by a patient to the detriment of a fellow-practitioner — even if he knows it to be true! — though the measure he metes may not be measured to him again, he will have the satisfaction of knowing that he has closed the ears of his soul to ninety-nine lies, and to have missed the hundredth truth will not hurt him.
Ibid., "On the Educational Value of the Medical Society"

Fully half of the quarrels of physicians are fomented by the tittle-tattle of patients.
Ibid., "Unity, Peace, and Concord"

Sir W. Arbuthnot Lane
[1856–1943]

If you get a rude letter, always send a polite one back. It's much better.
Quoted by W. E. Tanner in *Sir W. Arbuthnot Lane*, "Lane as I Knew Him"

"Mr. Lane, how do you get your doctors to submit their patients to such treatment?" His answer was: "Well, you see, some of them are intelligent!"
Idem

How hard it is for some people in authority to realize the folly of being overbearing and rude to those whom they can control!
Ibid., "Lane as a Ship's Surgeon"

William J. Mayo [1861–1939]

The surgeon is often intolerant and the internist self sufficient.
Surgery, Gynecology & Obstetrics 32:97, 1921

Oliver St. John Gogarty
[1878–1957]

Here [in London] the doctors are so kind and professional conduct is so nice that they never contradict each

other. To maintain this harmony it is taboo to make a diagnosis. In Dublin, where the conspiracy is unfriendly, it is necessary to keep the wits keen if one has to live on his professional brethren's repairs.
> *As I Was Going Down Sack-ville Street,* Ch. XVIII

Martin H. Fischer [1879–1962]

Empiricist and theorist — each has called the other a quack.
> Quoted by Howard Fabing and Ray Marr in *Fischerisms*

Hermann J. Muller [1890–1967]

I think that it is up to everyone in fields they're conversant with to speak up and try to work out the truths to-gether with others whose fields over-lap, and even with complete outsiders, because *only* with such free discussion, and not with dictatorship, can we ar-rive at the decisions that will benefit mankind.
> Dartmouth Convocation on *The Great Issues of Conscience in Modern Medicine* (1960), First Panel Discussion

Joyce Dennys [20th Cent.]

Of course everybody knows that Doc-tors never say anything unkind about each other, it is part of their Unwritten Law and a sore trial to nearly all of them.
> *The Over-Dose*

Polish Proverb

A beggar does not hate another beggar as much as one doctor hates another.

PROFESSIONS

See also MEDICINE, PHYSI-CIANS, RELIGION

Plato [427?–347 B.C.]

And he who has learned medicine is a physician, in like manner? He who

has learned anything whatever is that which his knowledge makes him.
> *Gorgias,* 460.B (tr. by Benja-min Jowett)

The surest sign of bad government and social anarchy is to find many judges and many physicians.

Philemon [361?–263? B.C.]

Only physicians and advocates can kill without being killed.
> Quoted by Stobaeus in *Flori-legium,* CII.6

Council of Ratisbon [877]

Monks shall not study law or medicine.

G. F. Poggio-Bracciolini [1380–1459]

Jurisprudence and medicine have this in common, that they are humiliating to contemplate.
> *A Disputation upon Law and Medicine*

Michel de Montaigne [1533–1592]

Lawyers and physicians are a bad pro-vision for a country.
> *Essays,* Bk. III, Ch. 13, "Of Experience" (tr. by Donald M. Frame)

Christopher Marlowe [1564–1593]

Philosophy is odious and obscure,
Both Law and Physicke are for pettie wits,
Divinitie is basest of the three,
Unpleasant, harsh, contemptible and vilde,
Tis Magicke, Magicke that hath rav-isht mee.
> *The Tragicall History of Doc-tor Faustus,* line 134

William Shakespeare [1564–1616]

He is the wiser man, Master Doctor. He is a curer of souls, and you a curer of bodies.
> *The Merry Wives of Windsor,* II, iii, 39

Thomas Fuller [1608–1661]

Commonly physicians, like beer, are best when they are old, and lawyers, like bread, when they are young and new.

The Holy State, Ch. XVI

Cyrano de Bergerac [1619–1655]

In fine, three sorts of people are sent into the world, purposely to martyrize man in this life; the Lawyer torments the purse, the Physician the Body, and the Divine the soul. . . . the Feavour assaults us, the Physician kills us, and the Priest sings.

Satyrical Characters and Handsome Descriptions in Letters, No. 33

Gabriel Thomas [fl. 1690]

Of *Lawyers* and *Physicians* I shall say nothing, because this Countrey is very Peaceable and Healthy; long may it so continue and never have occasion for the Tongue of the one, nor the Pen of the other, both equally destructive to mens Estates and Lives.

An Historical and Geographical Account of the Province and Country of Pennsylvania and of West-New-Jersey in America

Voltaire [1694–1778]

The art of war is like that of medicine, murderous and conjectural.

William Heberden [1710–1801]

Plutarch says that the life of a vestal virgin was divided into three portions; in the first she learned the duties of her profession, in the second she practiced them, and in the third she taught them to others. This is no bad model for the life of a physician: and as I have now passed through the two first of these times, I am willing to employ the remainder of my days in teaching what I know to any of my sons who may choose the profession of physic.

Commentaries on the History and Cure of Diseases, Preface

Sir William Blackstone [1723–1780]

For the gentlemen of the faculty of physic, I must frankly own that I see no special reason why they in particular should apply themselves to the study of law, unless . . . to complete the character of general and extensive knowledge; a character which their profession, beyond others, has remarkably deserved.

Commentaries on the Laws of England, Introduction, Sect. I

John Coakley Lettsom [1744–1815]

Knowing, as I do, the difficulties attendant on the medical profession, I confess I feel a reluctance in recommending the pursuit of it; and yet I can say, were I to commence life anew, I know of no profession, arduous as it is, that I should so cordially embrace.

Letter to a friend, September 6, 1791

Samuel Parr [1747–1825]

Of the three learned professions, in erudition, in science and in habits of deep and comprehensive thinking, the pre-eminence must be assigned in some degree to physicians.

Napoleon Bonaparte [1769–1821]

A physician and a priest ought not to belong to any particular nation, and be divested of all political opinions.

Quoted by Barry E. O'Meara in *Napoleon in Exile,* October 16, 1817

Sydney Smith [1771–1845]

There is only one rule of professional conduct. Do what you think right and take position and emoluments as an accident; all else is labour and sorrow.

Quoted by Lady Holland in *A Memoir of the Rev. Sydney Smith*

Peter Mere Latham [1789–1875]

I have a conservative jealousy of the rank due to my profession.
Lectures on Clinical Medicine, Lect. I

Oliver Wendell Holmes [1809–1894]

When lawyers take what they would give,
And doctors give what they would take.
Latter-day Warnings

If you would die fagged to death like a crow with the king birds after him, — be a schoolmaster; if you would wax thin and savage, like a half-fed spider, — be a lawyer; if you would go off like an opium-eater in love with your starving delusion, — be a doctor.
Letter to Phineas Barnes, March 1831

I warn you against all ambitious aspirations outside of your profession. Medicine is the most difficult of sciences and the most laborious of arts. It will task all your powers of body and mind if you are faithful to it. Do not dabble in the muddy sewer of politics, nor linger by the enchanted streams of literature, nor dig in far-off fields for the hidden waters of alien sciences. The great practitioners are generally those who concentrate all their powers on their business. If there are here and there brilliant exceptions, it is only in virtue of extraordinary gifts, and industry to which very few are equal.
Medical Essays, "The Young Practitioner"

The lawyers are the cleverest men, the ministers are the most learned, and the doctors are the most sensible.
The Poet at the Breakfast Table, Sect. V

George Eliot (Marian Evans Cross) [1819–1880]

The best augury of a man's success in his profession is that he thinks it the finest in the world.
Daniel Deronda, Ch. 58

Theodor Billroth [1829–1894]

Culture is always an aristocratic thing. The physician, the school teacher, the lawyer, the clergyman should be the best men of their village, of their city, of the circles in which they move. In order to be so they must have the super-power that comes with knowledge and skill, and this is acquired only through the hard work of study, and even more through the cultivation of the inner urge to study.
The Medical Sciences in the German Universities, Pt. 2

Abraham Jacobi [1830–1919]

Aims, methods, and persistency are common to the medical profession of all countries. On its flag is inscribed what should be the life rule of all nations: Fraternity and solidarity.

John Shaw Billings [1838–1913]

The public is not always sagacious, but in the long run, it does somehow contrive to find out who are the skilled lawyers and doctors.

Santiago Ramón y Cajal [1852–1934]

Only the doctor and the dramatist enjoy the rare privilege of charging us for the annoyance they give us.
Charlas de Café

Sir John Bland-Sutton [1855–1936]

I divided my life into three parts: in the first I learned my profession, in the second I taught it, in the third I enjoy it.
The Story of a Surgeon

Louis D. Brandeis [1856–1941]

A profession is an occupation for which the necessary preliminary training is

457

intellectual in character, involving knowledge and to some extent learning, as distinguished from mere skill. . . . It is an occupation which is pursued largely for others and not merely for one's self. . . . It is an occupation in which the amount of financial return is not the accepted measure of success.

Business — A Profession, Ch. 1

A. Lawrence Lowell [1856–1943]

It is hardly an exaggeration to summarize the history of four hundred years by saying that the leading idea of a conquering nation in relation to the conquered was, in 1600, to change their religion; in 1700, to change their trade; in 1800, to change their laws; and in 1900, to change their drainage. May we not, then, say that on the prow of the conquering ship in these four centuries first stood the priest, then the merchant, then the lawyer, and finally the physician?

George Bernard Shaw [1856–1950]

Nobody supposes that doctors are less virtuous than judges; but a judge whose salary and reputation depended on whether the verdict was for plaintiff or defendant, prosecutor or prisoner, would be as little trusted as a general in the pay of the enemy.

The Doctor's Dilemma, "Preface on Doctors"

Anton Chekhov [1860–1904]

Doctors are just the same as lawyers; the only difference is that lawyers merely rob you, whereas doctors rob you and kill you, too.

Ivanov, Act I (tr. by Elisaveta Fen)

I have made a point all my life of mistrusting all doctors, lawyers, and women. They are shammers and deceivers.

Ibid., Act II (tr. by Marian Fell)

You advise me not to hunt after two hares, and not to think of medical work. I do not know why one should not hunt two hares even in the literal sense. . . . I feel more confident and more satisfied with myself when I reflect that I have two professions and not one. Medicine is my lawful wife and literature my mistress. When I get tired of one I spend the night with the other. Though it's disorderly, it's not so dull, and besides neither of them loses anything from my infidelity. If I did not have my medical work I doubt if I could have given my leisure and my spare thoughts to literature.

Letter to A. S. Suvorin, September 11, 1888 (tr. by Constance Garnett)

William J. Mayo [1861–1939]

The church and the law with the yesterdays of life; medicine deals with the tomorrows.

Collected Papers of the Mayo Clinic and Mayo Foundation 23:1001, 1931

Harvey Cushing [1869–1939]

In spite of all the discouraging things they are permitted to learn about the units composing society, the doctor and the priest continue to have not only hope for but faith in their fellow men, and expect them, in spite of their frailties, to be unselfish and honest till they prove themselves otherwise; whereas in trade, politics, and the law, we are told, a man is primarily taken to be self-seeking until he proves the contrary.

The Medical Career, "Medicine at the Crossroads"

Samuel Hopkins Adams [1871–1958]

With the exception of lawyers, there is no profession which considers itself above the law so widely as the medical profession.

The Health Master, Ch. I

W. Somerset Maugham
[1874–1965]

Mrs. Carey thought there were only four professions for a gentleman, the Army, the Navy, the Law, and the Church. She had added medicine . . . but did not forget that in her young days no one ever considered the doctor a gentleman.
> *Of Human Bondage,* Ch.
> XXXIII

The medical profession is the only one which a man may enter at any age with some chance of making a living.
> *Ibid.,* Ch. LV

Albert Schweitzer [1875–1965]

I wanted to be a doctor that I might be able to work without having to talk. For years I had been giving myself out in words, and it was with joy that I had followed the calling of theological teacher and of preacher. But this new form of activity I could not represent to myself as being talking about the religion of love, but only as an actual putting it into practice.
> *Out of My Life and Thought,*
> Ch. 9 (tr. by C. T. Campion)

Martin H. Fischer [1879–1962]

The priest sees them half un-dressed; the doctor sees them naked. They lie to the former; they masquerade before the lawyer; they cannot deceive the discerning physician.
> Quoted by Howard Fabing and
> Ray Marr in *Fischerisms*

This is the trouble with us doctors: our talk is sloppy, like the preachers' — and the result is bad for both professions.
> *Idem*

José Ortega y Gasset [1883–1955]

The gentleman who professes to be a doctor, or magistrate, or general, or philologist, or bishop — that is, a person who belongs to the directive class of society — if he is ignorant of what the physical cosmos is today for the European man, is a perfect barbarian, however well he may know his laws, or his medicine, or his Holy Fathers.
> *Collected Works*

Alan Gregg [1890–1957]

Take as a career something that in its difficulty requires resolve, in its complexity brains, and in its accomplishment gives lasting satisfaction.
> Aphorism (Quoted by Wilder
> Penfield in *The Difficult Art of
> Giving,* Appendix A)

Anonymous

Physicians and politicians resemble one another in this respect, that some defend the constitution and others destroy it.
> *Acton or the Circle of Life*

The doctor sees men not at their best, as does the minister, nor at their worst, as does the lawyer; the doctor sees them as they are.
> Quoted by James B. Herrick in
> *Memories of Eighty Years,* Ch.
> IV

Proverb

War and physic are governed by the eye.

Chinese Proverb

Only the healing art enables one to make a name for himself and at the same time give benefit to others.

English Proverb

Few lawyers die well; few physicians live well.

Hungarian Proverb

The most over-populated professions: doctors, fools, advisers.

Indian (Marathi) Proverb

First farming, next trade, last service, or at least begging; if you cannot obtain alms, learn to be a doctor.

Italian Proverb

Deceive not thy physician, confessor, nor lawyer.

PROGNOSIS

See also DIAGNOSIS

Hippocrates [460?–377? B.C.]

In acute diseases it is not quite safe to prognosticate either death or recovery.
> *Aphorisms,* II.19 (tr. by Francis Adams)

It appears to me a most excellent thing for the physician to cultivate Prognosis; for by foreseeing and foretelling, in the presence of the sick, the present, the past, and the future, and explaining the omissions which patients have been guilty of, he will be the more readily believed to be acquainted with the circumstances of the sick; so that men will have confidence to intrust themselves to such a physician. And he will manage the cure best who has foreseen what is to happen from the present state of matters. . . . Thus a man will be the more esteemed to be a good physician, for he will be the better able to treat those aright who can be saved, from having long anticipated everything; and by seeing and announcing beforehand those who will live and those who will die, he will thus escape censure.
> *On the Prognostics,* I (tr. by Francis Adams)

It is impossible to make all the sick people well; this, indeed, would have been better than to be able to foretel what is going to happen.
> *Idem*

Hillel ben Samuel [ca. 1220–1295]

Promise to serve everyone who is ill with thy wisdom.
But do not promise to cure a physician.
> Introduction to his translation of Bruno de Lungoburgo's *Chirurgia Magna* (tr. by H. Friedenwald in *The Jews and Medicine,* Vol. I, Essay 5)

William Shakespeare [1564–1616]

His friends, like physicians,
Thrice give him over.
> *Timon of Athens,* III, iii, 11

Sir Thomas Browne [1605–1682]

'Tis as dangerous to be sentenced by a Physician as a Judge.
> *A Letter to a Friend*

Cyrano de Bergerac [1619–1655]

I am condemned (but 'tis only by the Physician) from which I can more easily appeale than from a Criminall decree. . . . This graduate notwithstanding tells me, that t'will be nothing and at the same time protests to every body else, that I cannot escape without a Miracle.
> *Satyrical Characters and Handsome Descriptions in Letters,* No. 33

Benjamin Rush [1745?–1813]

I do not think your disease should alarm you. By following *all* the above directions, I think your recovery is as certain as physicians dare to pronounce any events to be that relate to the issue of diseases.
> Postscript to letter to Mr. Walter Stone, January 5, 1791

Sir Walter Scott [1771–1832]

A doctor is like Ajax — give him light, and he may make battle with a disease; but, no disparagement to the Esculapian art, they are bad guessers.
> Letter to Lord Montagu, April 14, 1824

Charles Dickens [1812–1870]

Being promptly blooded, however, by a skilful surgeon, he rallied; and although the doctors all agreed, on his being attacked with symptoms of apoplexy six months afterwards, that he ought to die, and took it very ill that he did not, he remained alive — possibly on account of his constitutional slowness — for nearly seven years more, when he was one morning found speechless in his bed.
Barnaby Rudge, Chapter the Last

Sir John Bland-Sutton [1855–1936]

Forecasts of this kind have great charm for me. The really clever man, call him a prophet if you will, is he who can see a little further into the future than other men.
The Story of a Surgeon, Ch. IX

Sir Henry Howarth Bashford ("Peter Harding") [1880–1961]

If your news must be bad, tell it soberly and promptly.
The Corner of Harley Street, Ch. 26

Albert R. Lamb [1881–   ]

Patients and their families will forgive you for wrong diagnoses, but will rarely forgive you for wrong prognoses; the older you grow in medicine, the more chary you get about offering iron clad prognoses, good or bad.
Quoted in *Journal of Chronic Diseases* 16:441, 1963

Harold T. Hyman [1894–   ]

In individual prognosis, statistics function as a weathervane. From them the practitioner recognizes the wind direction; he knows nothing of wind velocity, or of weather conditions such as temperature, humidity or visibility.
Handbook of Treatment, "Psychotherapy"

George T. Pack [1898–   ]

The patient's family will never forgive a guarantee of cure that failed and the patient will not let the physician forget a pronouncement of incurability if he is so fortunate as to survive.
Annals of Surgery 127:1105, 1948

David Seegal [1899–   ]

Frailty, thy name is physician in the *over-exercise* of prognoses of longevity.
The Pharos of Alpha Omega Alpha 27:81, 1964

Lewis L. Robbins [1913–   ]

The antiquity of the art of prognosis dates back to the dawn of history, nay, to the beginning of the world. The Lord, the Great Physician, had problems. Thus, in the Bible we read that the Lord told Adam: "Of every tree you may freely eat but of the tree of the knowledge of good and evil thou shalt not eat of it, for in the day that thou eatest thereof, thou shalt surely die" and Adam we are informed, "lived 930 years thereafter." [1]
Archives of Internal Medicine 107:801, 1961

Anonymous

There are doctors who to show their worth and to be sure of an excuse make bad seem worse and of the worse make a disaster.

PROGRESS

Hieremias Martius [fl. 1568]

But what the present age now scorns and hates, a grateful posterity may perhaps find a worthy work.
Noni Medici Clarissimi de omnium particularium morborum curatione, "Interpres ad Zoilum"

[1] *Genesis* 2:16 and 5:5.

Sir Francis Bacon [1561–1626]

Medicine is a science which hath been (as we have said) more professed than laboured, and yet more laboured than advanced; the labour having been, in my judgment, rather in circle than in progression. For I find much iteration, but small addition.
> *The Advancement of Learning,* Bk. II

Surely every medicine is an innovation; and he that will not apply new remedies must expect new evils; for time is the greatest innovator, and if time of course alter things to the worse, and wisdom and counsel shall not alter them to the better, what shall be the end?
> *Essays,* "Of Innovations"

Augustin Belloste [1654–1730]

That which is New at this time, will one day be Ancient; as what is Ancient was once New. It is not Length of Time which can give Value to Things, it is only their own Excellency.
> *The Hospital Surgeon*

William Heberden [1710–1801]

I please myself with thinking that the method of teaching the art of healing is becoming every day more conformable to what reason and nature require; that the errors introduced by superstition and false philosophy are gradually retreating; and that medical knowledge, as well as all other dependent upon observation and experience, is continually increasing in the world. The present race of physicians is possessed of several most important rules of practice, utterly unknown to the ablest in former ages, not excepting Hippocrates himself, or even Aesculapius.
> Letter to Dr. Thomas Percival, October 15, 1794

William Shippen, Jr. [1736–1808]

All ages have agreed as to the danger of innovations: and the sanction derived from precedents, has generally been proportioned to their antiquity: but in this case, as in all other rules, there must be exceptions; and it need not be remarked that the wisest systems have grown to perfection by degrees, and that without the aid of innovations, no system almost would have deserved the epithet of wise.

Joseph Hodgson [1788–1869]

But let us look to the future. The time must surely come when the arts of destruction shall bend before the works of peace; when those pursuits which increase our powers, which avert or relieve our sufferings and which diffuse health and comfort among the people, shall occupy that position and that consideration which reason and right feeling justly accord to them.
> *The Hunterian Oration,* 1855

Elisha Bartlett [1804–1855]

In the infinite future, which will ever stretch out before the advancing progress of science and art, properties and relations of all forms of matter, now unimagined and undreamed of, may yet be discovered, by means and processes of investigation now wholly hidden, which shall utterly overthrow the present theory of light, beautiful and stable as it appears to be.
> *Philosophy of Medical Science,* Pt. I, Ch. 4

Oliver Wendell Holmes [1809–1894]

You have not learned all that art has to teach you, but you are safer practitioners to-day than were many of those whose names we hardly mention without a genuflection.
> *Medical Essays,* "The Young Practitioner"

I find the great thing in this world is not so much where we stand as in what direction we are moving.

Claude Bernard [1813–1878]

The progress of the experimental

method consists in this, — that the sum of truths grows larger in proportion as the sum of error grows less. But each one of these particular truths is added to the rest to establish more general truths. In this fusion, the names of promoters of science disappear little by little, and the further science advances, the more it takes an impersonal form and detaches itself from the past.

> *An Introduction to the Study of Experimental Medicine,* Pt. I, Ch. 2, Sect. iv (tr. by H. C. Greene)

Abraham Coles [1813–1891]

Believing needless ignorance a crime,
You strive to reach the summit of your time;
To old age learning up from early youth
Your life one long apprenticeship to truth:
Wisely suspicious sometimes of the new,
Ye give alert acceptance to the true:
Even though it make old science obsolete,
It with a thousand welcomes still you greet. . . .
Each Year adds something — many things ye know
Your sires knew not a Hundred Years ago.

> *The Microcosm,* "Physician's Character and Aims — Science Progressive"

Louis Pasteur [1822–1895]

[I am] a man whose invincible belief is that Science and Peace will triumph over Ignorance and War, that nations will unite, not to destroy, but to build, and that the future will belong to those who will have done most for suffering humanity.

> Speech at his Golden Jubilee, December 27, 1892 (tr. by René J. Dubos in *Pasteur and Modern Science*)

S. Weir Mitchell [1829–1914]

The true rate of advance in medicine is not to be tested by the work of single men, but by the practical capacity of the mass.

The truer test of national medical progress is what the country doctor is.

Frank Kittredge Paddock [1841–1901]

A grand hypothesis is not the usual path for the advancement of medical knowledge. As a rule, first comes a new or improved method whose application to a variety of problems sometimes leads unexpectedly to greater understanding.

> Aphorism

Sir William Osler [1849–1919]

Everywhere the old order changes and happy they who can change with it.

> *The Principles and Practice of Medicine* (1895)

William J. Mayo [1861–1939]

The glory of medicine is that it is constantly moving forward, that there is always more to learn.

> *National Education Association: Addresses and Proceedings* 66:163, 1928

Alfred North Whitehead [1861–1947]

Our rate of progress is such that an individual human being, of ordinary length of life, will be called upon to face novel situations which find no parallel in his past. The fixed person, for the fixed duties, who in older societies was such a godsend, in the future will be a public danger.

Sir Berkeley Moynihan [1865–1936]

Those who have learned from a great master must surely not be content to imitate his methods, but rather must

strive to capture his authentic spirit, and in that spirit to seek for new roads, and so to discover still firmer truths. Few virtues are nobler than loyalty to a great tradition. But such tradition is kept alive not by routine observance of ancient ceremony, nor by mute obedience to outworn creed, but by active faith for ever seeking new truths and exploring new paths, in conformity with the old spirit, and with unfaltering devotion to that great ideal which tradition enshrines.
Truants

Stephen B. Leacock [1869–1944]

The progress of medicine . . . is something wonderful. Any lover of humanity (or of either sex of it) who looks back on the achievements of medical science must feel his heart glow and his right ventricle expand with the pericardiac stimulus of a permissible pride.

Just think of it. A hundred years ago there were no bacilli, no ptomaine poisoning, no diphtheria, and no appendicitis. Rabies was but little known, and only imperfectly developed. All of these we owe to medical science. Even such things as psoriasis and parotitis and trypanosomiasis, which are now household names, were known only to the few, and were quite beyond the reach of the great mass of the people.
Literary Lapses, "How to Be a Doctor"

W. Wayne Babcock [1872–   ]

We shall not scorn what was done yesterday because we have something better today any more than our interest in the past will cause us to continue the practice of the past.
Textbook of Surgery, Preface

Sir Winston Churchill [1874–1965]

The whole prospect and outlook of mankind grew immeasurably larger, and the multiplication of ideas also pro-

ceeded at an incredible rate. This vast expansion was unhappily not accompanied by any noticeable advance in the stature of man either in his mental faculties or his moral character. His brain got no better; but it buzzed more.
Address in Massachusetts, March 31, 1949

Otto Weininger [1880–1903]

Definite scientific conceptions are preceded by anticipations. The process of clarification is spread over many generations.
Sex and Character, Pt. II, Ch. 3

Samuel Clark Harvey [1886–1953]

It is necessary in this time of conflict and confusion within society that medicine, if it is to survive as a profession, be not only on guard but energetically pressing forward all along the line.
Yale Journal of Biology and Medicine 5:323, 1933

Sir F. M. R. Walshe [1888–   ]

Medicine is the oldest learned profession in the world and it is rooted in its past. Each successive generation of doctors stands, as it were, upon the shoulders of its predecessors, and the fair perspectives that are now opening before you are largely the creation of those who have gone before you. It is therefore reasonable to think that anyone who has spent a long professional life in medicine must have something to hand on — however small or modest.
Canadian Medical Association Journal 67:395, 1952

Sir James Learmonth [1895–1967]

Progress in science, and particularly in medical science, is both continuous and episodic, episodic progress depending on the genius of men and of women and on the possibilities of putting promising therapeutic agents to properly controlled clinical trial. . . . in its time the invention of the wheel was more revolutionary than was the more recent invention of television.

Lancet 2:303, 1947

William Dock [1898–   ]

The physician must look beyond the picture, now widely cherished, of the lonely, great-hearted doctor, bowed impotent beside the dying child. Modern transportation, modern methods of communication, and modern techniques of diagnosis and treatment, have made that picture as obsolete as the village blacksmith at his charcoal forge.

The Next Half Century in Medicine (Symposium)

Prince Philip, Duke of Edinburgh [1921–   ]

Progress is undiscriminating. Progress gives us better medical science, but it also gives us better bombs. How do you relate computers to compassion?

Speech (Quoted by Alden Hatch in *The Mountbattens,* Pt. III, Ch. 6)

PSYCHIATRY

See also INSANITY, MIND, PSYCHOANALYSIS, PSYCHOLOGY, PSYCHOSOMATICS, PSYCHOTHERAPY

John Hunter [1728–1793]

Perhaps there is nothing in Nature more pleasing than the study of the human mind, even in its imperfections or depravities; for, although it may be more pleasing to a good mind to contemplate and investigate the application of its powers to good purposes, yet as depravity is an operation of the same mind, it becomes at least equally necessary to investigate, that we may be able to prevent it.

Surgical Observations, Vol. I

John Aikin [1747–1822]

In particular, one whose office it is to apply *medicine to the mind,* must, as well as the physician of the body, conquer his reluctance to give temporary pain, for the sake of affording lasting benefit.

Letters from a Father to His Son, Letter II, "On Strength of Character"

Aloysius Sieffert [fl. 1858]

The care of the human mind is the most noble branch of medicine.

Medical and Surgical Practitioner's Memorandum

Sigmund Freud [1856–1939]

Now and then occasions arise in which the physician is bound to take up the position of teacher and mentor, but it must be done with great caution, and the patient should be educated to liberate and to fulfil his own nature and not to resemble ourselves.

Pierre Marie Félix Janet [1859–1947]

If a patient is poor he is committed to a public hospital as "psychotic"; if he can afford the luxury of a private sanitarium, he is put there with the diagnosis of "neurasthenia"; if he is wealthy enough to be isolated in his own home under constant watch of nurses and physicians he is simply an indisposed "eccentric."

La Force et la faiblesse psychologiques

Alfred North Whitehead [1861–1947]

The ideas of Freud were popularized by people who only imperfectly understood them, who were incapable of the great effort required to grasp them in their relationship to larger truths, and who therefore assigned to them a prom-

inence out of all proportion to their true importance.
> *Dialogues,* Dialogue XXVIII (June 3, 1943)

W. Somerset Maugham [1874-1965]

The mystic sees the ineffable, and the psycho-pathologist the unspeakable.
> *The Moon and Sixpence,* Ch. I

Hughes Mearns [1875–   ]

As I was going up the stair
I met a man who wasn't there,
He wasn't there again to-day.
I wish, I wish he'd stay away.
> *The Psychoed*

Lord Robert Webb-Johnstone [1879–   ]

A neurotic is the man who builds a castle in the air. A psychotic is the man who lives in it. And a psychiatrist is the man who collects the rent.
> *Collected Papers*

Samuel Goldwyn [1] [1882–   ]

Anyone who spends money on a psychiatrist should have his head examined.

Sir F. M. R. Walshe [1888–   ]

Certainly psychiatry had not then [1910] shown signs of those cannibal tendencies to devour the whole of medicine from which we have so constantly to defend ourselves and our students today.
> *Canadian Medical Association Journal* 67:395, 1952

Carl Binger [1889–   ]

To see another human being with any understanding involves a relationship, and into this relationship our feelings will inevitably enter. The important thing is for us to try to become aware of our feelings, and when they are so intense that they cloud or distort

[1] Attributed to Samuel Goldwyn.

our judgment or lead us into blunders, we must try to face ourselves squarely and look for the trouble spots there.
> *Harper's Magazine,* June 1964, "Psychiatrist in a Looking Glass"

Lawrence S. Kubie [1896–   ]

There is no heterodoxy, only an array of fighting orthodoxies [among the various schools of psychiatry]. Each group tends all too rapidly to become formula-ridden and hidebound. Each develops a tendency to outlaw the data and theories from the other schools, and to view them with angry rejection and suspicion. . . . What all behavioral science needs . . . is the heterodoxy of the fully informed and erudite scholar who rebels against orthodoxy within himself and within his own camp.
> *Journal of Nervous and Mental Disorders* 137:311, 1963

Bertram D. Lewin [1896–   ]

The heat which arises from so many useless clashes between the proponents of "organic" and "psychological" medicine might not appear, if it were realized that the main issue was a matter of preference, an emotional preference for the dead or the live patient.
> *Psychosomatic Medicine* 8:195, 1946

Walter Lincoln Palmer [1896–   ]

Don't refer a patient to a psychiatrist as if you are telling him to go to hell.
> Aphorism

Al Capp [1909–   ]

Psychiatrists are often amusing company, especially when they are drunk.
> *Tufts Folia Medica* 9:97, 1963

Edwin McH. Dunlop [1917–   ]

With the drugs we now have available, the GP can and should be the frontline psychiatrist. The sooner this happens, the quicker we can stop the psychiatric landslide threatening to bury us all.

> *Medical World News* 3 (No. 11):27, 1962

Jane Merchant [1919–   ]

Good sirs, pray tell
In accents calm
Why Adam fell
Who had no mom.

> *To Certain Psychiatrists*

Philip Rieff [1922–   ]

The significance of Freud's life and thought is too important, as a historical expression of forces deeper than Freud himself realized, to be left to the Freudians.

> Review of Giovanni Costigan's *Sigmund Freud* in *The New York Times Book Review*, May 30, 1965

Harry Wiener [1924–   ]

Schizophrenia . . . splits psychiatrists into two cultures, the psychologic (psychodynamic) and the organic (somatic). Each group ignores the other and wishes it would go away.

> *Journal of the American Medical Association* 197:1046, 1966

Anonymous

The new definition of psychiatry is the care of the id by the odd.

The psychiatrist is the obstetrician of the mind.

PSYCHOANALYSIS

See also INSANITY, MIND, PSYCHIATRY, PSYCHOTHERAPY

Sir Francis Bacon [1561–1626]

Let a full and careful treatise be constructed . . . that so we may have a scientific and accurate dissection of minds and characters, and the secret dispositions of particular men may be revealed; and that from the knowledge thereof better rules may be framed for the treatment of the mind.

> *The Advancement of Learning,* Bk. VII, Ch. III

Sigmund Freud [1856–1939]

The poets and philosophers before me have discovered the unconscious; I have discovered the scientific method with which the unconscious can be studied.

> *Letter*

Bernard Berenson [1865–1959]

Psychoanalysts are not occupied with the minds of their patients; they do not believe in the mind but in a cerebral intestine.

> Quoted by Umberto Morra in *Conversations with Berenson,* February 8, 1931 (tr. by Florence Hammond)

G. K. Chesterton [1874–1936]

Psychoanalysis is confession without absolution.

Karl Kraus [1874–1936]

Psychoanalysis is the disease it purports to cure.

Thomas Mann [1875–1955]

Analysis as an instrument of enlightenment and civilization is good, in so far as it shatters absurd convictions, acts as a solvent upon natural prejudices, and undermines authority; good, in other words, in that it sets free, refines, humanizes, makes slaves ripe for freedom. But it is bad, very bad, in so far as it stands in the way of action, cannot shape the vital forces, maims life at its roots. Analysis can be a very unappetizing affair, as much so as death, with which it may well belong — allied to the grave and its unsavory anatomy.

> *The Magic Mountain*, Ch. V, "Freedom" (tr. by H. T. Lowe-Porter)

Clarence P. Oberndorf [1882–1954]

Progress and experience in psychoanalytic teaching have brought out the need to avoid the microscopic examination of individual symptoms and to correlate them instead with the overall picture of the mental disorder as a whole and its setting in the patient's environment and period of life.

> *Medicine and Other Disciplines*

Karen Horney [1885–   ]

Fortunately analysis is not the only way to resolve inner conflicts. Life itself still remains a very effective therapist.

> *Our Inner Conflicts*, Ch. XIII

Erich Fromm [1900–   ]

The minute study of the process of rationalization is perhaps the most significant contribution of psychoanalysis to human progress.

> *Psychoanalysis and Religion*, Ch. 3

Erik H. Erikson [1902–   ]

The moral idea was clearly stated for all to behold: the "classical arrangement" was only a means to an end — namely, a human relationship in which the observer who has learned to observe himself teaches the observed to become self-observant.

> *Childhood and Society*, Ch. 11

Jacques Barzun [1907–   ]

Psychoanalysis does not measure. But this turns out to be much less of a difference [from other sciences] when we know that in modern physics what can be measured is the statistical probability of action of a great many units. The single electron is as flighty and unpredictable as the compulsive neurotic in Freud's office — perhaps more so.

> *Harper's Magazine*, June 1949

Harley C. Shands [1916–   ]

The ambivalence of my feelings about psychoanalysis is clearly evident throughout this book, I think. The positive part of this ambivalence is directed towards the practice of psychotherapy, a development for which psychoanalysis is clearly responsible. The negative feelings are directed towards the restrictive and basically anti-scientific aspects of the "closed shop" of organized psychoanalysis.

> *Thinking and Psychotherapy*, Preface

Anonymous

Omniscient in your juggler's booth,
All is discovered through your patter
Except the simple obvious truth
Of what was actually the matter.

> Quoted in *Archives of Internal Medicine* 117:152, 1966

PSYCHOLOGY

See also BODY AND MIND, DREAMS, MIND, PSYCHIATRY

Aristotle [384–322 B.C.]

In children may be observed the traces and seeds of what will one day be settled psychological habits, though psychologically a child hardly differs for the time being from an animal.

> *Historia Animalium*, VIII.1 (tr. by D. W. Thompson)

John Stuart Mill [1806–1873]

Hardly any medical practitioner is a psychologist. Respecting the mental characteristics of women; their observations are of no more worth than those of common men.

> *The Subjection of Women*, Ch. I

Sir Frederick Walker Mott [1853–1926]

No progress was possible in the advancement of our knowledge of mental disease until we had shaken off the spell of metaphysical speculation . . . the doctrine that the mind is an invisible, intangible spirit with a separate existence in the body. We now recognize the brain as the seat of the psyche, but the functions of the mind are dependent upon the whole body and the harmonious interaction of all its parts.

> Quoted by W. S. Dawson in *Aids to Psychiatry*, Introduction

Sigmund Freud [1856–1939]

The economy of expenditure in psychic inhibition brought about by wit — small though it may be in comparison to the sum total of psychic expenditure — will remain a source of pleasure for us, because we thereby save a particular expenditure which we are wont to make, and which we were also ready to make this time.

> *Basic Writings*, "Motives of Wit as a Social Process" (tr. by A. A. Brill)

John Dewey [1859–1952]

Popular psychology is a mass of cant, of slush and of superstition worthy of the most flourishing days of the medicine man.

> *The Public and Its Problems*, Ch. 5

Bernard Berenson [1865–1959]

Each of us is in himself like such a building. In the lower storeys we live with our animal needs, animal greeds, and animal passions. Woe if we neglect the first, ignore the second, and pretend to be free from the last! No matter how high we rise we must never lose sight, never cease being aware, of the animal basis of our nature. If we do, we lose the sense of things. We get vapid, vague, hypocritical, arrogant, insolent. The tall structure that we have become turns into a tower of Babel, toppling over and confounding its builder.

> *Sketch for a Self-Portrait*, Pt. 3, Ch. 6

Wilfred Trotter [1872–1939]

This subconscious or subwaking self is regarded as embodying the "lower" and more obviously brutal qualities of man. It is irrational, imitative, credulous, cowardly, cruel, and lacks all individuality, will, and self-control. This personality takes the place of the normal personality during hypnosis and when the individual is one of an active crowd, as, for example, in riots, panics, lynchings, revivals, and so forth.

> *Instincts of the Herd in Peace and War*, Pt. I, Ch. 4

Nowhere has been and is the domination of the herd more absolute than in the field of speculation concerning man's general position and fate, and in consequence prodigies of genius have been expended in obscuring the simple truth that there is no responsibility for man's destiny anywhere at all outside his own responsibility, and that there is no remedy for his ills outside his own efforts.

> *Ibid.*, "Postscript of 1919"

Karl Kraus [1874–1936]

Psychology is as unnecessary as directions for using poison.

W. Somerset Maugham [1874–1965]

The unhappiness of Philip's life at school had called up in him the power of self-analysis; and this vice, as subtle as drug-taking, had taken possession

of him so that he had now a peculiar keenness in the dissection of his feelings.
> *Of Human Bondage,* Ch. I

Carl Jung [1875–1961]

The separation of psychology from the premises of biology is purely artificial, because the human psyche lives in indissoluble union with the body.
> *Factors Determining Human Behavior,* "Psychological Factors Determining Human Behavior"

What the physician observes of psychical manifestations is an infinitesimal part of the psychical world, and moreover often distorted by pathological conditions. . . . Just as human anatomy has a long evolution behind it, the psychology of modern man depends upon its historical roots, and can only be judged by its ethnological variants.
> Foreword to Frieda Fordham's *An Introduction to Jung's Psychology*

Edwin Bidwell Wilson [1879–1964]

It would be a pity if Wundt had taken Psychology from her mother Philosophy and married her to Science only to have her desert to a paramour Mathematics.
> *Psychometrika* 4:148, 1939

Everett Dean Martin [1880–1941]

A crowd is a device for indulging ourselves in a kind of temporary insanity by all going crazy together.
> *The Behavior of Crowds,* Ch. 2

Oswald Spengler [1880–1936]

I maintain that today many an inventor, many a diplomat, many a financier is a sounder philosopher than all those who practice the dull craft of experimental psychology.
> *Decline of the West,* Introduction, Sect. 15

Helene Deutsch [1884–   ]

We know that degree of normal psychic health is not determined by the absence of conflicts, but by the adequacy of the methods used to solve and master them.
> *The Psychology of Women,* Vol. I, Preface

W. Russell, Lord Brain [1895–1966]

Medical psychology is concerned with all kinds of abnormalities of human behaviour, and it was the study of this subject by Freud which produced a revolution in man's conception of himself. . . . Freud's discovery of unconscious motivation, and the importance of the experiences of early infancy for the subsequent development of the personality, has profoundly influenced our conception of human nature, and had lasting effects on ethics. To understand all may not be to forgive all, but at least it affects our attitude to condemnation and punishment, partly by increasing our understanding of the culprit, and partly by exposing the unconscious basis of our own mental attitudes. All these developments in medical psychology have therefore been a challenge to accepted ideas of criminal responsibility.
> *Doctors Past and Present,* "The Doctor's Place in Society"

Oscar Hammerstein [1895–1960]

You've got to be taught to hate and fear.
> *South Pacific,* "You've Got to Be Carefully Taught"

Helen Harris Perlman [1905–   ]

I never saw a person's id
I hope I never see one.
But I can tell you if I did
I'd clamp an ego as a lid
Upon the id to keep it hid,

Which is, I gather, what God did
When he first saw a free one.
*National Association of Social
Workers News* 9:2, 1964

W. I. B. Beveridge [1908–   ]

The work of some psychologists on
extrasensory perception and precogni-
tion may be a present-day example of
a discovery before its time. Most scientists have difficulty in accepting the
conclusions of these workers despite
apparently irrefutable evidence, because the conclusions cannot be reconciled with present knowledge of
the physical world.
*The Art of Scientific Investiga-
tion,* Ch. IX

Anonymous

Human nature can never be observed
as such, but only in its specific manifestations in specific situations. It is
a theoretical construction which can be
inferred from empirical study of the
behavior of man. In this respect, the
science of man in constructing a
"model of human nature" is no different from other sciences which operate
with concepts of entities based on, or
controlled by, inferences from observed
data and not directly observable themselves.

PSYCHOSOMATICS

See also BODY AND MIND,
HYPOCHONDRIA

Giorgio Baglivi [1669–1707?]

All Men have their own Cares, and
every one lies under a bitter Necessity of spending almost all the Periods
of his Life, in attending the doubtful
Events of his Labour. Now this being
true, 'tis equally a Truth obvious to
all Men, that a great Part of Diseases
either take their Rise from, or are fed
by that Weight of Care that hangs
upon every one's Shoulders.
The Practice of Physick, Ch. 14

Laurence Sterne [1713–1768]

He knew the fallacy of medicine to a
creature, whose ILLNESS HAS ARISEN
FROM THE AFFLICTION OF HER MIND.
Letters to Eliza, Letter IX

Tobias Smollett [1721–1771]

I have known a gentleman who was
paralytic to a deplorable degree, en-
raged to a perfect use of all his limbs
while his anger predominated.
*Essay on the External Use of
Water*

Johann Wolfgang von Goethe [1749–1832]

If you start to think about your physical or moral condition, you usually
find that you are sick.
Sprüche in Prosa, Pt. 1, Bk. II

James Currie [1756–1805]

There is a part of the philosophy of
medicine that has as yet been little
attended to; I mean that which treats
of the diseases of the mind, of the
influence of affections primarily mental,
on the corporeal functions, and particularly of the passions and emotions.
Letter to Dr. George Bell, October 20, 1781

Nathaniel Hawthorne [1804–1864]

A bodily disease, which we look upon
as whole and entire within itself, may,
after all, be but a symptom of some
ailment in the spiritual part.
The Scarlet Letter, Ch. 10

Mary Baker Eddy [1821–1910]

Disease is an experience of mortal
mind. It is fear made manifest on the
body.
Science and Health, Ch. XIV

Elie Metchnikoff [1845–1916]

The toxin of fatigue has been demonstrated; but the poisons generated by evil temper and emotional excess over non-essentials have not yet been determined, although without a doubt they exist.

Marcel Proust [1871–1922]

For one disorder that doctors cure with drugs (as I am told that they do occasionally succeed in doing) they produce a dozen others in healthy subjects by inoculating them with that pathogenic agent a thousand times more virulent than all the microbes in the world, the idea that one is ill.

> *The Guermantes Way,* Pt. I, "My Grandmother's Illness" (tr. by C. K. Scott-Moncrieff)

Frank Loesser [1910–   ]

The average unmarried female, basically insecure
Due to some long frustration, may react
With psychosomatic symptoms, difficult to endure,
Affecting the upper respiratory tract.
In other words, just from waiting around
For that plain little band of gold
A person . . . can develop a cold.

When they get on the train for Niagara and she can hear the churchbells chime;
The compartment is air-conditioned and the mood sublime;
Then they get off at Saratoga, for the fourteenth time,
A person . . . can develop la grippe,
La grippe, la postnasal drip.
With the wheezes and the sneezes
And a sinus that's really a pip.

From a lack of community property and a feeling she's getting too old,
A person . . . can develop a bad, bad cold.

> *Guys and Dolls,* "Adelaide's Lament"

PSYCHOTHERAPY

See also INSANITY, PSYCHIATRY, PSYCHOANALYSIS

Henri de Mondeville [1260–1320]

Keep up your patient's spirits by music of viols and ten-stringed psaltery, or by forged letters describing the death of his enemies, or by telling him he has been elected to a bishopric, if a churchman.

> *Treatise on Surgery*

Sir Francis Bacon [1561–1626]

How wisely and aptly can you speake and discerne of Phisicke ministred to the bodie, and consider not that there is the like occasion of physicke ministred to the mind.

> *Apology Concerning the Earl of Essex*

Thomas Jefferson [1743–1826]

If the appearance of doing something be necessary to keep alive the hope & spirits of the patient, it should be of the most innocent character.

> Letter to Dr. Caspar Wistar, June 21, 1807

Philippe Pinel [1745–1826]

Laborious employment . . . is not a little calculated to divert the thoughts of lunatics from their usual morbid channel, to fix their attention upon more pleasing objects, and by exercise to strengthen the functions of the understanding.

> *A Treatise on Insanity,* Sect. V, No. 94 (tr. by D. D. Davis)

John Conolly [1794–1866]

Restraint and neglect are synonymous. They are a substitute for the thousand attentions needed by a disturbed patient.

> *The Treatment of the Insane Without Mechanical Restraints*

Emile Coué [1857–1926]

Every day, in every way, I am getting better and better.
> General formula for auto-suggestion used at his clinic in Nancy (Quoted in *My Method*, Ch. III)

Carl Jung [1875–1961]

It is indeed high time for the clergyman and the psychotherapist to join forces.
> *Modern Man in Search of a Soul*, Ch. XI

James Bridie [1888–1951]

Calamy, laudamy, poultices, pills,
They are the stuff for bodily ills.
Thingummybobs of a different kind
Are the stuff for disorderliness of the mind.
When with distresses your psyche is wracked,
Relax. Think of nothing at all. Abreact.
Associate freely, sublimate
The origins of your anxiety state.
Snap your fingers, my dear, as I do,
At the tortuous twistings of your libido.
Away with repression and up with the Id.
Tell your medical man whatsoever you did.
Trust the Unconscious. And that I suppose is
How to get rid of hallucinoses
And pseudopathomorphic psychosomaticoses,
And lie on a perpetual bed of roses.
> *Tedious and Brief*, Pt. I, "A Change for the Worse"

Therese F. Benedek [1892–   ]

The therapist's personality (his emotional maturity, psychosexual stability and personal integrity) is the most important agent of the therapeutic process.
> *Bulletin of the Menninger Clinic* 17:201, 1953

Robert Graves [1895–   ]

A well chosen anthology is a complete dispensary of medicine for the more common mental disorders, and may be used as much for prevention as cure.
> *On English Poetry*, Ch. XXIX

Harley C. Shands [1916–   ]

To be maximally happy, the individual must learn to enjoy success by participating in that of the group. In Piaget's phrase, he has to "decentralize" himself; in Freud's statement, to abandon "narcissism." The more his capacity for establishing relationships of participation, the more his likelihood of satisfaction. This means that he must learn to enjoy the spectator aspect more than the actor aspect. . . . Performers are in active, vigorous competition, while the observer is able to abandon competitive goals in the interest of enjoyment within himself.
> *Thinking and Psychotherapy*, Ch. 1

PUBLIC HEALTH

See also HEALTH, OCCUPATIONAL DISEASE, PREVENTIVE MEDICINE, SOCIAL MEDICINE

Aristotle [384–322 B.C.]

Surely the members of a household must have health just as they must have life. And as from one point of view the master of the house and the ruler of the State have to consider about health, from another point of view not they but the physician.
> *Politics*, I.iii

Tobias Smollett [1721–1771]

When I see a number of well-dressed people, of both sexes, sitting on the covered benches, exposed . . . to the cold, raw, night air, devouring sliced

beef, and swilling port, and punch, and cider, I can't help compassionating their temerity, . . . but, when they course along those damp and gloomy walks, or crowd together upon the wet gravel, without any other cover than the cope of heaven, . . . how can I help supposing they are actually possessed by a spirit more absurd and pernicious than anything we meet with in the precincts of Bedlam? In all probability, the proprietors of this, and other public gardens of inferior note . . . are . . . connected with the faculty of physic, and the company of undertakers; for . . . I am persuaded that more gouts, rheumatisms, catarrhs, and consumptions are caught in these nocturnal pastimes, *sub dio,* than from all the risks and accidents to which a life of toil and danger is exposed.
> *The Expedition of Humphry Clinker,* Letter 30

Karl F. H. Marx [1796-1877]

That is the best country which has the fewest diseases, laws and crime.
> Quoted by F. H. Garrison in *Bulletin of the New York Academy of Medicine* 4:1001, 1928

Benjamin Disraeli, Lord Beaconsfield [1804-1881]

The health of a people is really the foundation upon which all their happiness and all their power as a State depend.
> Speech, June 23, 1877

Charles Dickens [1812-1870]

Some years ago, being in Scotland, I went with one of the most humane members of the humane medical profession, on a morning tour among some of the worst-lodged inhabitants of the old town of Edinburgh. In the closes and wynds of that picturesque place — I am sorry to remind you what fast friends picturesqueness and typhus often are — one saw more poverty and sickness in an hour than many people would believe in a life.
> Speech on behalf of the Hospital for Sick Children (Freemason's Hall), February 9, 1858

Florence Nightingale [1820-1910]

The first possibility of rural cleanliness lies in *water supply.*
> Letter to Medical Officer of Health, November 1891

Rudolf Virchow [1821-1902]

Medical instruction does not exist to provide individuals with an opportunity of learning how to make a living, but in order to make possible the protection of the health of the public.
> Address to medical students at the Pathological Institute, Berlin

Jakob Laurenz Sonderegger [1826-1896]

Each meal was a glittering feast. Yet, I had haunted, uneasy moments. Ghosts scurried about: children from the sulphur pits, peasants, hungry and ill, who worked in the rice paddies all day long to earn fifty centimes. Off and on, a subtle smell of beggars and wretched misery seemed to waft through the banquet hall which was elegantly perfumed. A glass of *Lacrimae Christi* appeased the soul. An old remedy.
> Speech to the Cholera Congress in Rome, 1885 (tr. by Max Samter)

Charles V. Chapin [1856-1941]

It will make no demonstrable difference in a city's mortality whether its streets are clean or not, whether the garbage is removed promptly or allowed to accumulate, or whether it has a plumbing law.
> *Papers,* "Dirt, Disease, and the Health Officer"

George Bernard Shaw [1856–1950]

When you are so poor that you cannot afford to refuse eighteenpence from a man who is too poor to pay you any more, it is useless to tell him that what he or his sick child needs is not medicine, but more leisure, better clothes, better food, and a better drained and ventilated house.

> *The Doctor's Dilemma,* "Preface on Doctors"

Hermann M. Biggs [1859–1923]

Public Health Is Purchasable. Within Natural Limitations Any Community Can Determine Its Own Death Rate.[1]

> *New York State Department of Health Monthly Bulletin* 9:45, 1914

William J. Mayo [1861–1939]

Of all coöperative enterprises public health is the most important and gives the greatest returns.

> *Collected Papers of the Mayo Clinic and Mayo Foundation* 11:1157, 1919

Charles H. Mayo [1865–1939]

Good health is an essential to happiness, and happiness is an essential to good citizenship.

> *Journal of the American Dental Association* 6:505, 1919

It is a poor government that does not realize that the prolonged life, health and happiness of its people are its greatest asset.

> *Journal of the American Medical Association* 73:411, 1919

Richard H. Tawney [1880–1962]

It is not till it is discovered that high individual incomes will not purchase the mass of mankind immunity from cholera, typhus, and ignorance, still less secure them the positive advan-

[1] This motto appeared on the title page of the journal.

tages of educational opportunity and economic security, that slowly and reluctantly, amid prophecies of moral degeneration and economic disaster, society begins to make collective provision for needs which no ordinary individual, even if he works overtime all his life, can provide himself.

> *Equality,* Ch. 5, Sect. ii

Franklin D. Roosevelt [1882–1945]

The old idea of the right of an individual to be sick or of a community to have epidemics no longer exists. That right has been turned around and transferred to the State. I mean by "State" the general governing agencies, and they undoubtedly have the right to insist on good health.

> *Address on Public Health and the Development of Saratoga Springs as a Health Center,* June 25, 1929

The State must protect them [the citizens], so far as lies in its power, from disease, from ignorance, from physical injury, and from old-age want.

> *Address Before the New York State Charities Aid Association,* January 17, 1930

Nothing can be more important to a State than its public health; the State's paramount concern should be the health of its people.

> *Report of the Special Health Commission Transmitted to the New York Legislature,* February 19, 1931

Public health is more than a local responsibility. Disease knows nothing about town lines, nor do bacilli undertake to inquire about local jurisdictions. Their carriers are on the public highways and riding in the railroad trains.

> *Address on the Excessive Costs and Taxes in Local Government,* July 6, 1931

The health of the people is a public concern; ill health is a major cause of suffering, economic loss, and dependency; good health is essential to the security and progress of the nation. . . .

I have been concerned by the evidence of inequalities that exist among the States as to personnel and facilities for health services. There are equally serious inequalities of resources, medical facilities and services in different sections and among different economic groups. These inequalities create handicaps for the parts of our country and the groups of our people which most sorely need the benefits of modern medical science.

> *Message to Congress on the National Health Program,* January 23, 1939

Harry S. Truman [1884–   ]

I believed that the United States should be the healthiest country in the world and lead in finding and developing new ways to improve the health of every citizen. . . . I proposed a national health program. President Roosevelt had set the stage for a health program in his "economic bill of rights," which included "the right to adequate medical care and the opportunity to achieve and enjoy good health."

> *Memoirs,* Vol. II, Ch. 1

"Socialized medicine" was constantly used by the opposition in an attempt to confuse the provisions of the national health insurance program.

> *Ibid.,* Ch. 30

Arnold Toynbee [1889–   ]

The twentieth century will be remembered chiefly, not as an age of political conflicts and technical inventions, but as an age in which human society dared to think of the health of the whole human race as a practical objective.

Henry E. Sigerist [1891–1957]

The organization of medical services

. . . is a world-wide development. In some countries the process is finished and services completely organized, others are halfway in the development, and in others it is just beginning, but no country can escape the trend.

> *Atlantic Monthly,* June 1939

We are told . . . that health conditions are better . . . than ever before in the history of the United States. . . . If health conditions are better here than in certain foreign countries, it is not because medical services are superior, but because this country was able to develop a higher standard of living.

> *Idem*

Health cannot be forced upon the people. It cannot be dispensed to the people. They must want it and be prepared to do their share and to cooperate fully in whatever health program a country develops.

> *Canadian Journal of Public Health* 35:253, 1944

We must never say that health conditions are good, but must rather ask ourselves constantly whether they are as good as they could be.

> *Civilization and Disease,* Ch. 12

Disease creates poverty and poverty disease. The vicious circle is closed.

> *Medicine and Human Welfare,* Ch. 1

There is an iron rule which is valid everywhere, namely, that no individual and no family can lead a decent and healthy life unless they have a certain minimum income. . . . If this is not done, people will of necessity become antisocial, may develop illness or break the law, and in such cases society must pay a far greater bill by erecting and operating hospitals and jails.

> *Idem*

The people's health is the concern of the people themselves. They must want

health. They must struggle for it and plan for it.
> *Ibid.*, Ch. 2

Education, general education and health education, represent the starting point of all health activities.
> *Proceedings of the American Philosophical Society* 90:275, 1946

All societies have a social organization to fight disease.
> Quoted in *Journal of the History of Medicine and Allied Sciences* 13:214, 1958

Wendell L. Willkie [1892–1944]

The real public-health problem, of course, is poverty.
> *One World,* Ch. 2

Sir Robert Platt [1900–   ]

Even in my own time the hospital population which I knew as a young man was inadequately clothed and fed and housed and usually dirty, ignorant and ill-informed.
> *Universities Quarterly* 17:327, 1963

René J. Dubos [1901–   ]

Physicians and public health officials, like soldiers, are always equipped to fight the last war.
> *The Dreams of Reason,* Ch. IV

John F. Kennedy [1917–1963]

The health of our nation is a key to its future — to its economic vitality, to the morale and efficiency of its citizens, to our success in achieving our own goals and demonstrating to others the benefits of a free society. Ill health and its harsh consequences are not confined to any State or region, to any race, age, or sex or to any occupation or economic level. This is a matter of national concern.
> *Message to Congress on a Health Program,* February 9, 1961

Good health is a prerequisite to the enjoyment of "pursuit of happiness." Whenever the miracles of modern medicine are beyond the reach of any group of Americans, for whatever reason — economic, geographic, occupational or other — we must find a way to meet their needs and fulfill their hopes. For one true measure of a nation is its success in fulfilling the promise of a better life for each of its members. Let this be the measure of our nation.
> *Message to Congress on the Nation's Health Needs,* February 27, 1962

The basic resource of a nation is its people. Its strength can be no greater than the health and vitality of its population. Preventable sickness, disability and physical or mental incapacity are matters of both individual and national concern.
> *Idem*

The dramatic results of new medicines and new methods — opening the way to a fuller and more useful life — are too often beyond the reach of those who need them most. Financial inability, absence of community resources, and shortages of trained personnel keep too many people from getting what medical knowledge can obtain for them.
> *Idem*

Good health for all our people is a continuing goal. In a democratic society where every human life is precious, we can aspire to no less. Healthy people build a stronger nation, and make a maximum contribution to its growth and development.
> *Message to Congress on a Health Program,* February 7, 1963

Our health can be no better than the knowledge and skills of the physicians,

dentists, nurses, and others to whom we entrust it.
Idem

Thomas A. Dooley [1927–1961]

Politics, like clouds and passing things, quickly scud by. The terrors of disease are always with us. Here is a challenge. It is flung at each of us individually. The response must come from each of us individually. This response is not the job of the government alone. A government can only go so far. It can never, it will never, replace the individual citizen's sense of responsibility for those in the world who "ain't got it so good."
Letter to Dr. William D. Snively, Jr., April 24, 1958

PULSE

See also BLOOD, CIRCULATION, HEART

William Shakespeare [1564–1616]

My pulse as yours doth temperately keep time
And makes as healthful music.
Hamlet, III, iv, 140

Your pulsidge beats as extraordinarily as heart would desire.
Henry IV, Part II, II, iv, 25

      But are you flesh and blood?
Have you a working pulse?
Pericles, V, i, 154

Peter Mere Latham [1789–1875]

The oracle of old made it the top of wisdom to know oneself, but did not fix the credit due to that fragment of self-knowledge which enables a man to keep count of his own pulse.
General Remarks on the Practice of Medicine, "The Heart and Its Affections," Ch. II

PURGATIVES

See also BOWELS

Charles Wriothesley [1508?–1562]

Some recken he [Cardinal Wolsey] killed himselfe with purgations.
Chronicle, "Henrici VIII, Anno 21"

William Shakespeare [1564–1616]

To prevent our maladies unseen,
We sicken to shun sickness when we purge.
Sonnet CXVIII

Robert Burton [1577–1640]

Purge downward rather than upward, use potions rather than pills, and when you begin physic, persevere and continue in a course; for as one observes, . . . to stir up the humour (as one purge commonly doth) and not to prosecute, doth more harm than good.
The Anatomy of Melancholy, Pt. 2, Sect. 4, Memb. 1, Subsect. 3

Oliver St. John Gogarty [1878–1957]

The Englishman . . . believes that a purgative can fatten or make him thin; he believes that either there is only one kind of ache or that one medicine can cure various kinds. His empty churches would be filled twice over by the faith he wastes on the permutations and importance of his lower bowel.
As I Was Going Down Sackville Street, Ch. III

QUACKS

See also NOSTRUMS

Cato [234–149 B.C.]

A quack's words are heard, but no one

trusts himself to him when he is sick.
Quoted by Aulus Gellius in *Attic Nights*, I.xv.9 (tr. by J. C. Rolfe)

Celsus [25 B.C.–A.D. 50]

It is like a montebank to exaggerate a small matter in order to enhance his own achievement.
De Medicina, V.26 (tr. by W. G. Spencer)

Sir Francis Bacon [1561–1626]

Nay, we see [the] weakness and credulity of men is such, as they will often prefer a montabank or witch before a learned physician. And therefore the poets were clear-sighted in discerning this extreme folly, when they made Aesculapius and Circe brother and sister, both children of the sun.
The Advancement of Learning, Bk. II

For in all times, in the opinion of the multitude, witches and old women and imposters have had a competition with physicians.
Idem

Philip Massinger [1583–1640]

           Your physicians are
Mere voice, and no performance; I have found
A man that can do wonders.
The Duke of Milan, Act V, Sc. ii

Philip Massinger [1583–1640] **and Thomas Dekker** [1572?–1632?]

           Out, you impostors!
Quacksalving, cheating mountebanks! your skill
Is to make sound men sick, and sick men kill.
The Virgin Martyr, Act IV, Sc. i

John Ford [1586?–1640?]

Mountebanks, empirics, quack-salvers, mineralists, wizards, alchemists, cast-

apothecaries, old wives and barbers, are all suppositors [1] to the right worshipful doctor.
The Lover's Melancholy, Act I, Sc. iii

Lady Mary Wortley Montagu [1689–1762]

We have no longer faith in miracles and relics, and therefore with the same fury run after recipes and physicians. The same money which three hundred years ago was given for the health of the soul is now given for the health of the body, and by the same sort of people — women and half-witted men.
Letter to Mr. Wortley Montagu, April 24, 1748

Benjamin Franklin [1706–1790]

Quacks are the greatest liars in the world except their patients.

Percivall Pott [1714–1788]

The desire of health and ease, like that of money, seems to put all understandings, and all men, upon a level; the avaricious are duped by every bubble; the lame and the unhealthy by every quack. Each party resigns his understanding; swallows greedily, and for a time believes implicitly, the most groundless, ill-founded, and delusory promises; and nothing but loss and disappointment ever produce conviction.
Chirurgical Works, Vol. I, "General Remarks on Fractures and Dislocations"

Horace Walpole [1717–1797]

By quack I mean imposter, not in opposition to but in common with physicians.

Tobias Smollett [1721–1771]

We have quacks in religion, quacks in physic, quacks in law, quacks in government — High German quacks, that

---

[1] suppositors = supporters.

have blistered, sweated, bled, and purged the nation into an atrophy.

> *The Adventures of Sir Launcelot Greaves,* Ch. 10

Oliver Goldsmith [1728–1774]

A quack, unable to distinguish the particularities in each disease, prescribes at a venture: if he finds such a disorder may be called by the general name of fever, for instance, he has a set of remedies which he applies to cure it, nor does he desist till his medicines are run out, or his patient has lost his life. But the skilful physician distinguishes the symptoms, manures the sterility of nature, or prunes her luxuriance; nor does he depend so much on the efficacy of medicines as on their proper application.

> Letter to Rev. Thomas Contarine, 1753

Jeremy Bentham [1748–1832]

A valetudinarian, who quacked himself to death.

George Crabbe [1754–1832]

There was a time, when we beheld the quack,
On public stage, the licensed trade attack;
He made his labour'd speech with poor parade;
And then a laughing zany lent him aid: . . .
  But now our quacks are gamesters, and they play
With craft and skill to ruin and betray;
With monstrous promise they delude the mind,
And thrive on all that tortures humankind.

> *The Borough,* Letter VII

From powerful causes spring th' empiric's gains,
Man's love of life, his weakness, and his pains;

These first induce him the vile trash to try,
Then lend his name, that other men may buy.

> *Idem*

A potent quack, long versed in human ills,
Who first insults the victim whom he kills;
Whose murd'rous hand a drowsy Bench protect,
And whose most tender mercy is neglect.

> *The Village,* Bk. I

Robert Southey [1774–1843]

Man is a dupable animal. Quacks in medicine, quacks in religion, and quacks in politics know this, and act upon that knowledge.

> *The Doctor,* Ch. 87

Charles C. Colton [1780?–1832]

It is better to have recourse to a quack, if he can cure our disorder, although he cannot explain it, than to a physician, if he can explain our disease, but cannot cure it.

> *Lacon,* Vol. I, Ch. CCCXXIII

Peter Mere Latham [1789–1875]

The practice of physic is jostled by quacks on the one side, and by science on the other.

> *Collected Works,* Vol. I, Sir Thomas Watson's "In Memoriam"

Thomas Carlyle [1795–1881]

Quackery gives birth to nothing; gives death to all things.

> *Heroes and Hero-Worship,* Lect. I

Henry Wadsworth Longfellow [1807–1882]

You behold in me
Only a travelling Physician;
One of the few who have a mission

To cure incurable diseases,
Or those that are called so.
> *Christus: A Mystery,* Pt. II,
> Sect. i

Frederick Saunders [1807–1902]

Empirics and charlatans are the excrescences of the medical profession.
> *Salad for the Social,* "The Mysteries of Medicine"

Oliver Wendell Holmes [1809–1894]

Quackery and idolatry are all but immortal.
> *Medical Essays,* "The Medical Profession in Massachusetts"

Abraham Coles [1813–1891]

The man of impure life and sordid aims
He smuts his office and his calling
shames:
Him you disown and place him under
ban
As nothing better than a charlatan.
> *The Microcosm,* "Physician's Character and Aims — Science Progressive"

Rudolf Virchow [1821–1902]

Imprisoned quacks are always replaced by new ones.
> Quoted by F. H. Garrison in *Bulletin of the New York Academy of Medicine* 4:995, 1928

Laws should be made, not against quacks but against superstition.
> *Idem*

Sir William S. Gilbert [1836–1911]

The advertising quack who wearies
  With tales of countless cures,
    His teeth, I've enacted,
    Shall all be extracted
  By terrified amateurs.
> *The Mikado,* Act II

Karl Sudhoff [1853–1938]

In essence, quackery is ever the same. In its "good" forms, it is simply an impudent abstraction from previous epochs of scientific medicine. In its worst forms, it is the degeneration and distortion of the borrowed material, of most exaggerated type, often completely reversing the original material or thought, with the most harmful consequences.
> *An Historical Museum of the Healing Art* (tr. by Herman T. Radin)

Robert Tuttle Morris [1857–1945]

The number of quacks in a locality is an index to the character of the regular medical profession in that locality.
> *Doctors Versus Folks,* Ch. 4

Anton Chekhov [1860–1904]

It would not have been so bad if he had simply been a quack, of whom there were plenty, but no — he was a quack who believed in himself, a quack who was furtively in revolt.
> *An Unpleasantness* (tr. by Avrahm Yarmolinsky in *The Unknown Chekhov*)

Martin H. Fischer [1879–1962]

Don't cry out against the quack; find out wherein his success lies — and be a better quack.
> Quoted by Howard Fabing and Ray Marr in *Fischerisms*

John F. Kennedy [1917–1963]

It has been estimated that consumers waste $500 million a year on medical quackery and another $500 million dollars annually on some "health foods" which have no beneficial effect. . . . Unnecessary deaths, injuries, and financial loss . . . can be expected to continue until the law requires adequate testing for safety and efficacy of products and devices before they are made available to consumers.
> *Message to Congress on Problems of the Aged,* February 21, 1963

Anonymous

Great outcry has been raised of late in the *Lancet* and other journals, against Quacks and Quackery. Let them not flatter themselves that it is possible to put either down. The Quack is a personage too essential to the comfort of a large class of society, to be deprived of his vocation. He is, in fact, the Physician of the Fools, — a body whose numbers and respectability are by far too great to admit of anything of the kind. We propose that every Quack should not only not be suffered to call himself what he is not, but should be compelled to call himself what he is.

> *Punch*, 1845, "A Dose for the Quacks"

The followers of quacks are the causes of quackery.

QUANTITATION

See also STATISTICS

Leonardo da Vinci [1452–1519]

No human investigation can be called true science without passing through mathematical tests.

> *Treatise on Painting*, Ch. 1 (tr. by Jean Paul Richter)

Sir Francis Bacon [1561–1626]

As Physic advances farther and farther every day and develops new axioms, it will require fresh assistance from Mathematic.

> *The Advancement of Learning*, Bk. III, Ch. VI

Stephen Hales [1677–1761]

Since we are assured that the all-wise Creator has observed the most exact proportions, of *number, weight and measure*, in the make of all things; the most likely way therefore, to get any insight into the nature of those parts of the creation, which come within our observation, must in all reason be to number, weigh and measure.

> *Vegetable Staticks*, Introduction

William Thomson, Lord Kelvin [1824–1907]

When you cannot measure it, when you cannot express it in numbers, — you have scarcely, in your thoughts, advanced to the stage of Science, whatever the matter may be.

George M. Beard [1839–1883]

As quantitative truth is of all forms of truth the most absolute and satisfying, so quantitative error is of all forms of error the most complete and illusory.

> *Popular Science Monthly* 14: 751, 1879

Martin H. Fischer [1879–1962]

Quibbling over hair-splitting qualitative differences is always an evidence of sophistry. Vital distinctions are quantitative.

> Quoted by Howard Fabing and Ray Marr in *Fischerisms*

Sir George P. Thomson [1892–]

To many people science is a matter of measurements carried out with meticulous accuracy. Such measurements play a great role in developing a discovery but they are rarely its cause.

> *The Inspirations of Science*

Loren Eiseley [1907–]

Today there is a tendency in some quarters to regard the physical sciences as superior in reliability to those in which precise mathematical adeptness has not been achieved. Without wishing to challenge this point of view, it may still be worth a chastening thought that, in this long controversy extending well over half a century, the physicists made extended use of mathematical techniques and still were hope-

lessly and, it must be added, arrogantly wrong.
Darwin's Century, Ch. 9

Dwight J. Ingle [1907–   ]

Science cannot be equated to measurement, although many contemporary scientists behave as though it can. For example, the editorial policies of many scientific journals support the publication of data and exclude the communication of ideas.
Principles of Research in Biology and Medicine

Anonymous

"Systems analysis" may be defined as quantitative common sense.

RABIES

Celsus [25 B.C.–A.D. 50]

When too little has been done for such a wound [bite of a mad animal], it usually gives rise to a fear of water which the Greeks call *hydrophobia*. . . . In these cases there is very little hope for the sufferer. But still there is just one remedy, to throw the patient unawares into a water tank which he has not seen beforehand. If he cannot swim, let him sink under and drink, then lift him out; if he can swim, push him under at intervals so that he drinks his fill of water even against his will; for so his thirst and dread of water are removed at the same time. Yet this procedure incurs a further danger, that a spasm of sinews, provoked by the cold water, may carry off a weakened body. Lest this should happen, he must be taken straight from the tank and plunged into a bath of hot oil.
De Medicina, V.27 (tr. by W. G. Spencer)

William Shakespeare [1564–1616]

The venom clamours of a jealous woman

Poisons more deadly than a mad dog's tooth.
The Comedy of Errors, V, i, 69

Oliver Goldsmith [1728–1774]

This dog and man at first were friends;
  But when a pique began,
The dog, to gain his private ends
  Went mad and bit the man. . . .

But soon a wonder came to light,
  That show'd the rogues they lied,
The man recovered of the bite,
  The dog it was that died.
Elegy on the Death of a Mad Dog

READING

See also LIBRARIES, LITERATURE

Andrew Boorde [1490–1549]

It is extremely difficult for a physician who puts too much trust in what he reads to form a proper decision from what he sees.

Edouard Auber [1804– ?]

Above all learn and know how to read before engaging in writing, and before so producing, understand how to choose and select, for many a time you will be judged by a plain stock-taking of your library, and one will say of you: — I know what you are and what you esteem, for I discern what it is that you read and what you approve of, enjoy and appreciate.
Bibliothèque de l'étudiant en médecine et du médecin practicien

Jacob M. Da Costa [1833–1900]

All that goes on in medicine is to be the chief matter of interest to you. Hence you must be busy readers; and, as habits form, you will learn to look to medical journals with avidity, and new publications will be examined with keen relish. But to become distinguished, nay, to become even respectable in your profession, you must be something more than readers, you must become active thinkers and sifters of knowledge, learn, as Bacon counsels, to weigh and consider books.

> Valedictory address, Jefferson Medical College, 1874

We are, I think, in this busy age of ours, in great danger of over-estimating the value of mere reading. It is often a lazy mode of half-culture, a kind of mental dissipation, relished the more because it is mingled with a feeling of self-satisfaction at following what seems an intellectual pursuit; a trouble-saving invention, indulged in fitfully, and without regard to its true purpose. That purpose is to make the knowledge sought completely our own, to examine it critically, and if fully satisfied with it, to adapt it so thoroughly as part of our mental organization, that we are not conscious of how it came there.

> *Idem*

Sir William Osler [1849–1919]

It is astonishing with how little reading a doctor can practise medicine, but it is not astonishing how badly he may do it.

> *Aequanimitas, with Other Addresses,* "Books and Men"

Do not waste the hours of daylight in listening to that which you may read by night.

> Quoted by W. S. Thayer in *Bulletin of the Johns Hopkins Hospital* 30:198, 1919

George Sarton [1884–1956]

The art of reading implies the art of non-reading, and more energy is sometimes needed in order to skip rather than continue useless drifting. Many would-be scholars never learn anything not only because they cannot read, but also because they cannot stop reading; they are like asses turning round and round in a mill with blinkers on their eyes.

> *Science* 131:1182, 1960

William S. Middleton [1890–   ]

Call it what you will, discriminating, purposeful reading is good medicine.

> *The Pharos of Alpha Omega Alpha* 22:211, 1959

Henry E. Sigerist [1891–1957]

One point I should like to mention . . . is the speed of reading. I know that American schools try to teach their students to read as quickly as possible. . . . If the physician can devote only two hours a day to reading, it is obviously important for him to be able to read much in a short time. I am a hopelessly slow reader and therefore probably prejudiced in the matter. When I read a book and a paragraph strikes me as particularly good I may read it several times and make notes about it. I wonder if studies have been made with quick readers to find out how much they remembered of what had particularly impressed them in a book, after five, ten or 15 years. Some books we wish to forget as soon as possible as they are not worth being remembered, but others we want to assimilate, want them to become part of ourselves, and this takes a certain time.

> *On the History of Medicine,* Ch. 4

Karl Sternberg [fl. 20th Cent.]

If you would read more you would invent and discover less.

> Aphorism

REASON

See also LOGIC, THINKING

Leonardo da Vinci [1452–1519]

Whoever in discussion adduces authority uses not intellect but rather memory.

> *Codice Atlantico,* 76 (tr. by Edward MacCurdy in *The Notebooks of Leonardo da Vinci,* Vol. I, Ch. II)

William Shakespeare [1564–1616]

My Reason, the physician to my Love,
Angry that his prescriptions are not
    kept,
Hath left me.
> *Sonnet CXLVII*

William Cullen [1710–1790]

The facts of physic are more frequently the inference of reason than the simple objects of sense.
> *First Lines of the Practice of Physic*

John Keats [1795–1821]

I have never yet been able to perceive how any thing can be known for truth by consequitive reasoning — and yet it must be.
> Letter to Benjamin Bailey, November 22, 1817

Hermann von Helmholtz [1821–1894]

The Critique of Pure Reason is a continual sermon against the use of the category of thought beyond the limits of actual experience.
> Quoted by F. H. Garrison in *Bulletin of the New York Academy of Medicine* 4:996, 1928

Santiago Ramón y Cajal [1852–1934]

That which enters the mind through reason can be corrected. That which is admitted through faith, hardly ever.
> *Charlas de Café*

Wilfred Trotter [1872–1939]

Now the faculty of reason in one aspect may be said to be the indispensable agent in everything man has accomplished. It enables him to learn, to add knowledge and preserve it, to build up arts, sciences, and civilizations without limit. Yet, in another aspect, this same implement can as it were, turn in his hand and become the enemy of all constructive activities.
> *Collected Papers,* "Has the Intellect a Function?"

Alexis Carrel [1873–1944]

A few observations and much reasoning leads to error; many observations and a little reasoning to truth.

Alan Gregg [1890–1957]

Making up your mind does not mean freeing yourself to believe what you want — but examining so closely that you know the result.
> Aphorism (Quoted by Wilder Penfield in *The Difficult Art of Giving,* Appendix A)

W. I. B. Beveridge [1908–   ]

A useful habit for scientists to develop is that of not trusting ideas based on reason only. . . . Practically all reasoning is influenced by feelings, prejudice and past experience, albeit often subconsciously.
> *The Art of Scientific Investigation,* Ch. VII

REDUCTIONISM

Baron Justus von Liebig [1803–1873]

A rational physiology cannot be founded on mere reactions, and the living body cannot be viewed as a chemical laboratory.
> *Organic Chemistry,* Preface

Elisha Bartlett [1804–1855]

Could the scalpel of the dissector, or the lenses of the optician, or the retort of the analyst, or all combined, have ever revealed to us the power of the liver to secrete bile, of the kidneys to secrete urine, of the mammary glands to secrete milk? Let us suppose that our anatomical knowledge of the brain had reached its ultimate limit of accuracy and perfection — that its complicated and delicate meshes of tubes and fibres had all been unravelled — that its intricate connexions and dependencies had all been ascertained — that no element or condition of its material organization had escaped us; — would all this knowledge have furnished us with any information as to the part which it plays, and the offices which it performs, in the living economy?

> *Philosophy of Medical Science,* Pt. II, Ch. 5

Homer W. Smith [1895–1962]

I would define mechanism, as we use the word today, as designating the belief that all the activities of the living organism are ultimately to be explained in terms of its component molecular parts. This was Descartes' greatest contribution to philosophy next to his principle of doubt. Abandon Cartesian mechanism and you will close up every scientific biological laboratory in the world at once, you will turn back the clock by three full centuries.

> *The Historical Development of Physiological Thought,* "The Biology of Consciousness"

René J. Dubos [1901–   ]

I believe that the acceptance of an oversimplified mechanistic theory of life has narrowed considerably the front of progress in biological sciences.
> *The Dreams of Reason,* Ch. V

The fact that Descartes's assumptions have led to such great scientific advances does not prove, however, that these assumptions are correct. . . . despite the triumphs of molecular biology, it has not yet been proven that the living body is only a machine and that life is merely a complex integra-

tion of known physicochemical forces. . . . I may seem to be reviving the vitalistic doctrine with all its false intellectual mysticism. . . . I am doing nothing of the sort. I am only emphasizing that the machine view of living things is buried so deep in the modern subconscious that few scientists ever try to bring it to the surface to examine its significance in the bright light of critical knowledge.
> *Idem*

Maurice B. Strauss [1904–1974]

A metaphysical concept prevalent among medical scientists is that the properties of a whole system can be fully derived from information about the behavior of its isolated parts. . . . This . . . assumption neglects the fact of organization — the first fact, indeed, that strikes one about organisms.
> *New England Journal of Medicine* 262:805, 1960

So far as organization exists in every system from that of the atom to the universe, and from that of the single cell to the society of nations, the properties of no system can be wholly deduced from a knowledge of its isolated parts.
> *Idem*

Herbert J. Muller [1905–   ]

To say, for example, that a man is made up of certain chemical elements is a satisfactory description only for those who intend to use him as a fertilizer.
> *Science and Criticism,* "Biology"

REGIMEN

See also HYGIENE, PREVENTIVE MEDICINE

Cicero [106–43 B.C.]

It is our duty, my young friends, to

resist old age; to compensate for its defects by a watchful care; to fight against it as we would fight against disease; to adopt a regimen of health; to practice moderate exercise; and to take just enough food and drink to restore our strength and not to overburden it.

> *On Old Age*, XI.35 (tr. by W. A. Falconer)

Epictetus [60?–120?]

Do you wish to win an Olympic victory? So do I, by the gods! for it is a fine thing. But consider the matters which come before that, and those which follow after, and only when you have done that, put your hand to the task. You have to submit to discipline, follow a strict diet, give up sweet cakes, train under compulsion, at a fixed hour, in heat or in cold; you must not drink cold water, nor wine just whenever you feel like it; you must have turned yourself over to your trainer precisely as you would to a physician.

> *Encheiridion*, 29 (tr. by W. A. Oldfather)

School of Salerno [1095–1224]

The *Salerne Schoole* doth by these lines impart
All health to *Englands King*, and doth advise
From care his head to keepe, from wrath his heart,
Drinke not much wine, sup light, and soon arise,
When meate is gone, long sitting breedeth smart:
And after-noone still waking keepe your eyes.
When mov'd you find your selfe to *Natures Needs*,
Forbeare them not, for that much danger breeds,
Use three Physicians still; first Doctor *Quiet*,
Next Doctor *Merry-man*, and Doctor *Dyet*. . . .[1]

[1] Cf. Proverb, p. 386b.

And here I cease to write, but will not cease
To wish you live in health, and die in peace:
And ye our Physicke rules that friendly read,
God grant that Physicke you may never need.

> *Regimen Sanitatis Salernitanum* (tr. by Sir John Harington as *The Englishman's Doctor*)

Ser Lapo Mazzei [1350–1412]

Let not the sun go down behind the hill, without your having gone forth; or if indeed you cannot, take before meals a little exercise to tire you, without however causing you to sweat. You should have a block of wood and a saw, and give a few strokes, or go speedily upstairs divers times. For your food has no help from nature, and even as embers die out if they are not stirred, so the food in your stomach is frozen, for lack of exercising your person. And after supper, wait for at least two hours before sleep, that the food can take shape; for, in good faith, the physicians will approve this more than so many clysters — that is, that you should take food easy to digest, and helpful to your bowels' functions. And it would help you much to drink a quarter of an hour ere your repast, a full half-glass of good red wine.

> Letter to Francesco di Marco Datini, 1400 (Quoted by Iris Origo in *The Merchant of Prato*)

Sir Edward Coke [1552–1634]

Sex horas somno, totidem des legibus aequis,
Quatuor orabis, des epulisque duas;
Quod superest ultra sacris largire camaenis.
[Six hours in sleep, in law's grave study six,
Four spend in prayer, the rest on Nature fix.]

> *First Institute of the Laws of England*, Bk. I, Ch. I

John Locke [1632–1704]

And thus I have done with what concerns the Body and Health, which reduces it self to these few and easily observable Rules. Plenty of open *Air, Exercise* and *Sleep;* Plain *Diet,* no *Wine* or *Strong Drink,* and very little or no *Physick;* not too Warm and straight *Clothing,* especially the *Head* and *Feet* kept cold, and the *Feet* often used to cold Water, and exposed to Wet.

> *Some Thoughts Concerning Education,* Sect. 30

Voltaire [1694–1778]

Regimen is superior to medicine.
> *A Philosophical Dictionary,* "Physicians"

Samuel Johnson [1709–1784]

I am much pleased that you are going [on] a very long journey, which may by proper conduct restore your health and prolong your life.
Observe these rules:
1. Turn all care out of your head as soon as you mount the chaise.
2. Do not think of frugality; your health is worth more than it can cost.
3. Do not continue any day's journey to fatigue.
4. Take now and then a day's rest.
5. Get a smart sea-sickness, if you can.
6. Cast away all anxiety, and keep your mind easy.
This last direction is the principal; with an unquiet mind, neither exercise, nor diet, nor physick can be of much use.

> Quoted by James Boswell in *Life of Samuel Johnson,* "To Mr. Perkins," July 28, 1782

Sir William Jones [1746–1794]

Seven hours to law, to soothing slumber seven
Ten to the world allot, and *all* to heaven.

> Lines in substitution for Sir Edward Coke's "Six hours in sleep" (Quoted by Lord Teignmouth in *Memoirs of the Life of Sir William Jones,* Vol. II)

John Redman Coxe [1773–1864]

The longer I live the less confidence I have in drugs and the greater is my confidence in the regulation and administration of diet and regimen.

> *A Short View of the Importance and Respectability of the Science of Medicine,* address to the Philadelphia Medical Society, February 7, 1800

Joseph Smith [1832–1914]

Strong drinks are not for the belly, but for the washing of your bodies.
And again, tobacco is not for the body, neither for the belly, and is not good for man, but is an herb for bruises and all sick cattle, to be used with judgment and skill.
And again, hot drinks are not for the body or belly.
And again, . . . all wholesome herbs God hath ordained for the constitution, nature and use of man. . . .
Yea, flesh also of beasts and of the fowls of the air, I, the Lord, have ordained for the use of man with thanksgiving; nevertheless, they are to be used sparingly.

> *The Doctrine and Covenants of the Church of Jesus Christ of Latter-Day Saints,* Sect. 89

Sir William Osler [1849–1919]

Patients should have rest, food, fresh air, and exercise — the quadrangle of health.

> Quoted by William B. Bean in *Sir William Osler: Aphorisms,* Ch. 3

Marcel Proust [1871–1922]

If there is one thing more difficult than submitting oneself to a regime it is refraining from imposing it upon other people.

> *Cities of the Plain,* Pt. II, Ch. 3 (tr. by C. K. Scott-Moncrieff)

Austen Fox Riggs [1876–1940]

Four habits of life — balanced living, with work, play and rest in proportion;

living in the present; accepting reality; directing one's energies with useful purpose.

Notebooks

Anonymous

Get up at five, have lunch at nine,
Supper at five, retire at nine.
And you will live to ninety-nine.[1]

Quoted by François Rabelais in *Works*, Bk. IV, Ch. 64 (tr. by Jacques Le Clercq)

To rise at six, to bed at ten,
Makes a man live for ten times ten.

Inscribed in Victor Hugo's house on the Isle of Guernsey [2]

REHABILITATION

See also SOCIAL MEDICINE

Hippocrates [460?–377? B.C.]

Use strengthens, disuse debilitates.

In the Surgery, XX (tr. by E. T. Withington)

Franklin D. Roosevelt [1882–1945]

For those who may no longer earn their daily bread, because of some swift-falling accident or slow incurable disease, we have provided, and we are providing, hospitals, sanitaria, and institutions where, so far as is humanly possible, they may be restored to useful life or, if that is not possible, receive care and comforts.

Address Before the New York Women's Trade Union League on Old-Age Security, June 8, 1929

This is a problem that demands a crusade. The progress of the past fifty years has been great, but we have marched only a short way. The extension of the work must go on until every child in the United States can be assured of the best that science, Government assistance and private aid can give.

Address on Rehabilitation of the Mentally and Physically Handicapped, July 13, 1929

The overwhelming majority of children who become crippled can with proper treatment be restored to a useful, active life in the community.

Radio Address on a Program of Assistance for the Crippled, February 18, 1931

I am in favor of war. I am very much in favor of the kind of war that we are conducting here at Warm Springs, the kind of war that, aided and abetted by what we have been doing at Warm Springs now for fourteen or fifteen years, is spreading all over the country — the war against the crippling of men and women and, especially, of children.

Remarks at Warm Springs, Georgia, November 23, 1939

RELIGION

See also FAITH, PRAYERS, PROFESSIONS

Michel de Montaigne [1533–1592]

The religion of my doctor or my lawyer cannot matter. That consideration has nothing in common with the functions of the friendship they owe me.

Essays, Bk. I, Ch. 28, "Of Friendship" (tr. by Donald M. Frame)

Jonathan Swift [1667–1745]

Physicians ought not to give their judgment of religion, for the same rea-

[1] The "canonical hours" for preserving health.
[2] To this inscription in his place of exile Hugo prefixed, "La vie est un exil" [Life is an exile].

son that butchers are not admitted to be jurors upon life and death.[1]

> *Thoughts on Various Subjects, Moral and Diverting*

Samuel Johnson [1709–1784]

It has been observed that physicians and lawyers are no friends to religion, and many conjectures have been formed to discover the reason. . . . The truth is, very few of them have thought about religion, but they have all seen a parson.

> *The Rambler*, No. 9 (April 17, 1750)

Hartley Coleridge [1796–1849]

There is a good deal of the mysterious in whatever is practical.

> *Lives of Northern Worthies,* "Dr. John Fothergill"

Henry Marshall[2] [early 19th Cent.?]

My religion consists mainly of wonder and gratitude.

> Quoted by John Brown in *Horae Subsecivae*, Series I, "Excursus Ethicus"

Ralph Waldo Emerson [1803–1882]

I knew a witty physician who found the creed in the biliary duct, and used to affirm that if there was disease in the liver, the man became a Calvinist, and if that organ was sound, he became a Unitarian.

> *Essays* (Second Series), "Experience"

Sir William Withey Gull [1816–1890]

Realize, if you can, what a paralyzing influence on all scientific inquiry the ancient belief must have had which attributed the operations of nature to the caprice not of one divinity only, but of many. There still remain vestiges of this in most of our minds, and the more distinct in proportion to our weakness and ignorance.

> *British Medical Journal* 2:425, 1874

Arthur Hugh Clough [1819–1861]

And almost every one when age,
  Disease, or sorrows strike him,
Inclines to think there is a God,
  Or something very like Him.

> *Dipsychus*, Pt. I, Sc. v

George Eliot (Marian Evans Cross) [1819–1880]

It is seldom a medical man has true religious views — there is too much pride of intellect.

> *Middlemarch*, Ch. 21

Louis Pasteur [1822–1895]

Happy is he who bears a god within himself, an ideal of beauty, and obeys him: an ideal of art, an ideal of science, an ideal of the nation, an ideal of the virtues of the Gospel. These are the living springs of great thoughts and great actions. All are illuminated by reflections of the infinite.

> Speech on his reception into the Académie Française, April 27, 1882

The Greeks have given us one of the most beautiful words of our language, the word "enthusiasm" — a God within. The grandeur of the acts of men is measured by the inspiration from which they spring. Happy is he who bears a God within!

> *Ibid.* (tr. by René J. Dubos)

It is because of having reflected and studied that I have the faith of a Breton. If I had reflected and studied more, I would have attained to the faith of a Bretoness.[1]

---

[1] Butchers were formerly excluded from juries in capital cases.

[2] Marshall was a Scottish physician.

[1] This was Pasteur's reply to a student who asked him how, as a scientific man, he could remain a Roman Catholic.

William E. Aughinbaugh
[1870–1940]

Each morning twelve [Burmese] women would be taken to the presence of the [white] elephant. Naked, they knelt before him in a long line, while the great beast, approaching languorously, stood behind them, passing his trunk over their naked shoulder, and one by one sucking their breasts dry. Then, nonchalantly, he would retire to his dais to munch a dessert of hay and fruit. In the meantime the physician in attendance had his hands full reviving the exhausted women, most of whom became hysterical after making their religious offering.
    I Swear by Apollo

W. Somerset Maugham
[1874–1965]

Perhaps religion is the best school of morality. It is like one of those drugs you gentlemen use in medicine which carries another in solution: it is of no efficacy in itself, but enables the other to be absorbed.
    Of Human Bondage, Ch. LXXXVIII

T. S. Eliot [1888–1965]

The wounded surgeon plies the steel
That questions the distempered part;
Beneath the bleeding hands we feel
The sharp compassion of the healer's
    art
Resolving the enigma of the fever
    chart.

Our only health is the disease
If we obey the dying nurse
Whose constant care is not to please
But to remind of our, and Adam's
    curse,
And that, to be restored, our sickness
    must grow worse.

The whole earth is our hospital
Endowed by the ruined millionaire,
Wherein, if we do well, we shall
Die of the absolute paternal care

That will not leave us, but prevents us
    everywhere.
    Four Quartets, "East Coker,"
    IV

Paul Reznikoff [1896–   ]

Conflict between science and religion should never exist. Their aims are entirely different — science tries to find out how, religion deals with why.
    Aphorism

Erich Fromm [1900–   ]

Whether we are religionists or not, whether we believe in the necessity for a new religion or in a religion of no religion or in the continuation of the Judaeo-Christian tradition, inasmuch as we are concerned with the essence and not with the shell, with the experience and not with the word, with man and not with the church, we can unite in firm negation of idolatry and find perhaps more of a common faith in this negation than in any affirmative statements about God. Certainly we shall find more of humility and of brotherly love.
    Psychoanalysis and Religion,
    Ch. 5

Medieval Proverb

Where there are three physicians there are two atheists.[1]

REMEDIES

See also CURES, DRUGS, NOSTRUMS, TREATMENT

Aeschylus [525–456 B.C.]

Hear the rest, and you will marvel even more at the crafts and resources I've contrived. Greatest was this: in the former times if a man fell sick he had no defense against the sickness, neither healing food nor drink, nor un-

---

[1] Ubi tres medici, duo athei.

guent; but through the lack of drugs men wasted away, until I showed them the blending of mild simples wherewith they drive out all manner of diseases.
> *Prometheus Bound*, 476 (tr. by D. Grene)

Sophocles [496?–406 B.C.]

A remedy too strong for the disease.
> *Tereus*, Fragment II.589

Euripides [484–406 B.C.]

For diverse ills are remedies diverse.
> *Fragments*, 962

Hippocrates [460?–377? B.C.]

Opposites are cures for opposites.[1]
> *Breaths*, I (tr. by W. H. S. Jones)

It is a good remedy sometimes to use nothing.
> *On Joints*, 40 (tr. by E. T. Withington)

Pien Ch'iao [ca. 225 B.C.]

Men worry over the great number of diseases; doctors worry over the small number of remedies.

Celsus [25 B.C.–A.D. 50]

A reckoning up of the cause often solves the malady.
> *De Medicina*, Prooemium (tr. by W. G. Spencer)

It is better to try a double-edged remedy than none at all.
> *Ibid.*, II.x

It is impossible to remedy a severe malady unless by a remedy likewise severe.
> *Ibid.*, II.xi.6

Why should a remedy be certain because it is unique?
> *Ibid.*, VII.xxii

[1] Cf. Samuel Hahnemann, p. 71a.

Seneca [4? B.C.–A.D. 65]

At the beginning no one tries extreme remedies.
> *Agamemnon*, 153

Remedies do not avail unless they remain in the system.
> *Moral Epistles to Lucilius*, XL (tr. by Richard M. Gummere)

Galen [fl. 2nd Cent.]

All who drink of this remedy recover in a short time, except those whom it does not help, who all die. Therefore it is obvious that it fails only in incurable cases.

Rhazes [850–923]

At the beginning of a disease choose such remedies as will not lessen the patient's strength.

Dante Alighieri [1265–1321]

To salve my sore there came the healing plaster.
> *The Divine Comedy*, "Hell," Canto XXIV (tr. by Dorothy L. Sayers)

Martin Luther [1483–1546]

'Tis wonderful how God has put such excellent physic in mere muck; we know by experience that swine's dung stints the blood; horse's serves for the pleurisy; man's heals wounds and black blotches; asses' is used for the bloody flux, and cow's with preserved roses, serves for epilepsy, or for convulsions of children.
> *Table-Talk*, XCII, "Of God's Works" (tr. by William Hazlitt)

Experience has proved the toad to be endowed with valuable qualities. If you run a stick through three toads, and, after having dried them in the sun, apply them to any pestilent tumour, they draw out all the poison, and the malady will disappear.
> *Ibid.*, DCCLXXX, "Of Sickness"

Paracelsus [1493?–1541]

Only he whose remedies are efficacious is a physician.
> *Die grosse Wundarznei*, Treatise II, Foreword (tr. by Norbert Guterman in *Selected Writings*)

Ambroise Paré [1517?–1590]

Better a tried remedy than a newfangled one.

Michel de Montaigne [1533–1592]

For the most violent diseases the most violent remedies.
> *Essays*, Bk. II, Ch. 3, "A Custom of the Island of Cea" (tr. by Donald M. Frame)

John Gerard [1545–1612]

The root of Solomons seale stamped while it is fresh and green, and applied, taketh away in one night, or two at the most, any bruise, blacke or blew spots gotten by fals or womens wilfulnesse, in stumbling upon their hasty husbands fists, or such like.
> *Herball or Generall Historie of Plantes*, Ch. 143

Sir Francis Bacon [1561–1626]

The remedy is worse than the disease.
> *Essays*, "Of Seditions and Troubles"

William Shakespeare [1564–1616]

Diseases desperate grown
By desperate appliance are reliev'd,
Or not at all.
> *Hamlet*, IV, iii, 9

I do beseech your Majesty may salve
The long-grown wounds of my intemperance.
> *Henry IV, Part I*, III, ii, 155

But let us hence, my sovereign, to provide
A salve for any sore that may betide.
> *Henry VI, Part III*, IV, vi, 87

My pity hath been balm to heal their wounds.
> *Ibid.*, IV, viii, 41

I'll fetch some flax and whites of eggs
To apply to his bleeding face.
> *King Lear*, III, vii, 106

I shall desire you of more acquaintance, good Master Cobweb. If I cut my finger, I shall make bold with you.
> *A Midsummer Night's Dream*, III, i, 185

To see the salve doth make the wound ache more.
> *The Rape of Lucrece*, line 1116

Your plantain leaf is excellent for . . . your broken shin.
> *Romeo and Juliet*, I, ii, 52

You rub the sore
When you should bring the plaster.
> *The Tempest*, II, i, 138

Ben Jonson [1573?–1637]

Many men have beene cur'd of diseases by Accidents; but they were not Remedies.
> *Discoveries*, "Beneficia"

'Tis an odious kinde of remedy,
To owe our health to a disease.
> *The New Inn*, Act IV, Sc. iv

Would you live free from all diseases?
Doe the act, your mistris pleases;
Yet fright all aches from your bones?
Here's a med'cine, for the nones.
> *Volpone*, Act II, Sc. ii

Baltasar Gracián
[1601–1658]

The best remedy for disturbances is to let them run their course, for so they quiet down.
> *The Art of Worldly Wisdom*, Maxim 138 (tr. by Joseph Jacobs)

Samuel Butler [1612–1680]

Learn'd he was in Med'c'nal Lore,
For by his side a Pouch he wore
Replete with strange Hermetick Powder,
That Wounds six Miles point-blank
would solder.
> *Hudibras,* Pt. I, Canto II

Duc François de La Rochefoucauld [1613–1680]

There are certain situations, as there are maladies, which the accepted remedies serve only to aggravate at times; a truly clever man will know when it is dangerous to apply them.
> *Maxims,* No. 288 (tr. by Constantine FitzGibbon)

We must deal with luck as with health: enjoy it when it is good, be patient when it is bad, and resort to extreme remedies only in extreme need.
> *Ibid.,* No. 392

Molière [1622–1673]

Most men die of their remedies, and not of their illnesses.
> *Le Malade Imaginaire,* Act III, Sc. iii

Clysterium donare
Postea seignare
Ensuita purgare.[1]
> *Ibid.,* Third Interlude

Thomas Sydenham [1624–1689]

The arrival of a good clown exercises a more beneficial influence upon the health of a town than of twenty asses laden with drugs.

John Ward [1629–1681]

A fellow is at Cambridge which cures agues by injecting somewhat into the veins, as Mr. Wren did into the veins of a dog.
> *Diary of the Reverend John Ward*

[1] Latin hodgepodge answer to question about remedies for "hydropisia": give an enema, then bleed, finally purge.

Samuel Pepys [1633–1703]

Now mighty well, and truly I cannot but impute it to my fresh hare's foote.
> *Diary,* January 21, 1665

John Radcliffe [1650–1714]

When a young physician he possessed twenty remedies for every disease, and at the close of his career he found twenty diseases for which he had not one remedy.
> Quoted by R. H. Campbell in *The Life of John Radcliffe,* Ch. 6

George Farquhar [1678–1707]

My constant Drink is Tea, or a little Wine and Water; 'tis prescrib'd me by the Physician for a Remedy against the Spleen.
> *The Beaux' Stratagem,* Act III

John Armstrong [1709–1779]

Music exalts each Joy, allays each Grief,
Expels Diseases, softens every Pain,
Subdues the rage of Poison and the Plague.
> *The Art of Preserving Health,* Bk. IV

William Withering [1741–1799]

It is much easier to write upon a disease than upon a remedy. The former is in the hands of nature and a faithful observer with an eye of tolerable judgment cannot fail to delineate a likeness. The latter will ever be subject to the whim, the inaccuracies and the blunders of mankind.

Sir Astley Paston Cooper [1768–1841]

If you are too fond of new remedies, first you will not cure your patients; secondly, you will have no patients to cure.

Charles C. Colton [1780?–1832]

No men despise physic so much as

physicians, because no men so thoroughly understand how little it can perform. They have been tinkering with the human constitution four thousand years, in order to cure about as many disorders. . . . It is true that each disorder has a thousand prescriptions, but not a single remedy.
> *Lacon,* Vol. I, Ch.
> CCCXXXVIII

Ann Taylor [1782–1866]

Kiss the place to make it well.
> *Original Poems for Infant Minds,*
> "My Mother"

Daniel Drake [1785–1852]

Among the therapeutic agents not to be found bottled up and labelled on our shelves, is Travelling; a means of prevention, of cure, and of restoration, which has been famous in all ages.
> *Western Medical and Physical Journal* 1:305, 1827

Peter Mere Latham [1789–1875]

You cannot be sure of the success of your remedy, while you are still uncertain of the nature of the disease.
> *Diseases of the Heart,* Lect. XIV

We must not make our ignorance of how the special remedy cures a bar to our use of it.
> *General Remarks on the Practice of Medicine,* Ch. III

Remedies, indeed, are our great analysers of disease.
> *Ibid.,* Ch. VII

Elisha Bartlett [1804–1855]

There is nothing in the whole range of medical history, which shows so miserable a logic, and so false a philosophy, as the introduction of this multitudinous assemblage of new remedies, *with the properties which are so confidently assigned to them.* But then the fault and the error are, — not that the remedies are new, — but that the evidence of their value and efficacy is so utterly wanting.
> *Philosophy of Medical Science,*
> Pt. II, Ch. 16

Sir William Withey Gull [1816–1890]

Make haste and use all new remedies before they lose their effectiveness.[1]

Lydia E. Pinkham [1819–1883]

A FEARFUL TRAGEDY
A clergyman of Stratford, Connecticut
KILLED BY HIS OWN WIFE,
Insanity Brought on by 16 Years of Suffering with
FEMALE COMPLAINTS THE CAUSE.
Lydia E. Pinkham's Vegetable Compound
The Sure Cure for These Complaints,
Would Have prevented this Direful **Deed.**
> Quoted by Stewart H. Holbrook
> in *The Golden Age of Quackery,*
> Pt. 3

Mary Baker Eddy [1821–1910]

Drugs, cataplasms, and whiskey are stupid substitutes for the dignity and potency of divine Mind, and its efficacy to heal.
> *Science and Health,* Ch. VI

Rudolf Virchow [1821–1902]

From the basic error that specific remedies were created for particular diseases came the notion that the whole course of a disease, or even its separate stages, could be annihilated by a single remedy. It was reserved for the ablest physicians of all time to perceive that identical remedies are good only for identical phases of different diseases and that for different phases of the same disease, different remedies are necessary.
> Quoted by F. H. Garrison in
> *Bulletin of the New York Academy of Medicine* 4:994, 1928

[1] Cf. William Heberden, p. 630a.

John Shaw Billings [1838–1913]

I am certain I shall never forget the effects of "Composition Powder," or of "Number Six," which was essentially a concentrated tincture of Cayenne pepper, and one dose of which was enough to make a boy willing to go to school for a month.

> *Boston Medical and Surgical Journal* 124:349, 1891

William Allen Jamieson [1839–1916]

Nine times out of ten our miscalled remedies are absolutely injurious to our patients, suffering under diseases of whose real character and cause we are most culpably ignorant.

> Quoted in *Vital Magnetic Cure*, "Contrast Between Medicine and Magnetism"

Sir Dyce Duckworth [1840–1928]

To employ newly introduced remedies with too great frequency is to be engaged in frivolous experimentation.

> *St. Bartholomew's Hospital Reports* 52:39, 1916

Sir William Osler [1849–1919]

The true polypharmacy . . . is the skillful combination of remedies.

> *British Medical Journal* 2:185, 1909

Marcel Proust [1871–1922]

Nature hardly seems capable of giving us any but quite short illnesses. But medicine has annexed to itself the art of prolonging them. Remedies, the respite that they procure, the relapses that a temporary cessation of them provokes, compose a sham illness to which the patient grows so accustomed that he ends by making it permanent, just as children continue to give way to fits of coughing long after they have been cured of the whooping cough. Then remedies begin to have less effect, the doses are increased, they cease to do any good, but they have begun to do harm thanks to that lasting indisposition.

> *The Captive*, Pt. I, Ch. 1 (tr. by C. K. Scott-Moncrieff)

Anonymous

If you want to be cured of I don't know what, take this herb of I don't know what name, apply it I don't know where, and you will be cured I don't know when.

> Medieval joke

For every ill beneath the sun
There is some remedy or none;
If there be one, resolve to find it;
If not, submit, and never mind it.

> Maxim (ca. 1843)

TO RESTORE FROM STROKE OF LIGHTNING. — Shower with cold water for two hours; if the patient does not show signs of life, put salt in the water, and shower an hour longer.

> *The Home Cookbook* (1877), "Medicinal Receipts"

Jack and Jill went up the hill
  To fetch a pail of water;
Jack fell down and broke his crown,
  And Jill came tumbling after.

Up Jack got, and home did trot,
  As fast as he could caper,
To old Dame Dob, who patched his nob
With vinegar and brown paper.

> *The Oxford Book of Nursery Rhymes*, No. 254

Proverb

There is a remedy for everything, could men find it.

Chinese Proverbs

A single untried popular remedy often throws the scientific doctor into hysterics.

It is easy to get a thousand prescriptions, but hard to get one single remedy.

English and German Proverb

There is a salve for every sore.

Indian (Tamil) Proverb

Whatever a physician prescribes is a remedy.

Latin Proverbs

A doubtful remedy is better than none.

No remedies cause so much pain as those which are efficacious.

There are some remedies worse than the disease.

Welsh Proverb

Three remedies of the physicians of Myddfai: water, honey, and labour.

RESEARCH

See also DISCOVERY, EXPERIMENTAL MEDICINE, HYPOTHESIS, INVESTIGATORS, SCIENTIFIC METHOD, THEORY, THEORY AND PRACTICE

I. GENERAL

Terence [185–159 B.C.]

Nothing is so difficult but that it may be found out by seeking.
> *Heauton Timorumenos*, Act IV

Marcus Aurelius [121–180]

Nothing is so conducive to greatness of mind as the ability to examine systematically and honestly everything that meets us in life.
> *Meditations*, III.11 (tr. by C. R. Haines)

Leonardo da Vinci [1452–1519]

Shun those studies in which the work that results dies with the worker.
> Forster Bequest MS. III, Victoria and Albert Museum (tr. by Edward MacCurdy in *The Notebooks of Leonardo da Vinci*, Vol. I, Ch. I)

It is by testing that we discern fine gold.
> Manuscript H, Library of the Institut de France (*ibid.*, Ch. II)

Michel de Montaigne [1533–1592]

There is no end to our researches; our end is in the other world.
> *Essays*, Bk. III, Ch. 13, "Of Experience" (tr. by Donald M. Frame)

Sir Francis Bacon [1561–1626]

We have also parks and inclosures of all sorts of beasts and birds, which we use not only for view or rareness, but likewise for dissections and trials; that thereby we may take light what may be wrought upon the body of man. . . . We try also all poisons and other medicines upon them, as well of chirurgery as physic.
> *New Atlantis*

The study of nature with a view to works is engaged in by the mechanic, the mathematician, the physician, the alchemist, and the magician; but by all (as things now are) with slight endeavour and scanty success.
> *Novum Organum*, "Aphorisms," V

The lame man who keeps the right road outstrips the runner who takes a wrong one. Nay, it is obvious that when a man runs the wrong way, the more active and swift he is the further he will go astray.
> *Ibid.*, LXI

William Harvey [1578–1657]

Nature is nowhere accustomed more openly to display her secret mysteries than in cases where she shows tracings of her workings apart from the beaten paths; nor is there any better way to advance the proper practice of medicine than to give our minds to the discovery of the usual law of nature, by careful investigation of cases of rarer forms of disease.

> Letter to John Vlackveld, April 24, 1657

Robert Herrick [1591–1674]

Attempt the end, and never stand to doubt;
Nothing's so hard, but search will find it out.

> *Hesperides,* "Seeke and finde"

René Descartes [1596–1650]

I have resolved to devote what time I may still have to live to no other occupation than of endeavouring to acquire some knowledge of Nature, which shall be of such a kind as to enable us therefrom to deduce rules in Medicine of greater certainty than those at present in use.

> *Discours de la Méthode,* Pt. VI
> (tr. by John Veitch)

P. A. Kirchner [1602– ?]

Nature often allows amazing miracles to be produced which originate from the most ordinary observations and which are, however, recognized only by those who are equipped with sagacity and research acumen, and who consult experience, the teacher of everything.

> Quoted by Wilhelm Conrad Roentgen in an address, December 28, 1895

Sir Thomas Browne [1605–1682]

The wisedome of God receives small honour from those vulgar heads, that rudely stare about, and with a grosse rusticity admire his workes; those highly magnifie him whose judicious enquiry into his acts, and deliberate research of his creatures, returne the duty of a devout and learned admiration.

> *Religio Medici,* Pt. I, Sect. 13

Marcello Malpighi [1628–1694]

Study with me, then, a few things in the spirit of truth alone, so that we may establish the manner of Nature's operations in the individual viscera as I have revealed it in the liver and other organs. . . . Do not stop to question whether these ideas are new or old, but ask, more properly, whether they harmonize with Nature. And be assured of this one thing, that I never reached my idea of the structure of the kidney by the aid of books, but by the long, patient and varied use of the microscope. I have gotten the rest by the deductions of reason, slowly, and with an open mind, as is my custom.

> *Exercitationes de Structura Viscerum,* "Proemium de Renibus"
> (tr. by J. M. Hayman, Jr.)

And since the manifestations of Nature's working are most varied, we may discover mechanisms which are unknown to us and whose operations we cannot understand.

> *Idem*

Jeremy Collier [1650–1726]

All Experiments are not worth the making. 'Tis much better to be ignorant of a Disease then to catch it. Who would wound himself for Information about Pain, or smell a Stench for the sake of the Discovery?

> *A Short View of the Immorality and Profaneness of the English Stage,* Ch. I

Mark Akenside [1721–1770]

Speak ye the pure delight, whose favour'd steps

The lamp of Science through the jealous maze
Of Nature guides, when haply you reveal
Her secret honours.
> *The Pleasures of Imagination,*
> Pt. II

Immanuel Kant [1724–1804]

To yield to every whim of curiosity, and to allow our passion for inquiry to be restrained by nothing but the limits of our ability, this shows an eagerness of mind not unbecoming to scholarship. But it is wisdom that has the merit of selecting from among the innumerable problems which present themselves, those whose solution is important to mankind.

John Hunter [1728–1793]

I think your solution is just, but why think? Why not try the experiment?
> Letter to Edward Jenner, August 2, 1775

Gotthold Lessing [1729–1781]

Not the possession of truth but the effort in struggling to attain to it brings joy to the researcher.

Sir Astley Paston Cooper
[1768–1841]

In the collecting of evidence upon any medical subject, there are but three sources from which we can hope to obtain it: viz. from observation of the living subject; from examination of the dead; and from experiment upon living animals.
> *Surgical Essays*

Baron Georges Cuvier [1769–1832]

The observer listens to Nature; the experimenter questions and forces her to unveil herself.

William Wordsworth [1770–1850]

Lost in a gloom of uninspired research.
> *The Excursion,* Bk. IV

Sydney Smith [1771–1845]

What does the world yet owe to American physicians or surgeons? What new substances have their chemists discovered? or what old ones have they analyzed?
> *Edinburgh Review,* January–May, 1820

Sir Humphry Davy [1778–1829]

I have heard of some experiments you have made on the action of digitalis, and other poisons, on yourself. I hope you will not indulge in trials of this kind. I cannot see any useful result that can arise from them. It is in states of disease, and not of health, that they are to be used; and you may injure your constitution without gaining any important result.
> Letter to medical student
> (Quoted by John Davy in *Life of Sir Humphry Davy,* Vol. I, Ch. 2)

William Beaumont [1785–1853]

Truth, like beauty, when "unadorned is adorned the most," and in prosecuting these experiments and inquiries I believe I have been guided by its light.
> *Experiments and Observations,*
> Sect. 5

Peter Mere Latham [1789–1875]

To those who walk about with their eyes open, objects often present themselves with a fidelity and truth which are too apt to suffer diminution and loss when the same objects are submitted to more curious experiments.
> *General Remarks on the Practice of Medicine,* "The Heart and Its Affections," Ch. II

John Henry, Cardinal Newman
[1801–1890]

To discover and to teach are distinct functions; they are also distinct gifts, and are not commonly found united in the same person.

> *On the Scope and Nature of University Education*, Preface

Elisha Bartlett [1804–1855]

So far as medical science has any just title to the appellation; and so far as medical art possesses any rules, sufficiently positive to be worth anything, it is owing, exclusively, to the diligent, unprejudiced, and conscientious study of the phenomena and relationships of disease.

> *Philosophy of Medical Science,* Pt. II, Ch. 12

Sir Richard Owen [1804–1892]

He becomes the true discoverer who establishes the truth; and the sign of the truth is the general acceptance. Whoever, therefore, resumes the investigation of neglected or repudiated doctrine, elicits its true demonstration, and discovers and explains the nature of the errors which have led to its tacit or declared rejection, may certainly and confidently await the acknowledgements of his right in its discovery.

> *Homologies of the Skeleton*

Charles Darwin [1809–1882]

I love fools' experiments. I am always making them.

> Quoted by Francis Darwin in *Charles Darwin*

Nature will tell you a direct lie if she can.[1]

Oliver Wendell Holmes [1809–1894]

I told him I liked to follow the workings of another mind through these minute teasing investigations, to see a relentless observer get hold of Nature and squeeze her until the sweat broke out all over her and Sphincters loos-

[1] Cf. Thomas Carlyle, p. 316b.

ened — but I could not bring my own mind to it.[1]

> Letter to S. Weir Mitchell, May 8, 1862

Robert Browning [1812–1889]

As is your sort of mind,
So is your sort of search — you'll find
What you desire.

> *Easter-Day*, Pt. VII

Claude Bernard [1813–1878]

[The science of life] is a superb and dazzlingly lighted hall which may be reached only by passing through a long and ghastly kitchen.

> *An Introduction to the Study of Experimental Medicine*, Pt. I, Ch. 1, Sect. iii (tr. by H. C. Greene)

If an idea presents itself to us, we must not reject it simply because it does not agree with the logical deductions of a reigning theory.

> *Ibid.*, Ch. 2, Sect. iii

It has often been said that to make discoveries, one must be ignorant. This opinion . . . means that it is better to know nothing than to keep in mind fixed ideas based on theories whose confirmation we constantly seek, neglecting meanwhile everything that fails to agree with them.

> *Idem*

Men who have excessive faith in their theories or ideas are not only ill prepared for making discoveries; they also make very poor observations.

> *Idem*

We must never make experiments to confirm our ideas, but simply to control them.

> *Idem*

[1] Relating a conversation with Professor Louis Agassiz.

Man can learn nothing except by going from the known to the unknown.
Ibid., Sect. v

Scholastics or Systematizers never question their starting point, to which they seek to refer everything; they have a proud and intolerant mind, and do not accept contradiction. . . . The experimenter, on the contrary, who always doubts and who does not believe that he possesses absolute certainty about anything, succeeds in mastering the phenomena which surround him, and in extending his power over nature.
Ibid., Sect. vi

Some physicians fear and avoid counterproof; as soon as they make observations in the direction of their ideas, they refuse to look for contradictory facts, for fear of seeing their hypothesis vanish.
Ibid., Sect. viii

It seems, indeed, a necessary weakness of our mind to be able to reach truth only across a multitude of errors and obstacles.
Ibid., Pt. III, Ch. 1, Sect. ii

We must . . . never be too much absorbed by the thought we are pursuing.
Idem

Let me assume that, instead of succeeding at once in making a rabbit diabetic, all the negative facts had first appeared; it is clear that, after failing after two or three times, I should have concluded . . . that the theory guiding me was false. . . . Yet I should have been wrong. How often must man have been and still must be wrong in this way! It even seems impossible absolutely to avoid this kind of mistake. We wish to draw from this experiment another general conclusion, . . . that negative facts when considered alone, never teach us anything.
Ibid., Ch. 2, Sect. i

The origin of an original work is always the pursuit of a fact which does not fit into accepted ideas.
Manuscript, Collège de France (Quoted in *Perspectives in Biology and Medicine* 8:30, 1964)

In pathology, as in physiology, the true worth of an investigator consists in pursuing not only what he seeks in an experiment, but also what he did not seek.

Emil Du Bois-Reymond [1818–1896]

I would much prefer a scholar who investigates and does excellent work in a limited field, to one whose knowledge may be extensive but who has accomplished nothing remarkable in any particular line.

Hermann von Helmholtz [1821–1894]

After previous investigation of the problem in all directions . . . happy ideas come unexpectedly without effort, like an inspiration.
Address, 1891

I am fain to compare myself with a wanderer on the mountains who, not knowing the path, climbs slowly and painfully upwards and often has to retrace his steps because he can go no further — then, whether by taking thought or from luck, discovers a new track that leads him on a little till at length when he reaches the summit he finds to his shame that there is a royal road, by which he might have ascended, had he only had the wits to find the right approach to it.
Quoted by L. Koenigsberger in *Hermann von Helmholtz* (tr. by F. A. Welby)

Louis Pasteur [1822–1895]

If you suppress laboratories, physical

science will be stricken with barrenness and death.

> *Some Reflections on Science in France*, Pt. I

Outside their laboratories, the physicist and chemist are soldiers without arms on the field of battle.

> *Idem*

Preconceived ideas are like searchlights which illumine the path of the experimenter and serve him as a guide to interrogate nature. They become a danger only if he transforms them into fixed ideas — this is why I should like to see these profound words inscribed on the threshold of all the temples of science: "The greatest derangement of the mind is to believe in something because one wishes it to be so."

> Speech to the French Academy of Medicine, July 18, 1876 (tr. by René J. Dubos)

When, after so many efforts, you have at last arrived at a certainty, your joy is one of the greatest which can be felt by a human soul.

> Speech at the Inauguration of the Pasteur Institute, November 14, 1888 (tr. by Mrs. R. L. Devonshire)

I am . . . most fearful of committing myself when I lack evidence. But on the contrary, no consideration can keep me from defending what I hold as true when I can rely on solid scientific proof.

> Quoted by René J. Dubos in *Louis Pasteur, Free Lance of Science*

To him who devotes his life to science, nothing can give more happiness than increasing the number of discoveries, but his cup of joy is full when the results of his studies immediately find practical applications.

> *Idem*

Theodor Billroth [1829–1894]

The principle, method and the goal of investigations is recognition of truth, even though the truth may be in conflict with our social, ethical and political circumstances.

> *The Medical Sciences in the German Universities*

Hughlings Jackson [1835–1911]

The study of the causes of things must be preceded by the study of things caused.

William Stanley Jevons [1835–1882]

So-called original research is now regarded as a profession, adopted by hundreds of men, and communicated by a system of training.

> *The Principles of Science*, Ch. XXVI

John Shaw Billings [1838–1913]

The results which we now have, can best be compared to those obtained by the young chemist who made an analysis of a rat — putting the entire animal into his crucible.

> *Public Health Reports* 2:47, 1874–75

Sir Francis Darwin [1848–1925]

But in science the credit goes to the man who convinces the world, not to the man to whom the idea first occurs.

> *Eugenics Review* 6:1, 1914

Sir William Osler [1849–1919]

Too often the reaper is not the sower. Too often the fate of those who labour at some object for the public good is to see their work pass into other hands, and to have others get the credit for enterprises which they have initiated and made possible.

> *Aequanimitas, with Other Addresses*, "Books and Men"

Ivan Pavlov [1849–1936]

Experiment alone crowns the efforts of medicine, experiment limited only by the natural range of the powers of the human mind. Observation discloses in the animal organism numerous phenomena existing side by side and interconnected now profoundly, now indirectly, or accidentally. Confronted with a multitude of different assumptions the mind must *guess* the real nature of this connection. Experiment, as it were, takes the phenomena in hand, sets in motion now one of them, now another, and thus, by means of artificial, simplified combinations, discovers the actual connection between the phenomena.

> *Experimental Psychology and Other Essays*, Pt. X, Essay 3 (tr. by S. Belsky)

William H. Welch [1850–1934]

America is now contributing her fair share to the advancement of medical science, whereas a quarter of a century ago almost no scientific work in medicine was done in this country. . . . Far more remains to be accomplished than has been done, but now that the public and men of wealth realize that medical education and institutions for research are worthy objects of endowment, and that advancement of medical and sanitary knowledge is of immense importance to the welfare of mankind, the outlook for the future is most hopeful.

> Quoted by Simon and James T. Flexner in *William Henry Welch and the Heroic Age of American Medicine*, Ch. 14

A. C. Bradley [1851–1935]

Research, though toilsome, is easy; imaginative vision, though delightful, is difficult.

> *Oxford Lectures on Poetry*, "Shakespeare's Theatre and Audience"

Santiago Ramón y Cajal [1852–1934]

I remember that once I spent twenty hours continuously at the microscope watching the movements of a sluggish leucocyte in its laborious efforts to escape from a blood capillary.

> *Recollections of My Life*, Pt. II, Ch. 1 (tr. by E. Horne Craige)

Sir Ronald Ross [1857–1932]

A witty friend of mine once remarked that the world thinks of the man of science as one who pulls out his watch and exclaims, "Ha! half an hour to spare before dinner: I will just step down to my laboratory and make a discovery." Who but men of science themselves are to blame for such a misconception? Out of the many memoirs which fill our libraries few recount the labours of investigators, even of those who seek to solve the secrets of the great maladies which annually destroy millions of us — surely a matter of interest to everyone. Our books of science are records of results rather than of that sacred passion for discovery which leads to them. Yet many discoveries have really been the climax of an intense drama, full of hopes and despairs, visions seen in darkness, many failures, and a final triumph: in which the protagonists are man and nature, and the issue a decision for all the ages.

> *Memoirs*, Preface

Theobald Smith [1859–1934]

Research is fundamentally a state of mind involving continual reexamination of the doctrines and axioms upon which current thought and action are based. It is, therefore, critical of existing practices.

> *American Journal of Medical Science* 178:741, 1929

The joy of research must be found in doing since every other harvest is uncertain.

> Letter to Dr. E. B. Krumbhaar, October 11, 1933 (Quoted in *Journal of Bacteriology* 27:19, 1934)

J. Chalmers Da Costa [1863–1933]

It is given to few to be Columbuses of great continents of surgery — given to but few to discover such a principle as antisepsis as did Lord Lister — but all of us have at times our small triumphs, all of us are workers in the cause and all of us add something to knowledge.

> *The Trials and Triumphs of the Surgeon,* Ch. 1

Some men are most ingenious in finding forgotten ideas and putting them forth as new and original. This process is, in reality, getting scientific eggs from cold storage and selling them as newly laid.

> *Ibid.,* "Stepping Stones and Stumbling Blocks"

Abraham Flexner [1866–1959]

Research, untrammeled by near reference to practical ends, will go on in every properly organized medical school; its critical method will dominate all teaching whatsoever; but under-graduate instruction will be throughout explicitly conscious of its professional end and aim.

> *Medical Education, A Comparative Study*

Charles Nicolle [1866–1936]

Chance favours only those who know how to court her.
> *Biologie de l'Invention,* Ch. 1

Ernest H. Starling [1866–1927]

Only . . . by way of experiment, can we hope to attain to a comprehension of the "wisdom of the body and the understanding of the heart," and thereby to the mastery of disease and pain, which will enable us to relieve the burden of mankind.

> *Lancet* 2:865, 1923

Walter B. Cannon [1871–1945]

While patience and tenacity in research are admirable, a situation may arise in which persistence is unwarranted. Then these admirable qualities may become mere obstinacy.

> *The Way of an Investigator,* "Fitness for the Enterprise"

The investigator may be made to dwell in a garret, he may be forced to live on crusts and wear dilapidated clothes, he may be deprived of social recognition, but if he has time, he can steadfastly devote himself to research. Take away his free time and he is utterly destroyed as a contributor to knowledge.

> *Ibid.*

Wilfred Trotter [1872–1939]

While it is to be insisted on that rationality is not the ultimate test of scientific truth, there is no reason to question the value of the rational process as an implement of research.

> *Collected Papers,* "Has the Intellect a Function?"

Hans Zinsser [1878–1940]

[Charles] Nicolle was one of those men who achieve their successes by long preliminary thought, before an experiment is formulated, rather than by the frantic and often ill-conceived experimental activities that keep lesser men in ant-like agitation.

> *As I Remember Him,* Ch. 19, Sect. 1

Men go into this branch of work [bacteriology] from a number of motives, the last of which is a self-conscious desire to do good. The point is that it remains one of the few sporting propositions left for individuals who feel the need of a certain amount of excitement. Infectious disease is one of the few genuine adventures left in the world.

> *Rats, Lice and History,* Ch. I, Pt. 3

Albert Einstein [1879–1955]

Do not stop to think about the reasons for what you are doing, about why you are questioning. Curiosity has its own reason for existence. One cannot help but be in awe when he contemplates the mysteries of eternity, of life, of the marvelous structure of reality. It is enough if one tries merely to comprehend a little of this mystery each day. Never lose a holy curiosity.

Martin H. Fischer [1879–1962]

A laboratory is only a place where one may better set up and control conditions.

> Quoted by Howard Fabing and Ray Marr in *Fischerisms*

All the world is a laboratory to the inquiring mind.
> *Idem*

As soon as you injure an animal, you remove it from the physiological conditions of its life, and the experiments performed upon it are worthless. The great discoveries in physiology are the result of work with sound organs in sound animals.
> *Idem*

Research is not a timeclock-monkey-wrench job.
> *Idem*

Research has been called good business, a necessity, a gamble, a game. It is none of these — it's a state of mind.
> *Idem*

The recognition of the existence of a problem is the first step in its solution.
> *Idem*

You can't organize research.
> *Idem*

Peyton Rous [1879–   ]

Flexner [1] showed that society would be more than wise to support men solely for what they might find out, however distant this appeared from stated medical needs; and that men of the right sort could be trusted to have better ideas than others could think up for them.
> *Science* 107:611, 1948

Sir Alexander Fleming [1881–1955]

The lone hand has advantages as well as the much-advertised team-work, but each in its own place.
> Presidential Address, Society for General Microbiology, February 16, 1945

Alphonse Raymond Dochez [1882–1964]

You do one experiment in medicine to convince yourself, then 99 more to convince others.
> Quoted in *P & S Quarterly* 11: 18, June 1966

J. Howard Brown [1884–   ]

A man may do research for the fun of doing it but he can not expect to be supported for the fun of doing it.
> *Journal of Bacteriology* 23:1, 1932

W. W. C. Topley [1886–1944]

Committees are dangerous things that need most careful watching. I believe that a research committee can do one useful thing and one only. It can find the workers best fitted to attack a particular problem, bring them together, give them the facilities they need, and leave them to get on with the work. It can review progress from time to time, and make adjustments;

[1] Simon Flexner, founder of the Rockefeller Institute of Medical Research.

but if it tries to do more, it will do harm.

Authority, Observation and Experiment in Medicine

Alan Gregg [1890–1957]

One wonders whether the rare ability to be completely attentive to, and to profit by, nature's slightest deviation from the conduct expected of her is not the secret of the best research minds and one that explains why some men turn to most remarkably good advantage seemingly trivial accidents. Behind such attention lies an unremitting sensitivity, analogous, I suspect, to that strange experience we all have of encountering a new word two or three times within the first week after we have learned it.

The Furtherance of Medical Research, Ch. 3

Emile F. Holman [1890–   ]

Contributions to medical literature may be the product of philosophic speculation, or they may follow observations in the experimental laboratory from which logical and orderly deductions may be made. The first method has frequently resulted in conclusions wholly unsupported by reality, as for example the curious conceptions emanating from Galen's fertile imagination concerning the circulation of blood. Despite their illogical assumptions, and their complete contravention of easily observed facts, these phantasies of Galen were universally accepted for an unforgivable period.

Surgery 26:889, 1949

Henry E. Sigerist [1891–1957]

One characteristic of American research is the cheerful optimism and a certain gay spirit of enterprise which animates the majority of scientists. They attack problems even when these offer slight prospect of solution, and when sensible people shake their heads. They try a shot and very frequently hit the mark.

American Medicine, Ch. 9 (tr. by Hildegard Nagel)

Dana W. Atchley [1892–   ]

No warm sympathetic person is frozen by research experience, nor is a cold tactless individual thawed by general practice.

Journal of Medical Education 34 (October, Pt. 2):17, 1959

Alan T. Waterman [1892–1967]

If one feels he must make a psychiatric test of an individual to determine why he wants to do a piece of research, then it is undoubtedly basic.[1]

Symposium on Basic Research (ed. by D. Wolfle), "Basic Research in the United States"

James B. Conant [1893–   ]

Remember that you are dealing in your laboratories with the application of science; you must look to the universities for the fundamental advances which you later apply. Secondly, you must each year look to the universities for trained men. Therefore, if you raid the university staffs and pick off the promising young professors for your work, you are endangering your greatest assets.

Address to the American Chemical Society

Albert Szent-Györgyi [1893–   ]

Somehow, problems get into my blood and they don't give me peace, they torture me. I have to get them out of my system, and there is but one way to get them out — by solving them. A problem solved is no problem at all, it just disappears.

Perspectives in Biology and Medicine 5:173, 1962

[1] This premise is employed by the National Science Foundation in determining "investigation motives."

Francis Heed Adler [1895–   ]

The faculties developed by doing research are those most needed in diagnosis.

> *Transactions of the American Academy of Ophthalmology and Otolaryngology* 70:17, 1966

Dickinson W. Richards [1895–   ]

The word πεῖρα, *peira*, is not "experiment" in the modern sense. Hippocrates was not an experimental scientist, he was an observer and a doer, discerning, effective, practical, the supreme clinician. The word comes from πειράω, to try or to attempt. So πεῖρα is simply a trial of any kind: medicine, or other treatment, in clinical practice.

> *Perspectives in Biology and Medicine* 4:62, 1961

The problems are the ones that we have always known. The little gods are still with us, under different names. There is conformity: of technique, leading to repetition; of language, encouraging if not imposing conformity of thought. There is popularity: it is so easy to ride along on an already surging tide; to plant more seed in an already well-ploughed field; so hard to drive a new furrow into stony ground. There is laxness: the disregard of small errors, of deviations, of the unexpected response; the easy worship of the smooth curve. There is also fear: the fear of speculation; the overprotective fear of being wrong. We are forgetful of the curious and wayward dialectic of science, whereby a well-constructed theory even if it is wrong, can bring a signal advance.

> *Transactions of the Association of American Physicians* 75:1, 1962

Homer W. Smith [1895–1962]

One of the rough spots of modern medical research is that many young men, interested, willing, and competent, come and go through our laboratory portals, spending at the most two or three years in research before launching into a career in which they are all too frequently engulfed by other professional or administrative duties.

> *Circulation of the Blood* (ed. by A. P. Fishman and D. W. Richards), Ch. 9

Profitable is the course of science when a man is moved, by whatever considerations, to drift a bit, to leave his laboratory and mingle with colleagues working on seemingly unrelated experiments.

> *Idem*

On every scientist's desk there is a drawer labeled UNKNOWN in which he files what are at the moment unsolved questions, lest through guesswork or impatient speculation he come upon incorrect answers that will do him more harm than good. Man's worst fault is opening the drawer too soon. His task is not to discover final answers but to win the best partial answers that he can, from which others may move confidently against the unknown, to win better ones.

> *From Fish to Philosopher*, Ch. 13

Howard, Lord Florey [1898–1968]

The historical lesson of twentieth century medical science is that the application of experiment will unlock many doors, that experiment is the most efficient method of acquiring new knowledge that we know of, and that all our efforts should be devoted to expanding its scope in the laboratory and in the clinic.

> *Yale Journal of Biology and Medicine* 33:212, 1961

David Seegal [1899–   ]

Progress in medical science depends chiefly on the uncommon man, pos-

sessed of that rare asset, a brain so beautifully integrated with the retina, that when he looks, he perceives.
> *Journal of Medical Education* 39:321, 1964

David and Beatrice C. Seegal
[1899–   ] [1898–   ]

In the course of carrying out procedures in the . . . laboratories you will note reactions which represent *exceptions* to the anticipated result. No one can tell which of these exceptions represents the seed of a new and sometimes important observation. . . . Variations from the expected theme may be a nuisance to the routinist, but to the trained and the prepared mind, they may be the stimulus for a new symphony.
> *The Diplomate* 22:125, 1950

William H. George [fl. 20th Cent.]

Scientific research is not itself a science; it is still an art or craft.
> *The Scientist in Action*, Ch. 1, Sect. 4

Sir Robert Platt [1900–   ]

A conclusion based upon a badly conceived experiment is usually further from the truth than one based on clinical observation.
> *Universities Quarterly* 17:327, 1963

Above all it [the Royal College of Physicians] must concern itself with ethical standards and morale. It should help in the promotion of research but should not itself be a research institute, for the research of a physician emanates from the problems he sees at the bedside and its laboratory is in a hospital.
> *Idem*

René J. Dubos [1901–   ]

The history of experimental science is far too short to permit an adequate perspective of its true relation to hu-

man welfare and to the understanding of the universe.
> *Louis Pasteur, Free Lance of Science*, Ch. I

All natural phenomena can be profitably investigated at different levels of integration.
> *Ibid.*, Ch. VII

The few who reach the intuitive perception of truth must be preceded by the host of workers, most of them forgotten, whose role it has been to accumulate the facts that constitute the raw material of successful working hypotheses, of the intuitions of discovery. The immense wastefulness of organic life, which demands that thousands of germs perish so that one may live, has its counterpart in the processes of intellectual life; many must run, so that one or a few may reach the goal.
> *Ibid.*, Ch. XIII

Harold L. Mason [1901–   ]

The pursuit of excellence too often loses in the scramble for funds, recognition and prestige.
> *Journal of Clinical Endocrinology and Metabolism* 24:1214, 1964

Jacques Barzun [1907–   ]

Thousands of young men are at work on little papers; thousands more are racking their brains to think of an experiment or study. Most of them worry more about the acceptability of the subject in academic eyes than about their chances of doing and saying something useful.
> *The House of Intellect*, Ch. 9

W. I. B. Beveridge [1908–   ]

A well-known scientist told me once that he purposely leaves his research students alone for some time to give them an opportunity to find their own feet. Such a policy may have its advantages in selecting those that are worthwhile, on a sink or swim principle, but to-day there are better methods of teaching swimming than the primitive one of throwing the child into water.

The Art of Scientific Investigation, Preface

Elaborate apparatus plays an important part in the science of to-day, but I sometimes wonder if we are not inclined to forget that the most important instrument in research must always be the mind of man.

Idem

After a problem has been selected the next procedure is to ascertain what investigations have already been done on it.

Ibid., Ch. I

People whose minds are not disciplined by training often tend to notice and remember events that support their views and forget others.

Idem

Some scientists . . . contend that reading what others have written on the subject conditions the mind to see the problem in the same way and makes it more difficult to find a new and fruitful approach.

Idem

The rôle of reason in research is not so much in exploring the frontiers of knowledge as in developing the findings of the explorers.

Ibid., Ch. VII

Developmental type of research is more often carried on by the very methodical type of scientist who is content to consolidate the advances, to search over the newly won country for more modest discoveries, and to exploit fully the newly gained territory by putting it to use.

Ibid., Ch. X

Brilliant examinees are sometimes no good at research, while on the other hand some famous scientists have made a poor showing at examinations. Paul Ehrlich only got through his final medical examinations by the grace of the examiners who had the good sense to give recognition to his special talents, and Einstein failed at the entrance examination to the Polytechnic School.

Ibid., Ch. XI

Until recent times research was carried on only by the devotees, because the material rewards were so poor, but nowadays research has become a regular profession.

Idem

Edmund D. Pellegrino
[1920–   ]

Investigators seem to have settled for what is measurable instead of measuring what they would really like to know.

Clinical Research 12:421, 1964

William R. Best [1922–   ]

No amount of brilliant programming will make fruit salad out of garbage when data is being processed.

Journal of the American Medical Association 182:994, 1962

The Bible

Seek, and ye shall find.

Matthew 7:7

Prove all things; hold fast that which is good.

I Thessalonians 5:21

Anonymous

Much of medical research can be termed *conceptual,* that is, the search for a concept to explain a chance observation or to exploit a new technique on the one hand, or the effort to validate a concept serendipitously derived by devising proper experiments, on the other.

Three children: one baptized; one circumcised; one kept as control.

English Proverb

Seek till you find and you'll not lose your labour.

Spanish Proverb

He that seeks finds.[1]

II. RESEARCH FINANCING

William Stanley Jevons
[1835–1882]

Public opinion however is not discriminating and is likely to interpret the agitation for the endowment of science as meaning that science can be had for money.

The Principles of Science, Ch. XXVI

Hans Zinsser [1878–1940]

One reads the increasing mass of literature on the origins of the great American Fortunes of the nineteenth century, and one takes bicarbonate of soda. But however one feels about that, one must acknowledge that the preëminent position of American medicine to-day would have been impossible without a certain amount of rich malefaction in the eighties and nineties.

As I Remember Him, Ch. 10

Arlie V. Bock [1888–   ]

Then [1911–1917], any man found to be interested in real research was thought to be a bit queer; today, in the absence of flair, geist, or aptitude, dollars by the billion lure men into the new world of "research."

Harvard Medical Alumni Bulletin 40:2, Fall 1965

Alan Gregg [1890–1957]

I believe that endowment, whether from government or private sources, is

the soundest way to secure optimum results when it is certain the work to be done is needed. The steady confidence that is conferred by endowment calls out from scientists honesty and steadfastness of purpose: the hesitant uncertainty of short-term grants all but insults the intelligence, if not the sincerity, of the recipient and certainly makes a mockery of long-term planning.

Address at opening of McConnell Wing, Montreal Neurological Institute, 1953

I take it as likely that I shall not die before my sixty-fifth year, nor be seriously ill. That means that many things undertaken can be of three to five years' duration. If the trustees of the [Rockefeller] Foundation would only see the importance of endowing a few big things instead of frittering away the money in many small projects, I could finish a few of the really significant undertakings . . . with endowments, instead of grants.

Notes (Quoted by Wilder Penfield in *The Difficult Art of Giving*, Ch. 19)

Some people seem to think that the meetings of our Trustees [of the Rockefeller Foundation] can be described as disburse and disperse!

William S. Middleton [1890–   ]

Naively the laity cherishes the belief that money will purchase the answer to all the secrets of nature and the shibboleth has loosened the purse-strings of the nation. As might be anticipated, qualitative results have not regularly attended quantitative effort.

The Pharos of Alpha Omega Alpha 29:120, 1966

Anonymous

The hypothesis is unencumbered by any supporting evidence. The budget

---

[1] Italian Proverb: He that seeks finds and sometimes what he would rather not.

is the only part of the application which seems to have any substance whatsoever.[1]

REST

Sophocles [496?–406 B.C.]

Who in season labors best,
His labors ended, has the sweetest rest.
> *Philoctetes*, 637 (tr. by F. Storr)

Michel de Montaigne [1533–1592]

I have always liked to rest, whether lying or sitting, with my legs as high as my seat or higher.
> *Essays*, Bk. III, Ch. 13, "Of Experience" (tr. by Donald M. Frame)

Voltaire [1694–1778]

Repose . . . is sometimes, just between us, so like boredom, that one could easily mistake the one for the other.
> Letter, September 1716

Benjamin Franklin [1706–1790]

He that can take rest is greater than he that can take cities.
> *Poor Richard's Almanack*, 1737

Thomas Carlyle [1795–1881]

Rest is for the dead.
> *Journal*, June 22, 1830

Sir John Lubbock, Baron Avebury [1834–1913]

The idle man does not know what it is to rest. Hard work, moreover, tends not only to give us rest for the body, but, what is even more important, peace to the mind.
> *The Pleasures of Life*, Pt. II, Ch. X

---

[1] Comment by a reviewing member of a National Institutes of Health study section on an application for funds.

Thomas Mann [1875–1955]

I have the feeling that once I am at home again I shall need to sleep three weeks on end to get rested from the rest I've had!
> *The Magic Mountain*, Ch. IV, "The Thermometer" (tr. by H. T. Lowe-Porter)

Logan Clendening [1884–1945]

Immature faddists are continuously proclaiming the value of exercise: four people out of five are more in need of rest than exercise.
> *Modern Methods of Treatment*, Ch. 1

Rest in bed will do more for more diseases than any other single procedure.
> *Idem*

Wilder Penfield [1891–   ]

Rest, with nothing else, results in rust. It corrodes the mechanisms of the brain. The rhubarb that no one picks goes to seed.
> *The Second Career*, Ch. I

The Bible

Come unto me, all ye that labour and are heavy laden, and I will give you rest.
> *Matthew* 9:28

Anonymous

Bed is a good thing; if one does not sleep, one rests on it.

German Proverb

If I rest, I rust.[1]

Irish Proverb

Change of work is equivalent to rest.

Italian Proverb

Bed is a medicine.

---

[1] Rast ich, so rost ich.

RETIREMENT

Samuel Johnson [1709–1784]

Don't think of retiring from the world until the world will be sorry that you retire.

William Heberden [1710–1801]

I have entered my eighty-fifth year; and when I retired a few years ago from the practice of physic, I trust it was not a wish to be idle, which no man capable of being usefully employed has a right to be; but because I was willing to give over before my presence of thought, judgment and recollection was so impaired that I could not do justice to my patients. It is more desirable for a man to do this a little too soon, than a little too late; for the chief danger is on the side of not doing it soon enough.
Letter, 1794

Oliver Goldsmith [1728–1774]

O blest retirement, friend to life's decline,
Retreats from care that never must be mine,
How happy he who crowns in shades like these,
A youth of labour with an age of ease.
The Deserted Village

William Cowper [1731–1800]

Absence of occupation is not rest,
A mind quite vacant is a mind distress'd.
Retirement

But few, that court Retirement, are aware
Of half the toils they must encounter there.
Idem

Thomas Jefferson [1743–1826]

There is a time to retire from labor, and that time has come for me.

Charles Lamb [1775–1834]

Let me caution persons grown old in active business, not lightly, nor without weighing their own resources, to forego their customary employment all at once, for there may be danger in it.
The Last Essays of Elia, "The Superannuated Man"

Harvey Cushing [1869–1939]

Why not put the surgical age of retirement for the attending surgeon at sixty and the physician at sixty-three or sixty-five, as you think best? I have an idea that the surgeon's fingers are apt to get a little stiff and thus make him less competent before the physician's cerebral vessels do. However, as I told you, I would like to see the day when somebody would be appointed surgeon somewhere who had no hands, for the operative part is the least part of the work. Then, of course, many of us may get vascularly speaking, a little inelastic well on this side of sixty, or may remain in this respect as youthful at seventy as are others at fifty. This is all a lottery of inheritance and habits, and I shall be very glad, for one, to have legislated to stop active work at sixty.
Letter to Dr. Henry Christian, November 20, 1911

Stephen B. Leacock [1869–1944]

Let me give a word of advice to you young fellows around fifty who have been looking forward to retirement: Have nothing to do with it. Listen: it's like this. Have you ever been out for a late autumn walk in the closing part of the afternoon, and suddenly looked up to realize that the leaves have practically all gone? And the sun has set and the day gone before you knew it — and with that a cold wind blows across the landscape? That's retirement.
Address

Béla Schick [1877–1967]

Every Chief of Service should have a pet dog, like Ulysses had. When he retires from the hospital he should leave his dog on the floor of the department he served, because when he returns the only one who will recognize him will be his dog.

> Quoted by I. J. Wolf in *Aphorisms and Facetiae of Béla Schick,* "Early Years"

John F. Kennedy [1917–1963]

Retirement . . . should be through choice, not through compulsion due to the lack of employment opportunities.

> *Message to Congress on Problems of the Aged,* February 21, 1963

RHEUMATIC FEVER

Jean Baptiste Bouillaud [1796–1881]

The coincidence [of rheumatic heart disease and rheumatic fever] is the rule, and noncoincidence is the exception.

> *Law of Coincidence*

Ernest Charles Laségue [1816–1883]

Pathologists have long known . . . that rheumatic fever "licks at the joints, but bites at the heart."

> Quoted by Alvan R. Feinstein in *Annals of Internal Medicine* 61:27, 1964

RHEUMATISM

See also SCIATICA

William Shakespeare [1564–1616]

This raw rheumatic day.

> *The Merry Wives of Windsor,* III, i, 47

Rheumatic diseases do abound.
And thorough this distemperature we see
The seasons alter.

> *A Midsummer Night's Dream,* II, i, 105

John Taylor ("The Water Poet") [1580–1653]

Some men ('gainst Raine) doe carry in their backs
Prognosticating Aching Almanacks;
Some by a painefull elbow, hip or knee
Will shrewdly guesse, what weather's like to be.

> *Drink and Welcome*

Anton van Leeuwenhoek [1632–1723]

As to my health, thanks be to God, as long as I sit still I am without any pain, but if I do but walk a little I have pains in my legs, but that is, I think, caused by former colds and because they have carried my body so long.

> Letter to J. Chamberlayne, May 17, 1707

Cotton Mather [1663–1728]

It is possible at the same Time there may be found out, some *internal Antiarthritic,* which may at the same Time inwardly concur to sweeten the Mass of Blood, and otherwise dispose of the ill-figured Particles floating in it, and at once dissolve the thickened Moisture in the Joint, and carry off the Humour from the Blood by some other Channels. *Who can tell?* Gentlemen *Physicians,* employ yett more of your *Studies* and your *Prayers* on this Occasion! We hope 'tis not come to a *ne plus ultra,* with you.

> *The Angel of Bethesda,* Ch. XII

Philip Stanhope, Lord Chesterfield [1694–1773]

I have now been here [at Bath] near a month, bathing and drinking the waters, for complaints much of the same kind as yours; I mean pains in my legs, hips, and arms. . . . I wish it were a declared gout, which is the distemper of a gentleman; whereas the rheumatism is the distemper of a hackney-coachman or chairman, who are obliged to be out in all weathers and at all hours.

> Letter to his son, November 28, 1765

William Heberden [1710–1801]

The rheumatism is a common name for many aches and pains, which have yet got no peculiar appellation, though owing to very different causes.

> *Commentaries on the History and Cure of Diseases*, Ch. 79

John Bell [1796–1872]

Of the two forms of *arthritis* or articular inflammation, rheumatism is the tax most frequently paid by the vulgar dram and grog drinker; gout, that incurred by the genteel and sometimes the literary wine-bibber.

> *Lectures on the Theory and Practice of Physic*, Lect. CLXVII

Ralph Waldo Emerson [1803–1882]

We do not believe the less in astronomy and vegetation, because we are writhing and roaring in our beds with rheumatism.

> *Lectures,* "The Sovereignty of Ethics"

John W. Strutt, Baron Rayleigh [1842–1919]

I cannot conceive why we who are composed of over 90 per cent water should suffer from rheumatism with a slight rise in the humidity of the atmosphere.

> Letter

J. Chalmers Da Costa [1863–1933]

Appearances are deceptive. I knew a man who acquired a reputation for dignity because he had muscular rheumatism in the neck and back.

> *The Trials and Triumphs of the Surgeon*, Ch. 1

SALT

Huang Ti (The Yellow Emperor) [2697–2597 B.C.]

Hence if too much salt is used in food, the pulse hardens.

> *Nei Ching Su Wên*, Bk. 3, Sect. 10 (tr. by Ilza Veith in *The Yellow Emperor's Classic of Internal Medicine*)

Homer [ca. 850 B.C.]

Until thou comest to men that know naught of the sea and eat not of food mingled with salt.

> *Odyssey*, XI.121 (tr. by A. T. Murray)

John Florio [1553?–1625]

Salt savoureth, and seasoneth all things.

> *Second Frutes*, Folio 53

Nathaniel Hawthorne [1804–1864]

Salt is white and pure, — there is something holy in salt.

> *American Notebooks*, October 4, 1840

Wallace O. Fenn [1893–   ]

Potassium is of the soil and not the sea; it is of the cell but not the sap.

> *Physiological Reviews* 20:377, 1940

The Bible

Can that which is unsavoury be eaten without salt? or is there any taste in the white of an egg?

> *Job* 6:6

Ye are the salt of the earth: but if the salt have lost his savour, wherewith shall it be salted?
　　　Matthew 5:13

Salt is good: but if the salt have lost his saltness, wherewith will ye season it?
　　　Mark 9:50

Anonymous

Salt is what makes things taste bad when it isn't in them.

Proverbs

The best smell is bread, the best savour salt, the best love that of children.

Hebrew Proverb

If you take away the salt, you may throw the flesh to the dogs.

Latin Proverbs

Nothing more useful than the sun and salt.[1]

With a grain of salt.

Sanskrit Proverb

There are six flavors, and of them all salt is the chief.

SCARS

See also WOUNDS

William Shakespeare [1564–1616]

A scar nobly got, or a noble scar, is a good liv'ry of honour.
　　　All's Well That Ends Well, IV, v, 105

[1] Nil sole et sale utilius.

Scratch thee but with a pin, and there remains
Some scar of it.
　　　As You Like It, III, v, 21

MENENIUS:　Where is he wounded?
VOLUMNIA:　I' th' shoulder and i' th' left arm. There will be large cicatrices to show the people.
　　　Coriolanus, II, i, 161

George Gordon, Lord Byron
[1788–1824]

What deep wounds ever closed without a scar?
　　　Childe Harold's Pilgrimage, Canto III, Stanza 84

English Proverb

Though the wound be healed yet the scar remains.

SCHOLARSHIP

See also STUDENTS

Oliver Wendell Holmes
[1809–1894]

The world's great men have not commonly been great scholars, nor its great scholars great men.
　　　The Autocrat of the Breakfast Table, Sect. VI

SCIATICA

William Shakespeare [1564–1616]

Which of your hips has the most profound sciatica?
　　　Measure for Measure, I, ii, 58

　　　　　Thou cold sciatica,
Cripple our senators, that their limbs may halt
As lamely as their manners!
　　　Timon of Athens, IV, i, 23

SCIENCE

See also RESEARCH, SCIENCE AND ART, SCIENTIFIC METHOD, SCIENTISTS, THEORY AND PRACTICE

Hippocrates [460?–377? B.C.]

Science is the father of knowledge, but opinion breeds ignorance.
> *The Canon* [*Law*], IV (tr. by John Chadwick and W. N. Mann)

Geoffrey Chaucer [1340?–1400]

For out of olde feldes, as men seyth,
Cometh al this newe corn from yer to yere,
And out of olde bokes, in good feyth,
Cometh al this newe science that men lere.
> *The Parliament of Fowls*

François Rabelais [1494?–1553]

Science without conscience is the death of the soul.

Sir Francis Bacon [1561–1626]

Books must follow sciences, and not sciences books.
> *A Proposition . . . Touching Amendment of the Laws of England*

Thomas Hobbes [1588–1679]

Science [is] knowledge of the truth of Propositions, and how things are called.
> *Human Nature*, Ch. VI

Science is the knowledge of consequences, and dependance of one fact upon another.
> *Leviathan*, Pt. I, Ch. 5

Blaise Pascal [1623–1662]

Physical science will not console me for the ignorance of morality in the times of affliction. But the science of ethics will always console me for the ignorance of the physical sciences.
> *Pensées*, Sect. II, No. 67 (tr. by W. F. Trotter)

John Dryden [1631–1700]

Science distinguishes a Man of Honour from one of those Athletick Brutes whom undeservedly we call Heroes.
> *Fables Ancient and Modern*, Dedication

Is it not evident, in these last hundred years when the Study of Philosophy has been the business of all the *Virtuosi* in *Christendome* that almost a new Nature has been reveal'd to us? that more errours of the School have been detected, more useful Experiments in Philosophy have been made, more Noble Secrets in Opticks, Medicine, Anatomy, Astronomy, discover'd, than in all those credulous and doting Ages from *Aristotle* to us? so true it is that nothing spreads more fast than Science, when rightly and generally cultivated.
> *Of Dramatick Poesie*

Stanislas I (Leszczyński) of Poland [1677–1766]

Science when well digested is nothing but good sense and reason.
> *Oeuvres du Philosophe Bienfaisant*, Maxim 43

Samuel Johnson [1709–1784]

There prevails among men of letters an opinion, that all appearance of science is particularly hateful to women.
> *The Rambler*, No. 173 (November 12, 1751)

Laurence Sterne [1713–1768]

Sciences may be learned by rote, but Wisdom not.
> *Tristram Shandy*, Bk. V, Ch. 32

Mark Akenside [1721–1770]

Science! thou fair effusive ray
From the great source of mental day,
  Free, generous, and refin'd!
Descend with all thy treasures fraught,
Illumine each bewilder'd thought,
  And bless my labouring mind.
      Hymn to Science

That last best effort of thy skill,
To form the life, and rule the will,
  Propitious Power! impart:
Teach me to cool my passion's fires,
Make me the judge of my desires,
  The master of my heart.

Raise me above the vulgar's breath,
Pursuit of fortune, fear of death,
  And all in life that's mean;
Still true to reasons be my plan,
Still let my actions speak the man,
  Through every various scene.
      Idem

Adam Smith [1723–1790]

Science is the great antidote to the poison of enthusiasm and superstition.
      The Wealth of Nations, Bk. V,
      Ch. 1, Pt. 3, Article 3

Thomas Paine [1737–1809]

It is a fraud of the Christian system to call the sciences *human invention;* it is only the applications of them that is human. Every science has for its basis a system of principles as fixed and unalterable as those by which the universe is regulated and governed. Man cannot make principles, he can only discover them.
      The Age of Reason, Pt. I

Thomas Jefferson [1743–1826]

I am for encouraging the progress of science in all it's branches; and not for . . . awing the human mind by stories of raw-head & bloody bones to a distrust of its own vision & to repose implicitly on that of others.
      Letter to Elbridge Gerry, January 26, 1799

The main object of all science is the freedom and happiness of man.
      Quoted by Philip A. Bruce in
      History of the University of Virginia, Vol. I, Introduction, Ch. IV

Johann Wolfgang von Goethe [1749–1832]

Thus I saw that most men only care for science so far as they get a living by it, and that they worship even error when it affords them a subsistence.
      Quoted by Johann Peter Eckermann in *Conversations with Goethe,* October 15, 1825 (tr. by J. Oxenford)

Science has been seriously retarded by the study of what is not worth knowing, and of what is not knowable.

Charles Lamb [1775–1834]

In every thing that relates to *science,* I am a whole Encyclopaedia behind the rest of the world.
      The Essays of Elia, "The Old and the New Schoolmaster"

William Hazlitt [1778–1830]

The origin of all science is in the *desire to know causes;* and the origin of all false science and imposture is in the desire to accept false causes rather than none; or, which is the same thing, in the unwillingness to acknowledge our own ignorance.
      The Atlas, February 15, 1829, "Burke and the Edinburgh Phrenologists" [1]

George Gordon, Lord Byron [1788–1824]

      Knowledge is not happiness,
        and science
But an exchange of ignorance for that
Which is another kind of ignorance.
      Manfred, Act II, Sc. iv

[1] This article is unsigned in *The Atlas,* but it appears in P. P. Howe's *New Writings by William Hazlitt* (London, 1925).

John Clare [1] [1793–1864]

Science finds out ingenious ways to kill
Strong men, and keep alive the weak
　　and ill —
That these a sickly progeny may breed,
Too poor to tax, too numerous to feed.
　　　The Spectator

William Hickling Prescott [1796–1859]

It is the characteristic of true science,
to discern the impassable, but not very
obvious, limits which divide the province of reason from that of speculation.
Such knowledge comes tardily. How
many ages have rolled away in which
powers, that, rightly directed, might
have revealed the great laws of nature,
have been wasted in brilliant, but
barren, reveries on alchemy and as-
trology!
　　　*History of the Conquest of
　　　Mexico,* Bk. I, Ch. 4

Ralph Waldo Emerson [1803–1882]

Men love to wonder, and that is the
seed of our science.[2]
　　　Society and Solitude, "Works
　　　and Days"

Oliver Wendell Holmes [1809–1894]

SCIENCE is the topography of ignorance. . . . The best part of our
knowledge is that which teaches us
where knowledge leaves off and ignorance begins.
　　　Medical Essays, "Border Lines
　　　of Knowledge in Some Prov-
　　　inces of Medical Science"

Science is a first-rate piece of furniture
for a man's upper chamber, if he has
common sense on the ground floor.
　　　*The Poet at the Breakfast Ta-
　　　ble,* Sect. V

[1] Attributed to John Clare.
[2] Cf. William Temple, p. 522a.

Alfred, Lord Tennyson [1809–1892]

Science moves, but slowly slowly,
　　creeping on from point to point.
　　　Locksley Hall

James Anthony Froude [1818–1894]

The superstition of science scoffs at
the superstition of faith.
　　　Eclectic Review, February
　　　1852, "The Lives of the Saints"

Charles Kingsley [1819–1875]

Science is, I verily believe, like virtue,
its own exceeding great reward.
　　　Health and Education, "Sci-
　　　ence"

Herbert Spencer [1820–1903]

Science is organized knowledge.
　　　Education, Ch. 2

Science is for Life, not Life for Science.

Hermann von Helmholtz [1821–1894]

I consider the study of medicine to
have been that training which preached
more impressively and more convinc-
ingly than any other could have done,
the everlasting principles of all scientific work; principles which are so
simple and yet are ever forgotten
again, so clear and yet always hidden
by a deceptive veil.
　　　Das Denken in der Medizin (tr.
　　　by E. Atkinson in *Popular Lec-
　　　tures on Scientific Subjects*)

Rudolf Virchow [1821–1902]

The task of science, therefore, is not
to attack the objects of faith, but to
establish the limits beyond which
knowledge cannot go and to found a
unified self-consciousness within these
limits.
　　　Disease, Life, and Man, "On
　　　Man" (tr. by L. J. Rather)

There can be no scientific dispute with respect to faith, for science and faith exclude one another.
Idem

Science in itself is nothing, for it exists only in the human beings who are its bearers. . . . the idea "science for its own sake" . . . recalls the non-human conception in which man regards his soul as the true reality, as his real essence, where he "knows himself only as spirit and has not yet come to value his corporeal part."
Ibid., "Standpoints in Scientific Medicine"

The touchstone of true science is power of performance, for it is a truism that what can, also will, and thus attains to real existence.

Louis Pasteur [1822–1895]

No category of sciences exists to which one could give the name of applied sciences. *There are science and the applications of science,* linked together as fruit is to the tree that has borne it.
Pourquoi la France n'a pas trouvé d'hommes supérieurs au moment de péril, Sect. IV

I am imbued with two deep impressions; the first, that science knows no country; the second, which seems to contradict the first, although it is in reality a direct consequence of it, that science is the highest personification of the nation. Science knows no country because knowledge belongs to humanity, and is the torch which illuminates the world. Science is the highest personification of the nation because that nation will remain the first which carries the furthest the works of thought and intelligence.
Toast at banquet of the International Congress of Sericulture, Milan, Italy, 1876 (tr. by René J. Dubos)

It is characteristic of experimental science that it opens ever-widening horizons to our vision.
Quoted by René J. Dubos in *Louis Pasteur, Free Lance of Science*

Paul Broca [1824–1880]

If science must be the slave of either, a philosophical system opposed to religious dogma is just as objectionable as that dogma itself.
Bullétin de la Société Anthropologique 5:168, 1870

Private practice and marriage — those twin extinguishers of science!
Letter, April 10, 1851

Thomas Huxley [1825–1895]

Science . . . commits suicide when it adopts a creed.
Darwiniana, "The Darwin Memorial"

Science has fulfilled her function when she has ascertained and enunciated truth.
Man's Place in Nature, Ch. II

Science is, I believe, nothing but *trained and organised common sense,* differing from the latter only as a veteran may differ from a raw recruit: and its methods differ from those of common sense only as far as the guardsman's cut and thrust differ from the manner in which a savage wields his club.
Science and Education, "On the Educational Value of the Natural History Sciences"

Count Leo Tolstoy [1828–1910]

What is called science today consists of a haphazard heap of information, united by nothing, often utterly unnecessary, and not only failing to present one unquestionable truth, but as often as not containing the grossest errors today put forward as truths, and tomorrow overthrown.

> *What Is Religion?*, Ch. 1 (tr. by V. Tchertkoff and A. C. Fifield)

William Stanley Jevons
[1835–1882]

Science arises from the discovery of Identity amidst Diversity.

> *The Principles of Science,* Ch. I

Mark Twain (Samuel L. Clemens)
[1835–1910]

There is something fascinating about science. One gets such wholesome returns of conjectures out of such trifling investment of fact.

Sir Clifford Allbutt [1836–1925]

In science, law is not a rule imposed from without, but an expression of an intrinsic process.

> Quoted by F. H. Garrison in *Bulletin of the New York Academy of Medicine* 4:1000, 1928

We find, in ruling classes, and in social circles which put on aristocratical fashions, that ideas, and especially scientific ideas, are held in sincere aversion and in simulated contempt.

> *Idem*

Anatole France [1844–1924]

I hate science . . . for having loved it too much, after the manner of voluptuaries who reproach women with not having come up to the dream they formed of them.

> *The Opinions of Jérôme Coignard,* Ch. 9 (tr. by Mrs. Wilfred Jackson)

The sciences are beneficent. They prevent men from thinking.

Sir William Osler [1849–1919]

Who can doubt that the leaven of science, working in the individual, leavens in some slight degree the whole social fabric. Reason is at least free, or nearly so; the shackles of dogma have been removed, and faith herself, freed from a morganatic alliance, finds in the release great gain.

> *Aequanimitas, with Other Addresses,* "The Leaven of Science"

The future belongs to science. More and more she will control the destinies of the nations. Already she has them in her crucible and on her balances.

> Foreword to René Vallery-Radot's *Life of Pasteur*

Charles V. Chapin [1856–1941]

Science can never be a closed book. It is like a tree, ever growing, ever reaching new heights. Occasionally the lower branches, no longer giving nourishment to the tree, slough off. We should not be ashamed to change our methods; rather we should be ashamed never to do so.

> *Papers,* "Science and Public Health"

George Bernard Shaw [1856–1950]

Science is always wrong. It never solves a problem without creating ten more.

Karl Pearson [1857–1936]

When every fact, every present or past phenomenon of [the whole physical] universe, every phase of present or past life therein, has been examined, classified, and co-ordinated with the rest, then the mission of science will be completed. What is this but saying that the task of science can never end till man ceases to be, till history is no longer made, and development itself ceases?

> *The Grammar of Science,* Ch. I, Sect. 5

Max Planck [1858–1947]

A new scientific truth does not triumph by convincing its opponents and making them see the light, but rather because its opponents eventually die, and a new generation grows up that is familiar with it.
> *Scientific Autobiography* (tr. by Frank Gaynor)

Science cannot exist without some small portion of metaphysics.
> *The Universe in the Light of Modern Physics*, Ch. 7 (tr. by W. H. Johnston)

Scientific discovery and scientific knowledge have been achieved only by those who have gone in pursuit of it without any practical purpose whatsoever in view.
> *Where Is Science Going?*, Ch. IV (tr. by J. Murphy)

Science cannot solve the ultimate mystery of nature. And that is because, in the last analysis, we ourselves are part of nature and therefore part of the mystery that we are trying to solve.
> *Ibid.*, Epilogue

Miguel de Unamuno [1864–1936]

Science robs men of wisdom and usually converts them into phantom beings loaded up with facts.
> *Essays and Soliloquies*, "Some Arbitrary Reflections Upon Europeanization" (tr. by J. E. Crawford Flitch)

Wisdom is to science what death is to life, or, if you prefer it, wisdom is to death what science is to life.
> *Idem*

Marie Curie [1867–1934]

In science we must be interested in things, not in persons.
> Quoted by Eve Curie in *Madame Curie*, Ch. XVI (tr. by Vincent Sheean)

Richard Clarke Cabot [1868–1939]

Ethics and Science need to shake hands.
> *The Meaning of Right and Wrong*, Introduction

Max Neuburger [1868–1955]

Doctrinaire formula-worship, that is our real enemy.

Wilfred Trotter [1872–1939]

In science the primary duty of ideas is to be useful and interesting even more than to be 'true.'
> *Collected Papers*, "The Functions of the Human Skull," Sect. 1

Sir Winston Churchill [1874–1965]

Science bestowed immense new powers on man, and, at the same time, created conditions which were largely beyond his comprehension and still more beyond his control.
> Speech at Massachusetts Institute of Technology, March 31, 1949

Sir Charles Singer [1876–   ]

Our knowledge of health and of disease thus depends on the sciences as a whole — nay, on Knowledge as a whole. Those who would promote the health of mankind would do well if they sought to encourage not so much the medical sciences as Science as a whole, or rather Learning as a whole, for Science is a way of life which may penetrate into all departments of Learning, and is something far greater than those discrete accumulations of knowledge that we call "the sciences." The Sciences, working out their destiny, must in the end come together again.
> *A Short History of Medicine*, Epilogue

Martin H. Fischer [1879–1962]

Facts are not science—as the dictionary is not literature.
> Quoted by Howard Fabing and Ray Marr in *Fischerisms*

William Temple, Archbishop of Canterbury [1881–1944]

Science has its being in a perpetual mental restlessness.[1]
> *Essays and Studies by Members of the English Association,* Vol. XVII, "Poetry and Science"

J. Frank Dobie [1888–1964]

Putting on the spectacles of science in expectation of finding the answer to everything looked at signifies inner blindness.
> *The Voice of the Coyote,* Introduction

Emil Brunner [1889–   ]

Science knows what it is, it does not know what it ought to be. . . . science in our day claims more room in the totality of human life than it is entitled to.
> *Christianity and Civilization,* Pt. II, Sect. II

Wilder Penfield [1891–   ]

The trouble is not in science but in the uses men make of it. Doctor and layman alike must learn wisdom in their employment of science, whether this applies to atom bombs or blood transfusion.
> *The Second Career,* "A Doctor's Philosophy"

Henry E. Sigerist [1891–1957]

The technology of medicine has outrun its sociology.
> *Medicine and Human Welfare,* Ch. 3

[1] Cf. Ralph Waldo Emerson, p. 518a.

J. B. S. Haldane [1892–1964]

Science is vastly more stimulating to the imagination than are the classics.
> *Daedalus*

Paul Reznikoff [1896–   ]

Conflict between science and religion should never exist. Their aims are entirely different — science tries to find out how, religion deals with why.
> Aphorism

Ashley Montagu [1905–   ]

As the god of contemporary man's idolatry, science is a two-handed engine, and as such science is too important a human activity to leave to the scientists.
> Quoted in *New York Times Book Review,* April 26, 1964, advertisement of Jacques Barzun's *Science: The Glorious Entertainment*

Dwight J. Ingle [1907–   ]

Science cannot be equated to measurement, although many contemporary scientists behave as though it can. For example, the editorial policies of many scientific journals support the publication of data and exclude the communication of ideas.
> *Principles of Research in Biology and Medicine,* Ch. 1

Francis L. K. Hsu [1909–   ]

To achieve popular acceptance, magic has to be dressed like science in America, while science has to be cloaked as magic in Hsi-ch'eng [China].
> *Health, Culture and Community* (ed. by B. D. Paul), Pt. 2

Kenneth E. Boulding [1910–   ]

Science might almost be defined as the process of substituting unimportant questions which can be answered for important questions which cannot.
> *The Image,* Ch. 11

Spanish Proverb

Science is madness if good sense does not cure it.

SCIENCE AND ART

See also SCIENCE

Michel de Montaigne [1533–1592]

The sciences and arts are not cast in a mold, but are formed and shaped little by little, by repeated handling and polishing, as the bears lick their cubs into shape at leisure.

> *Essays,* Bk. II, Ch. 12, "Apology for Raymond Sebond" (tr. by Donald M. Frame)

Sir Francis Bacon [1561–1626]

If the debasement of arts and sciences to purposes of wickedness, luxury, and the like, be made a ground of objection, let no one be moved thereby. For the same may be said of all earthly goods.

Alexander Pope [1688–1744]

One Science only will one genius fit,
So vast is Art, so narrow human wit.
> *An Essay on Criticism,* Pt. I

Johann Wolfgang von Goethe [1749–1832]

Science and art belong to the whole world, and the barriers of nationality vanish before them.

Benjamin Disraeli, Lord Beaconsfield [1804–1881]

What Art was to the ancient world, Science is to the modern.
> *Coningsby,* Bk. IV, Ch. 1

John Brown [1810–1882]

Science and Art are the offspring of light and truth, of intelligence and will; they are the parents of philosophy — that its father, this its mother. Art comes up out of darkness, like a flower, — is there before you are aware, its roots unseen, not to be meddled with safely. . . . It draws its nourishment from all its neighborhood, taking this, and rejecting that, by virtue of its elective instinct knowing what is good for it; it lives upon the débris of former life. Science comes from the market; it is sold, can be measured and weighed, can be handled and gauged. It is full of light; but is lucid rather than luminous; it is, at its best, food, not blood, much less muscle — the fuel, not the fire.

> *Horae Subsecivae,* Series I, "Art and Science"

Your well-informed, merely scientific, men are all alike. Set one agoing at any point, he brings up as he revolves the same figures, the same thoughts, or rather ghosts of thoughts, as any ten thousand others. Look at him on one side, and, like a larch, you see his whole; every side is alike. Look at the poorest hazel, holding itself by its grappling talons on some gray rock, and you never saw one like it; you will never see one like it again; it has more sides than one; it has had a discipline, and has a will of its own; it is self-taught, self-sufficient.

> *Idem*

Claude Bernard [1813–1878]

A contemporary poet has characterized this sense of the personality of art and of the impersonality of science in these words, — "Art is myself; science is ourselves. "

> *An Introduction to the Study of Experimental Medicine,* Pt. I, Ch. 2, Sect. iv (tr. by H. C. Greene)

Joseph Roux [1834–1886]

Science is for those who learn; poetry, for those who know.
> *Meditations of a Parish Priest,* Ch. I, No. LXXI (tr. by Isabel F. Hapgood)

John Fiske [1842–1901]

All human science is but the increment of the power of the eye, and all human art is the increment of the power of the hand.

> *The Destiny of Man,* Ch. VII

Detlev W. Bronk [1897–   ]

Science, like art, music and poetry, tries to reduce chaos to the clarity and order of pure beauty.

> Quoted in *Journal of the American Medical Association* 191:991, 1965

SCIENTIFIC METHOD

See also DISCOVERY, EMPIRICISM, HYPOTHESIS, INVESTIGATORS, RESEARCH, SCIENCE, THEORY

Aristotle [384–322 B.C.]

To be matter of scientific knowledge a truth must be demonstrated by deduction from other truths.

> *Nicomachean Ethics,* VI.vi (tr. by H. Rackham)

Leonardo da Vinci [1452–1519]

But first I will make some experiment before proceeding farther because it is my intention first to cite experience then to show by reasoning why this experience is constrained to act in this manner. And this is the rule according to which speculators as to natural effects have to proceed. And although nature commences with reason and ends in experience it is necessary for us to do the opposite, that is to commence as I said before with experience and from this to proceed to investigate the reason.

> Manuscript E, Library of the Institut de France (tr. by Edward MacCurdy in *The Notebooks of Leonardo da Vinci,* Vol. I, Ch. XIX)

Sir Francis Bacon [1561–1626]

Now what the sciences stand in need of is a form of induction which shall analyse experience and take it to pieces, and by a due process of exclusion and rejection lead to an inevitable conclusion. . . . To the immediate and proper perception of the sense therefore I do not give much weight; but I contrive that the office of the sense shall be only to judge of the experiment, and that the experiment itself shall judge of the thing.

> *The Great Instauration,* "The Plan of the Work"

Although the roads to human power and to human knowledge lie close together, and are nearly the same, nevertheless on account of the pernicious and inveterate habit of dwelling on abstractions, it is safer to begin and raise the sciences from those foundations which have relation to practice, and to let the active part itself be as the seal which prints and determines the contemplative counterpart.

> *Novum Organum,* "Aphorisms," IV

It would be an unsound fancy and self-contradictory to expect that things which have never yet been done can be done except by means which have never yet been tried.

> *Ibid.,* VI

Moreover the works already known are due to chance and experiment rather than to sciences; for the sciences we now possess are merely systems for the nice ordering and setting forth of things already invented; not methods of invention or directions for new works.

> *Ibid.,* VIII

The men of experiment are like the ant; they only collect and use: the reasoners resemble spiders, who make cobwebs out of their own substance. But the bee takes a middle course; it

gathers its material from the flowers of the garden and of the field, but transforms and digests it by a power of its own.
Ibid., XCV

"*Experimenta lucifera*," experiments of *light*, . . . have one admirable property and condition; they never miss or fail. For since they are applied, not for the purpose of producing any particular effect, but only of discovering the natural cause of some effect, they answer the end equally well whichever way they turn out; for they settle the question.
Ibid., XCIX

Our road does not lie on a level, but ascends and descends; first ascending to axioms, then descending to works.
Ibid., CIII

For my way of discovering sciences goes far to level men's wits, and leaves but little to individual excellence; because it performs everything by the surest rules and demonstrations.
Ibid., CXXII

René Descartes [1596–1650]

Like those who walk alone and after nightfall, I resolved to proceed so slowly, and with such meticulous circumspection, that if my advance was but small, I should at least guard myself from falling.
Discours de la Méthode, Pt. II (tr. by Norman K. Smith)

Lazzaro Spallanzani [1729–1799]

If I set out to prove something, I am no real scientist — I have to learn to follow where the facts lead me — I have to learn to whip my prejudices.

Antoine Lavoisier [1743–1794]

We must trust to nothing but facts: These are presented to us by Nature, and cannot deceive. We ought, in every instance, to submit our reasoning to the test of experiment, and never to search for truth but by the natural road of experiment and observation.
Elements of Chemistry, Preface (tr. by Robert Kerr)

Alexander M'Call [early 19th Cent.]

Medical theory is truly useful, only when its practical results are beneficial. To judge correctly of these results, we must have recourse to the phenomena presented to clinical observers. It is by inductive reasoning thus experimentally obtained, that we can be prepared to detect the fallacy of each protean medical theory, whose shadowy being might long elude any other species of investigation.
American Medical Recorder 6:254, 1823

Elisha Bartlett [1804–1855]

Certainly, there is no conceivable process of inductive reasoning, by which the mind of Sir Isaac Newton could have arrived at the knowledge of the heterogeneous and compound nature of light. It was with the prism, and his eyes, and not by any magic of his great intellect, that the web of its homogeneous rays was first unwoven and analyzed, and its composition ascertained.
Philosophy of Medical Science, Pt. I, Ch. 2

Charles Darwin [1809–1882]

I must begin with a good body of facts and not from a principle (in which I always suspect some fallacy) and then as much deduction as you please.
Letter to J. Fiske, December 8, 1874

Science consists in grouping facts so that general laws or conclusions may be drawn from them.
Quoted by Francis Darwin in *Charles Darwin*, Ch. 2

Claude Bernard [1813–1878]

Good methods can teach us to develop and use to better purpose the faculties with which nature has endowed us, while poor methods may prevent us from turning them to good account. Thus the genius of inventiveness, so precious in the sciences, may be diminished or even smothered by a poor method, while a good method may increase and develop it. . . . In biological sciences, the rôle of method is even more important than in other sciences, because of the immense complexity of the phenomena and the countless sources of error which complexity brings into experimentation.

> *An Introduction to the Study of Experimental Medicine*, Pt. I, Ch. 2, Sect. ii (tr. by H. C. Greene)

In science, the best precept is to alter and exchange our ideas as fast as science moves ahead.

> *Ibid.*, Sect. iv

Science rejects the indeterminate.

> *Ibid.*, Sect. vi

True science teaches us to doubt and, in ignorance, to refrain.

> *Idem*

All natural philosophy is summarized in *knowing the law of phenomena*. The whole experimental problem may be reduced to foreseeing and directing phenomena.

> *Ibid.*, Sect. viii

Particular facts are never scientific; only generalization can establish science.

> *Ibid.*, Pt. II, Ch. 2, Sect. i

In experimentation it is always necessary to start from a particular fact and proceed to the generalization. . . . But above all one must observe.

> Manuscript, Collège de France (Quoted in *Perspectives in Biology and Medicine* 8:30, 1964)

Put off your imagination, as you take off your overcoat, when you enter the laboratory; but put it on again, as you do your overcoat, when you leave the laboratory. Before the experiment and between whiles, let your imagination wrap you round; put it right away from you during the experiment itself lest it hinder your observing power.

John Ruskin [1819–1900]

The work of science is to substitute facts for appearances, and demonstrations for impressions.

> *Stones of Venice*, Vol. III, Ch. II

Herbert Spencer [1820–1903]

Every science begins by accumulating observations, and presently generalizes these empirically; but only when it reaches the stage at which its empirical generalizations are included in a rational generalization, does it become developed science.

> *The Data of Ethics*, Ch. IV

Louis Pasteur [1822–1895]

Science proceeds by successive answers to questions more and more subtle, coming nearer and nearer to the very essence of phenomena.

> *Études sur la bière*, Ch. VI, Sect. vi (tr. by Réne J. Dubos)

The great art consists in devising decisive experiments, leaving no place to the imagination of the observer. Imagination is needed to give wings to thought at the beginning of experimental investigations on any given subject. When, however, the time has come to conclude, and to interpret the facts derived from observations, imagination must submit to the factual results of the experiments.

> Quoted by René J. Dubos in *Louis Pasteur, Free Lance of Science*

Thomas Huxley [1825–1895]

Sit down before fact as a little child, be prepared to give up every preconceived notion, follow humbly wherever and to whatsoever abysses Nature leads, or you shall learn nothing.

> Letter to Charles Kingsley, September 23, 1860

My business is to teach my aspirations to conform themselves to fact, not to try to make facts harmonise with my aspirations.

> *Idem*

The man of science has learned to believe in justification, not by faith, but by verification.

> *On the Advisableness of Improving Natural Knowledge*

Theodor Billroth [1829–1894]

Solitary, meditative observation is the first step in the poetry of research, in the formation of scientific phantasies, the reality of which we then test with the tools of logic, mathematics, physics and chemistry.

> *The Medical Sciences in the German Universities*, Pt. II

The method of research, however, of positing the questions and solving the questions posited, is invariably the same, whether we have before us a blooming rose, a diseased grape-vine, a shining beetle, the spleen of a leopard, a bird's feather, the intestines of a pig, the brain of a poet or a philosopher, a sick poodle, or an hysterical princess.

> *Idem*

Robert G. Ingersoll [1833–1899]

Reason, Observation, and Experience — the Holy Trinity of Science.

> *The Gods*

Emile Duclaux [1840–1904]

A series of judgments, revised without ceasing, goes to make up the incontestable progress of science.

> *Pasteur*, Pt. III, Ch. 7

William James [1842–1910]

Many persons nowadays seem to think that any conclusion must be very scientific if the arguments in favor of it are derived from twitching of frogs' legs — especially if the frogs are decapitated — and that — on the other hand — any doctrine chiefly vouched for by the feelings of human beings — with heads on their shoulders — must be benighted and superstitious.

> *Pragmatism*

Science like life feeds on its own decay. New facts burnst old rules; then newly developed concepts bind old and new together into a reconciling law.

> *The Will to Believe*

Louis A. Duhring [1845–1913]

Science is classified knowledge, and development of any science depends upon improved methods of classification.

> *Epitome of Diseases of the Skin*, "Classification"

Sir William Richard Gowers [1845–1915]

In the present state of my ignorance it seems more useful to gather facts than to formulate hypotheses.

Paul Ehrlich [1854–1915]

Much testing; accuracy and precision in experiment; no guesswork or self-deception.

> Quoted by Martha Marquardt in *Paul Ehrlich*, Ch. XIII

Try to analyse striking experimental facts . . . difficult to understand and by so analysing to find the laws that govern the action.

George Bernard Shaw [1856–1950]

It does happen exceptionally that a practising doctor makes a contribution to science. . . . but it happens much oftener that he draws disastrous conclusions from his clinical experience because he has no conception of scientific method, and believes, like any rustic, that the handling of evidence and statistics needs no expertness.

> *The Doctor's Dilemma,* "Preface on Doctors"

George Santayana [1863–1952]

Science is nothing but developed perception, interpreted intent, common sense rounded out and minutely articulated.

> *The Life of Reason: Reason in Science,* Ch. 11

Abraham Flexner [1866–1959]

Science is essentially a matter of observation, inference, verification, generalization. The mind of Sydenham, interested in a sick child and humanely preoccupied with its cure, did not, insofar as it functioned scientifically, operate differently from that of Galileo, interested in cosmic physics. Both alike observed, reflected, verified, generalized.

> *Medical Education, A Comparative Study,* Ch. 1

The investigator, obviously, observes, experiments and judges; so do the physician and surgeon who practise their art in the modern spirit. At bottom the intellectual attitude and processes of the two are — or should be — identical: neither investigator nor practitioner should be blinded by prejudice or jump at conclusions; both should observe, reflect, conclude, try, and, watching results, continuously reapply the same method until the problem in hand has been solved or abandoned.

> *Idem*

Walter B. Cannon [1871–1945]

Investigators are commonly said to be engaged in a search for the truth. I think they themselves would usually state their aims less pretentiously. What the experimenter is really trying to do is to learn whether facts can be established which will be recognized as facts by others and which will support some theory that in imagination he has projected. But he must be ingenuously honest. He must face facts as they arise in the course of experimental procedure, whether they are favorable to his idea or not. In doing this he must be ready to surrender his theory at any time if the facts are adverse to it.

> *The Way of an Investigator,* "Fitness for the Enterprise"

Wilfred Trotter [1872–1939]

Although rational and imaginative speculation is of the greatest general value to science in keeping it from going dry and orthodox, as an actual implement of research it has not very much to its credit.

> *Collected Papers,* "Has the Intellect a Function?"

Hans Zinsser [1878–1940]

The preparatory accumulation of minor discoveries and of accurately observed details . . . is, in scientific pursuits, almost as important for the mobilization of great forward drives as the periodic correlation of these disconnected observations into principles and laws by the vision of genius.

> *As I Remember Him,* Ch. X

Max Born [1882–   ]

There are two objectionable types of believers: those who believe the incredible and those who believe that 'belief' must be discarded and replaced by 'the scientific method.'

> *Natural Philosophy of Cause and Chance,* Appendix One

Dickinson W. Richards [1895–   ]

It should be noted, also, that conceptual disorder is by no means always a bad thing. It has, in fact, been highly recommended — by Henderson, White-

head, and others — in that a conscious and sustained "muddleheadedness" is a very proper state of mind in the slow and deliberate evolution of a difficult idea. One insists on keeping one's self confused until the right answer forces a clear solution. Perhaps this is one part of the "gradualness" which Pavlov recommended to his students.[1]
> *Perspectives in Biology and Medicine* 3:238, 1960

SCIENTISTS

See also INVESTIGATORS, RESEARCH, SCIENCE, SCIENTIFIC METHOD

Moses ben Maimon (Maimonides) [1135–1204]

The soul is subject to health and disease, just as is the body. The health and disease of both . . . undoubtedly depend upon beliefs and customs, which are peculiar to mankind. Wherefore I call senseless beliefs and degenerate customs . . . diseases of humanity.

Within the sum total of these diseases there is one which is widespread, and from which men rarely escape. This disease varies in degree in different men, just as all bodily . . . diseases vary. . . . I refer to this: that every person thinks his mind . . . more clever and more learned than it is. . . . I have found that this disease has attacked many an intelligent person . . . who is well-versed in physical science, or mechanical art, or one of the positive sciences. And they . . . express themselves (not only) upon the science with which they are familiar, but upon other sciences (as well) about which they know nothing. . . . If (they are) met with applause . . . and (their) words are heeded . . . so

[1] Cf. Ivan Pavlov, p. 575b.

does the disease itself become aggravated.
> *Aphorisms According to Galen* (Quoted in *Bulletin of the Institute of the History of Medicine* 3:555, 1935)

Georg Christoph Lichtenberg [1742–1799]

I have traveled the way of science in the manner of dogs that go for a walk with their masters, a hundred times backward and forward, and when I arrived I was weary.
> *Aphorismen* (1789–1793)

Charles C. Colton [1780?–1832]

Professors in every branch of the sciences prefer their own theories to truth: the reason is that their theories are private property but the truth is common stock.
> *Lacon*

Coffinhal [fl. 1794]

The Republic has no need for scientists.
> Comment while presiding at trial of Antoine Lavoisier before the Revolutionary Tribunal in Paris, 1794

Winthrop Mackworth Praed [1802–1839]

Of science and logic he chatters,
  As fine and as fast as he can;
Though I am no judge of such matters,
  I'm sure he's a talented man.
> *Poems of Life and Manners,* "The Talented Man"

Claude Bernard [1813–1878]

It is in the darker regions of science that great men are recognized; they are marked by ideas which light up phenomena hitherto obscure and carry science forward.
> *An Introduction to the Study of Experimental Medicine,* Pt. I, Ch. 2, Sect. iv (tr. by H. C. Greene)

Louis Pasteur [1822–1895]

It is not without utility to show to the man of the world, and to the practical man, at what cost the scientist conquers principles, even the simplest and the most modest in appearance.
> Quoted by René J. Dubos in *Louis Pasteur, Free Lance of Science*

When moving forward toward the discovery of the unknown, the scientist is like a traveler who reaches higher and higher summits from which he sees in the distance new countries to explore.
> *Idem*

Mark Twain (Samuel L. Clemens) [1835–1910]

Scientists have odious manners, except when you prop up their theory; then you can borrow money of them.
> *What Is Man and Other Essays,* "The Bee"

Samuel J. Meltzer [1851–1921]

I think the Young Turks are getting rather old.[1]
> *The Association of American Physicians: Its First Seventy-Five Years*

Jules Henri Poincaré [1854–1912]

The scientist does not study nature because it is useful to do so. He studies it because he takes pleasure in it, and he takes pleasure in it because it is beautiful.
> *Science and Method,* Vol. I, Ch. I (tr. by Francis Maitland)

Georgi Plekhanov [1857–1918]

Bourgeois scientists make sure that

---

[1] Meltzer made this remark in 1921 about his brainchild, the American Society for Clinical Investigation, which was founded as an outlet for young investigators in 1907–1908. Its members were nicknamed the "Young Turks" from the nationalist rebellion in Turkey at that time.

their theories are not dangerous to God or to capital.
> *Karl Marx*

August Bier [1861–1949]

Medical scientists are nice people, but you should not let them treat you.
> Aphorism

Charles H. Mayo [1865–1939]

The scientist is not content to stop at the obvious.
> *Collected Papers of the Mayo Clinic and Mayo Foundation* 18:1093, 1926

Ross Granville Harrison [1870–1959]

Wilhelm Ostwald (1853–1932), in his interesting book on great men of science, classified them, according to their talents, as romantics and classics. . . . To the romantic, ideas come thick and fast; they must find quick expression. His first care is to get a problem off his hands to make room for the next. The classic is more concerned with the perfection of his product, with setting his ideas in the proper relation to each other and to the main body of science. His impulse is to work over his subject so exhaustively and perfectly that no contemporary is able to improve upon it. . . . It is the romantic that revolutionizes, while the classic builds from the ground up.
> *American Scientist* 53:304, 1965

Bertrand Russell [1872–   ]

All the conditions of happiness are realized in the life of the man of science.
> *The Conquest of Happiness,* Ch. X

Sir Winston Churchill [1874–1965]

Scientists should be on tap, but not on top.
> Quoted by Randolph S. Churchill in *Twenty-one Years,* Epilogue

Albert Einstein [1879–1955]

Many kinds of men devote themselves to Science, and not all for the sake of Science herself. There are some who come into her temple because it offers them the opportunity to display their particular talents. To this class of men science is a kind of sport in the practice of which they exult, just as an athlete exults in the exercise of his muscular prowess. There is another class of men who come into the temple to make an offering of their brain pulp in the hope of securing a profitable return. These men are scientists only by the chance of some circumstance which offered itself when making a choice of career. . . . it is clear that if the men who have devoted themselves to science consisted only of the two categories I have mentioned, the edifice could never have grown to its present proud dimensions. . . . I am inclined to agree with Schopenhauer in thinking that one of the strongest motives that lead people to give their lives to art and science is the urge to flee from everyday life, with its drab and deadly dullness, and thus to unshackle the chains of one's own transient desires, which supplant one another in an interminable succession so long as the mind is fixed on the horizon of daily environment.
> Prologue to Max Planck's
> *Where Is Science Going?*

Sir F. M. R. Walshe [1888–   ]

It often is the cloistered scientist who knows least about men who is apt to pontificate most loudly and confidently about Man. Beware of him when he assures you that he knows all the answers about us, for too often he is one of those Peter Pans of science that every generation produces: a clever boy who hasn't grown up.
> *Canadian Medical Association Journal* 67:395, 1952

Homer W. Smith [1895–1962]

A scientist is one who, when he does not know the answer, is rigorously disciplined to speak up and say so unashamedly; which is the essential feature by which modern science is distinguished from primitive superstition, which knew all the answers except how to say, "I do not know."
> *From Fish to Philosopher,* Ch. 13

D. J. van Lennep [1898–   ]

"Achievers" work persistently and reliably on problems set for them, using established methods and not requiring initiative or original thought. They think their work useful to society and prefer regular step-by-step techniques. They do not think or worry about their work after hours.

"Creators" work independently without terms of reference on problems of their own choosing for which methodology is not existent. Older concepts exist only to be remolded. They are rebellious and do not care if their work is useful to society. They are enthusiasts; they talk about their results too soon; they often omit steps.

"Problem-solvers" bring to solution projects which are clearly formulated but for which no methodology exists. They feel their results justify their existence. They do not talk or publish too soon; they do not omit steps; they do not repeat others' work because of ignorance of it.[1]
> Address at Bedford College, University of London, May 6, 1959

Sir Robert Platt [1900–   ]

The unprecedented development of science and technology [has been] so rapid that it is said that 90 per cent of the scientists which this country has ever produced are still living today.
> *Universities Quarterly* 17:327, 1963

[1] The main concepts of Professor van Lennep's address were summarized thus in *Lancet* 1:1039, 1959.

René J. Dubos [1901–   ]

Like other men, scientists become deaf and blind to any argument or evidence that does not fit into the thought pattern which circumstances have led them to follow.
>Louis Pasteur, Free Lance of Science, Ch. VII

Karl R. Popper [1902–   ]

It is not his *possession* of knowledge, of irrefutable truth, that makes the man of science, but his persistent and recklessly critical *quest* for truth.
>The Logic of Scientific Discovery, Ch. 10

Sir C. P. Snow [1905–   ]

It is not enough for scientists to make statements of the greatest possible truth; they must have the courage to carry those statements through because they alone know enough to be able to impress their authority upon a world which is anxious to hear, if it can only find voices which can speak with enough clarity and, I think I must say, enough noise.
>Address at Dartmouth Convocation on *The Great Issues of Conscience in Modern Medicine,* September 8–10, 1960

Jacob Bronowski [1908–   ]

At bottom, the society of scientists is more important than their discoveries. What science has to teach us here is not its techniques but its spirit: the irresistible need to explore.
>Science and Human Values, Ch. 3

Anonymous

I do not think that he should cut off his ear for posterity.
>Comment concerning an egotistical medical scientist

SCRATCHING

See also ITCH

Michel de Montaigne [1533–1592]

Scratching is one of the sweetest gratifications of nature, and as ready at hand as any.
>Essays, Bk. III, Ch. 13, "Of Experience" (tr. by Donald M. Frame)

Anonymous

'Tis better than riches
To scratch when it itches.

Proverb

Scratching is bad; because it begins with pleasure, and ends with pain.

Russian Proverb

He who scratches a scar is wounded twice.

SCURVY

Richard Mead [1673–1754]

That experienced and brave admiral, Sir Charles Wager, once told me . . . his sailors were terribly afflicted with the Scurvy. . . . Recollecting, from what he had often heard, how effectual these fruits [oranges and lemons] were in the cure of this distemper, he ordered a chest of each to be brought upon deck, and opened every day. The men, besides eating what they would, mixed the juice in their beer. It was also their constant diversion to pelt one another with the rinds; so that the deck was always strewed and wet with the fragrant liquor. The happy effect was, that he brought his sailors home in good health.
>Medical Works, "A Discourse on the Scurvy",

James Lind [1716–1794]

Armies have been supposed to lose more of their men by sickness, than by the sword. But this observation has been much more verified in our fleets and squadrons; where the scurvy alone, during the last war, proved a more destructive enemy, and cut off more valuable lives, than the united efforts of the *French* and *Spanish* arms.
> *A Treatise of the Scurvy,* Preface

SEASICKNESS

William Shakespeare [1564–1616]
> Why look you pale?
> Seasick, I think, coming from Muscovy.
> *Love's Labour's Lost,* V, ii, 392

John Donne [1573–1631]
> He's one that goes
> To sea for nothing but to make him sick.
> *Elegies,* XVIII

George Gordon, Lord Byron [1788–1824]

The best of remedies is a beef-steak
   Against seasickness: try it, sir, before
You sneer.
> *Don Juan,* Canto II, Stanza 13

Henry Wheeler Shaw ("Josh Billings") [1818–1885]

One ov the best temporary cures for pride and affektashun that i hav ever seen tried is sea sickness; a man who wants tew vomit never puts on airs.
> *Works,* "Ods and Ens"

Samuel Butler [1835–1902]

How holy people look when they are sea-sick! There was a patient Parsee near me who seemed purified once and for ever from all taint of the flesh. Buddha was a low, worldly-minded, music-hall comic singer in comparison. He sat for a long time until . . . and he made a noise like cows coming home to be milked on an April evening.
> *Note-Books,* "The Channel Passage"

Mark Twain (Samuel L. Clemens) [1835–1910]

If there is one thing that will make a man peculiarly and insufferably self-conceited, it is to have his stomach behave itself, the first day at sea, when nearly all his comrades are seasick.
> *The Innocents Abroad,* Ch. III

We all like to see people seasick when we are not, ourselves.
> *Idem*

Sir William S. Gilbert [1836–1911]

And I'm never, never sick at sea!
What, never?
No, never!
What, *never?*
Hardly, ever!
> *H.M.S. Pinafore,* Act I

English Sailors' Proverb

The only cure for seasickness is to sit on the shady side of an old brick church in the country.

SEIZURES

Hippocrates [460?–377? B.C.]

It is better that a fever succeed to a convulsion, than a convulsion to a fever.
> *Aphorisms,* II.26 (tr. by Francis Adams)

Celsus [25 B.C.–A.D. 50]

Some have freed themselves from such a disease [epilepsy] by drinking the hot blood from the cut throat of a glad-

iator: a miserable aid made tolerable by a malady still more miserable.
> *De Medicina*, III.xxiii.7 (tr. by W. G. Spencer)

Dante Alighieri [1265–1321]

As one who falls, nor knows how the fit comes,
By diabolic power, or oppilation
That chokes the brain with stupefying fumes,

Who, when he rises, stares in consternation
All round, bewildered by his late hard throes,
With rolling eyes and anguished suspiration.

> *The Divine Comedy*, "Hell," Canto XXIV (tr. by Dorothy L. Sayers)

William Shakespeare [1564–1616]

CASCA: He fell down in the market place and foam'd at mouth and was speechless.
BRUTUS: 'Tis very like. He hath the falling sickness. . . .
CASCA: . . . When he came to himself again, he said, if he had done or said anything amiss, he desir'd their worships to think it was his infirmity.
> *Julius Caesar*, I, ii, 254

IAGO: My lord is fall'n into an epilepsy.
This is his second fit; he had one yesterday.
CASSIO: Rub him about the temples.
IAGO: No, forbear.
The lethargy must have his quiet course.
If not, he foams at mouth, and by-and-by
Breaks out to savage madness.
> *Othello*, IV, i, 51

William Heberden [1710–1801]

The epilepsy may be called the reproach of physicians as well as the gout; for it was well known before the writing of the most ancient medical books, and yet no certain method of cure has been discovered.
> *Commentaries on the History and Cure of Diseases*, Ch. 33

The fit makes the patient fall down senseless; and without his will or consciousness presently every muscle is put in action, as if all the powers of the body were exerted to free itself from some great violence. In these strong and universal convulsions, the urine, excrements, and seed, are sometimes forced away, and the mouth is covered with foam, which will be bloody, when the tongue has been bitten, as it often is in the agony.
> *Idem*

Thomas Carlyle [1795–1881]

A man is not strong who takes convulsion-fits; though six men cannot hold him then.
> Lecture in London, May 19, 1840

SELF-MEDICATION

See also TREATMENT

Voltaire [1694–1778]

I constantly hear used a most false and fatal argument. "Such and such a man," it is said, "has been cured by such and such a means: I have his complaint, so I must try his remedy." How many people have died for having reasoned thus! People do not choose to see that the complaints which afflict us are as different as the features of our faces.
> Letter to Louis de Breteuil, baron de Preuilly, ca. December 5, 1723 (tr. by S. G. Tallentyre)

Benjamin Franklin [1706–1790]

It is ill Jesting with the Joiner's Tools, worse with the Doctor's.
> *Poor Richard's Almanack*, 1752

Sir William Osler [1849–1919]

A physician who treats himself has a fool for a patient.
> Quoted by William B. Bean in *Sir William Osler: Aphorisms,* Ch. 1

Dexter Masters [1908–   ]

A good many of the ailments . . . are more annoying than dangerous, more a bother than a threat. They are part of the occupational hazard of living, and it is likely that, left to our own devices, we would be quite capable of getting along with them during their comings and goings. But we are not left to our own devices. Indeed, we are all but overwhelmed with the devices of others, the popular products which have occupied the drugstores, which stare at us from advertisements in the newspapers and magazines, and which give us our instructions from the television screens they now command.
> *The Medicine Show,* Introduction

Proverbs

Every one is a fool or a physician to himself after thirty.

He who physics himself poisons a fool.

Indian (Tamil) Proverb

Domestic medicine is preferable to that of a physician.

SENILITY

See also LONGEVITY, OLD AGE: BAD ASPECTS

Aristophanes [448?–380? B.C.]

Old age is but a second childhood.
> *Clouds,* 1417 (tr. by Thomas Mitchell)

Menander [343?–291? B.C.]

Old men are children for the second time.
> *Fragments,* 517 (tr. by F. G. Allinson)

Plautus [254?–184 B.C.]

Once a man gets old and reaches the senseless, witless stage, they do say he's apt to have a second childhood.
> *Mercator,* II.ii.295 (tr. by P. Nixon)

Cicero [106–43 B.C.]

Senile debility, usually called "dotage," is a characteristic, not of all old men, but only of those who are weak in mind and will.
> *On Old Age,* XI.36 (tr. by W. A. Falconer)

William Shakespeare [1564–1616]

> Last scene of all,
That ends this strange eventful history,
Is second childishness and mere oblivion,
Sans teeth, sans eye, sans taste, sans everything.
> *As You Like It,* II, vii, 163

Jonathan Swift [1667–1745]

Tho' it is hardly understood
Which way my death can do them good,
Yet thus, methinks, I hear 'em speak:
"See, how the Dean begins to break!
Poor gentleman, he droops apace!
You plainly find it in his face.
That old vertigo in his head
Will never leave him till he's dead.
Besides, his memory decays:
He recollects not what he says;
He cannot call his friends to mind:
Forgets the place where last he din'd;
Plyes you with stories o'er and o'er;
He told them fifty times before. . . ."
> *On the Death of Dr. Swift*

Samuel Johnson [1709–1784]

There is a wicked inclination in most people to suppose an old man decayed in his intellects. If a young or middle-aged man, when leaving a company, does not recollect where he laid his hat, it is nothing; but if the same inattention is discovered in an old man, people will shrug up their shoulders and say, "His memory is going."
> Quoted by James Boswell in *Life of Samuel Johnson*, 1783

Thomas Jefferson [1743–1826]

Bodily decay is gloomy in prospect, but of all human contemplations the most abhorrent is body without mind.
> Letter to John Adams, August 1, 1816

William Hazlitt [1778–1830]

The worst old age is that of the mind.
> *The Monthly Magazine*, July 1829, "The Prose Album" [1]

Joel Chandler Harris [1848–1908]

I [am] . . . in the prime of senility.
> Quoted by Julia C. Harris in *Life and Letters*, Ch. 27

Santiago Ramón y Cajal [1852–1934]

Like an earthquake, true senility announces itself by trembling and stammering.
> *Charlas de Café*

Eugen Bleuler [1857–1939]

Senility often becomes a disease only as a result of the sudden cessation of the ordinary attractions of life.
> *Textbook of Psychiatry*, Ch. XII, Pt. V (tr. by A. A. Brill)

[1] This article is unsigned in *The Monthly Magazine,* but it appears in P.P. Howe's *New Writings by William Hazlitt* (London, 1925).

SENSES

See also HEARING, SIGHT

Pliny the Elder [23–79]

The brain . . . is the citadel of sense-perception.
> *Natural History*, XI.49 (tr. by H. Rackham)

Dante Alighieri [1265–1321]

When some one faculty, by its apprehension
Of pain or pleasure, grows so clamorous
That it commands the soul's entire attention,

Of all powers else the soul's oblivious —
Which goes to show how false is the surmise
That soul is kindled above soul in us.
> *The Divine Comedy*, "Purgatory," Canto IV (tr. by Dorothy L. Sayers)

Leonardo da Vinci [1452–1519]

The common sense is that which judges the things given to it by the other senses.
> *Codice Atlantico*, 90 (tr. by Edward MacCurdy in *The Notebooks of Leonardo da Vinci*, Vol. I, Ch. V)

Blaise Pascal [1623–1662]

Our senses perceive no extreme. Too much sound deafens us; too much light dazzles us; too great distance or proximity hinders our view. Too great length and too great brevity of discourse tend to obscurity; too much truth is paralysing.
> *Pensées*, Sect. II (tr. by W. F. Trotter)

We feel neither extreme heat nor extreme cold. Excessive qualities are prejudicial to us and not perceptible by the senses; we do not feel but suffer them.
> *Idem*

Samuel Johnson [1709–1784]

The senses have not only that advantage over conscience, which things necessary must always have over things chosen, but they have likewise a kind of prescription in their favour.
> *The Rambler*, No. 7 (April 10, 1750)

David Hume [1711–1776]

The examination of our sensations belongs more to anatomists and natural philosophers than to moral.
> *A Treatise of Human Nature*, Bk. I, Ch. I, Sect. 2

William Blake [1757–1827]

If Perceptive Organs vary, Objects of Perception seem to vary:
If the Perceptive Organs close, their Objects seem to close also.
> *Jerusalem*, Ch. II, Sect. 24

Charles Lamb [1775–1834]

I have my sight, hearing, taste, pretty perfect; and can read the Lord's Prayer in common type, by the help of a candle, without making many mistakes.
> Letter to Mr. and Mrs. J. D. Collier, January 6, 1823

Peter Mere Latham [1789–1875]

The knowledge of the senses is the best knowledge; but delusions of the senses are the worst delusions.
> *Diseases of the Heart*, Lect. IV

It is safer to appeal to men's perceptions than to their logic.
> *General Remarks on the Practice of Medicine*, Ch. XIV

Elisha Bartlett [1804–1855]

The senses, even when aided by all the means and appliances of science and art, reveal to us only a part, and probably a small part of the properties, phenomena, and relations, of the substances and agencies, which go to make up the material universe.
> *Philosophy of Medical Science*, Pt. I, Ch. 4

Sir Clifford Allbutt [1836–1925]

The infinite delicacy of the educated senses is almost more incredible than the compass of the imagination. When they unite in creation, no shadow is too fleeting, no line too exquisite for their common engagement and mutual reinforcement.

Christopher Burney [1917–   ]

We need the constant ebb and flow of wavelets of sensation, thought, perception, action and emotion, lapping on the shore of our consciousness. . . . We are narrow men, twisted men, smooth and nicely rounded men, and poets; but whatever we are, we have our shape, and we preserve it best in the experience of many things.
> *Solitary Confinement*

SEX

See also ADULTERY, CONCEPTION, IMPOTENCE, VENEREAL DISEASE, VIRGINITY

Lactantius Firmianus [ca. 306]

Everyone should bear in mind that the union of the two sexes is given to living beings for procreation, and that these passions are subject to the law that they must beget offspring.
> *Divine Institutions*, VI.xxiii

St. Augustine [354–430]

I have decided that there is nothing I

should avoid so much as marriage. I know of nothing which brings the manly mind down from the heights more than a woman's caresses and that joining of bodies without which one cannot have a wife.

> *Soliloquies,* I.x.17 (tr. by T. F. Gilligan)

Moses ben Maimon (Maimonides) [1135–1204]

Effusion of semen represents the strength of the body and its life, and the light of the eyes. Whenever it [semen] is emitted to excess, the body becomes consumed, its strength terminates, and its life perishes. . . . He who immerses himself in sexual intercourse will be assailed by [premature] aging. His strength will wane, his eyes will weaken, and a bad odor will emit from his mouth and his armpits. . . . His teeth will fall out and many maladies other than these will afflict him. The wise physicians have stated that one in a thousand dies from other illnesses and the [remaining 999 in the thousand] from excessive sexual intercourse. Therefore, a man must be cautious in this matter if he wishes to live wholesomely. He should not cohabit unless his body is healthy and very strong and he experiences many involuntary erections. . . . Such a person requires coitus and it is therapeutic for him to have sexual intercourse.

A person should not cohabit when he is satiated nor when he is hungry but after the food is digested in his intestines. He should examine whether need for excretion [of urine or feces] exists before coitus and after coitus. One should not have sexual intercourse standing or sitting and not in a bathhouse nor on the day when he takes a bath nor on the day of phlebotomy nor on the day when setting out on a journey nor on the previous or following [days of such occurrences].

> *Mishneh Torah,* "Hilchoth

De'oth," Ch. IV, No. 19 (tr. by Fred Rosner in *Annals of Internal Medicine* 62:372, 1965)

Leonardo da Vinci [1452–1519]

The act of procreation and the members employed therein are so repulsive, that if it were not for the beauty of the faces and the adornments of the actors and the pent-up impulse, nature would lose the human species.

> *Dell' Anatomia,* Fogli A (tr. by Edward MacCurdy in *The Notebooks of Leonardo da Vinci,* Vol. I, Ch. III)

Martin Luther [1483–1546]

Men have broad and large chests, and small narrow hips, and more understanding than women, who have but small and narrow breasts, and broad hips, to the end they should remain at home, sit still, keep house, and bear and bring up children.

> *Table-Talk,* DCCXXV, "Of Marriage and Celibacy" (tr. by William Hazlitt)

William Shakespeare [1564–1616]

For your physicians have expressly charg'd,
In peril to incur your former malady,
That I should yet absent me from your bed.

> *The Taming of the Shrew,* Induction, ii, 123

Sir Thomas Browne [1605–1682]

I could be content that we might procreate like trees, without conjunction, or that there were any way to perpetuate the world without this triviall and vulgar way of coition; It is the foolishest act a wise man commits in all his life, nor is there any thing that will more deject his coold imagination, when hee shall consider what an odde and unworthy piece of folly hee hath committed.

> *Religio Medici,* Pt. II, Sect. 9

John Armstrong [1709–1779]

> Shun the soft Embrace
> Emasculant, till twice ten years and
>   more
> Have steeled thy Nerve, and let the
>   holy Rite
> License the Bliss.
>   *The Economy of Love*

Tobias Smollett [1721–1771]

> Eternal infamy his name surround,
> Who planted first that vice [homo-
>   sexuality] on British ground!
> A vice that spite of sense and nature
>   reigns,
> And poisons genial love, and manhood
>   stains! . . .
> Let Chardin with a chaplet round his
>   head,
> The taste of Maro and Anacreon plead,
> "Sir, Flaccus knew to live as well as
>   write,
> And kept, like me, two boys array'd
>   in white."
>   *Advice: A Satire*

Pierre de Beaumarchais
[1732–1799]

That which distinguishes man from
the beast is drinking without being
thirsty and making love at all seasons.
   Le Mariage de Figaro, Act II,
   Sc. xxi

Thomas Jefferson [1743–1826]

He [the American Indian] is neither
more defective in ardor, nor more impotent with his female, than the white
reduced to the same diet and exercise.[1]
   Notes on the State of Virginia,
   Query VI

William Blake [1757–1827]

What is it men in women do require?
The lineaments of Gratified Desire.
What is it women do in men require?

[1] Jefferson is answering Buffon's argument
that the American environment causes animals and humans to degenerate.

The lineaments of Gratified Desire.
   The Question Answer'd

Thomas Malthus [1766–1834]

I think I may fairly make two postulata.
   First, That food is necessary to the
existence of man.
   Secondly, That the passion between
the sexes is necessary, and will remain
nearly in its present state.
   *An Essay on the Principle of
   Population* (1798), Ch. 1

Samuel Taylor Coleridge
[1772–1834]

The man's desire is for the woman;
but the woman's desire is rarely other
than for the desire of the man.
   Table Talk, July 23, 1827

Honoré de Balzac [1799–1850]

Physically, a man is a man for a much
longer time than a woman is a woman.
   The Physiology of Marriage

Sir William Osler [1849–1919]

The natural man has only two primal
passions, to get and beget.
   Science and Immortality

Sir John Bland-Sutton
[1855–1936]

After Eve disregarded the prohibition
of the Appletree a peculiar dislike to
complete nakedness overcame civilized
men and women. Clothes are necessary
for protection against weather and for
decency; moreover, in civilized communities they help men and women to
be attractive to each other.
   The Story of a Surgeon, Ch.
   VIII

George Santayana [1863–1952]

Friends are generally of the same sex,
for when men and women agree, it is
only in their conclusions; their reasons
are always different. So that while intellectual harmony between men and

women is easily possible, its delightful and magic quality lies precisely in the fact that it does not arise from mutual understanding, but is a conspiracy of alien essences and a kissing, as it were, in the dark.

> *The Life of Reason: Reason in Society*, Ch. VI

Arthur Guiterman [1871–1943]

Amoebas at the start
Were not complex;
They tore themselves apart
And started Sex.

> *The Light Guitar*, "Sex"

Otto Weininger [1880–1903]

The statements that men have stronger sexual impulses than women, or that women have them stronger than men, are false. The strength of the sexual impulse in a man does not depend upon the proportion of masculinity in his composition, and in the same way the degree of femininity of a woman does not determine her sexual impulse. These differences in mankind still await classification.

> *Sex and Character*, Pt. II, Ch. 2

The condition of sexual excitement is the supreme moment of a woman's life. The woman is devoted wholly to sexual matters, that is to say, to the spheres of begetting and of reproduction.

> *Idem*

The sexual instinct is always active in woman whilst in man it is at rest from time to time.

> *Idem*

Man possesses sexual organs; her sexual organs possess woman.

> *Idem*

Alfred Kreymborg [1883–   ]

Some sexes
change their
sexes now
and make a

mere man wonder
how.

> *The Little World*, "Outmoded"

Alan Gregg [1890–1957]

One of the impressions from the East is that, in the West, we are obsessed with sex and romance [in our] plays, stories, songs, poetry, social customs.

> Aphorism (Quoted by Wilder Penfield in *The Difficult Art of Giving*, Appendix A)

Samuel Hoffenstein [1890–1947]

Breathes there a man with hide so
 tough
Who says two sexes aren't enough?

> *Poems in Praise of Practically Nothing*, "Love Songs, At Once Tender and Informative"

James Thurber [1894–1961] and E. B. White [1899–   ]

Is Sex Necessary?

> Title of a book

Margaret Mead [1901–   ]

I have suggested that certain human traits have been socially specialized as the appropriate attitudes and behaviour of only one sex, while other human traits have been specialized for the opposite sex. This social specialization is then rationalized into a theory that the socially decreed behaviour is natural for one sex and unnatural for the other, and that the deviant is a deviant because of glandular defect, or developmental accident.

> *Sex and Temperament in Three Primitive Societies*, Ch. 18

William H. Masters [1915–   ] and Virginia E. Johnson [1925–   ]

If problems in the complex field of human sexual behavior are to be attacked successfully, psychologic theory and sociologic concept must at times find support in physiologic fact. Without adequate support from basic sexual physiology, much of psychologic theory

will remain theory and much of sociologic concept will remain concept. . . .
There is no man or woman who does
not face in his or her lifetime the concerns of sexual tensions. Can that one
facet of our lives, affecting more people
in more ways than any other physiologic response other than those necessary to our very existence, be allowed
to continue without benefit of objective, scientific analysis?

> *Human Sexual Response,* Pref-
> ace

The functioning role of the penis is as
well established as that of any other
organ in the body. Ironically, there
is no organ about which more misin-
formation has been perpetrated. The
penis constantly has been viewed but
rarely seen. . . . Our culture has been
influenced by and has contributed to
manifold misconceptions of the functional role of the penis. These "phallic
fallacies" have colored our arts and,
possibly of even more import to our
culture, influenced our behavioral and
biologic sciences.

> *Ibid.,* Ch. 12, Sect. 2

Anonymous

O! Cupid! Cast away your bow and
quiver —
Statistics prove your method inexact.
O Donne! Go take a jump into the
river:
You hymned the essence, but ignored
the fact.

Locked in some cool aseptic heaven
above,
Trained statisticians painlessly inquire
Into the quaint geometry of love,
The quantitative aspects of desire;
Observe the conduct of the lovesick
male
(Not passionate, not noble, not ob-
scene),
And plot it on a logarithmic scale,
Noting a random scatter round the
mean.

O monumental volume, smug and fat!

Did Man, who wrote the Song of
Songs, write this?
O God! O Kinsey! O Jehoshaphat!

> *Lancet* 2:431, 1948, "On Read-
> ing Professor Kinsey's Survey
> of Sexual Behavior in the Hu-
> man Male"

German Proverb

Man without woman is head without
body; woman without man is body
without head.

Latin Proverb

Every animal is sad after intercourse.

SICKNESS

See also DISEASE, INVALID,
PATIENTS

Huang Ti (The Yellow Emperor) [2697–2597 B.C.]

Illness is comparable to the root; good
medical work is comparable to the
topmost branch or a beacon. If this
root is not reached, the evil influences
cannot be subjugated.

> *Nei Ching Su Wên,* Bk. 4, Sect.
> 14 (tr. by Ilza Veith in *The
> Yellow Emperor's Classic of In-
> ternal Medicine*)

Euripides [484–406 B.C.]

A weary thing is sickness and its
pains!

> *Hippolytus,* 176 (tr. by D.
> Grene)

Herophilus [fl. 300 B.C.]

To lose one's health renders science
null, art inglorious, strength effortless,
wealth useless and eloquence powerless.

> Quoted by Sextus Empiricus in
> *Adversus Ethicus,* XI.50

Pliny the Elder [23–79]

In sickness the mind reflects upon itself.

> *Natural History,* VII

Pliny the Younger [62–113]

We are never so virtuous as when we are in sickness. . . . [A man] resolves that if he has the luck to recover, his life will be passed in luxurious ease, that is, in harmless happiness.
>   *Epistles,* VII.26 (tr. by W. Melmoth)

Gabriel Harvey [1545?–1630?]

Sicke, as a Dog.
>   *Foure Letters and Certaine Sonnets,* First Letter

William Shakespeare [1564–1616]

The more one sickens, the worse at ease he is.
>   *As You Like It,* III, ii, 24

A sick man's appetite . . . desires most that
Which would increase his evil.
>   *Coriolanus,* I, i, 182

For suddenly a grievous sickness took him
That makes him gasp and stare and catch the air.
>   *Henry VI, Part II,* III, ii, 370

He fell sick suddenly and grew so ill
He could not sit his mule.
>   *Henry VIII,* IV, ii, 15

But where the greater malady is fix'd,
The lesser is scarce felt.
>   *King Lear,* III, iv, 8

As testy sick men, when their deaths be near,
No news but health from their physicians know.
>   *Sonnet CXL*

John Donne [1573–1631]

There are more *sicknesses* than *names.*
>   *Devotions Upon Emergent Occasions,* IX

Francis Rous [1579–1659]

Now death his servant Sickness forth hath sent.
>   *Thule, or Vertues Historie,* Bk. II, Canto IV

Sir Thomas Browne [1605–1682]

Every sickness will tell you you cannot well do without health.
>   *Christian Morals,* Pt. I, Sect. 4

Men that looke no further than their outsides thinke health an appertinance unto life, and quarrell with their constitutions for being sick; but I that have examined the parts of man, and know upon what tender filaments that Fabricke hangs, doe wonder that we are not always so; and considering the thousand dores that lead to death doe thanke my God that we can die but once.
>   *Religio Medici,* Pt. I, Sect. 44

Samuel Butler [1612–1680]

And out of his own Bowels spins
A Rack and Torture for his Sins.
>   *Satyr Upon the Weakness and Misery of Man*

Matthew Prior [1664–1721]

All covet Life, yet call it Pain:
All feel the Ill, yet shun the Cure.
>   *Written in the Beginning of Mezeray's History of France*

Jonathan Swift [1667–1745]

We are so fond of one another, because our ailments are the same.
>   Letter to Stella, February 1, 1711

Stanislas I (Leszczyński) of Poland [1677–1766]

Long ailments wear out pain, and long hopes joy.
>   *Oeuvres du Philosophe Bienfaisant*

Philip Stanhope, Lord Chesterfield [1694–1773]

Physical ills are the taxes laid upon this wretched life; some are taxed higher, and some lower, but all pay something.
> Letter to the Bishop of Waterford, November 22, 1757

Benjamin Franklin [1706–1790]

Be not sick too late, nor well too soon.
> *Poor Richard's Almanack*, 1734

Samuel Johnson [1709–1784]

It is so *very* difficult for a sick man not to be a scoundrel.
> Quoted by Hester Lynch Piozzi in *Anecdotes of the Late Samuel Johnson*

Jean Jacques Rousseau [1712–1778]

In regard to sickness, I shall not repeat the vain and false declamations made against medicine by most men in health.
> *A Discourse Upon the Origin and the Foundation of the Inequality Among Mankind*, Pt. I

Tobias Smollett [1721–1771]

A seasonable fit of illness is an excellent medicine for the turbulence of passion. Such a reformation had the fever produced in the economy of his thoughts, that he moralised like an apostle and projected several prudential schemes for his future conduct.
> *The Adventures of Peregrine Pickle*, Ch. 79

Very subject to rheums, accompanied with fever, dejection and difficulty in breathing. The least alteration of the weather towards cold or moisture, change of dress, the smallest excess in point of exercise, whether on foot or horseback, or in a carriage, occasions fresh commotions in the animal economy. The nervous system, being extremely irritable, undergoes a variety of spasms . . . and all night long the heat, restlessness, anxiety and asthma prevail. . . . The patient's flesh wastes apace, and his strength continues to decay.
> Letter to Dr. Fizès, November 1763

Johann Wolfgang von Goethe [1749–1832]

If man thinks about his physical or moral state he usually discovers that he is ill.
> *Sprüche in Prosa*, Pt. I, Bk. II

William Dunlap [1766–1839]

He seems a little under the weather, somehow; and yet he's not sick.
> *The Memoirs of a Water Drinker*, Vol. I, Ch. VIII

John Quincy Adams [1767–1848]

He [Andrew Jackson] is one of our tribe of great men who turn disease to commodity. . . . He is so ravenous of notoriety that he craves the sympathy for sickness as a portion of his glory.
> *Diary*, June 27, 1833

Sir Walter Scott [1771–1832]

What poor things does a fever-fit or an overflowing of the bile make of the master of creation.
> *Journal*, January 10, 1826

Sydney Smith [1771–1845]

I have gout, asthma, and seven other maladies, but am otherwise very well.
> Letter to Mrs. Meynell, December 1841

Charles Lamb [1775–1834]

How sickness enlarges the dimensions of a man's self to himself! he is his own exclusive object. . . . He has nothing to think of but how to get well.
> *The Last Essays of Elia*, "The Convalescent"

If there be a regal solitude, it is a sick bed.
> *Idem*

Thomas Carlyle [1795–1881]

I am always sick; I am sicker and worse in body and mind, a little, for the present; but it has no deep significance: it is *weariness* merely.
> Letter to Ralph Waldo Emerson, November 5, 1836

Ralph Waldo Emerson [1803–1882]

There is one topic peremptorily forbidden to all well-bred, to all rational mortals, namely, their distempers.
> *The Conduct of Life,* Ch. V

It is dainty to be sick, if you have leisure and convenience for it.
> *Journals,* February 7, 1839

A person seldom falls sick but the by-standers are animated with a faint hope that he will die.

If a man is sick, is unable, is mean-spirited and odious, it is because there is so much of his nature which is un-lawfully withholden from him.

Samuel Bartlett Parris [1806–1827]

Go to the sick man's bedside — mark how dim
The eye, once bright with meaning; and the limb
Once strung with nature's firmest energies,
See how unnerved and impotent it lies!
Where are the kindlings of the mighty soul,
Whose daring independence scorn'd control?
Where are the quick sensations, once alive
To all the rapture, life can ever give?
Dead to delight, he loathing turns aside

From ev'ry luxury, kindness can provide;
His aching temples throb with furious beat,
Flushed in his burning cheek with fev'rish heat;

To his parch'd mouth, his tongue, un-moisten'd, cleaves,
Refreshing sleep his wakeful eyelids leaves;
Or if a moment they may chance to close,
'Tis not to slumber in a calm repose,
But in distempered and delirious dreams,
Beset with foes and fears and death, he seems,
Till waked with horror, he affrighted springs,
Glad to escape those dark imaginings.
To him more painful is the sun's glad light
Than all the horrors of the darkest night.
> *Anticipations and Recollections,* Pt. I

John Brown [1810–1882]

Many a man's life is lengthened by a sharp illness; and this is in several ways. In the first place he is laid up, out of reach of all external mischief and exertion, he is like a ship put in the dock for repairs; time is gained. A brisk fever clarifies the entire man, if it is beaten and does not beat; it is like cleaning a chimney by setting it on fire; it is perilous but thorough. Then the effort to throw off the disease often quickens and purifies and cor-roborates the central powers of life; the flame burns more clearly; there is a cleanness, so to speak, about all the wheels of life.
> *Horae Subsecivae,* "Letter to John Cairns"

Charles Dickens [1812–1870]

There is something in sickness that breaks down the pride of manhood.

Henri Amiel [1821–1881]

There is no curing a sick man who believes himself in health.
> *Journal Intime,* February 6, 1877 (tr. by Mrs. Humphrey Ward)

Charles Baudelaire [1821–1867]

Illness and Death make ashes of all
> the fire that flamed for us.
> *Les Fleurs du Mal,* "Le Portrait" (tr. by M. Colum)

Jean Martin Charcot [1825–1893]

In dealing with a nervous patient, you should regard the malady before you merely as an episode. Thus, in a case of chorea, it is only necessary to inquire how long it has existed. The condition of the patient is only an accident in the history of the disease, just as each of us is only an accident in the history of humanity.
> *De l'expectation en médecine*

C. H. Spurgeon [1834–1892]

As sick as a cat.
> *John Ploughman's Talk,* Ch. 20

Samuel Butler [1835–1902]

It came out that illness of any sort was considered in Erewhon to be highly criminal and immoral; and that I was liable, even for catching cold, to be had up before the magistrates and imprisoned for a considerable period.
> *Erewhon,* Ch. VIII

In that country if a man falls into ill health, or catches any disorder, or fails bodily in any way before he is seventy years old, he is tried before a jury of his countrymen, and if convicted is held up to public scorn and sentenced more or less severely as the case may be. There are subdivisions of illnesses into crimes and misdemeanours as with offences amongst ourselves — a man being punished very heavily for serious illness, while failure of eyes

or hearing in one over sixty-five, who has good health hitherto, is dealt with by fine only, or imprisonment in default of payment.
> *Ibid.,* Ch. X

Hence though they conceal ill health by every cunning and hypocrisy and artifice which they can devise, they are quite open about the most flagrant mental diseases, should they happen to exist, which to do the people justice is not often.
> *Idem*

I reckon being ill as one of the greatest pleasures of life, provided one is not too ill and is not obliged to work till one is better.
> *The Way of All Flesh,* Ch. LXXX

Friedrich Nietzsche [1844–1900]

The sick are the greatest danger for the healthy; it is not from the strongest that harm comes to the strong, but from the weakest.
> *Genealogy of Morals,* Essay 3, Sect. 14 (tr. by Horace B. Samuel)

Robert Louis Stevenson [1850–1894]

When I was sick and lay a-bed,
I had two pillows at my head,
And all my toys beside me lay
To keep me happy all the day.
> *A Child's Garden of Verses,* "The Land of Counterpane"

You must not fancy I am sick, only over-driven and under the weather.
> *The Wrecker,* Ch. 4

Oscar Wilde [1854–1900]

Nor do I in any way approve of the modern sympathy with invalids. I consider it morbid. Illness of any kind is hardly a thing to be encouraged in others.
> *The Importance of Being Earnest,* Act I

Marcel Proust [1871–1922]

But it is rarely that these grave maladies, like that which now at last had struck her full in the face, do not take up their abode in the sick man for a long time before killing him, during which time they make haste, like a "sociable" neighbour or tenant, to introduce themselves to him. A terrible acquaintance, not so much from the sufferings that it causes as from the strange novelty of the definite restriction which it imposes upon life.

> *The Guermantes Way,* Pt. II, "My Grandmother's Illness" (tr. by C. K. Scott-Moncrieff)

It is in moments of illness that we are compelled to recognise that we live not alone but chained to a creature of a different kingdom, whole worlds apart, who has no knowledge of us and by whom it is impossible to make ourselves understood: our body. . . . to ask pity of our body is like discoursing before an octopus, for which our words can have no more meaning than the sound of the tides, and with which we should be appalled to find ourselves condemned to live.

> *Idem*

Thomas Mann [1875–1955]

Illness so adjusted its man that it and he could come to terms; there were sensory appeasements, short circuits, a merciful narcosis; nature came to the rescue with measures of spiritual and moral adaptation and relief, which the sound person naively failed to take into account. There could be no better illustration than the case of all this tuberculous crew up here, with their reckless folly, light-headedness and loose morals, and their total lack of desire for health. In short, let the sound man with all his respect for illness once fall ill himself, and he would soon see that being ill is a state of being in itself — no very honourable one either — and that he had been taking it a good deal too seriously.

> *The Magic Mountain,* Ch. VI, "Operationes Spirituales" (tr. by H. T. Lowe-Porter)

Sir Henry Howarth Bashford ("Peter Harding") [1880–1961]

There comes a period in most illnesses, I think, sometimes during a temporary respite, more often perhaps at the first dawn of convalescence, when one becomes extraordinarily conscious, yet without discomfort, of the almost trivial delicacy of one's surrounding tissue. . . . Yet I suppose we do forget it, most of us, and probably quite healthily, when once the dwelling is bricked up again, and the new paint is on, and it stands foursquare to winds that may not enter now. And yet again, if the message has once been heard . . . I don't believe it is ever entirely lost. And there, perhaps, may even lie the key to all the mystery; so that when the last storm blows, and Nature must shake her head, and let the frail house fall, its tenant may not go out altogether unprepared.

> *The Corner of Harley Street,* Letter 19

Virginia Woolf [1882–1941]

Considering how common illness is, how tremendous the spiritual change that it brings, how astonishing, when the lights of health go down, the undiscovered countries that are then disclosed, what wastes and deserts of the soul a slight attack of influenza brings to view, what precipices and lawns sprinkled with bright flowers a little rise of temperature reveals, what ancient and obdurate oaks are uprooted in us by the act of sickness, how we go down into the pit of death and feel the waters of annihilation close above our heads and wake thinking to find ourselves in the presence of the angels and the harpers when we have a tooth out and come to the surface in the dentist's arm-chair and confuse his "Rinse the mouth—rinse the mouth" with the greeting of the Deity stooping from the floor of Heaven to welcome us—when we think of this, as we are so frequently forced to think of it, it becomes strange indeed that illness has not taken its place with love and battle and jealousy among the prime themes of literature.

> *The Moment and Other Essays,* "On Being Ill"

John W. Boylan [1914–   ]

Some people get sick and some do not.
> Letter to Maurice B. Strauss, September 22, 1964

The Bible

They that be whole need not a physician, but they that are sick.
> *Matthew* 9:12

The Talmud

Rather any complaint, but not a complaint of the bowels; any pain, but not heart pain; any ache, but not head ache; any evil, but not an evil wife!
> *Shabbath,* I.11a (tr. by H. Freedman)

Proverbs

An ill man is worst when he appeareth good.

As sick as a horse.

He who was never sick dies the first fit.

Sickness is better than sadness.

Sickness is felt, but health not at all.[1]

Sickness soaks the purse.

[1] Dutch Proverb: An ounce of illness is felt more than an hundredweight of health.

Dutch Proverb

Sickness comes on horseback and departs on foot.[1]

English Proverbs

The chamber of sickness is the chapel of devotion.

We are usually the best men when in the worst health.

Italian Proverb

Illnesses tell us what we are.

Scottish Proverb

Be long sick that you may be soon well.

SIGHT

See also BLINDNESS, EYE

I. GENERAL

Huang Ti (The Yellow Emperor) [2697–2597 B.C.]

The number of those who are confused and dim of vision is like the number of atoms and hair. Their number can be judged to be one hundred times ten

[1] Chinese Proverb: The appearance of a disease is swift as an arrow; its disappearance slow, like a thread.
  Creole Proverb: Sickness comes riding upon a hare, but goes away riding upon a tortoise.
  English Proverb: Agues come on horseback, but go away on foot.
  Estonian Proverb: Diseases come on couriers' horses, but go away on tired oxen.
  French Proverb: All sicknesses arrive on wings and depart limpingly.
  Indian (Sindhi) Proverb: Diseases come swift as horses and go back slow as lice.
  Romanian Proverb: Illness comes in a coach and goes away through the eye of a needle.
  Russian Proverb: Health goes in puds [40 Russian lbs.] and comes back in zolotniks [1/96 lb.].

thousand, and even this can be increased.

> *Nei Ching Su Wên,* Bk. 3, Sect. 8 (tr. by Ilza Veith in *The Yellow Emperor's Classic of Internal Medicine*)

Cicero [106–43 B.C.]

The keenest of all our senses is the sense of sight.

> *On the Orator,* II.lxxxvii.357 (tr. by E. W. Sutton)

Seneca [4? B.C.–A.D. 65]

Letters, however small and dim, are comparatively large and distinct when seen through a glass globe filled with water.

> *Questiones Naturales,* I.vi (tr. by John Clarke)

Pliny the Elder [23–79]

Some people have long sight but others can only see things brought close to them. The sight of many depends on the brilliance of the sun, and they cannot see clearly on a cloudy day or after sunset; others have dimmer sight in the day time but are exceptionally keen-sighted at night.

> *Natural History,* XI.54 (tr. by H. Rackham)

Leonardo da Vinci [1452–1519]

The pupil of the eye which receives through a very small round hole the images of bodies situated beyond this hole always receives them upside down and the visual faculty always sees them upright as they are. And this proceeds from the fact that the said images pass through the centre of the crystalline sphere situated in the middle of the eye.

> Manuscript D, Library of the Institut de France (tr. by Edward MacCurdy in *The Notebooks of Leonardo da Vinci,* Vol. I, Ch. IX)

Joseph Addison [1672–1719]

Our Sight is the most perfect and most delightful of all our Senses.

> *The Spectator,* Vol. VI, No. 411 (June 21, 1712)

Adelbert Ames [1835–1933]

The things we see are the mind's best bet as to what is out front.

Walter B. Cannon [1871–1945]

The near point of clear vision recedes until with unaided eyes the elderly person, holding the page at arm's length in order to see it clearly, is bothered by the indistinctness due to distance; caught between these troubles of too near and too far, he moves the page back and forth — as Holmes put it, he has reached the "trombone age"!

> *The Way of an Investigator,* "The Fruitful Years"

II. EYEGLASSES

William Cowper [1731–1800]

Between Nose and Eyes a strange contest arose,
  The spectacles set them unhappily wrong;
The point in dispute was, as all the world knows,
  To which the said spectacles ought to belong.

> *Report of an Adjudged Case, Not to Be Found in Any of the Books*

Thomas Jefferson [1743–1826]

I received safely the spectacles & glasses you were so kind as to send me by Mr. Mackie, and now inclose you a 20.Dollar bill of the bank of the U.S., the amount of their cost. The smallest pair of spectacles I am charmed with; they answer perfectly my wish. The other pair with double glasses I have not yet had time to try sufficiently and get them to fit my eye exactly. I have

no doubt they also will answer my expectation.
>Letter to John McAllister

Dorothy Parker [1893–1967]

Men seldom make passes
At girls who wear glasses.
>*Enough Rope,* "News Item"

Anne Hollander [1956–   ]

How could you find your glasses if you didn't have them on to see them if they were there?
>Comment to Maurice B. Strauss, October 19, 1965

SKEPTICISM

Moses ben Maimon (Maimonides) [1135–1204]

If anyone declares to you that he has actual proof, from his own experience, of something which he requires for the confirmation of his theory, — even though he be considered a man of great authority, truthfulness, earnest words and morality, yet, just because he is anxious for you to believe his theory, you should hesitate.
>*Aphorisms According to Galen* (Quoted in *Bulletin of the Institute of the History of Medicine* 3:555, 1935)

Prosper Alpinus [1553–1617]

Excuse my incredulity, but I do not wish to deceive myself.
>*Annotationes,* III.16 (tr. by Max Samter)

Thomas Jefferson [1743–1826]

The natural course of the human mind is certainly from credulity to scepticism.
>Letter to Dr. Caspar Wistar, June 21, 1807

Edward Jenner [1749–1823]

The scepticism that appeared, even among the most enlightened of medical men when my sentiments on the important subject of the cow-pox were first promulgated, was highly laudable. To have admitted the truth of a doctrine, at once so novel and so unlike any thing that ever had appeared in the annals of medicine, without the test of the most rigid scrutiny, would have bordered upon temerity.
>*A Continuation of Facts and Observations Relative to the Variolae Vaccinae, or Cow-Pox*

Baron Ernst von Feuchtersleben [1806–1849]

Half-informed physicians are generally skeptics.
>*Dietetics of the Soul,* XII, Entry 27 (tr. by G. Pollak)

Oliver Wendell Holmes [1809–1894]

The solemn scepticism of science has replaced the sneering doubts of witty philosophers. The more positive knowledge we gain, the more we incline to question all that has been received without absolute proof.
>*Medical Essays,* "Currents and Counter-Currents in Medical Science"

Claude Bernard [1813–1878]

The doubter is a true man of science; he doubts only himself and his interpretations, but he believes in science.
>*An Introduction to the Study of Experimental Medicine,* Pt. I, Ch. 2, Sect. vi (tr. by H. C. Greene)

Jean Martin Charcot [1825–1893]

Common-place skepticism, which is so readily opposed to all progress of the human mind, is a convenient pillow for lazy heads; but in this epoch there is no longer time to go to sleep.

> *Leçons cliniques sur les maladies des vieillards et les maladies chroniques,* Introduction, Sect. 5

Alfred North Whitehead [1861–1947]

The guiding motto in the life of every natural philosopher should be, Seek simplicity and distrust it.

> *The Concept of Nature,* Ch. VII

Miguel de Unamuno [1864–1936]

True science teaches, above all, to doubt and to be ignorant.

> *The Tragic Sense of Life,* Ch. V

Bertrand Russell [1872–   ]

The scepticism that I advocate amounts only to this: (1) that when the experts are agreed, the opposite opinion cannot be held to be certain; (2) that when they are not agreed, no opinion can be regarded as certain by a non-expert; and (3) that when they all hold that no sufficient grounds for a positive opinion exist, the ordinary man would do well to suspend his judgment.

> *Sceptical Essays,* Ch. 1

SKIN

William Shakespeare [1564–1616]

On her left breast
A mole cinque-spotted, like the crimson drops
I' th' bottom of a cowslip.

> *Cymbeline,* II, ii, 37

Under her breast
(Worthy the pressing) lies a mole, right proud
Of that most delicate lodging.

> *Ibid.,* II, iv, 134

Now, the dry suppeago [1] on the subject.

> *Troilus and Cressida,* II, iii, 80

Louis A. Duhring [1845–1913]

The power of making a correct diagnosis is the key to all success in the treatment of skin diseases; without this faculty, the physician can never be a thorough dermatologist, and therapeutics at once cease to hold their proper position, and become empirical.

> *American Journal of Syphilography and Dermatology* 2:104, 1871

The skin and subcutaneous tissue, composing the integument, should be regarded as part of the body rather than as an independent organ. The skin possesses the closest relations with the general economy, as shown by the observation that there are comparatively few so-called general diseases in which it . . . is not at some period involved in a slight or a marked degree.

> *Cutaneous Medicine,* Pt. I, Preface

The skin calls for faculty of close observation and attention to detail.

> Valedictory address, University of Pennsylvania Medical School, June 7, 1894

Sir William Osler [1849–1919]

In its more aggravated forms diffuse scleroderma is one of the most terrible of all human ills. Like Tithonus (who was a Greek mythological hero) to "wither slowly" and like him to be "beaten down and marred and wasted" until one is literally a mummy, encased in an evershrinking, slowly contracting skin of steel, is a fate not pictured in any tragedy, ancient or modern.

> *Journal of Cutaneous Diseases* 16:49, 1898

[1] suppeago = serpigo.

Anonymous

A mole on the neck,
You shall have money by the peck.
   Old English rhyme

If you've got a mole above your chin,
You'll never be beholden to any of
   your kin.
   Idem

Dermatology is the best speciality. The
patient never dies — and never gets
well.

American Proverb

It will never get well if you pick it.

Venetian Proverb

Woolen clothing keeps the skin healthy.

SLEEP

See also DREAMS, SLEEP AND
DEATH

I. GENERAL

Homer [ca. 850 B.C.]

There is weariness even in too much
sleep.
   Odyssey, XV.394 (tr. by A. T.
   Murray)

Sophocles [496?–406 B.C.]

Sleep's the only medicine that gives
ease.
   Philoctetes, 766 (tr. by F.
   Storr)

Euripides [484–406 B.C.]

Dear spell of sleep, assuager of disease.
   Orestes, 211 (tr. by A. S. Way)

Hippocrates [460?–377? B.C.]

In whatever disease sleep is laborious,
it is a deadly symptom; but if sleep
does good, it is not deadly.
   Aphorisms, II.1 (tr. by Francis
   Adams)

When sleep puts an end to delirium, it
is a good symptom.
   Ibid., II.2

Sleep and watchfulness, both of them,
when immoderate, constitute disease.
   Ibid., VII.72

Plautus [254?–184 B.C.]

Sleep after luncheon is not good.
   Mostellaria, III.ii.697

Ovid [43 B.C.–A.D. 17?]

That which lacks its alternations of
repose will not endure; this is what repairs the strength and renews the
wearied limbs.
   The Heroides, IV.89

O Sleep, thou rest of all things, Sleep
mildest of the gods, balm of the soul.
who puttest care to flight, soothest our
bodies, worn with hard ministries, and
preparest them for toil again!
   Metamorphoses, XI.623 (tr. by
   F. J. Miller)

Even that sleep which is food to a
slender frame does not support as it
should my impoverished body.
   Pontic Epistles, I.x.21 (tr. by
   A. L. Wheeler)

School of Salerno [1095–1224]

Long sleepe at after-noones by stirring
   fumes,
Breeds Slouth, and Agues, Aking heads
   and Rheumes.
   Regimen Sanitatis Salernita-
   num (tr. by Sir John Harington
   as *The Englishman's Doctor*)

Moses ben Maimon (Maimonides)
[1135–1204]

The day and night consist of 24 hours.
It is sufficient for a person to sleep

one third thereof which is eight hours. These should [preferably] be at the end of the night so that from the beginning of his sleep until the rising of the sun will be eight hours. Thus he will arise from his bed before the sun rises.

> *Mishneh Torah,* "Hilchoth De'oth," Ch. IV, No. 4 (tr. by Fred Rosner in *Annals of Internal Medicine* 62:372, 1965)

A person should not sleep on his face nor on his back but on his side; at the beginning of the night, on the left side and at the end of the night on the right side. Further he should not go to sleep shortly after eating but should wait approximately three or four hours after a meal. One should not sleep during the day.

> *Ibid.,* No. 5

John Russell [fl. 1450]

For much sleep is not medicinal in middle of the day.

> *Book of Nurture*

Andrew Boorde [1490–1549]

To bedwarde be you mery, or have mery company aboute you, so that, to bedwarde, no anger nor hevynes, sorowe, nor pencyfulnes, do trouble or disquyet you. . . . In the nyght, let the wyndowes of your howse, specially of your chambre, be closed. . . . Let your nyght-cap be of skarlet. . . . Olde auncyent doctours of Physycke sayth, viii houres of slepe in Sommer, and ix houres of slepe in wynter, is suffycyent for any man, but I do thynke that slepe ought to be taken as the complexyon of man is. Whan you do ryse in the morenynge, ryse with myrth, and remembre God.

> *A Dyetary of Helth,* Ch. VIII

Miguel de Cervantes [1547–1616]

Sleep . . . covers a Man all over, Thoughts and all, like a Cloak; 'tis Meat for the Hungry, Drink for the Thirsty, Heat for the Cold, and Cold for the Hot.

> *Don Quixote,* Pt. II, Ch. 68 (tr. by Peter Motteux)

Edmund Spenser [1552?–1599]

Sleepe after toyle, port after stormie seas,
Ease after warre, death after life, does greatly please.

> *The Faerie Queene,* Bk. I, Canto IX

Henry IV of France [1553–1610]

Great eaters and great sleepers are incapable of anything else that is great.

Sir Philip Sidney [1554–1586]

Come, Sleepe! O Sleepe, the certaine knot of peace,
The baiting-place of wit, the balme of woe,
The poore man's wealth, the prisoner's release,
Th' indifferent judge betweene the high and low.

> *Astrophel and Stella,* Sonnet 39

William Shakespeare [1564–1616]

For some must watch, while some must sleep:
  Thus runs the world away.

> *Hamlet,* III, ii, 284

          Oppressed nature sleeps.
This rest might yet have balm'd thy broken senses,
Which, if convenience will not allow,
Stand in hard cure.

> *King Lear,* III, vi, 103

Sleep that knits up the ravell'd sleave of care,
The death of each day's life, sore labour's bath,
Balm of hurt minds, great nature's second course,
Chief nourisher in life's feast.

> *Macbeth,* II, ii, 37

A great perturbation in nature, to re-

ceive at once the benefit of sleep and do the effects of watching!
> *Ibid.*, V, i, 10

John Northbrooke [fl. 1568–1579]

When we sleepe too muche, all the moystures and humors of the bodie, with the naturall heate, retire to the extreme parts thereof, no where purging or evacuating whatsoever is redundant.
> *Spiritus est vicarius Christi in terra,* Ch. 1

Thomas Dekker [1572?–1632?]

Sleep is that golden chaine that ties health and our bodies together.
> *The Guls Horn-Booke,* Ch. II

Sir William Davenant [1606–1668]

I shall sleep like a top.
> *The Rivals,* Act III

John Milton [1608–1674]

            His sleep
Was Aerie light from pure digestion bred.
> *Paradise Lost,* Bk. V

Joseph Addison [1672–1719]

What means this heaviness that hangs
     upon me?
This lethargy that creeps through all
     my senses?
Nature, oppress'd and harass'd out
     with care,
Sinks down to rest.
> *Cato,* Act V, Sc. i

Sweet are the slumbers of the virtuous man!
> *Ibid.,* Sc. iv

Edward Young [1683–1765]

Tired Nature's sweet restorer, balmy
     Sleep!
> *Night Thoughts,* Night I

All the wild trash of sleep, without the
     rest.
> *Ibid.,* Night VIII

James Thomson [1700–1748]

For is there aught in sleep can charm
     the wise?
To lie in dead oblivion, losing half
The fleeting moments of too short a
     life, —
Total extinction of the enlightened
     soul!
Or else to feverish vanity alive,
Wildered, and tossing through distempered dreams!
Who would in such a gloomy state remain
Longer than Nature craves?
> *The Seasons,* "Summer"

Samuel Johnson [1709–1784]

Preserve me from unseasonable and immoderate sleep.
> *Prayers and Meditations,* January 1, 1767

I never take a nap after dinner but when I have had a bad night, and then the nap takes me.
> Quoted by James Boswell in *Life of Samuel Johnson,* 1775

Laurence Sterne [1713–1768]

Of all the soft, delicious functions of nature this is the chiefest; what a happiness it is to man, when the anxieties and passions of the day are over.

Jean Paul Richter [1763–1825]

Sleep, riches, and health, are only truly enjoyed after they have been interrupted.
> *Flower, Fruit and Thorn Pieces,* Ch. 8

Arthur Wellesley, Duke of Wellington [1769–1852]

When it is time to turn over, it is time to turn out.
> *Maxims and Table-Talk*

Sir Walter Scott [1771–1832]

The half hour between waking and rising has all my life proved propitious to any task which was exercising my invention. . . . It was always when I first opened my eyes that the desired ideas thronged upon me.

Letter to a friend

Samuel Taylor Coleridge [1772–1834]

Visit her, gentle Sleep! with wings of healing.
Dejection: An Ode

Oh sleep! it is a gentle thing,
Beloved from pole to pole!
The Rime of the Ancient Mariner, Pt. V

Robert Southey [1774–1843]

Thou hast been call'd, O Sleep! the friend of Woe;
But 'tis the happy who have call'd thee so.
The Curse of Kehama, Canto XV, Stanza 12

Charles Lamb [1775–1834]

We have had a sick child, who sleeping, or not sleeping, next me with a pasteboard partition between, killed my sleep. The little bastard is gone.
Letter to Edward Moxon, April 27, 1833

Daniel Drake [1785–1852]

It is bad enough to sleep in feathers in summer, when one lives far in the north; but to be delivered over to such a fate in the latitude of 34° is deplorable. Every where in this region, the taverns, and, in general, the houses of the people, are furnished with feather beds, for June, July and August, not less than for January. The medical gentlemen of this country should raise their voices against this absurd and enervating custom. A hard bed for hot weather referring rather to health or comfort, should be the motto of the whole South.
Western Journal of Medicine and Surgery, 1844

John Keats [1795–1821]

O magic sleep! O comfortable bird,
That broodest o'er the troubled sea of the mind
Till it is hush'd and smooth! O unconfin'd
Restraint! imprisoned liberty!
Endymion, Bk. I

My spirit is too weak — mortality
Weighs heavily on me like unwilling sleep.
On Seeing the Elgin Marbles

Honoré de Balzac [1799–1850]

He . . . went to bed, and slept the sleep of the dissipated, which, for some queer reason — of which no rhymer has yet taken advantage — is as profound as that of innocence.
The Girl with the Golden Eyes (tr. by Ellen Marriage and Ernest Dowson)

Charles Dickens [1812–1870]

I was tired now, and, getting into bed again, fell — off a tower and down a precipice — into the depths of sleep.
David Copperfield, Ch. 55

Sir William Withey Gull [1816–1890]

I do not know what a brain is, and I do not know what sleep is, but I do know that a well-fed brain sleeps well.
Quoted in *St. Bartholomew's Hospital Reports* 52:45, 1916

Herman Melville [1819–1891]

The native strength of [the Marquesans'] constitution is no way shown more emphatically than in the quantity of sleep they can endure. To many of them, indeed, life is little else than an often interrupted and luxurious nap.
Typee, Ch. XX (Ch. XIX in 1847 and 1850 eds.)

Mark Twain (Samuel L. Clemens)
[1835–1910]

There ain't no way to find out why a snorer can't hear himself snore.
Tom Sawyer Abroad, Ch. 10

Thomas Bailey Aldrich
[1836–1907]

What probing deep
Has ever solved the mystery of sleep?
Quatrains, "Human Ignorance"

Friedrich Nietzsche [1844–1900]

No small art is it to sleep: it is necessary for that purpose to keep awake all day.
Thus Spake Zarathustra, Pt. I, Ch. 2 (tr. by Oscar Levy)

William Sharp ("Fiona Macleod")
[1855–1905]

By the Gate of Sleep we enter the Enchanted Valleys.
Through the Ivory Gate, Pt. V

George Bernard Shaw [1856–1950]

A nap, my friend, is a brief period of sleep which overtakes superannuated persons when they endeavor to entertain unwelcome visitors or to listen to scientific lectures.
Back to Methuselah, Pt. IV, "Tragedy of an Elderly Gentleman," Act I

James Bridie [1888–1951]

He [man] can lie on his back, a posture long sustained by no other uncarapaced animal except in death. It is little wonder that his sleep is the amazement of the animal kingdom. It is superior to the long unconsciousness of hibernating animals. They curl their vegetative organs into the smallest bulk, and lie in an uncomfortable tight knot in a condition near to death. How different is man! Man's great lungs heave and blow, his noble heart thuds merrily, and his marvellous bowels continue in gentle peristalsis, his brain is the house of a thousand lovely fancies, his liver, his blood, his glands, transform the dead cells of his food into the living elements of his body and slay his myriad of airy foes. He is badly constructed for locomotion by road or by tree. The slowest fish swims faster. He is adapted primarily for rest.
Tedious and Brief, Pt. II, "The Umbilicus"

Thomas Wolfe [1900–1938]

Sleep lay upon the wilderness, it lay across the faces of nations, it lay like silence on the hearts of sleeping men; and low upon lowlands, and high upon hills, flowed gently sleep, smooth-sliding sleep — sleep — sleep.
Of Time and the River, Bk. I, Pt. IV

Ogden Nash [1902–   ]

Sleep is perverse as human nature,
Sleep is perverse as a legislature,
Sleep is as forward as hives or goiters,
And where it is least desired, it loiters.
The Face Is Familiar, "Read This Vibrant Exposé"

Cyril Connolly [1903–   ]

I believe in sleep: the time spent in sleep (the time when we are out of trouble) is not charged to our account but is handed back to us in later life to use as we please.
Encounter, April 1961

The Bible

I will not give sleep to mine eyes, or slumber to mine eyelids.
Psalms 132:4

Yet a little sleep, a little slumber, a little folding of the hands to sleep.
Proverbs 6:10 and 24:33

The sleep of a labouring man is sweet, whether he eat little or much: but the abundance of the rich will not suffer him to sleep.
Ecclesiastes 5:12

The Bible: Apocrypha

Sound sleep cometh of moderate eating: he riseth early, and his wits are with him.
>   *Ecclesiasticus* 31:20

Proverb

One hour's sleep before midnight is worth three after.[1]

English Proverbs

Nature requireth five hours sleep;
    Custom taketh seven;
Idleness takes nine;
    And wickedness eleven.

Six hours' sleep for a man, seven for a woman, and eight for a fool.

Sleep is better than medicine.

Irish Proverb

The beginning of health is sleep.

Latin Proverb

He sleeps well who knows not that he sleeps ill.

Spanish Proverb

In sleep we are all equal.

Welsh Proverb

Disease and sleep keep far apart.

II. INSOMNIA

Tibullus [54?–18? B.C.]

Sleep vanishes before the house of care.
>   *Elegies,* III.iv.20 (tr. by J. P. Postgate)

Sir Thomas Wyatt [1503?–1542]

The waky nights.
>   *Complaint upon Love to Reason*

---

[1] One hour's sleep before midnight's worth two hours after.

William Shakespeare [1564–1616]

I have not slept one wink.
>   *Cymbeline,* III, iv, 103

>   O sleep, O gentle sleep!
> Nature's soft nurse, how have I
>   frighted thee,
> That thou no more wilt weigh my
>   eyelids down
> And steep my senses in forgetfulness?
>   *Henry IV, Part II,* III, i, 5

> Our foster nurse of nature is repose,
> The which he lacks. That to provoke
>   in him
> Are many simples operative, whose
>   power
> Will close the eye of anguish.
>   *King Lear,* IV, iv, 12

Giddy for lack of sleep.
>   *The Taming of the Shrew,* IV, iii, 9

Antonio de Escobar y Mendoza [1589–1669]

If a man cannot sleep without taking supper, is he bound to fast? By no means.
>   *Universae theologiae moralis receptiores sententiae,* I, Exam. 13, Ch. 3

Sir John Suckling [1609–1642]

> Sleep is as nice as woman: the more I
>   court it,
> The more it flies me.
>   *The Tragedy of Brennoralt,* Act II, Sc. i

George Gordon, Lord Byron [1788–1824]

> My slumbers — if I slumber — are
>   not sleep,
> But a continuance of enduring thought.
>   *Manfred,* Act I, Sc. i

>   Sleep,
> Which will not be commanded.
>   *Marino Faliero,* Act IV, Sc. i

In vain from side to side he throws
His form, in courtship of repose.
The Siege of Corinth, Stanza 13

William Arthur Dunkerley
("John Oxenham") [1852–1941]

Thank God for sleep!
And, when you cannot sleep,
Still thank Him that you live
To lie awake.
The Sacrament of Sleep

Elbert G. Hubbard [1856–1915]

Insomnia never comes to a man who
has to get up exactly at six o'clock.
Insomnia troubles only those who can
sleep any time.
The Philistine, August 1907,
"In Re Muldoon"

John Bruce MacCallum
[1876–1906]

Long have I wooed thee through the
  slow winged hours,
O sleep, and in the darkness past the
  lone,
Dim shadows of a dying day have
  flown,
Dreams of a restless life, and hills,
  and flowers,
And shining clouds that float across
  the sky;
And then, again, the drift of hurrying
  feet,
Long rows of houses in a dusty street,
With moving men and ceaseless din
  and cry.

O sleep, I cannot rest. Mine eyes
  are dim,
And o'er the bourneless tide of time
  and space
My soul must wander till it finds a
  place
Of comfort, past the ocean's utmost
  rim.
O sleep, I would thy poppy-scented
  breath

Might give me rest, or bring me dream-
  less death.
Sleep (Quoted by Archibald
Malloch in *The Life and Let-
ters of John Bruce MacCallum,
M.D.*, Ch. 1)

Sir Henry Howarth Bashford
("Peter Harding") [1880–1961]

Sleeplessness *per se* has never killed
anybody yet.
The Corner of Harley Street,
Ch. 16

Franklin P. Adams (F.P.A.)
[1881–1960]

If, my dear, you seek to slumber,
Count of stars an endless number;
If you still continue wakeful,
Count the drops that make a lakeful;
Then, if vigilance yet above you
Hover, count the times I love you;
And if slumber still repel you,
Count the times I do not tell you.
The Melancholy Lute, "Lul-
laby"

F. Scott Fitzgerald [1896–1940]

It appears that every man's insomnia is
as different from his neighbor's as are
their daytime hopes and aspirations.
The Crack-up (ed. by Edmund
Wilson), "Sleeping and Waking"

Irwin Shaw [1913–   ]

Sleep . . . is the first great natural
resource to be exhausted by modern
man. The erosion of the nerves, not
to be halted by any reclamation project, public or private.
The New Yorker, April 2,
1949, "The Climate of In-
somnia"

The Bible

When I lie down, I say, When shall
I arise, and the night be gone? and I
am full of tossings to and fro unto the
dawning of the day.
Job 7:4

SLEEP AND DEATH

See also DEATH, SLEEP

Homer [ca. 850 B.C.]

Sleep and Death, who are twin brothers.
> *Iliad,* XVI.681 (tr. by R. Lattimore)

Aristophanes [446–380 B.C.]

Perhaps death is life, and life is death,
And victuals and drink an illusion of the senses;
For what is Death but an eternal sleep?
And does not Life consist in sleeping and eating?
> *Frogs,* 1477 (tr. by John Hookham Frere)

Virgil [70–19 B.C.]

That sweet, deep sleep, so close to tranquil death.
> *Aeneid,* VI.522 (tr. by T. C. Williams)

Ovid [43 B.C.–A.D. 17?]

What else is sleep but the image of chill death?
> *The Amores,* II.x.41 (tr. by G. Showerman)

St. John Chrysostom [345?–407]

What is death at most? It is a journey for a season; a sleep longer than usual. If thou fearest death, thou shouldest also fear sleep.
> *Homilies on the Statutes,* Homily V (tr. by John H. Parker)

Leonardo da Vinci [1452–1519]

As a well-spent day brings happy sleep, so life well used brings happy death.
> *Codice Trivulziano,* 28a (tr. by Edward MacCurdy in *The Notebooks of Leonardo da Vinci,* Vol. I, Ch. I)

Thomas Sackville, Earl of Dorset [1536–1608]

Heavy Sleep, the cousin of Death.
> *The Mirror for Magistrates,* Pt. III, "Master Sackville's Induction"

Edmund Spenser [1552?–1599]

For next to death is Sleepe to be compard.
> *The Faerie Queene,* Bk. II, Canto VII

Robert Southwell [1561?–1595]

Sleep, death's ally.
> *St. Peter's Complaint,* Sect. 20

Samuel Daniel [1562–1619]

Care-charmer Sleepe, sonne of the sable night,
Brother to death, in silent darknes born.
> *Sonnets to Delia,* LIV

William Shakespeare [1564–1616]

O sleep, thou ape of death.
> *Cymbeline,* II, ii, 31

> To die — to sleep —
No more; and by a sleep to say we end
The heartache, and the thousand natural shocks
That flesh is heir to. 'Tis a consummation
Devoutly to be wish'd. To die — to sleep.
To sleep — perchance to dream: ay, there's the rub!
For in that sleep of death what dreams may come
When we have shuffled off this mortal coil,
Must give us pause.
> *Hamlet,* III, i, 59

Phineas Fletcher [1582–1650]

Sleep's but a shorter death, death's but a longer sleep.
> *Apollyonists,* Canto I, Stanza 6

Sir Thomas Browne [1605–1682]

Sleepe . . . is that death by which
we may be literally said to die daily,
a death which *Adam* died before his
mortality; a death whereby we live a
middle and moderating point betweene
life and death; in fine, so like death,
I dare not trust it without my prayers,
and an halfe adiew unto the world.
Religio Medici, Pt. II, Sect. 12

Sleepe is a death, O make me try,
By sleeping what it is to die.
And down as gently lay my head
Upon my Grave, as now my bed.
Idem

Samuel Butler [1612–1680]

And Sleep, Death's Brother, yet a
    Friend to Life,
Gave weary'd Nature a Restorative.
*Repartees Between Cat and
    Puss at a Caterwalling in the
    Modern Heroic Way*

Edward Young [1683–1765]

                Each night we die,
Each morn are born anew: Each day,
    a life!
Night Thoughts, Night II

John Wolcot ("Peter Pindar")
[1738–1819]

How sweet, though lifeless, yet with
    life to lie!
And, without dying, O how sweet to
    die.
Epigram on Sleep

George Gordon, Lord Byron
[1788–1824]

Death, so call'd, is a thing which
    makes men weep,
And yet a third of life is pass'd in
    sleep.
Don Juan, Canto XIV, Stanza 3

Percy Bysshe Shelley [1792–1822]

How wonderful is Death,
Death and his brother Sleep!
Queen Mab, Sect. I

Heinrich Heine [1797–1856]

For Sleep is good, but Death is better
    still —
The best is never to be born at all.
Romaniero, "Morphine" (tr. by
    Louis Untermeyer)

Thomas Hood [1799–1845]

Our very hopes belied our fears,
    Our fears our hopes belied —
We thought her dying when she slept,
    And sleeping when she died!
The Death-Bed

Ralph Waldo Emerson
[1803–1882]

Out of sleeping a waking,
Out of waking a sleep.
The Sphinx

Henry Wadsworth Longfellow
[1807–1882]

O peaceful Sleep! until from pain re-
    leased
    I breathe again uninterrupted
    breath!
Ah, with what subtile meaning did the
    Greek
    Call thee the lesser mystery, at the
    feast
    Whereof the greater mystery is
    death!
    Sleep

Alfred, Lord Tennyson
[1809–1892]

When in the down I sink my head,
Sleep, Death's twin-brother, times my
    breath.
In Memoriam, Sect. LXVIII

The Bible

The maid is not dead, but sleepeth.
Matthew 9:24

Anonymous

He shall sleepe the Iron sleep of death.
The Tragedie of Nero, Act III

SMALLPOX

See also VACCINATION

Avicenna [980–1037]

The physical signs of measles are nearly the same as those of smallpox, but nausea and inflammation is more severe, though the pains in the back are less. The rash of measles usually appears at once, but the rash of small-pox spot after spot.
> *The Canon,* Bk. IV

Voltaire [1694–1778]

Smallpox is, in a simple form, merely the blood ridding itself of its impurities, and positively paves the way to more vigorous health.
> Letter to Louis de Breteuil, baron de Preuilly, ca. December 5, 1723 (tr. by S. G. Tallentyre)

Oliver Goldsmith [1728–1774]

That dire disease whose ruthless power
Withers the beauty's transient flower.
> *Double Transformation*

Thomas Jefferson [1743–1826]

The Small-pox, at this time in many parts of the Commonwealth is likely to spread and become general, and it hath been proved by incontestible experience that the late discovery's and Improvements therein have produced great Benefits to Mankind, by rendering a Distemper, which taken in the common way is always dangerous and often fatal, comparatively mild and safe by Inoculation.
> *Bill Concerning Inoculation for Smallpox,* December 27, 1777

Medicine has never before produced any single improvement of such utility. . . . You have erased from the calendar of human afflictions one of its greatest. Yours is the comfortable reflection that mankind can never forget that you have lived. Future nations will know by history only that the loathsome small-pox has existed and by you has been extirpated.
> Letter to Dr. Edward Jenner, May 14, 1806 [1]

George Gordon, Lord Byron [1788–1824]

I said the small pox has gone out of late;
Perhaps it may be follow'd by the great.
> *Don Juan,* Canto I, Stanza 130

Chinese Proverb

Starve the measles, and nourish the smallpox.

Pashto Proverb

Until he gets over small-pox, parents do not count their child their own.

SNEEZING

Frances (Fanny) Burney [1752–1840]

You must not sneeze. If you have a vehement cold, you must take no notice of it; if your nose-membranes feel a great irritation, you must hold your breath; if a sneeze still insists upon making its way, you must oppose it, by keeping your teeth grinding together; if the violence of the repulse breaks some blood-vessel, you must break the blood-vessel — but not sneeze.[2]
> Letter to Esther Burney, December 17, 1785

Lewis Carroll (Charles L. Dodgson) [1832–1898]

Speak roughly to your little boy,
    And beat him when he sneezes:

[1] See note, p. 26a.
[2] Directions for coughing, sneezing, or moving before the King and Queen.

He only does it to annoy,
  Because he knows it teases.
    *Alice's Adventures in Wonder-
    land,* Ch. 6

David McCord [1897–   ]

I recommend for plain dis-ease
A good post-operandum sneeze;
You might as well be on the rack
When every stitch takes up its slack.
    And What's More, "Convales-
    cence"

Proverb

He hath sneezed thrice; turn him out
of the hospital.

SOCIAL MEDICINE

See also PREVENTIVE MEDI-
CINE, PUBLIC HEALTH, RE-
HABILITATION

Rudolf Virchow [1821–1902]

Medicine is a social science in its very
bone marrow. . . . No physiologist or
practitioner ought ever to forget that
medicine unites in itself all knowledge
of the laws which apply to the body
and the mind.
    Disease, Life, and Man, "Sci-
    entific Method and Therapeutic
    Standpoints" (tr. by L. J.
    Rather)

Should medicine ever fulfill its great
ends, it must enter into the larger political and social life of our time; it must
indicate the barriers which obstruct the
normal completion of the life-cycle
and remove them. Should this ever
come to pass, Medicine, what ever it
may then be, will become the common
good of all. It will cease to be medicine
and will be absorbed into that general
body of knowledge which is identifi-
able with power. Then will Bacon's
prediction be accomplished fact: what

seemed causal in theory will become
established rule in practice.
    *De Einheitsbestrebunger in der
    Wissenschaftlichen Medizin*

The physicians are the natural attor-
neys of the poor and the social problems should largely be solved by them.
    Quoted by Erwin H. Acker-
    necht in *Rudolf Virchow,* "The
    Doctor"

S. Weir Mitchell [1829–1914]

All the vast hygienic, social and moral
problems of our restless, energetic
labor-saving race are, in some degree,
those of the future student of disease
in America.

Elie Metchnikoff [1845–1916]

Ought we to listen to the cry of humanity that life is too short and that
it would be well to prolong it? Already
it is complained that the burden of
supporting old people is too heavy, and
statesmen are perturbed by the enormous expense which will be entailed by
state support of the aged.
    The Prolongation of Life (ed.
    by P. Chalmers Mitchell), Pt.
    4, Ch. 1

Henry Baird Favill [1860–1916]

The pathology of society is as much
the function of the medical man as the
pathology of human disease.
    *Medicine in the Scheme of Con-
    servation*

Charles H. Mayo [1865–1939]

Medicine is a profession for social service and it developed organization in
response to social need.
    *Collected Papers of the Mayo
    Clinic and Mayo Foundation*
    23:1020, 1931

Ida M. Cannon [1877–   ]

So it is that medicine is surely deeply
involved in the social organization of

our life, and that, if there is meaning in the phrase "doctor-patient relation," this meaning implies the recognition of the patient as a social being who lives in a network of relations, and not in the chance isolation of sickness.
On the Social Frontier of Medicine, Ch. 24

Walton H. Hamilton [1881–1958]

Although "the personal choice of a physician" is an excellent ideal, it does not, under current conditions, work well in practice. An old maxim, long known to every student of social philosophy, calls for a restriction of personal choice when "the consumer is not a proper judge of the quality of the ware." The art of medicine is intricate; the relation of the treatment of the sick to results obtained cannot be appraised by a layman; in medicine, almost more certainly than anywhere else, the patient has not the knowledge requisite for judgment.
Dissenting Opinion on the Report of the Committee on American Medicine, 1932

If we are to make the most of our human resources, for work and for life, it is necessary that our facilities for health shall be just as available for all who need them as are the schools and the churches. Nor should the matter of a membership in a health service be left to the free choice of the individual. The "reasonable man" of our ancestors, who was prudent and provident and would always seek his own best advantage, now lives only as a fiction.
Idem

Henry E. Sigerist [1891–1957]

The task of medicine is to promote health, to prevent disease, to treat the sick when prevention has broken down and to rehabilitate the people after they have been cured. These are highly social functions and we must look at medicine as basically a social science.
Civilization and Disease, Ch. 12

[Physicians] should know social conditions best as their profession takes them into the homes of all social classes, and it is their duty to work for the improvement of conditions. It is the duty of all of us as we practice not only psychosomatic but also social medicine.
International Record of Medicine 168:383, 1955

The tasks assigned [to the physician] . . . are determined primarily by the social and economic structure of society and by the technical and scientific means available to medicine at the time.
Medicine and Human Welfare, Ch. 3

Medicine . . . is a social science.
Proceedings of the American Philosophical Society 90:275, 1946

We see the physician as scientist, educator and social worker, ready to cooperate in teamwork, in close touch with the people he disinterestedly serves, a friend and leader . . . the social physician protecting the people and guiding them to a healthier and happier life.
Idem

Patients must be adjusted socially as well as medically. The physicians must thus also play a social role.
Quoted in *Journal of the History of Medicine and Allied Sciences* 13:214, 1958

Curtis Bok [1897–1962]

We are convinced that the only genuine medical insurance for this country lies in making the benefits of science available to all practitioners and to all patients.
Foreword to *Medical Research, A Midcentury Survey*

Carl J. Gilbert [1906–   ]

I believe there is too strong a tendency

on the part of so-called laymen to defer to the medical profession in regard to the [social] problems of medical care.

> *Health for the American People* (Symposium), "Community Action for Health"

SORROW

See also MELANCHOLY

St. Augustine [354–430]

Why does man like to be made sad when viewing doleful and tragical scenes, which yet he himself would by no means suffer? And yet he wishes, as a spectator, to experience from them a sense of grief, and in this very grief his pleasure consists. What is this but wretched insanity? . . . Howsoever, when he suffers in his own person, it is the custom to style it "misery"; but when he feels pity for others, then it is styled "mercy."

> *Confessions*, III.2 (tr. by J. G. Pilkington)

William Shakespeare [1564–1616]

Some griefs are med'cinable.
> *Cymbeline*, III, ii, 33

Great griefs, I see, med'cine the less.
> *Ibid.*, IV, ii, 243

Give sorrow words; the grief that does not speak
Whispers the o'erfraught heart and bids it break.
> *Macbeth*, IV, iii, 209

Fell sorrow's tooth doth never rankle more
Than when he bites, but lanceth not the sore.
> *Richard II*, I, iii, 302

William Cowper [1731–1800]

Grief is itself a medicine.
> *Charity*

Italian Proverb

Sighing is no medicine.

SPECIALIST

See also CONSULTATION

Herodotus [484–424 B.C.]

The art of medicine in Egypt is thus exercised: one physician is confined to the study and management of one disease; there are of course a great number who practice this art; some attend to the disorders of the eyes, others to those of the head, some take care of the teeth, others are conversant with all diseases of the bowels; whilst many attend to the cure of maladies which are less conspicuous.

> *Histories*, II.84 (tr. by William Beloe)

Thomas Bartholin [1616–1680]

Unfortunately, there are enough people who are so infatuated with their specialized studies that they are ignorant and unaware of other disciplines. If fate happens to lead them to fields other than their own, they are helpless and lost. May God protect you from an infection with the germs of haughty contempt for the efforts of scientists in other branches of science. Your country demands more than one-sided proficiency. Only the correlation of extensive knowledge will bring us closer to actual wisdom.

> *De theologiae et medicinae affinitate* (tr. by Max Samter)

Alexander Pope [1688–1744]

One Science only will one genius fit:
So vast is Art, so narrow human wit.
> *An Essay on Criticism*, Pt. I

John Morgan [1735–1789]

Whilst Medicine from the greatness of its object, the preservation of the species, is one of the most useful subjects of knowledge to a state, and at the same time one of the most extensive and difficult; we must regret that the very different employment of a Physician, Surgeon, and Apothecary, should be promiscuously followed by any one man, however great his abilities. They certainly require very different talents.

> *A Discourse Upon the Institution of Medical Schools in America*

If Physic, Surgery, and Pharmacy were in different hands, practitioners would then enjoy much more satisfaction in practice. They would commonly be less burdened with an over hurry of business, and have an opportunity of studying the cases of the sick at more leisure. Would not this tend to the more speedy relief of diseases and the perfection of medical science, as every Physician would have more time by study, observation, and experience united, to cultivate that knowledge which is the only foundation of practice?

> *Idem*

Sydney Smith [1771–1845]

There is always some man, of whom the human viscera stand in greater dread than of any other person, who is supposed, for the time being, to be the only person who can dart his pill into their inmost recesses; and bind them over, in medical recognisance, to assimilate and digest.

> Quoted in *The Wit and Wisdom of the Rev. Sydney Smith*

Thomas De Quincey [1785–1859]

A due balance and equilibrium of the mind is best preserved by a large and multiform knowledge: but knowledge itself is best served by an exclusive (or at least paramount) dedication of one mind to one science.

> *London Magazine*, July 1824, "Superficial Knowledge"

Oliver Wendell Holmes [1809–1894]

Specialized knowledge will do a man no harm if he also has common sense, but if he lacks this, it can only make him more dangerous to his patients.

Theodor Billroth [1829–1894]

The cases of throat, lung, brain, spinal and nerve diseases must not be taken from the general medical clinics, in order to supply the special clinics. The student ought not to become accustomed to hearing the professor say every day "You are hoarse? Go to the throat clinic," or "You are coughing? Go to the ward for lung cases!" Such a scattering of medical thought and action is sure to make a very bad impression on the students. They will accustom themselves not to examine and treat every case to the best of their ability, but on the contrary, they will think, "Well, if even the professor can't handle this case, what shall I do later on in my practice?"

> *The Medical Sciences in the German Universities*, Pt. II

Sir Clifford Allbutt [1836–1925]

The harm of "specialisation," the scorn of "the school of infinitesimal research," lies not in Nature but in narrowness of the student's mind, be he old or young. Enter into the realm of nature by whatsoever gate you please, you will find yourself in the presence of infinity.

> *British Medical Journal* 2:407, 1922

The harm of specialism lies then not in a limited field, this it is not; no side or adit of nature is limited; but because the specialism is reached not by carrying the whole into the part, but by stopping short at the turn.

> *Idem*

The barriers of convention . . . have split up medicine into fractions. As physic was divorced from surgery and mind from body, so the diseases of animals and plants were separated from those of mankind. The folly of the division of the medicine of the hand from the medicine of the bottle has now become so glaring that our next festival may be on the blowing up of this rampart; indeed, the gynaecologists have exploded their end of it already. But it is a big business to transform a medieval castle, with its baileys, barbicans and keep, into a modern domain.

> *Proceedings of the Royal Society of Medicine* (Section of Comparative Medicine) 17:1, 1923

Frank Kittredge Paddock
[1841–1901]

A general practitioner can no more become a specialist than an old shoe can become a dancing slipper. Both have developed habits which are immutable.
> Aphorism

Sir William Osler [1849–1919]

The extraordinary development of modern science may be her undoing. Specialism, now a necessity, has fragmented the specialties themselves in a way that makes the outlook hazardous. The workers lose all sense of proportion in a maze of minutiae.
> Address, Classical Association, Oxford, May 16, 1910

The incessant concentration of thought upon one subject, however interesting, tethers a man's mind in a narrow field.
> *Aequanimitas, with Other Addresses*, "Chauvinism in Medicine"

Philip A. Bruce [1856–1933]

He [Thomas Jefferson] had none of the spirit of the specialist, which would have given a preponderance to some one province in which he happened to be learned.
> *History of the University of Virginia*, "Fourth Period"

August Bier [1861–1949]

Patients consult so-called authorities. And I have become one also. Yet, we don't know more than the others. We are only the prey of hypochondriacs.
> Aphorism

William J. Mayo [1861–1939]

Given one well-trained physician of the highest type he will do better work for a thousand people than ten specialists.

Alfred North Whitehead
[1861–1947]

Each science confines itself to a fragment of the evidence and weaves its theories in terms of notions suggested by that fragment. Such a procedure is necessary by reason of the limitations of human ability. But its dangers should always be kept in mind. For example, the increasing departmentalization of universities during the last hundred years, however necessary for administrative purposes, tends to trivialize the mentality of the teaching profession.
> *Nature and Life*, Ch. 1

Nicholas Murray Butler
[1862–1947]

An expert is one who knows more and more about less and less.
> Commencement address, Columbia University

Charles H. and Charles W. Mayo
[1865–1939]　　[1898–　　]

The definition of a specialist as one who "knows more about less and less" is good and true. Its truth makes essential that the specialist, to do efficient work, must have some association with others who, taken altogether,

represent the whole of which the specialty is only a part.
Modern Hospital 51:68, 1938

Hilaire Belloc [1870–1953]

He sought a Specialist, who said:
"You have a swelling in the head:
Your Larynx is a thought relaxed
And you are greatly over-taxed. . . .
Come! Here's the treatment! I insist!
To Bed! to Bed! And do not speak
A single word till Wednesday week,
When I will come and set you free
(If you are cured) and take my fee."
Cautionary Verses, "Lord Roehampton"

Martin H. Fischer [1879–1962]

The specialist is a man who fears the other subjects.
Quoted by Howard Fabing and Ray Marr in *Fischerisms*

Harry E. Mock [1880–　]

To my sons: Whatever specialty they follow, may they never forget to be doctors.
Skull Fractures and Brain Injuries, Dedication

Geoffrey Fisher, Archbishop of Canterbury [1887–　]

Consultant specialists are a degree more remote (like bishops!); and therefore (again like bishops) they need a double dose of Grace to keep them sensitive to the personal and the pastoral.
Lancet 2:775, 1949

John A. Ryle [1889–1950]

There is a tendency diffused through the profession, more evident perhaps today than thirty years ago, to imbibe and to retain the influences of physical and chemical method, of the dissecting-room and the laboratory, of the operating theatre and the X-ray department at the expense of those other influences which are derived from the older naturalist school. The naturalist school, while eager for all forms of evidence, has always based its doctrine on close observation and that intimate form of human understanding which is best conveyed by the Greek word sympathy. . . . A study of man and his symptoms was what Hippocrates required of us, and all unwittingly in the present era we are tending to replace it with an elaboration of techniques. . . . The necessary but too rapid subdivision into specialisms and growing competition in every branch have, it would seem, been good for the technique but bad for the soul of medicine.
Fears May Be Liars, Ch. 6

Wilder Penfield [1891–　]

Every specialist, whatever his profession, skill or business may be, can improve his performance by broadening his base.
The Second Career, "The Use of Idleness"

Henry E. Sigerist [1891–1957]

Medicine has become highly specialized and access to it is uneven.
Quoted in *Journal of the History of Medicine and Allied Sciences* 13:214, 1958

William B. Castle [1897–　]

An expert is a man who tells you a simple thing in a confused way in such a fashion as to make you think the confusion is your own fault.
Quoted in *Harvard Medical Alumni Bulletin* 29:18, July 1955

George A. Perera [1911–　]

Specialization is the natural consequence of an expanding body of knowledge.
Annals of Internal Medicine 59:959, 1963

Robert H. Ebert [1914–   ]

There are probably as many "kindly old specialists" as there are "kindly old family physicians."
>Address to the National Tuberculosis Association, May 30, 1965

Anonymous

Choose your specialist and you choose your disease.
>*The Westminster Review,* May 18, 1906

The chief objection brought against specialties is, that they operate unfairly toward the general practitioner, in implying that he is incompetent to properly treat certain classes of diseases, and narrowing his field of practice.
>*Transactions of the American Medical Association* 20:111, 1869

An internist is someone who knows everything and does nothing.
>A surgeon is someone who does everything and knows nothing.
>A psychiatrist is someone who knows nothing and does nothing.
>A pathologist is someone who knows everything and does everything too late.

Legal Maxim

Every skilled person is to be believed with reference to his own art.

SPEECH

Thomas Carlyle [1795–1881]

A stammering man is never a worthless one. Physiology can tell you why. It is an excess of delicacy, excess of sensibility to the presence of his fellow-creature, that makes him stammer.
>Letter to Ralph Waldo Emerson, November 17, 1843

Sören Kierkegaard [1813–1855]

If I were a pagan I should say that an ironical deity had given men the gift of speech in order that he may be entertained by their self-deceit.
>*Journal,* Vol. XI, Pt. I, Entry 139 (tr. by Ronald G. Smith)

Sir William Osler [1849–1919]

Look wise, say nothing, and grunt. Speech was given to conceal thought.
>Quoted by William B. Bean in *Sir William Osler: Aphorisms,* Ch. 5

James Thurber [1894–1961]

If we went out on the street dressed the way we talk, we should be arrested for indecent exposure.

SPEECHES

See also COMMUNICATION, WRITING

Plato [427?–347 B.C.]

On several occasions I have been with my brother Herodicus or some other physician to see one of his patients, who would not allow the physician to give him medicine, or apply the knife or hot iron to him; and I have persuaded him to do for me what he would not do for the physician just by the use of rhetoric. And I say that if a rhetorician and a physician were to go to any city, and had there to argue in the Ecclesia or any other assembly as to which of them should be elected state-physician, the physician would have no chance; but he who could speak would be chosen if he wished.
>*Gorgias,* 456.B (tr. by Benjamin Jowett)

Jackson A. Smith [1917–   ]

Many physicians would prefer passing

a small kidney stone to presenting a paper.
> *Journal of the American Medical Association* 174:292, 1960

There are many ways to deliver papers; the best way is to toss them on the front porch before sunup.
> *Idem*

Anonymous

Speeches are like babies — easy to conceive but hard to deliver.

SPINE

Anonymous

The spine is a series of bones running down your back. You sit on one end of it and your head sits on the other.

SPLEEN

Plato [427?–347 B.C.]

The neighbouring organ [the spleen] is situated on the left-hand side, and is constructed with a view of keeping the liver bright and pure, — like a napkin, always ready prepared and at hand to clean the mirror.
> *Timaeus,* 72.C (tr. by Benjamin Jowett)

William Shakespeare [1564–1616]

You shall digest the venom of your spleen,
Though it do split you.
> *Julius Caesar,* IV, iii, 47

STAMMERING

See SPEECH

STARVATION

See HUNGER

STATISTICS

See also QUANTITATION

Thomas Carlyle [1795–1881]

A judicious man . . . looks at Statistics, not to get knowledge, but to save himself from having ignorance foisted on him.
> *Critical and Miscellaneous Essays,* "Chartism," Ch. II

Sir Francis Galton [1822–1911]

The object of statistical science is to discover methods of condensing information concerning large groups of allied facts into brief and compendious expressions suitable for discussion. The possibility of doing this is based on the constancy and continuity with which objects of the same species are found to vary.
> *Inquiries Into Human Faculty and Its Development,* "Statistical Methods"

John Shaw Billings [1838–1913]

Statistics are somewhat like old medical journals, or like revolvers in newly opened mining districts. Most men rarely use them, and find it troublesome to preserve them so as to have them easy of access; but when they do want them, they want them badly.
> *Medical Record* 36:589, 1889

Andrew Lang [1844–1912]

He uses statistics as a drunken man uses lampposts — for support rather than for illumination.

Charles V. Chapin [1856–1941]

We cannot expect that figures will ever cease to lie, but we may hope that vital statisticians will.
> *Papers,* "Pleasures and Hopes of the Health Officer"

August Bier [1861–1949]

Every sensible person promptly associates the term "statistics" with the thought: "This is a bunch of lies."
    Aphorism

Sir Berkeley Moynihan [1865–1936]

Statistics . . . will prove anything, even the truth.
    Addresses on Surgical Subjects, "Cancer and How to Fight It"

Edwin Bidwell Wilson [1879–1964]

The investigator reported that one-third of the rats were improved on the experimental medication, one-third remained the same and the other third couldn't be reported on because *that* rat got away.

Fiorello La Guardia [1882–1947]

Statistics are like alienists — they will testify for either side.
    Liberty, May 13, 1933

John Punnett Peters [1887–1955]

The statistical correlation of two variables does not *ipso facto* signify that either one is the cause or effect of the other.
    Yale Journal of Biology and Medicine 26:179, 1953

H. Bartels [20th Cent.]

Good correlations do not necessarily offer proof of causal relationships: the birth rate per family in Germany has decreased with a high coefficient of correlation to the decrease in the stork population; but the latter event has not caused the former!
    Development of the Lung (ed. by A. V. S. de Reuck and Ruth Porter), "Carriage of Oxygen in the Blood of the Foetus"

M. J. Moroney [20th Cent.]

Had it not been for the statisticians

Christ would have been born in the modest comfort of a cottage in Nazareth instead of in a stable at Bethlehem.
    Facts from Figures, Ch. 1

A statistical analysis, properly conducted, is a delicate dissection of uncertainties, a surgery of suppositions.
    Idem

Anonymous

Medical statistics are like a bikini. What they reveal is interesting but what they conceal is vital.

The figure of 2.2 children per adult female was felt to be in some respects absurd, and a Royal Commission suggested that the middle classes be paid money to increase the average to a rounder and more convenient number.
    Punch

STATUS QUO

Martin H. Fischer [1879–1962]

If you do not agree with the prevalent point of view, be ready to explain why.
    Quoted by Howard Fabing and Ray Marr in *Fischerisms*

Elsworth Amidon [1906–   ]

[When asked the reason for conditions at Mary Fletcher Hospital, Burlington, Vermont:] Well, things always have to be somehow, and right now they are this way.
    Comment on ward rounds

STERILITY

Elizabeth I of England [1533–1603]

The Quen of Scotlandis is leichter of a fair sonne, and I am bot a barren stok.
    Quoted in *Memoirs of Sir James Melville*, June 1566

William Shakespeare [1564–1616]

Hear, Nature, hear! dear goddess, hear!
Suspend thy purpose, if thou didst intend
To make this creature fruitful.
Into her womb convey sterility;
Dry up in her the organs of increase;
And from her derogate body never spring
A babe to honour her!
King Lear, I, iv, 297

STERILIZATION

Pope Pius XI [1857–1939]

Public magistrates have no direct power over the bodies of their subjects; therefore, where no crime has taken place and there is no cause present for grave punishment, they can neither directly harm or tamper with the integrity of the body, either for the reasons of eugenics or for any other reason.
Casti connubii (December 31, 1930), Sect. 70

German Law

Any person suffering from a hereditary disease may be rendered incapable of procreation by means of a surgical operation if the experience of medical science shows that it is highly probable that his descendants would suffer from some serious physical or mental hereditary defect.
For the Prevention of Hereditarily Diseased Offspring, July 14, 1933

STETHOSCOPE

René Laënnec [1781–1826]

In 1816 I was consulted by a young woman labouring under general symptoms of diseased heart, and in whose case percussion and the application of the hand were of little avail on account of the great degree of fatness. The other method just mentioned [direct auscultation] being rendered inadmissable by the age and sex of the patient, I happened to recollect a simple and well-known fact in acoustics, . . . the great distinctness with which we hear the scratch of a pin at one end of a piece of wood on applying our ear to the other. Immediately, on this suggestion, I rolled a quire of paper into a kind of cylinder and applied one end of it to the region of the heart and the other to my ear, and was not a little surprised and pleased to find that I could thereby perceive the action of the heart in a manner much more clear and distinct than I had ever been able to do by the immediate application of the ear.
Auscultation Mediate (tr. by John Forbes)

Dickinson W. Richards [1895–   ]

In order for the stethoscope to function, two things have to happen. *There has to be, by God, a sick man at one end of it and a doctor at the other!* The doctor has to be within thirty inches of his patient.
Transactions of the Association of American Physicians 75:1, 1962

Look at it as it hangs on its hook, with its ears up and its rubber legs twisted. Has anyone ever commented how remarkably in this posture it simulates the snakes of the caduceus, the symbol of our old friend Aesculapius?
Idem

STOMACH

See also BELLY, BOWELS, GASTROINTESTINAL TRACT, INDIGESTION

Aesop [fl. 550 B.C.]

The members of the Body rebelled

against the Belly, and said, "Why should we be perpetually engaged in administering to your wants, while you do nothing but take your rest, and enjoy yourself in luxury and self-indulgence?" The members carried out their resolve, and refused their assistance to the Body. The whole Body quickly became debilitated, and the hands, feet, mouth, and eyes, when too late, repented of their folly.

> *Fables,* "The Belly and the Members" (tr. by George Fyler Townsend)

Plutarch [46?–120?]

Menenius Agrippa . . . concluded his discourse with a celebrated fable. He said, namely, that all the other members of man's body once revolted against the belly, and accused it of being the only member to sit idly down in its place and make no contribution to the common welfare, while the rest underwent great hardships and performed great public services only to minister to its appetites; but that the belly laughed at their simplicity in not knowing that it received into itself all the body's nourishment only to send it back again and duly distribute it among the other members.

> *Lives,* "Coriolanus," VI.3 (tr. by B. Perrin)

William Shakespeare [1564–1616]

There was a time when all the body's members
Rebell'd against the belly; thus accus'd it:
That only like a gulf it did remain
I' th' midst o' th' body, idle and unactive,
Still cupboarding the viand, never bearing
Like labour with the rest; where th' other instruments
Did see and hear, devise, instruct, walk, feel,
And, mutually participate, did minister

Unto the appetite and affection common
Of the whole body. The belly answered. . . .
'True is it, my incorporate friends,' quoth he,
'That I receive the general food at first
Which you do live upon; and fit it is,
Because I am the storehouse and the shop
Of the whole body. But, if you do remember,
I send it through the rivers of your blood
Even to the court, the heart, to th' seat o' th' brain,
And, through the cranks and offices of man,
The strongest nerves and small inferior veins
From me receive that natural competency
Whereby they live.'

> *Coriolanus,* I, i, 99

William Hunter [1718–1783]

Some physiologists will have it that the stomach is a mill, others that it is a fermenting vat, others again that it is a stewing pan; but, in my view of the matter, it is neither a mill, a fermenting vat, nor a stew pan, but a stomach, gentlemen, a stomach.

John Hunter [1728–1793]

The secretion of gastric juice is increased in proportion to the call for nourishment in the body.

> *Observations on Digestion*

The stomach is more affected from the internal economy of the animal than from external influence, which is the reverse of the brain.

> *Principles of Surgery,* Ch. V

The stomach is the distinguishing part between an animal and a vegetable; for we do not know any vegetable that has a stomach nor any animal without one.

> *Idem*

STROKES

William Shakespeare [1564–1616]

This apoplexy, as I take it, is a kind of lethargy, an't please your lordship; a kind of sleeping in the blood, a whoreson tingling. . . . It hath it original from much grief, from study and perturbation of the brain. I have read the cause of his effects in Galen. It is a kind of deafness.
Henry IV, Part II, I, ii, 126

WARWICK: You do know these fits
Are with his Highness very ordinary.
Stand from him, give him air; he'll
    straight be well.
CLARENCE: No, no! he cannot long
    hold out these pangs.
Th' incessant care and labour of his
    mind
Hath wrought the mure that should
    confine it in
So thin that life looks through, and
    will break out. . . .
GLOUCESTER: This apoplexy will cer-
    tain be his end.
Ibid., IV, iv, 114

Oft have I seen a timely-parted ghost,
Of ashy semblance, meagre, pale, and
    bloodless,
Being all descended to the labouring
    heart,
Who, in the conflict that it holds with
    death,
Attracts the same for aidance 'gainst
    the enemy,
Which with the heart there cools, and
    ne'er returneth
To blush and beautify the cheek again.
Henry VI, Part II, III, ii, 161

Gilles Ménage [1613–1692]

A mild attack of apoplexy may be called death's retaining fee.
Menagiana, Pt. II

Thomas Willis [1621–1675]

For in as much as the Carotidick Arteries do communicate between themselves in various places, and are mutually ingrafted; from thence a double benefit results, though of a contrary effect: because by this one and the same means care is taken, both lest the brain should be defrauded of its due watring of the blood, and also lest it should be overwhelmed by the too impetuous flowing of the swelling stream or torrent. As to the first, lest that should happen, one of the *Carotides* perhaps being obstructed, the other might supply the provision of both; then, lest the blood rushing with too full a torrent should drown the chanels and little Ponds of the brain, the flood is chastised or hindred by an opposite Emissary, as it were a Floodgate, and so is commanded to return its flood, and haste backward by the same ways, and to run back with an ebbing Tide.
Practice of Physick, "Of the Anatomy of the Brain," Ch. IV

William Heberden [1710–1801]

The inability to speak is owing sometimes not to the paralytic state of the organs of speech only, but to the utter loss of the knowledge of language and letters; which some have quickly regained, and others have recovered by slow degrees, getting the use of the smaller words first, and being frequently unable to find the word they want, and using another for it of a quite different meaning, as if it were a language which they had once known, but by long disuse had almost forgotten.
Commentaries on the History and Cure of Diseases, Ch. 69

STUDENTS

See also EDUCATION, LEARNING, MEDICAL SCHOOLS, TEACHERS, TEACHING

Sushruta [5th Cent.? B.C.]

A pupil who is pure, obedient to his

preceptor, applies himself steadily to his work, and abandons laziness and excessive sleep, will arrive at the end of the science [he has been studying].
> *Sushruta-Samhitá,* "Sutrasthánam," Ch. 3 (tr. by K. K. L. Bhishagratna)

Thomas Bond [1712–1784]

When I consider the unskillful hands the practice of physic and surgery has of necessity been committed to in many parts of America, it gives me pleasure to behold so many worthy young men training up in those professions which from the nature of their objects are the most interesting to their community.
> *The Utility of Clinical Lectures*

William Shippen, Jr. [1736–1808]

It may also be worthy of observation, that a young student is never so well qualified to pass the necessary examinations for a doctor's degree, as just after he has been industriously employed in the medical schools.
> Quoted by Betsy Copping Corner in *William Shippen, Jr.*

Johann Wolfgang von Goethe [1749–1832]

To grasp the spirit of Medicine is easy:
Learn of the great and little world your fill,
To let it go at last, so please ye,
Just as God will!
In vain that through the realms of science you may drift;
Each one learns only — just what learn he can:
Yet he who grasps the Moment's gift,
He is the proper man.
> *Faust, Part I,* Act I, Sc. iv (tr. by Bayard Taylor)

William Beaumont [1785–1853]

Of all the lessons which a young man entering upon the profession of medicine needs to learn, this is perhaps the first — that he should resist the fascination of doctrines and hypotheses till he has won the privilege of such studies by honest labor and faithful pursuit of real and useful knowledge.
> *Notebook* (ed. by J. S. Myers in *Life and Letters,* Ch. 3)

Daniel Drake [1785–1852]

The student is liable to have his mind bent upon practical matters, long before he is able to comprehend their rationale; by which his attention is diverted from elementary studies, and a foundation laid for empiricism. Of the different modes of generating quacks, this is the most prolific; and, as they bear the external marks of legitimacy, the most pernicious to society.
> *Practical Essays on Medical Education and the Medical Profession in the U.S.*

Peter Mere Latham [1789–1875]

I know that much disquietude, if not unhappiness, has been felt by students, and especially by the best informed and best disposed, when, at the entrance of their profession, they have been met by obstacles which seem insurmountable.
> *Lectures on Clinical Medicine,* Lect. I

Armand Trousseau [1801–1867]

Take care not to fancy that you are physicians as soon as you have mastered scientific facts; they only afford to your understandings an opportunity of bringing forth fruit, and of elevating you to the high position of a man of art.
> *Clinical Medicine,* Vol. I, Introduction

Oliver Wendell Holmes [1809–1894]

MEDICAL STUDENTS . . . naturally have faith in their instructors, turning to them for truth, and taking what they may choose to give them; babes in knowledge, not yet able to tell the breast from the bottle, pumping away for the milk of truth at all that offers, were it nothing better than a Professor's shrivelled forefinger.

> *Medical Essays,* "The Contagiousness of Puerperal Fever"

Charles Dickens [1812–1870]

"These here ones as is below, though, ain't reg'lar thorough-bred Sawbones; they're only in trainin'." . . . Mr. Benjamin Allen was a coarse, stout, thick-set young man, with black hair cut rather short, and a white face cut rather long. . . . He presented, altogether, rather a mildewy appearance, and emitted a fragrant odour of full-flavoured Cubas. Mr. Bob Sawyer . . . had about him that sort of slovenly smartness, and swaggering gait, which is peculiar to young gentlemen who smoke in the streets by day, shout and scream in the same by night, call waiters by their Christian names, and do various other acts and deeds of an equally facetious description. . . . [He] looked, upon the whole, something like a dissipated Robinson Crusoe.

> *Pickwick Papers,* Ch. 30

Alfred Stillé [1813–1900]

[The recent medical graduate] should never forget that . . . however closely related the several branches of medicine are to one another, each one in its turn is best learned by an almost exclusive devotion to it for a time, and when his barns are filled to bursting with his harvest, let him not forget that the grain has still to be winnowed. His fan must be in his hand to purge the threshing-floor of the dead, the unessential, the hypothetical, the fanciful, and above all, the false. In all things truth must be his object, his inspiration, and his guide.

> *Medical News* 44:433, 1884

Sir James Paget [1814–1899]

In remembering those with whom I was year after year associated, and whom it was my duty to study, nothing appears more certain than that the personal character, the very nature, the will, of each student had far greater force in determining his career than any helps or hinderances whatever. All my recollections would lead me to tell that every student may draw from his daily life a very likely forecast of his life in practice, for it will depend on himself a hundredfold more than on circumstances. The time and the place, the work to be done, and its responsibilities, will change; but the man will be the same, except in so far as he may change himself.

> *St. Bartholomew's Hospital Reports* 5:238, 1869

Louis Pasteur [1822–1895]

Young men, have faith in those powerful and safe methods, of which we do not yet know all the secrets. And, whatever your career may be, do not let yourselves be discouraged by the sadness of certain hours which pass over nations. Live in the serene peace of laboratories and libraries.

> Speech at his Golden Jubilee, December 27, 1892 (tr. by René J. Dubos)

Joseph, Lord Lister [1827–1912]

The profession to which I have the great honour to belong is, I firmly believe, on the average, the most humane of all professions. The medical student may be sometimes a rough diamond; but when he comes to have personal charge of patients, and to have the life and health of a fellow-creature depending on his individual care, he becomes a changed man, and from that day forth his life becomes a constant exercise of beneficence. With that beneficence there is associated benevolence; and in that practical way

our profession becomes the most benevolent of all.
> *British Medical Journal* 1:317,
> 1897

Daniel Coit Gilman [1831–1908]

The medical student is likely to be one son of the family too weak to labour on the farm, too indolent to do any exercise, too stupid for the bar and too immoral for the pulpit.

John Homans [1836–1903]

I prefer to be called a fool for asking the question, rather than to remain in ignorance.[1]
> Quoted in *Boston Medical and Surgical Journal* 87:1, 1872

Sir William Osler [1849–1919]

There are also the two great types, the student-lark who loves to see the sun rise, who comes to breakfast with a cheerful morning face, never so "fit" as at 6 a.m. We all know the type. What a contrast to the student-owl with his saturnine morning face, thoroughly unhappy, cheated by the wretched breakfast bell of the two best hours of the day for sleep, no appetite, and permeated with an unspeakable hostility to his *vis-à-vis*, whose morning garrulity and good humour are equally offensive. Only gradually, as the day wears on and his temperature rises, does he become endurable to himself and to others. But see him really awake at 10 p.m. while our blithe lark is in hopeless coma over his books, from which it is hard to rouse him sufficiently to get his boots off for bed, our lean owl-friend, Saturn no longer in the ascendant, with bright eyes and cheery face, is ready for four hours of anything you wish — deep study or "Heart affluence in discursive talk," and by 2 a.m. he will undertake to unsphere the spirit of Plato. In neither

[1] Retort made as a medical student in 1860 to "an upbraiding professor."

a virtue, in neither a fault, we must recognize these two types of students, differently constituted, owing possibly — though I have but little evidence for the belief — to thermal peculiarities.
> *The Student Life*

Ivan Pavlov [1849–1936]

What can I wish to the youth of my country who devote themselves to science? *Firstly,* gradualness.[1] . . . Never begin the subsequent without mastering the preceding. . . . Try to penetrate the secret of their occurrence, persistently search for the laws which govern them.

Secondly, modesty. . . . Do not allow haughtiness to take you in possession. Due to that you will be obstinate where it is necessary to agree, . . . you will lose your objectiveness. *Thirdly,* passion. Remember that science demands from a man all his life. . . . Be passionate in your work and your searchings.
> *Bequest to the Academic Youth of Soviet Russia,* February 27, 1936

School yourself to demureness and patience. Learn to innure yourself to drudgery in science. Learn, compare, collect the facts.
> *Idem*

S. Squire Sprigge [1860–1937]

First, the [medical] student must be honest, then he may get honour; and lastly, though it does not follow, he will get on.

J. Chalmers Da Costa [1863–1933]

What will become of the students? We all know in a general way. All will die sooner or later. All will get more or less happiness and prosperity. Some will become rich. Most will continue poor. Some will remain bachelors. Most will marry and breed children

[1] Cf. Dickinson W. Richards, p. 529a.

for good or ill. Most will cleave to the profession for life. . . . A very few will become eminent, but a majority will not. Some will rise as the soaring eagle, others will mount as the mousing owl. Some will snatch at comets and grasp them. Others will only pick up jelly fish and be stung for their pains. Some will set traps for birds of paradise and catch skunks. Some will dwell upon the muck heap. Others will move among the constellations of profundity, drinking in as mother's milk the glory of the stars.

> *The Trials and Triumphs of the Surgeon,* Ch. 1

Chevalier Jackson [1865–1958]

In teaching the medical student the primary requisite is to keep him awake.

> *The Life of Chevalier Jackson,* Ch. 16

Abraham Flexner [1866–1959]

The student is to collect and evaluate facts. The facts are locked up in the patient. To the patient, therefore, he must go. Waiving the personal factor, always important, that method of clinical teaching will be excellent which brings the student into close and active relations with the patient: close, by removing all hindrance to immediate investigation; active, in the sense, not merely of offering opportunities, but of imposing responsibilities.

> *Medical Education, A Comparative Study*

David Riesman [1867–1940]

If you want to get out of medicine the fullest enjoyment, be students all your lives.

Martin H. Fischer [1879–1962]

There are no dark horses. Every great man in medicine was known as a yearling.

> Quoted by Howard Fabing and Ray Marr in *Fischerisms*

Alan Gregg [1890–1957]

The chief hindrance to creativeness is the lack of convictions big enough and deep enough to give a lasting pattern to your professional life. Don't plan your future like a pontoon bridge, each petty span no longer than its predecessor.

> Graduation address, University of Texas Medical School, June 5, 1953

Wilder Penfield [1891–   ]

The undergraduate usually prefers brief and positive statements of the "facts" made by a professor who hides his doubts beneath a mantle of shining authority. It gives the student such a sense of security, especially in regard to examinations.

> *The Second Career,* "Sir Charles Sherrington"

Dickinson W. Richards [1895–   ]

The key to learning by episode is observation, close, accurate, and thorough. What of our students: are they good observers? In my experience, they are not. They can often make single keen observations, but they are not good observers. They miss too many things. In a word, they need to be taught.

> *Transactions of the American Clinical and Climatological Association* 65:91, 1953

David Seegal [1899–   ]

The apprentice in the various trades is not permitted advancement until his special line of duties has been rigorously tested under close inspection. Certainly no lesser criterion should prevail for the medical student.

> *Journal of the American Medical Association* 180:476, 1962

A characteristic which makes the doctor an effective and successful physician . . . is *compulsiveness,* or better stated, a *controlled compulsiveness*. The student exhibiting this quality in college may elicit unfavourable reactions from his classmates and receive low scholastic ratings from some of his instructors. Such a student is wont to raise more questions than his more amenable associates, he may express undue skepticism about apparently proved doctrines; and he may *check and recheck not only his data but those of his confreres and his instructors*.

> *Journal of Chronic Diseases* 17:105, 1964

The involved student may thus come to appreciate that work, work, and more work plus a sense of proportion will ease him over the unexpected and man-made hurdles during his career in medical school. By reading the autobiographies and biographies of men in medicine, he will learn that his own experiences are not unique and were faced by many other members of the profession. Disappointments, anxieties, periods of depression, self-depreciation, uncertainty and even fear abound in the early lives of many giants of medicine.

> *Journal of Medical Education* 38:605, 1963

Alexander Lenard [1910–   ]

The new doctor isn't worth very much. I went into his room, and you know what he has hidden there? Books! He still has his books! He is only a student!

> *The Valley of the Latin Bear,* Ch. 8

Robert H. Ebert [1914–   ]

For many years the teaching of medicine was authoritarian; and it was more important for the student to know what the professor thought than what was right. This was particularly true of clinical medicine; and it was unwise for the student to question the evidence presented by his clinical teacher if the student wished to graduate.

> Address to the National Tuberculosis Association, May 30, 1965

I also remain unmoved by the argument that the student has been artificially removed from the environment in which he will practice. I would remind you that this removal was accomplished over a century ago because it was found that the apprenticeship system did not provide a satisfactory educational experience, and the hospital did.

> *Idem*

The result [of current training programs] has been a curious system of dual standards within the same institution. There may, for example, be the most careful scrutiny of candidates for medical school, internship, and residency at the same time that fellows are chosen with almost no consideration except possibly insistence on the ability to read and write English. The result has been the training of many individuals in the specialties of medicine who are second-rate people with second-rate research training. These are misplaced people who would never have entered research training had there not been so much money available for research and research training.

> *Idem*

Louis Lasagna [1923–   ]

Does it seem too farfetched to picture the young Helen Keller as the symbol par excellence of every student that ever lived? We are all Helen Kellers in some degree — vision beclouded, ears undiscriminating, speech uncertain and untrue. We have all needed at one time or another, to have TRUTH spelled out slowly for us, to have our capabilities redefined and reevaluated, and the limitations of our sensations and perceptions suggested.

> *Great Teachers* (ed. by H. Peterson), Introduction

Anonymous

Gaudeamus igitur,
Juvenes dum sumus:
Post jucundam juventutem,
Post molestam senectutem
Nos habebit humus.

[Let us live then and be glad
While young life's before us.
After youthful pastime had,
After old age hard and sad,
Earth will slumber o'er us.]

> Students' song, based on a 13th-century poem (tr. by John Symonds in *Wine, Women, and Song,* No. 60)

SUCCESS

See also FAME

George Bernard Shaw [1856–1950]

A serious illness or a death advertizes the doctor exactly as a hanging advertizes the barrister who defended the person hanged. Suppose, for example, a royal personage gets something wrong with his throat, or has a pain in his inside. If a doctor effects some trumpery cure . . . nobody takes the least notice of him. But if he operates on the throat and kills the patient, or extirpates an internal organ and keeps the whole nation palpitating for days whilst the patient hovers in pain and fever between life and death, his fortune is made.

> *The Doctor's Dilemma,* "Preface on Doctors"

Charles R. Stockard [1879–1939]

Success in life depends upon the three

I's, Integrity, Intelligence and Industry.

> Aphorism

Alan Gregg [1890–1957]

There is a danger in the great rewards of success, preeminence and popularity. Perhaps success in medicine is selfish, but great impartial power used for others is not selfish.

> Aphorism (Quoted by Wilder Penfield in *The Difficult Art of Giving,* Appendix A)

SUFFERING

See also PAIN

Virgil [70–19 B.C.]

I learn to relieve the suffering. [Miseris succurrere disco.] [1]

> *Aeneid,* I.630

Dio Chrysostom [40?–115?]

Generally speaking, men are too cowardly to be willing to undergo severe suffering, since they fear death and pain, but they highly prize being mentioned as having so suffered.

> *Eleventh (Trojan) Discourse,* X (tr. by J. W. Cohoon)

Alfred de Vigny [1797–1863]

I love the majesty of human suffering.
> *La Maison du Berger*

Victor Hugo [1802–1885]

If we must suffer, let us suffer nobly.[2]
> *Contemplations,* "Les Malheureux"

John Greenleaf Whittier [1807–1892]

It is the special vocation of the doctor to grow familiar with suffering.

[1] Motto on the seal of the New Jersey College of Medicine.
[2] Souffrons, mais souffrons sur les cimes.

Louis Pasteur [1822–1895]

One does not ask of one who suffers: What is your country and what is your religion? One merely says: You suffer, this is enough for me: you belong to me and I shall help you.
>> Speech at the opening of the Philanthropic Society's Refuge for Mothers, June 8, 1886 (tr. by René J. Dubos)

William J. Mayo [1861–1939]

It is easy to philosophize; the philosopher is said to be one who bears with equanimity the sufferings of others.
>> *Minnesota Medicine* 19:468, 1936

W. Somerset Maugham [1874–1965]

I knew that suffering did not ennoble; it degraded. It made men selfish, mean, petty and suspicious. It absorbed them in small things. . . . it made them less than men; and I wrote ferociously that we learn resignation not by our own suffering, but by the suffering of others.
>> *The Summing Up,* Sect. xix

It is easy to bear others' misfortunes with fortitude, and the more remote your position, the easier it is.

French Proverb

He who fears to suffer, suffers from fear.

SUICIDE

Socrates [470–399 B.C.]

There is a doctrine whispered in secret that man is a prisoner who has no right to open the door and run away; this is a great mystery which I do not quite understand. Yet I too believe that the gods are our guardians, and that we men are a possession of theirs. . . . Then if we look at the matter thus, there may be reason in saying that a man should wait, and not take his own life until God summons him, as he is now summoning me.
>> Quoted by Plato in *Phaedo*, 62.B (tr. by Benjamin Jowett)

Cicero [106–43 B.C.]

The god who rules within us forbids us to go hence without his command.
>> *Tusculan Disputations,* I.xxx.74 (tr. by Andrew P. Peabody)

Seneca [4? B.C.–A.D. 65]

Just as I shall select my ship when I am about to go on a voyage, or my house when I propose to take a residence, so I shall choose my death when I am about to depart from life.
>> *Moral Epistles to Lucilius,* LXX.xi (tr. by Richard M. Gummerè)

Pliny the Elder [23–79]

Amid the miseries of our life on earth, suicide is God's best gift to man.
>> *Natural History,* II

St. Augustine [354–430]

If a parricide be on that account more wicked than any homicide, because he kills not merely a man but a near relative; and among parricides too, the nearer the person killed, the greater criminal he is judged to be: without doubt worse still is he who kills himself, because there is none nearer to a man than himself.
>> *Treatise on Patience* (tr. by Rev. H. Browne)

William Shakespeare [1564–1616]

>   Against self-slaughter
There is a prohibition so divine
That cravens my weak hand.
>> *Cymbeline,* III, iv, 78

O that this too too solid flesh would melt,
Thaw, and resolve itself into a dew!

Or that the Everlasting had not fix'd
His canon 'gainst self-slaughter!
         Hamlet, I, ii, 129

To be, or not to be — that is the question:
Whether 'tis nobler in the mind to suffer
The slings and arrows of outrageous fortune
Or to take arms against a sea of troubles,
And by opposing end them.
         Ibid., III, i, 56

For who would bear the whips and scorns of time,
Th' oppressor's wrong, the proud man's contumely,
The pangs of despis'd love, the law's delay,
The insolence of office, and the spurns
That patient merit of th' unworthy takes,
When he himself might his quietus make
With a bare bodkin?
         Ibid., III, i, 70

Philip Massinger [1583–1640]

                              He
That kills himself to avoid misery, fears it,
And, at the best, shews but a bastard valour.
         Maid of Honor, Act IV, Sc. iii

Sir Thomas Browne [1605–1682]

Hee forgets that hee can die who complaines of misery; wee are in the power of no calamitie while death is in our owne.
         Religio Medici, Pt. I, Sect. 44

Daniel Defoe [1659?–1731]

Self-destruction is the effect of cowardice in the highest extreme.
         An Essay Upon Projects, "Of Projectors"

Eustace Budgell [1686–1737]

What Cato did, and Addison approv'd
Cannot be wrong.
         Lines found on his desk after his suicide, May 4, 1737 (Quoted by Theophilus Cibber in *Lives of the Poets,* Vol. V, Ch. 1)

Voltaire [1694–1778]

Not that suicide always comes from madness. There are said to be occasions when a wise man takes that course: but, generally speaking, it is not in an access of reasonableness that people kill themselves.
         Letter to James Marriott, 1767

Tobias Smollett [1721–1771]

Being taken with a suppression of urine, in imitation of Pomponius Atticus, [he resolved] to take himself off by abstinence; and this resolution he executed like an ancient Roman. He saw company to the last, cracked his jokes, conversed freely, and entertained his guests with music. On the third day of his fast, he found himself entirely freed of his complaint; but refused taking sustenance. He said, the most disagreeable part of the voyage was past, and he should be a cursed fool indeed to put about ship when he was just entering the harbour. In these sentiments he persisted, without any marks of affectation; and thus finished his course with such ease and serenity, as would have done honour to the firmest stoic of antiquity.
         The Expedition of Humphry Clinker, Letter 48

Georg Christoph Lichtenberg [1742–1799]

It would be of little use if suicides could often give their reasons in precise terms, for each hearer reduces them to his own language and does not so much invalidate them as make something completely different out of them.
         Aphorismen (1764–1771)

Daniel Webster [1782–1852]

There is no refuge from confession but suicide; and suicide is confession.
> *The Murder of Captain Joseph White: Argument on the Trial of John Francis Knapp*

R. H. Barham ("Thomas Ingoldsby") [1788–1845]

She drank Prussic acid without any water,
And died like a Duke-and-a-Duchess's daughter!
> *The Ingoldsby Legends,* "The Tragedy"

Thomas Hood [1799–1845]

One more Unfortunate,
Weary of breath,
Rashly importunate,
Gone to her death!
> *The Bridge of Sighs*

George Borrow [1803–1881]

If you must commit suicide . . . always contrive to do it as decorously as possible; the decencies, whether of life or of death, should never be lost sight of.
> *Lavengro,* Ch. XXIII

Henry Wadsworth Longfellow [1807–1882]

Ah, yes! the sea is still and deep,
All things within its bosom sleep!
A single step, and all is o'er;
A plunge, a bubble, and no more.
> *Christus: A Mystery,* Pt. II, Sect. v

Henry Wheeler Shaw ("Josh Billings") [1818–1885]

Hav yu ever committed suiside, and if so, how did it seem to affect yu?
> *Josh Billings: His Sayings,* Ch. 2

James A. Garfield [1831–1881]

Suicide is not a remedy.
> Inaugural address, March 4, 1881

Friedrich Nietzsche [1844–1900]

The thought of suicide is a great consolation: by means of it one gets successfully through many a bad night.
> *Beyond Good and Evil,* Ch. IV, Sect. 157 (tr. by Helen Zimmern)

Prevention of Suicide. — There is a justice according to which we may deprive a man of life, but none that permits us to deprive him of death: that is merely cruelty.
> *Human, All Too Human,* Ch. II, Sect. 88 (tr. by Alexander Harvey)

One should die proudly when it is no longer possible to live proudly.
> *The Twilight of the Idols,* "Skirmishes in a War with the Age" (tr. by Anthony Ludovici)

Churton Collins [1848–1908]

Suicide is the worst form of murder, because it leaves no opportunity for repentance.
> Quoted by L. C. Collins in *Life and Memoirs of John Churton Collins,* Appendix VII

Woodrow Wilson [1856–1924]

I am inclined to follow the course suggested by a friend . . . who says that he has always followed the rule never to murder a man who is committing suicide.
> Letter to Bernard Baruch, August 19, 1916

Havelock Ellis [1859–1939]

The prevalence of suicide . . . without doubt, is a test of height in civilization; it means that the population is winding up its nervous and intellectual system to the utmost point of tension and that sometimes it snaps.
> *The Dance of Life,* Ch. 7

Charlotte Perkins Stetson Gilman [1860–1935]

Human life consists in mutual service. No grief, pain, misfortune, or "broken heart," is excuse for cutting off one's life while any power of service remains. But when all usefulness is over, when one is assured of an unavoidable and imminent death, it is the simplest of human rights to choose a quick and easy death in place of a slow and horrible one.

> Note written before her suicide, August 17, 1935

W. Somerset Maugham [1874–1965]

Putting aside those who regard suicide as sinful because it breaks a divine law, I think the reason of the indignation which it seems to arouse in so many is that the suicide flouts the life-force, and by setting at naught the strongest instinct of human beings casts a terrifying doubt on its power to preserve them.

> *The Summing Up,* Sect. lxxiii

Don Marquis [1878–1937]

a suicide is a person who has
considered his own case and decided
that he is worthless and who acts
as his own judge jury and executioner
and he probably knows better
than anyone else whether there is justice
in the verdict

> *the lives and times of archy and
> mehitabel: archy does his part,*
> "now look at it"

Emil Ludwig [1881–1948]

Nature puts upon no man an unbearable burden; if her limits be exceeded, man responds by suicide. I have always respected suicide as a regulator of nature.

> Untitled essay in *I Believe* (ed. by Clifton Fadiman)

Dorothy Parker [1893–1967]

Razors pain you;
Rivers are damp;
Acids stain you;
And drugs cause cramp.
Guns aren't lawful;
Nooses give;
Gas smells awful;
You might as well live.

> *Enough Rope,* "Résumé"

Svend Ranulf [1894–   ]

Statistical evidence shows that the greater the intellectual freedom, and the higher the general average of intelligence in a community, the greater is also the number of suicides.

> *The Jealousy of the Gods and
> Criminal Law at Athens,* Ch. II

SURGEONS

See also PHYSICIANS, SURGERY

Hippocrates [460?–377? B.C.]

He who wishes to be a surgeon should go to war.

> *About the Physician*

Celsus [25 B.C.–A.D. 50)

Now a surgeon should be youthful or at any rate nearer youth than age; with a strong and steady hand which never trembles, and ready to use the left hand as well as the right; with vision sharp and clear, and spirit undaunted; filled with pity, so that he wishes to cure his patient, yet is not moved by his cries, to go too fast, or cut less than is necessary; but he does everything just as if the cries of pain cause him no emotion.

> *De Medicina,* VIII, Prooemium
> (tr. by W. G. Spencer)

Henri de Mondeville [1260–1320]

It is impossible to know perfectly the

part, if one is not acquainted with the whole, even in a gross way (grosso modo); so it is impossible to be a good surgeon if one is not familiar with the foundations and generalizations of medicine. On the other hand, as it is impossible to know the whole perfectly if we are not acquainted in a certain measure with each of its parts, it is impossible for anyone to be a good physician who is absolutely ignorant of the art of surgery, with a knowledge of its possibilities and its limitations.
Treatise on Surgery (tr. by J. J. Walsh)

Many more surgeons know how to cause suppuration than to heal a wound.
Idem

The characteristics of a good surgeon are that he should be moderately bold, not given to disputations before those who do not know medicine, operate with foresight and wisdom, not beginning dangerous operations until he has provided himself with every thing necessary for lessening the danger. He should have well shaped members, especially hands with long slender fingers mobile and not tremulous, and with all his members strong and healthy, so that he may perform all the proper operations without disturbance of mind. He must be highly moral, should care for the poor for God's sake, see that he makes himself well paid by the rich, should comfort his patients by pleasant discourse and always accede to their requests if these do not interfere with the cure of the disease.
Idem

You, Surgeons, if you have operated in the homes of the rich for an adequate sum, and in the homes of the poor for charity, you should fear neither fire, nor rain, nor wind; you have no need of going into religious places nor of making penitential pilgrimages, because by your science you are able to save your souls, to live not in poverty, and to die in your own homes, to live in peace and in joy, and to exult because your recompense is grand in Paradise.
Idem

Lanfranc of Milan [d. 1315]

It is necessary that a surgeon should have a temperate and moderate disposition. That he should have well-formed hands, long slender fingers, a strong body, not inclined to tremble, and with all his members trained to the capable fulfillment of the wishes of his mind. He should be well grounded in natural science, and should know not only medicine but every part of philosophy; should know logic well, so as to be able to understand what is written; to talk properly, and to support what he has to say by good reasons.
Chirurgia Magna (tr. by J. J. Walsh)

Why, in God's name, in our days, is there such a great difference between the physician and the surgeon? The physicians have abandoned operative procedures to the laity, either, as some say, because they disdain to operate with their hands, or rather, as I think, because they do not know how to perform operations. Indeed, this abuse is so inveterate that the common people look upon it as impossible for the same person to understand both surgery and medicine. It ought, however, to be understood that no one can be a good physician who has no idea of surgical operations, and that a surgeon is nothing if ignorant of medicine. In a word one must be familiar with both departments of Medicine.
Idem

Guy de Chauliac [1300–1370]

The conditions necessary for the surgeon are four: first, he should be learned: second, he should be expert: third, he must be ingenious, and fourth, he should be able to adapt himself. It is required for the first that the surgeon should know not only the principles of surgery, but also those of medicine in theory and practice; for the second, that he should have seen others operate; for the third, that he should be ingenious, of good judgment and memory to recognize conditions; and for the fourth, that he be adaptable and able to accommodate himself to circumstances. Let the surgeon be bold in all sure things, and fearful in dangerous things; let him avoid all faulty treatments and practices. He ought to be gracious to the sick, considerate to his associates, cautious in his prognostications. Let him be modest, dignified, gentle, pitiful, and merciful; not covetous nor an extortionist of money; but rather let his reward be according to his work, to the means of the patient, to the quality of the issue, and to his own dignity.

> *Ars Chirurgica,* Introduction
> (tr. by W. A. Brennan)

A blind man works on wood the same way as a surgeon on the body, when he is ignorant of anatomy.

> *Chirurgia Magna,* Treatise I, Doctrine I, Ch. 1

Paracelsus [1493?–1541]

These are the qualifications of a good surgeon:
Regarding his innate temper:
A clear conscience,
Desire to learn and to gather experience,
A gentle heart and a cheerful spirit,
Moral manner of life and sobriety in all things,
Greater interest in being useful to his patient than to himself,
He must not be married to a bigot. . . .
He should not be a runaway monk,
He should not practise self-abuse,
He must not have a red beard,
He must not act without judgment,
He must not accept belief without understanding,
He must scorn the workings of chance,
He must not boast of knowing anything without experience,
He must never boast or praise himself,
He must despise no one.

> *Notes for the "Antimedicus"*
> (tr. by Norbert Guterman in *Selected Writings*)

Thomas Gale [1507?–1586?]

The Chirurgian must also in theis his operations observe five thynges principally. First, that he doeth it safelye, and that wythout hurte and damage to the pacient. Secondly that he do not detracte tyme or let slepe good occasions offered in workyng, but with suche spede as arte wyll soffer, let hym finishe his cure. Therdly, that he work jently, courtyously, and wyth so lytle payne the pacient, as conveniently you may, and not roughly, butcherly, rudlye, and wythoute a comblenes. Forthly, that he be as free from crafte and deceyte in all his workynges, as the East is from the Weaste. Fiftly, that he taketh no cure in the hande for lucre or gaynes sake only, but rather for an honest and competent rewarde, with a godly affection, to doe his diligence. Laste of all, that he maketh no warrantyse of suche sicknes, as are incurable, as to cure a Cancer or ulcerate, or elephantiasis confirmed; but circumspectlye to consider what the effecte is, and promyse no more then arte can performe.

> *Certain Works of Chirurgie,* "A Institution of a Chirurgian"

John Halle [1529–1568]

A chirurgien should have three dyvers properties in his person. That is to saie, a harte as the harte of a lyon, his eyes like the eyes of an hawke, and his handes the handes of a woman.

> *Epistle to the Reader* in his translation of Lanfranc's *Chirurgia Parva*

William Clowes [1544–1604]

Then rises out of his chair, fleering and jeering, this miraculous Surgeon, floriously glittering like the man in the moon, with his bracelet about his arms, . . . his fingers full of rings, a silver case with Instruments hanging at his girdle . . . and said unto me that he would open the wound, and if it were before my face. 'For,' said he, 'my business lies not in London but abroad in the country, and with such persons that I cannot or will not tarry for you nor for no other whatsoever.' And now here he did begin to brag and boast as though all the keys of knowledge did hang at his girdle.

> *A Proved Practise for All Young Chirurgeons* (ed. by F. N. L. Poynter in *Selected Writings,* Ch. 12)

Guillaume de Salluste, Seigneur du Bartas [1544–1590]

Even as a Surgion, minding off to cut
Some cure-lesse limbe; before in use he put
His violent Engines on the vicious member,
Bringeth his Patient in a sense-lesse slumber,
And grief-lesse then (guided by use and Art)
To save the whole; sawes off th' infected part.

> *Devine Weekes and Workes,* "The Sixth Day of the First Weeke" (tr. by Joshua Sylvester)

William Shakespeare [1564–1616]

> Let me have a surgeon;
I am cut to th' brains.
> *King Lear,* IV, vi, 196

With the help of a surgeon he might yet recover.

> *A Midsummer Night's Dream,* V, i, 316

For the love of God, a surgeon! Send one presently to Sir Toby. . . . Has broke my head across, and has given Sir Toby a bloody coxcomb too. For the love of God, your help!

> *Twelfth Night,* V, i, 176

John Marston [1575?–1634]

A pitiful surgeon makes a dangerous sore.

> *The Malcontent,* Act IV, Sc. ii

John Selden [1584–1654]

If a Man had a sore Leg, and he should go to an Honest Judicious Chirurgeon, and he should only bid him keep it warm, and anoint with such an Oil (an Oil well known) that would do the cure, haply he would not much regard him, because he knows the Medicine beforehand an ordinary Medicine. But if he should go to a Surgeon that should tell him, your Leg will Gangrene within three days, and it must be cut off, and you will die, unless you do something that I could tell you, what listening there would be to this Man!

> *Table-Talk,* "Damnation"

Robert Herrick [1591–1674]

'Tis the Chyrurgions praise, and height of Art,
Not to cut off, but cure the vicious part.

> *Hesperides,* "Lenitie"

John Earle [1601?–1665]

His gaines are very ill got, for he lives by the hurts of the Common-wealth. He differs from a physician as a sore do's from a disease or the sicke from those that are not whole, the one distempers you within, the other blisters you without. . . . The rareness of his custome makes him pittiless when it comes: and he holds a Patient longer then our Courts a Cause.

> *Microcosmographie,* Ch. 42

John Jones [1729–1791]

The mind . . . must be prepar'd before its entrance into the study of sur-

gery, by a previous acquisition of those branches of knowledge, which form the rules by which we ought to conduct ourselves in the cure of diseases. 'Tis to such cultivated geniuses, that surgery owes its greatest progress — such were a Serverinus, a Fallopius, a Hildanus, a Vesalius, a Scultetus, a Le Dran, a Wiseman, a Cheselden, a Monro, a Sharp. These illustrious surgeons, whose minds were prepar'd by the study of the learn'd languages, cultivated by the belles lettres, and enrich'd with the knowledge of Philosophy, have hung up the best lights to conduct us through the dark and intricate windings of our art.
Introductory Lecture to His Course in Surgery

John Pearson [1758–1826]

He who reduces the province of a Surgeon to the performance of operations, and consequently directs his attention in a transient and careless manner to the less splendid parts of his profession, may learn the art of mutilating his fellow creatures, but will never deserve to be treated as a good Surgeon.
Principles of Surgery, Preface

Sir Astley Paston Cooper [1768–1841]

I have made many mistakes myself; in learning the anatomy of the eye I dare say, I have spoiled a hatful; the best surgeon, like the best general, is he who makes the fewest mistakes.
Lectures on Surgery

It is the surgeon's duty to tranquillize the temper, to beget cheerfulness, and to impart confidence of recovery.
Ibid., Lect. I

My lectures were highly esteemed, but I am of opinion my operations rather kept down my practice.
Quoted by F. H. Garrison in *Bulletin of the New York Academy of Medicine* 5:155, 1929

Ephraim McDowell [1771–1830]

[Mechanical surgeons] have been the *bane* of the science; intruding themselves into the ranks of the profession, with no other qualification but boldness in undertaking, ignorance of their responsibility, and indifference to the lives of their patients; proceeding according to the special dictates of some author, as mechanical as themselves, they cut and tear with fearless indifference, utterly incapable of exercising any judgment of their own in cases of emergency; and sometimes, without possessing even the slightest knowledge of the anatomy of the parts concerned. The preposterous and impious attempts of such pretenders, can seldom fail to prove destructive to the patient, and disgraceful to the science. It is by such this noble science has been degraded in the minds of many, to the rank of an art.
The Eclectic Repertory and Analytical Review, Medical and Philosophical 9:546, 1819

Sir Charles Bell [1774–1842]

The public, who are so ready to determine on the merits of our profession, and even the patients who are to suffer, are surprisingly ignorant both of the Surgeon's motives for what he does, and the propriety of the methods he puts in practice. He is continually operating in secret as a matter of necessity. The most sensible give the decision up to him; so that he is answerable to his own conscience, and to that alone.
Illustrations of the Great Operations in Surgery, Preface

Valentine Mott [1785–1865]

We regard those as surgeons, and those alone, who have by conscientious devotion to the study of our science, and the daily habitual discharge of its multifarious duties, acquired that knowledge which renders the mind of the practitioner serene, his judgement sound, and his hand skillful while it holds out to the patient rational hopes for amended health and prolonged life.

> Quoted in *Annals of Surgery* 107:644, 1938

Honoré de Balzac [1799–1850]

The glory of surgeons is like that of actors, who exist only in their lifetime and whose talent is no longer appreciable once they have disappeared.

> *The Atheist's Mass* (tr. by Francis T. Furey)

Alexandre Dumas père [1802–1870]

A good surgeon operates with his hand, not with his heart.

Alfred, Lord Tennyson [1809–1892]

Our doctor had call'd in another, I
  never had seen him before,
But he sent a chill to my heart when I
  saw him come in at the door,
Fresh from the surgery-schools of
  France and of other lands —
Harsh red hair, big voice, big chest,
  big merciless hands! . . .

Wonderful cures he had done, O yes,
  but they said too of him
He was happier using the knife than in
  trying to save the limb,
And that I can well believe, for he
  look'd so coarse and so red,
I could think he was one of those who
  would break their jests on the
  dead.
> *In the Children's Hospital*

Sir George Murray Humphry [1820–1896]

In surgery, eyes first and most; fingers next and little; tongue last and least.

Joseph, Lord Lister [1827–1912]

To intrude an unskilled hand into such a piece of Divine mechanism as the human body is indeed a fearful responsibility.

> *Lister and the Lister Ward in the Royal Infirmary of Glasgow*, Ch. 1

George G. Ross [1834–1892]

Any fool can cut off a leg — it takes a surgeon to save one.

Henry Maudsley [1835–1918]

A possible apprehension now is that the surgeon be sometimes tempted to supplant instead of aiding Nature.

Sir Clifford Allbutt [1836–1925]

From the time of Hippocrates surgery has ever been the salvation of inner medicine. In inner medicine physicians have dwelt too much on dogmas, opinions and speculations; and too often their errors passed undiscovered to the grave. The surgeon, for his good, has had a sharper training on facts; his errors hit him promptly in the face.

> *Lancet*, 1922

Maurice Richardson [1851–1912]

The surgeon reviewing his active years of practice cannot but be impressed by the responsibilities of his profession. He recalls the frequent misgivings with which, on the strength of his fallible opinion, he has advised and performed operations; the excitement of a critical operation and the deep breath of thankfulness when he has succeeded in averting some grave complication; his forebodings become realities; the too often useless struggle against overwhelming odds; the distressful death; the severe self-criticism and biting regrets. And is not the surgeon, appreciating his own unfitness in spite of years of devotion, in the position to condemn those who lightly take up such burdens without preparation and too often without conscience?

> *Journal of the American Medical Association* 61:161, 1913

William Stewart Halsted
[1852–1922]

Not so very long ago a surgeon requested me to assist him to perform a circular suture of the intestine (end to end anastomosis) upon one of his patients. He readily consented to practice the operation upon dogs. At first his dogs died. He finally succeeded in saving more than 50 per cent of the dogs operated upon. The operation upon his patient required five hours, but was successful. It is not difficult to predict what the result would have been if the practice on dogs had been omitted. . . .

I believe that the license to practice general surgery should be withheld from those who have not practiced on animals the operations for circular suture of the intestine and intestinal anastomosis.

> Surgical Papers, Vol. I, "Inflated Rubber Cylinders for Circular Suture of the Intestine"

Stephen Paget [1855–1926]

You cannot be a perfect surgeon, till you have enjoyed in your own person some surgical experience.[1]

> Confessio Medici, Ch. 7

Robert Tuttle Morris [1857–1945]

A vain surgeon is like a milking stool, of no use except when sat upon.

Rudolph Matas [1860–1957]

He needs the broad vision, the cultivated imagination, the catholicity of artistic taste and human sentiment, that give to his manual accomplishments the attributes and qualities that glorify the hand in the higher arts. To *do* all this and to *be* all this, the Master Surgeon must be a man of mind, a man of thought, a man who knows his prov-

[1] Cf. Chinese Proverb, p. 415b; Proverb, p. 592b.

ince, the human body, as a whole and not only one of its parts.

> Introduction to W. S. Halsted's *Surgical Papers*

It is the harmonious unison of mind and the senses, the hand and the head, science and craft, exhibited in the supermen who have exalted the fine art, from antiquity to the present time, that we find the ideal, difficult to attain it is true, that should be in the mind of those who aspire to the mastery of our profession.

> *Idem*

John Hammond Bradshaw
[1861–1943]

Now the welfare of the patient is our first consideration, not the welfare of our pockets, or our fame as an operator. In order best to conserve that welfare in our surgical work, we must always keep in mind that every wound of the human body is like a sensitive plant. It responds to gentle treatment and resents brutality. It is, moreover, in our own interest to be gentle, for we shall find that we get full compensation for value received: our wounds will heal better, our results will be better, our reputations will be better, and we shall have better satisfaction with ourselves and our work.

In a few words, therefore, we should be gentle-men!

> Surgery, Gynecology & Obstetrics 45:804, 1927

William J. Mayo [1861–1939]

The surgeon is often intolerant and the internist self sufficient.

> Surgery, Gynecology & Obstetrics 32:97, 1921

I think all of us who have worked years in the profession understand that many very skillful operators are not good surgeons.

> Ibid., 67:535, 1938

J. Chalmers Da Costa [1863–1933]

It is the solemn and imperative duty of a surgeon to give to able and worthy young men a chance to become surgeons. He should train them — weed out the unfit — stimulate and encourage the fit — stand by them till they can go it alone. Next to a good name there is no heritage I would so much like to leave as a group of fine young surgeons to whom I had had the good fortune to open doors of opportunity. Think of the benefit to humanity of such a heritage. Think of those men remembering the man who helped them with enduring affection.

The Trials and Triumphs of the Surgeon, Ch. 1

Most medical students are attracted to surgery. Its positive results please them. The bloody drama of the operation fascinates them, the dramatic force of some great operator stirs their admiration. They note decisive achievements and wonderful successes. They hear little of failures. They know nothing of the haunting anxieties, the keen disappointments, the baffling perplexities, the dread responsibilities, and the numerous self-reproaches of one who spends his life as an operating surgeon. Yet few even of these admiring students become surgeons. Some suffer disenchantment during their student days. Many lack the necessary qualities. Many shrink from the responsibility. Some never get an opportunity. Many find an opening in general practice and seize it for a livelihood. The very best minds in the class seldom lean to surgery. This is a sad admission, but it is true. Men with deep, broad, philosophic minds usually tend to laboratory science and experimental medicine. That such minds are apt to be repelled by surgery is often the fault of the teacher.

Idem

We waste much time blushing for the evil things done by our friends. In fact, the wisdom of some surgeons consists in knowing with certainty what other surgeons should or should not have done.

Idem

Sir Berkeley Moynihan [1865–1936]

The surgeon may in some degree share his responsibilities with others, but the chief responsibility must always lie with him, and being his must be exercised not only during the operation but also before, perhaps long before, and also after, perhaps long after, the operation is performed. The operation itself is but one incident, no doubt the most dramatic, yet still only one in the long series of events which must stretch between illness and recovery.

Lancet 2:789, 1926

Now of operators there are many types, and, like every other work of art, an operation is the expression of a man's temperament and character. There are still among us "brilliant" operators, from whom I pray to be spared when my hour has come. For them it is the mere quality of effort that counts. Their ideal of operative surgery is something swift and infinitely dexterous, something to dazzle the beholder, and excite his wonder that such things can so be done by human hands. The body of a man is the plastic material in which an artist works, and no art is worthy of such a medium unless it has in it something of a sacrament. Surgery of the "brilliant" kind is a desecration. Such art finds its proper scope in tricks with cards, in juggling with billiard balls, and nimble encounters with bowls of vanishing goldfish.

Surgery, Gynecology & Obstetrics 31:549, 1920

Robert B. Greenough [1871–1937]

The science and art of medicine is of necessity so little understood by the laity that they are obliged to entrust their lives and their welfare to the physician rather upon faith in his character and reputation than upon actual experience of his abilities. Thus, conscience becomes one of the most important elements in the character of the physician. Especially is this true as regards the surgeon, for his activities are carried on largely in the seclusion of the operating room and often only his colleagues and his assistants are in a position to judge intelligently whether his ministrations to the sick and injured are as efficient as the existing state of surgical knowledge and resources will permit. It is this fact that seems to justify a review of some of the features of the practice of surgery, which require a keen conscience on the part of the surgeon and a definite sense of responsibility to his patient, to his hospital, to his colleagues, and to the whole community.

> *Surgery, Gynecology & Obstetrics* 62:390, 1936

Russell John Howard
[1875–1942]

The first attribute of a surgeon is an insatiable curiosity.

> Quoted by F. G. St. Clair Strange in *The Hip*, Ch. 2

A surgeon has very little influence on the course of a deep suppuration.

> *Ibid.*, Ch. 8

Speed in operating should be the achievement, not the aim, of every surgeon.

> *Ibid.*, Ch. 9

Martin H. Fischer [1879–1962]

A good surgeon is a good medical man who can cut.

> Quoted by Howard Fabing and Ray Marr in *Fischerisms*

René Leriche [1879–　]

The individual on whom we operate is more than a physiological mechanism.

He thinks, he fears, his body trembles if he lacks the comfort of a sympathetic face. For him nothing will replace the salutary contact with his surgeon, the exchange of looks, the feeling that the doctor has taken charge, with the certainty, at least apparent, of winning. These are the imponderables which we have no right to sacrifice.

> *La Philosophie de la Chirurgie*, Foreword (tr. by Roberta Hurwitz)

Every surgeon carries about him a little cemetery, in which from time to time he goes to pray, a cemetery of bitterness and regret, of which he seeks the reason for certain of his failures.

> *Ibid.*, Pt. II, Ch. 1

Sir Harold Gillies [1882–1960]
and
D. Ralph Millard, Jr. [1919–　]

There is no better training for a surgeon than to be taught observation by a physician.

> *The Principles and Art of Plastic Surgery*, Vol. I, Ch. 2

Surgical style is the expression of personality and training exhibited by the movements of the fingers; its hallmark — dexterity and gentleness.

> *Idem*

Evarts A. Graham [1883–1957]

In many respects surgery is like music which has its great artists and its great composers. The great musical artists are like the great practical surgeons. They perform frequently before large audiences with a high degree of skill, and they make large incomes. But what they render is the work of the composers, the thoughtful men who have made it possible for them to perform and who too often have received but little financial reward. At the present time surgery needs more men of the composer type.

> *Southern Medical Journal* 18: 864, 1925

John J. Morton [1886–   ]

When a medical student puts years of his life into training to become a surgeon he has a right to ask what attributes should be possessed by the surgeon who is responsible for his training.

Surgery 44:927, 1958

Sir Heneage Ogilvie [1887–   ]

The surgeon who is his own physician, though he often has a fool for a colleague, has the happiness of working in an atmosphere of mutual confidence and admiration.

Lancet 2:1, 1948

Edwin P. Lehman [1888–1954]

Courage is often necessary to maintain equanimity or to exercise complete intellectual honesty, but as a separate entity it has characteristics of its own. It is the quality that enables the surgeon to assume responsibility for the remote chance of helping the desperately ill patient no matter what the risk. It is the quality that refuses to consider mortality rates or public reaction. It is fearlessness of any consequence except harm to the patient.

Annals of Surgery 129:545, 1949

Ben Hecht [1894–1964]

His wide mouth smiled quickly and abstractedly, as is often the case with surgeons who train their reactions not to interfere with their concentration.

Miracle of the Fifteen Murderers

Owen H. Wangensteen [1898–   ]

Because of the very nature of the cares and heavy responsibilities shared by surgeons, they come to have a certain preoccupation of mind. Try as we may, it is not easy to disguise completely our feelings when vexed with anxieties over ill patients. Those who know us best seem to be able to divine our true state of mind. The cares of patients weigh heavily upon the mind of the surgeon and it is understandable that his spirits may exhibit some of the fluctuations of a barometer contingent upon how the patients under his care are getting on. Who among us has not felt a certain buoyancy of spirit when a very ill postoperative patient takes a turn for the better?

Surgery, Gynecology & Obstetrics 84:567, 1947

For the difficult surgery of today, a sturdy pair of legs is also an indispensable necessity!

Idem

John S. Lockwood [1907–1950]

A major difference between responsibility of pilot and surgeon is that the former shares directly in the consequences of his error or neglect, while the latter does not. . . . the question might be asked as to whether the individual patient is any better able to judge the competence of a surgeon than is the passenger to select his pilot. In both cases selection must be based upon the judgment of competent examiners rather than incompetent consumers of the specialist's services. Here again the pilot is by circumstances allowed only one serious mistake, while the surgeon may commit many and not even recognize his own errors as such.

Annals of Surgery 130:589, 1949

Everett Idris Evans [1909–1954]

These surgeons of conscience (though perhaps relatively few in number) if left unfettered in our free society, will in time leaven the entire profession.

Annals of Surgery 132:315, 1950

Stanley O. Hoerr [1909–   ]

The surgeon is a man of action. By

temperament and by training he prefers to serve the sick by operating on them, and he inwardly commiserates with a patient so unfortunate as to have a disease not suited to surgical treatment. Young surgeons, busy mastering the technicalities of the art, are particularly alert to seize every legitimate opportunity to practice technical maneuvers, the more complicated the better.
American Journal of Surgery
103:411, 1962

We should always let our judgments and recommendations be guided by the fact that we operate on patients, not on diseases.
Idem

Francis D. Moore [1913–   ]

The surgical investigator must be a bridgetender, channeling knowledge from biologic science to the patient's bedside and back again. He traces his origin from both ends of the bridge. He is thus a bastard, and is called this by everybody. Those at one end of the bridge say that he is not a very good scientist, and those at the other end say he does not spend enough time in the operating room.
Surgery 44:1, 1958

Dylan Thomas [1914–1953]

When *I* take up assassination, I shall start with the surgeons in this city and work *up* to the gutter.
The Doctor and the Devils, Sc. 88

Lloyd G. Stevenson [1918–   ]

America, it has been said, was a land of practical men, of artisans and mechanics, of doers rather than theorizers. It was therefore a land of surgeons. The same ingenuity in mechanical contrivance which was proving so beneficial in industry was exhibited

also in the operating room. Americans were also thought to be impatient, prone to gamble, willing to take a risk. They were consequently ready to perform, or willing to submit to, heroic operative procedures.
Yale Journal of Biology and Medicine 33:159, 1960

John Le Carré [1931–   ]

He is like the surgeon who has grown tired of blood. He is content that others should operate.
The Spy Who Came In from the Cold

Charles Brook [fl. 1945]

It can be reasonably supposed that the average person, if asked to define the difference between a physician and a surgeon, would reply "a surgeon uses the knife while the physician prescribes medicines," but the real distinction is that the physician and the surgeon belong to entirely different schools of medical thought. The good physician is a disciple of Paracelsus, who was a sceptic, while the good surgeon is a disciple of Galen, who was a good dogmatist.
Battling Surgeon, Ch. 1

Anonymous

The egotistical surgeon is like a monkey; the higher he climbs the more you see of his less attractive features.[1]

Proverb

The best surgeon is he that has been well hacked himself.[2]

Arabic Proverb

The surgeon practices on the orphan's head.

[1] English Proverb: The higher the ape goes the more he shows his tail.
[2] Cf. Chinese Proverb, p. 415b; Stephen Paget, p. 588a.

SURGERY

See also MEDICINE, OPERA-
TIONS, SURGEONS

Sushruta [5th Cent.? B.C.]

All hold this Tantram [surgery] to be
most important of all the other
branches of the Áyurveda [science of
medicine], in as much as instantaneous
actions can be produced. . . . Hence
it is the highest in value of all the
medical Tantras. It is eternal and a
source of infinite piety, imparts fame
and opens the gates of Heaven to its
votaries, prolongs the durations of
human existence on earth, and helps
men in successfully fulfilling their mis-
sions, and earning a decent competence, in life.
> *Sushruta-Samhitá,* "Sutrasthá-
> nam," Ch. 1 (tr. by K. K. L.
> Bhishagratna)

Sophocles [496?–406 B.C.]

No good physician quavers incanta-
tions
When the malady he's treating needs
the knife.
> *Ajax,* 582 (tr. by J. Moore)

Callicter

Agelaus by operating killed Aces-
torides, for he said, "If he had lived
the poor fellow would have been
lame."
> *Greek Anthology,* XI.121 (tr.
> by W. R. Paton)

Galen [fl. 2nd Cent.]

Surgery is the ready motion of steady
and experienced hands.
> *Definitiones Medicae,* XXXV

Henri de Mondeville [1260–1320]

Surgery undoubtedly is superior to
medicine for the following reasons: 1.

Surgery cures more complicated maladies, such as toward which medicine
is helpless. 2. Surgery cures diseases
that cannot be cured by any other
means, not by themselves, not by nature, nor by medicine. Medicine indeed
never cures a disease so evidently that
one could say that the cure is due to
medicine. 3. The doings of surgery
are visible and manifest, while those
of medicine are hidden, which is very
fortunate for many physicians. If they
have made a mistake, it is not apparent and if they kill the patient, it
will not be done openly. But if the
surgeon commits an error while performing an incision on the hand or
arm, this is seen by everybody present
and could not be attributed to nature
nor to the constitution of the patient.
> *Treatise on Surgery*

Lanfranc of Milan [d. 1315]

All practice is theory; all surgery is
practice; ergo, all surgery is theory.
> *Chirurgia Magna*

Guy de Chauliac [1300–1370]

Think what a precious thing you work
upon. It is the temple of God, his own
image, the most precious creature that
ever God made.
> *Guydos Questions,* Preface

I have shewed the young Chirurgion
the meanes to doe it safely, without
tormenting the patients for nothing.

John of Mirfield [1362–1407]

The Surgeon, however, should leave
the sick man alone rather than operate, if he is in any doubt: for it is
safer to leave a man in the hands of
his Creator, than to put trust in surgery or medicine concerning which
there is any manner of doubt.
> *Floriarum Bartholomei,* "De
> Medicis et Eorum Medicinis"

Ambroise Paré [1517?–1590]

Five things are proper to the duty of a Chirurgian; To take away that which is superfluous; to restore to their places such things as are displaced; to separate those things which are joined together; to join those that are separated; and to supply the defects of nature.
> *Works,* Bk. I, Ch. 2 (tr. by T. H. Johnson)

William Clowes [1544–1604]

Indeed, it is, I suppose unpossible in the whole course of man's life that he is able without great care, study, and much diligence, to labour commendably, and with a good conscience to work in the Vineyard of Surgery.
> *Treatise on Struma* (ed. by F. N. L. Poynter in *Selected Writings,* Ch. 1)

William Shakespeare [1564–1616]

Can honour set to a leg? No. Or an arm? No. Or take away the grief of a wound? No. Honour hath no skill in surgery then? No.
> *Henry IV, Part I,* V, i, 133

Ben Jonson [1573?–1637]

Th' incurable cut off, the rest reforme.
> *Cynthia's Revels,* Act V, Sc. xi

Percivall Pott [1714–1788]

If practitioners, since the time of Albucasis, had been contented with his doctrine, and never had ventured to think for themselves, surgery had not been what it now is, and its great merit would still have consisted in the multiplicity of its hot irons.
> *Chirurgical Works,* Vol. I, "General Remarks on Fractures and Dislocations"

Many and great are the improvements which the chirurgic art has received within these last fifty years; and many thanks are due to those who have contributed to them: but when we reflect how much still remains to be done, it should rather excite our industry than inflame our vanity.
> *Ibid.,* Vol. III, "Chirurgical Observations Relative to the Cataract . . ."

John Hunter [1728–1793]

One gentleman said 'he did not choose to lose any reputation he might have in surgery by giving lectures,' which was at least modest. Talking of the improvement of the art, one of the surgeons confessed that 'He did not see where the art could be improved.' The natural conclusion from this declaration was that such a man would never improve it.[1]
> Letter, 1793

This last part of surgery, namely, operations, is a reflection on the healing art; it is a tacit acknowledgement of the insufficiency of surgery. It is like an armed savage who attempts to get that by force which a civilized man would get by stratagem.
> *Principles of Surgery,* Introduction

The principles of our art are not less necessary to be understood than the principles of the other sciences.
> *Ibid.,* Ch. 1

John Hilton [1804–1878]

It would be well, I think, if the surgeon would fix upon his memory, as the first professional thought which should accompany him in the course of his daily occupation, this physiological truth — that Nature has a constant tendency to repair the injuries to which her structures may have been subjected, whether those injuries be the result of fatigue or exhaustion, of inflammation or acci-

---

[1] Hunter was explaining in this letter the ineffectual teaching at St. George's Hospital, London.

dent. Also that this reparative power becomes at once most conspicuous when the disturbing cause has been removed: thus presenting to the consideration of the physician and surgeon a constantly recurring and sound principle for his guidance in his professional practice.

On Rest and Pain, Lect. 3

Bernhard von Langenbeck [1810–1887]

It is less important to invent new operations and new techniques of operating than to find ways and means to avoid surgery. Yet, it has become increasingly difficult to keep abreast of and to assimilate the investigative reports which accumulate day after day. Albrecht von Grafe, my unforgettable friend, was ill at ease because he felt unable to control even the area of his own discipline; one suffocates, he once told me, through exposure to the massive body of rapidly growing information.

Address at the First Congress of Surgery, April 10, 1872 (tr. by Max Samter)

Sir John Erichsen [1818–1896]

There must be a final limit to the development of manipulative surgery. The knife cannot always have fresh fields for conquest; and although methods of practice may be modified and varied, and even improved to some extent, it must be within a certain limit. That this limit has nearly, if not quite, been reached will appear evident if we reflect on the great achievements of modern operative surgery.

Lancet 2:489, 1873

Theodor Billroth [1829–1894]

One may perform surgical procedures only if there is a little chance of success. To operate without having a chance means to prostitute the beautiful art and science of surgery.

Robert Lawson Tait [1845–1899]

When in doubt, drain.

Quoted in *Archives of Surgery* 89:686, 1964

Sir William Osler [1849–1919]

The surgical cycle in woman: Appendix removed, right kidney hooked up, gall-bladder taken out, gastro-enterostomy, clean sweep of uterus and adnexa.

Quoted by William B. Bean in *Sir William Osler: Aphorisms,* Ch. 5

William Stewart Halsted [1852–1922]

The only weapon with which the unconscious patient can immediately retaliate upon the incompetent surgeon is hemorrhage.

Bulletin of the Johns Hopkins Hospital 23:191, 1912

In a wound that is perfectly dry, and in tissues never permitted to become even stained by blood, the operator, unperturbed, may work for hours without fatigue. The confidence gradually acquired from masterfulness in controlling hemorrhage gives to the surgeon the calm which is so essential for clear thinking and orderly procedure at the operating table.

The Johns Hopkins Hospital Reports 19:71, 1920

In ligating the first portion of the left subclavian within the chest the operator may not, as formerly, be more greatly impressed by the magnitude and cleverness of his performance than by the miraculous effect of the ligation of the artery upon the great, pulsating tumor which with each beat of the heart jarred the whole frame of the sufferer. The moment of tying the ligature is indeed a dramatic one. The monstrous, booming tumor is stilled

by a tiny thread, the tempest silenced by the magic wand.
> *Surgical Papers*, Vol. I, "Ligations of the Left Subclavian Artery in Its First Portion"

Robert Tuttle Morris [1857–1945]

The greatest triumph of surgery today . . . lies in finding ways for avoiding surgery.
> *Doctors Versus Folks*, Ch. 3

Allow patients to escape with the slightest attack of surgery your skill can supply.

August Bier [1861–1949]

The surgeon should not make beautiful anatomical preparations because he would destroy the natural arrangements.

Sir Berkeley Moynihan [1865–1936]

As art surgery is incomparable in the beauty of its medium, in the supreme mastery required for its perfect accomplishment, and in the issues of life, suffering, and death which it so powerfully controls.
> *Addresses on Surgical Subjects*, "The Approach to Surgery"

No training of the surgeon can be too arduous, no discipline too stern, and none of us may measure our devotion to our cause. For us an operation is an incident in the day's work, but for our patients it may be, and no doubt it often is, the sternest and most dreaded of all trials, for the mysteries of life and death surround it, and it must be faced alone.
> *Idem*

Surgery, after all, is an affair of the spirit; it is a fierce test of a man's technical skill, sometimes, but, in a grim or long fight, it is above all a trial of the spirit; and there are few things that can not be conquered if a man's heart is set on victory.
> Letter to Dr. Charles M. Graney

Every operation in surgery is an experiment in bacteriology. The success of the experiment in respect to the salvation of the patient, the quality of healing in the wound, the amount of local or constitutional reaction, the discomforts during the days following operation, and the nature and severity of any possible sequels, depend not only on the skill but also upon the care exercised by the surgeon in the ritual of the operation.

Harvey Cushing [1869–1939]

I would like to see the day when somebody would be appointed surgeon somewhere who had no hands, for the operative part is the least part of the work.
> Letter to Dr. Henry Christian, November 20, 1911

William D. Haggard [1872–1940]

In the other fine arts, art is justified for the sake of art. In surgery it is a real need because upon the finesse and perfection of its artistry, the success of a surgical procedure largely and sometimes entirely depends. It is the art of the sculptor rendered with the heroism and skill of a lifesaver.
> *Surgery, Queen of the Arts*, Ch. 1

Russell John Howard [1875–1942]

The most important person in the operating theatre is the patient.
> Quoted by F. G. St. Clair Strange in *The Hip*, Ch. 3

Martin H. Fischer [1879–1962]

The practice of medicine is a thinker's art, the practice of surgery a plumber's.
> Aphorism

Sir Harold Gillies [1882–1960]
and
D. Ralph Millard, Jr. [1919–]

There is little that can be called original since a sharp flint opened an abscess and some horsehair threaded through the first thorn needle sewed up a wound. Yet it all goes on, bit by bit, and the wheel of progress turns just a little in any man's lifetime.

The Principles and Art of Plastic Surgery, Acknowledgments

Logan Clendening [1884–1945]

Surgery does the ideal thing — it separates the patient from his disease. It puts the patient back to bed and the disease in a bottle.

Modern Methods of Treatment, Ch. 1

Edwin P. Lehman [1888–1954]

The great brake upon unnecessary operations by unscrupulous or incompetent operators has been in the past the fear of fatality. The extraordinary developments of surgery in the past ten years have almost removed this brake. The modern methods of protecting the patient by adequate preoperative preparation, properly chosen and skillfully administered anesthesia, continuous support on the operating table, and alert, postoperative care are available to the unjust as well as to the just. It is easy to remove a normal gall-bladder or a normal uterus if only one in 200 will succumb. How different it was in the days when one in ten or even one in five could be expected to die. Now the operator can be reasonably certain that his reputation for serving his patients is secure. How simple it has been made for him! This fact alone makes it urgent at all cost to salvage the good name of surgery.

Surgery 28:595, 1950

William E. Tanner [1889–]

Surgery is one of the humanities be-cause it must always take into account the nature peculiar to the human being.

Sir W. Arbuthnot Lane, Epilogue

Isidor S. Ravdin [1894–]

The surgeons of the future will not tolerate the divorce of the hand from the brain, and the surgery of the future will not again be merely a handicraft. . . . In the surgery of the future the individualist will be left by the roadside, for after all surgery is part of that broader field of experimental pathology to which all the medical sciences belong.

Annals of Surgery 127:666, 1948

Edward D. Churchill [1895–]

Surgery is in large part a handicraft with elaborate technics that may be grouped as Technology. . . . if one be honest . . . he cannot fail to see that Surgery is seeded with *ad hoc* hypotheses, or, in more frank terms, empiricisms and irrational beliefs.

Annals of Surgery 126:381, 1947

Warren H. Cole [1898–]

Too often, surgical therapy for elective conditions is postponed in elderly patients, in the hope, I presume, that the patient will die of some other disease before the present one threatens his life.

Annals of Surgery 138:145, 1953

A. Gerard Brom [1915–]

It is with coarctation surgery as with love: rather easy to do but difficult to understand.

Journal of Thoracic and Cardiovascular Surgery 50:166, 1965

John Rowan Wilson [1919–   ]

I've always said that the most useful equipment for a successful surgeon is a pessimistic pathologist.
Hall of Mirrors, Pt. III, Ch. 7

Arthur H. Keeney [1920–   ]

Pray before surgery, but remember God will not alter a faulty incision.
Aphorism

Anonymous

Thou shouldst cleanse [it] for him [with] two plugs of linen. Thou shouldst place two [other] plugs of linen saturated with grease in the inside of his two nostrils. Thou shouldst put [him] at his mooring stakes until the swelling is reduced [lit. drawn out]. Thou shouldst apply for him stiff rolls of linen by which his nose is held fast. Thou shouldst treat him afterward [with] grease, honey [and] lint, every day until he recovers.[1]
Edwin Smith Surgical Papyrus, Vol. I, Case 11 (tr. by J. H. Breasted)

Proverb

Lose a leg rather than life.

Montenegrin Proverb

In a good hand every sword cuts well.

SURVIVAL

See EVOLUTION

SWEAT

Seneca [4? B.C.–A.D. 65]

It is not manly to fear sweat.
Moral Epistles to Lucilius, XXXI.vii.31

[1] This treatment for a broken nose is part of the oldest record of surgical teaching, dating to around 3000 B.C.

What have I to do with those hot baths or with the sweating-room where they shut in the dry steam which is to drain your strength? Perspiration should flow only after toil.
Ibid., LI.vi (tr. by Richard M. Gummere)

William Shakespeare [1564–1616]

SYRACUSE DROMIO: She sweats a man may go over shoes in the grime of it.
SYRACUSE ANTIPHOLUS: That's a fault that water will mend.
SYRACUSE DROMIO: No, sir, 'tis in grain.
The Comedy of Errors, III, ii, 105

> Falstaff sweats to death
And lards the lean earth as he walks along.
Henry IV, Part I, II, ii, 115

John Ford [1586?–1640?]

> Sweats hot as sulpher
Boil through my pores!
The Broken Heart, Act IV

St. Jean Baptiste de la Salle [1651–1719]

When excessive perspiration makes it needful to wipe the face, it ought to be done with a handkerchief, and not with the hand, except in the case of extreme necessity; by attending to this, serious inconvenience may be avoided, for the rubbing of the hand on the face may give rise to ringworm, pimples, etc.
The Rules of Christian Manners and Civility, I

Henry Wadsworth Longfellow [1807–1882]

His brow is wet with honest sweat.
The Village Blacksmith

Thomas Dwight [1843–1911]

None but [Oliver Wendell] Holmes could have compared the microscopical

coiled tube of the sweat gland to a fairy's intestine.
Scribner's Magazine, January 1895

The Bible

They shall not gird themselves with any thing that causeth sweat.
Ezekiel 44:18

His [Jesus'] sweat was as it were great drops of blood falling down to the ground.
Luke 22:44

SWEATING SICKNESS

See also EPIDEMICS, PLAGUE

John Caius [1510–1573]

For this [the plague] commonly giveth three or four, often seven, sometimes nine, . . . sometimes eleven, and sometimes fourteen days' respect to whom it vexeth. But that [the sweating sickness] immediately killed some in opening their windows, some in playing with children in their street doors, some in one hour, many in two it destroyed, and at the longest, to they that merrily dined, it gave a sorrowful supper.
Works, "A Book or Counsel Against the Disease Commonly Called the Sweat or Sweating Sickness"

SYMPTOMS

See also DIAGNOSIS, PROGNOSIS

Thomas Sydenham [1624–1689]

Nature, in the production of disease, is uniform and consistent, so much so, that for the same disease in different persons the symptoms are for the most part the same; and the selfsame phenomena that you would observe in the sickness of a Socrates you would observe in the sickness of a simpleton.
Medical Observations (3rd ed.), Preface (tr. by R. G. Latham in *Works,* Vol. I)

Elisha Bartlett [1804–1855]

Almost all diseases are occasionally so impressed and modified, by inappreciable or unknown influences, that their usual diagnostic signs are wanting, or very much obscured, — the diseases being latent, as it is called.
Philosophy of Medical Science, Pt. II, Ch. 10

Certainly, it is by their signs and symptoms, that internal diseases are revealed to the physician. But daily observation shows, that there is no uniform and invariable relationship between the extent and intensity of disease, and its external signs. The prominency, the number, and the combination, of these, depend upon many circumstances beside the disease with which they are connected.
Ibid., Ch. 12

John Brown [1810–1882]

Symptoms are the body's mother tongue; signs are in a foreign language.
Horae Subsecivae, Series I, Introduction

Jean Martin Charcot [1825–1893]

Symptoms, then, are in reality nothing but the cry from suffering organs.
Leçons cliniques sur les maladies des vieillards et les maladies chroniques, Introduction, Sect. 1

S. Weir Mitchell [1829–1914]

It is . . . useless to be constantly digging up a person's symptoms to see if they are better.
Doctor and Patient, Introduction

TEA

William Cowper [1731–1800]

The cups
That cheer but not inebriate.
The Task, Bk. IV

Sydney Smith [1771–1845]

Thank God for tea! What would the world do without tea? how did it exist? I am glad I was not born before tea.
Quoted by Lady Holland in *A Memoir of the Rev. Sydney Smith*, Ch. 11

Thomas De Quincey [1785–1859]

Tea, though ridiculed by those who are naturally of coarse nerves . . . will always be the favourite beverage of the intellectual.
Confessions of an English Opium-Eater, Pt. II

Jesse Torrey [1787–1834]

Tea possesses an acrid astringent quality, peculiar to most leaves and exterior bark of trees, and corrodes and paralyzes the nerves.
The Moral Instructor, Pt. IV, Sect. II, Ch. 11

TEACHERS

See also EDUCATION, MEDICAL SCHOOLS, STUDENTS, TEACHING

Geoffrey Chaucer [1340?–1400]

And gladly wolde he lerne and gladly teche.
The Canterbury Tales, "Prologue"

Oliver Wendell Holmes [1809–1894]

A good clinical teacher is himself a Medical School.
Medical Essays, "Scholastic and Bedside Teaching"

The dullest of teachers is the one who does not know what to omit.
Idem

Hermann von Helmholtz [1821–1894]

A teacher who retains convictions foreign to himself is all well enough for pupils who depend upon authority as the source of their knowledge, but not for such as require basic convictions of the utmost depth.
Quoted by F. H. Garrison in *Bulletin of the New York Academy of Medicine* 4:996, 1928

Sir William Osler [1849–1919]

I have learned since to be a better student, and to be ready to say to my fellow students "I do not know."
Aequanimitas, with Other Addresses, "After Twenty-Five Years"

I desire no other epitaph — no hurry about it, I may say — than the statement that I taught medical students in the wards, as I regard this as by far the most useful and important work I have been called upon to do.
Ibid., "The Fixed Period"

The very best instructor for students may have no conception of the higher lines of work in his branch, and contrariwise, how many brilliant investigators have been wretched teachers?
Ibid., "Teaching and Thinking"

In the hurly-burly of to-day, when the competition is so keen and there are so many seeking the bubble reputation at the eye-piece and the test tube, it is well for young men to remember that no bubble is so irridescent or floats longer than that blown by the successful teacher. A man who is not fond of students and who does not suffer their foibles gladly, misses the greatest zest in life; and the teacher who wraps himself in the cloak of his researches, and lives apart from

the bright spirits of the coming generation, is very apt to find his garment the shirt of Nessus.
> *Glasgow Medical Journal* 76: 321, 1911

The successful teacher is no longer on a height, pumping knowledge at high pressure into passive receptacles. . . . he is a senior student anxious to help his juniors.
> *The Student Life*

August Bier [1861–1949]

A professor is a gentleman who has a different opinion.
> Aphorism

If there weren't so many professors, medicine would be much easier.
> Aphorism

Charles H. Mayo [1865–1939]

The safest thing for a patient is to be in the hands of a man engaged in teaching medicine. In order to be a teacher of medicine the doctor must always be a student.
> Quoted in *Proceedings of the Staff Meetings of the Mayo Clinic* 2:233, 1927

Thomas G. Orr [1884–1955]

Students must tolerate tiresome speakers because they cannot help themselves by walking out. In this respect students are often more courteous than their teachers. To teach properly is no easy task and cannot be done by haphazard methods. In my own experience as a medical student I recall that we had a very brilliant medical scholar as a teacher who could not make his talks interesting. His ward rounds were called by facetious students "shifting dullness."
> *The American Surgeon* 17:33, 1951

David Seegal [1899–   ]

The preceptor, trying to instill educa-

tive principles in his students, cannot foretell how far a beam his tiny light will throw. Aesculapius couldn't guess; Hippocrates couldn't guess; neither can he. But it is probable that some of the medical students he educated to teach will, in life, have their eyes more lifted to the stars and later find a grateful, smiling Hippocrates waiting to greet them in some Medical Elysium.
> *Journal of Medical Education* 39:1030, 1964

During their active years, full-time or part-time members of university medical schools may assist in the education of some 5,000 individuals as medical students, members of house staffs, peers, or ancillary members of the profession. This responsibility now extends to clinicians in a variety of other institutions such as community hospitals. Thus, the batons in the educational relay race are passed to many hands.
> *Idem*

W. H. Auden [1907–   ]

A professor is one who talks in someone else's sleep.

Thomas Szasz [1920–   ]

We can conclude that — the psychology of human relationships being what it is — in adult education there is an inverse relationship between "power" and "learning." Only the "weak" can teach. If the teacher comes into too much power, he ceases to be a "teacher" and becomes instead a religious or political (or other "group") "leader."
> *Psychoanalytic Training*, Vol. 39, 1958

Louis Lasagna [1923–   ]

Does it seem too farfetched to picture the young Helen Keller as the symbol par excellence of every student that ever lived? We are all Helen Kellers in some degree — vision beclouded, ears undiscriminating, speech uncertain and untrue. We have all needed at one time or another, to have TRUTH spelled out slowly for us, to have our capabilities redefined and reevaluated, and the limitations of our sensations and perceptions suggested. It is no mean epitaph for any teacher to have it said of him that "he rendered all whom he taught less deaf, less dumb, less blind."

> *Great Teachers* (ed. by H. Peterson), Introduction

Anonymous

If I were summing up the qualities of a good teacher of medicine, I would enumerate human sympathy, moral and intellectual integrity, enthusiasm, and ability to talk, in addition, of course, to knowledge of his subject.

TEACHING

See also EDUCATION, KNOWLEDGE, LEARNING, LECTURE, MEDICAL SCHOOLS, STUDENTS, TEACHERS

Peter Mere Latham [1789–1875]

Here is a great hospital; and here I hold that all teaching by lectures should have for its first and principle purpose to give effect to that self-teaching, which, from the objects which surround us, all may practise and profit by who have eyes and ears and a docile mind. Do not believe a word that I say until you have gone into the wards and proved it. There you will find your great book of instruction. I only pretend to supply a key, a glossary, or an index to it. Use that book as you ought, and then, though in the end you and I may have the same knowledge, it will not be because it has passed from my mind to yours, but, being gained by your own observation, ratified by your own proofs, and matured by your own

thought, you will have it and hold it as your own independent possession.

> *Diseases of the Heart,* Lect. IV

If I undertake to instruct you out of my little book of experience, I hold it but honesty to read it straight through. There is no such thing as turning practical medicine into a well-told tale.

> *Ibid.,* Lect. XI

It is one thing for a man to understand a matter for himself and for his own use, and another thing to understand it and explain it for the use of others.

> *General Remarks on the Practice of Medicine,* "The Heart and Its Affections," Ch. I

It requires some courage to talk gravely and with a purpose of instruction about common things. For either people do not listen at all, expecting to hear nothing new; or they listen reluctantly, not liking to be schooled about what they understand perfectly (they think) already.

> *Idem*

John Henry, Cardinal Newman [1801–1890]

To discover and teach are distinct functions; they are also distinct gifts, and are not commonly found united in the same person.

> *On the Scope and Nature of University Education,* Preface

Oliver Wendell Holmes [1809–1894]

The bedside is always the true centre of medical teaching.[1]

> *Medical Essays,* "Scholastic and Bedside Teaching"

Hermann von Helmholtz [1821–1894]

Whoever desires to give his hearers a perfect conviction of the truth of his principles must, first of all, know from

[1] Cf. Oliver Wendell Holmes, p. 137a.

his own experience how conviction is acquired and how not. He must have known how to acquire conviction where no predecessor has been before him, i.e., he must have worked on the confines of human knowledge and have conquered for it new territory.

> Quoted by F. H. Garrison in *Bulletin of the New York Academy of Medicine* 4:996, 1928

S. Weir Mitchell [1829–1914]

I must have told my story ill if to every physician who hears me its illustrations have not the invigorating force of moral tonics.

> *Transactions of the College of Physicians of Philadelphia* 9: 337, 1887

Jacques Loeb [1859–1924]

I cannot answer your question, because I have not yet read that chapter in the text-book myself, but if you will come to me to-morrow I shall then have read it and I may be able to answer you.

> Quoted by T. Brailsford Robinson in *The Spirit of Research*, "The Life and Work of Jacques Loeb"

Franklin P. Mall [1862–1917]

Nobody teaches anybody anything, at first every student's scalpel is dull and then later every student's scalpel is sharp, and nobody has taught anybody anything.

> Comment to Gertrude Stein (Quoted by Donald Fleming in *William H. Welch and the Rise of Modern Medicine*, Ch. 8)

Sir Robert Hutchison [1871–1960]

Those of us who have the duty of training the rising generation of doctors . . . must not inseminate the virgin minds of the young with the tares of our own fads. It is for this reason that it is easily possible for teaching to be too "up to date." It is always well, before handing the cup of knowledge to the young, to wait until the froth has settled.

> *British Medical Journal* 1:995, 1925

Martin H. Fischer [1879–1962]

Of course, I teach you only the truth — but that shouldn't make you believe it.

> Quoted by Howard Fabing and Ray Marr in *Fischerisms*

Dickinson W. Richards [1895–]

The primary requisites for clinical teaching are a sick man, a student, and a teacher, regardless of where they are located, or what the surrounding aura of sentimental values. And the student can be taught, not only what to learn, but also how to learn it.

> *Transactions of the American Clinical and Climatological Association* 65:94, 1953

David Seegal [1899–]

Many of those who can teach, can do, and do do.

> *The Pharos of Alpha Omega Alpha* 26:82, 1963

Sir Robert Platt [1900–]

The human lessons which medical practice teaches are great and should be passed on to our pupils.

> *Universities Quarterly* 17:327, 1963

Maurice B. Strauss [1904–1974]

If they are not interested in the care of the patient, in the phenomena of disease in the sick, they should not be in the clinical department of medicine, since they cannot teach students clinical medicine.

> *Medicine* 43:619, 1964

Edward A. Gall [1906–   ]

A teacher is paid to teach, not to sacrifice rats and hamsters.
> *Journal of Medical Education*
> 36:275, 1961

TEETH

I. GENERAL

Martial [fl. 1st Cent.]

Thais has black, Laecania white teeth; what is the reason? Thais has her own, Laecania bought ones.
> *Epigrams*, V.43 (tr. by H. G. Bohn)

Miguel de Cervantes [1547–1616]

Every Tooth in a Man's Head is more valuable than a Diamond.
> *Don Quixote*, Pt. I, Bk. III, Ch. IV (tr. by P. A. Motteux)

William Shakespeare [1564–1616]

'Twas full two years ere I could get a tooth.
> *Richard III*, II, iv, 29

Ben Jonson [1573?–1637]

>   What diseases,
> And putrefactions in the gummes are bred,
> By those [toothpicks] are made of adultrate, and false wood?
> *The Devil Is an Ass*, Act IV, Sc. ii

St. Jean Baptiste de la Salle [1651–1719]

It is necessary to clean the teeth frequently, more especially after meals, but not on any account with a pin, or the point of a penknife, and it must never be done at table.
> *The Rules of Christian Manners and Civility*, I

Jonathan Swift [1667–1745]

Sweet things are bad for the teeth.
> *Polite Conversation*, Dialogue II

Philip Stanhope, Lord Chesterfield [1694–1773]

I hope you take great care of your mouth and teeth, and that you clean them well every morning with a sponge and tepid water, with a few drops of arquebusade water dropped into it; besides washing your mouth carefully after every meal. I do insist upon your never using those sticks, or any hard substance whatsoever, which always rub away the gums, and destroy the varnish of the teeth.
> Letter to his son, February 15, 1754

Benjamin Franklin [1706–1790]

Hot things, sharp things, sweet things, cold things
All rot the teeth, and make them look like old things.
> *Poor Richard's Almanack*, 1734

Thomas Hood [1799–1845]

The best of friends fall out, and so His teeth had done some years ago.
> *A True Story*

Henry Wadsworth Longfellow [1807–1882]

>   Heaven gives almonds
> To those who have no teeth. That's nuts to crack.
> *The Spanish Student*, Act III, Sc. v

Mark Twain (Samuel L. Clemens) [1835–1910]

Adam and Eve had many advantages, but the principal one was that they escaped teething.
> *The Tragedy of Pudd'nhead Wilson*, Ch. 4, "Pudd'nhead Wilson's Calendar"

Ambrose Bierce [1842–1914?]

DENTIST, n. A prestidigitator who, putting metal into your mouth, pulls coins out of your pocket.
The Devil's Dictionary

Martin H. Fischer [1879–1962]

I find that most men would rather have their bellies opened for five hundred dollars than have a tooth pulled for five.
Quoted by Howard Fabing and Ray Marr in *Fischerisms*

The Bible

I am escaped with the skin of my teeth.
Job 19:20

The fathers have eaten sour grapes, and the children's teeth are set on edge.[1]
Ezekiel 18:2

Anonymous

Removing the teeth will cure something, including the foolish belief that removing the teeth will cure everything.

English Proverb

He looks like a tooth-drawer, i.e., very thin and meagre.

II. TOOTHACHE

William Shakespeare [1564–1616]

He that sleeps feels not the toothache.
Cymbeline, V, iv, 177

BENEDICK: I have the toothache.
DON PEDRO: Draw it.
Much Ado About Nothing, III, ii, 21

For there was never yet philosopher
That could endure the toothache patiently.
Ibid., V, i, 35

[1] Cf. Hungarian Proverb, p. 606a.

Being troubled with a raging tooth,
I could not sleep.
Othello, III, iii, 414

Richard Baxter [1615–1691]

An aching tooth is better out than in,
To loose a rotting member is a gain.
Poetical Fragments, "Man"

John Josselyn [fl. 1630–1675]

For the Toothach I have found the following medicine very available, Brimstone and Gunpower compounded with butter, rub the mandible with it, the outside being first warm'd.
An Account of Two Voyages to New-England, "The Second Voyage"

Jonathan Swift [1667–1745]

A coming shower your shooting corns presage,
Old a-ches throb, your hollow tooth will rage.
A Description of a City Shower

Robert Burns [1759–1796]

My curse upon your venom'd stang,
That shoots my tortur'd gooms alang,
An' thro' my lug [1] gies monie a twang
Wi' gnawing vengeance,
Tearing my nerves wi' bitter pang,
Like racking engines!
Address to the Toothache

Thomas Hood [1799–1845]

Of all our pains, since man was curst,
I mean of body, not the mental,
To name the worst, among the worst,
The dental sure is transcendental;
Some bit of masticating bone,
That ought to help to clear a shelf:
But lets its proper work alone,
And only seems to gnaw itself.
A True Story

One tooth he had with many fangs,
That shot at once as many pangs. . . .

[1] lug = ear.

One touch of that ecstatic stump
Could jerk his limbs, and make him
  jump.
          Idem

George Bernard Shaw [1856–1950]

The man with toothache thinks everyone happy whose teeth are sound.
          Man and Superman, "Maxims
          for Revolutionists"

W. Somerset Maugham
[1874–1965]

It is curious to notice that when they
speak of evil, philosophers so often use
toothache as their example. . . . In
their sheltered, easy lives it looks as
though this were the only pain that
had much afflicted them and one might
almost conclude that with the improvement of American dentistry the whole
problem could be conveniently shelved.
          The Summing Up, Sect. lxviii

Proverbs

Music helps not the toothache.

The tongue is ever turning to the aching tooth.

English Proverb

Who hath aching teeth hath ill tenants.

Hungarian Proverb

Adam has eaten the apple, and our
teeth ache from it.[1]

TELEOLOGY

Sir Charles Bell [1774–1842]

If we select any object from the whole
extent of animated nature, and contemplate it fully and in all its bearings,
we shall certainly come to this conclusion: that there is Design in the mechanical construction, Benevolence in

----

[1] Cf. German Proverb, p. 181b; The Bible,
Ezekiel 18:2, p. 605a.

the endowments of the living properties, and that Good on the whole is the
result.
          *The Hand, Its Mechanism and
          Vital Endowments as Evincing
          Design,* Ch. 1

Sir William Withey Gull
[1816–1890]

The foundation of the study of Medicine, as of all scientific inquiry, lies in
the belief that every natural phenomenon, trifling as it may seem, has a
fixed and invariable meaning.
          Published Writings, "Study of
          Medicine"

Ernst Wilhelm von Brücke
[1819–1892]

Teleology is a lady without whom no
biologist can live. Yet he is ashamed
to show himself with her in public.[1]
          Quoted by Sir Hans A. Krebs in
          *Bulletin of the Johns Hopkins
          Hospital* 95:45, 1954

Walter B. Cannon [1871–1945]

My first article of belief is based on the
observation, almost universally confirmed in present knowledge, that what
happens in our bodies is directed toward a useful end.
          The Way of an Investigator,
          "Some Working Principles"

W. I. B. Beveridge [1908–   ]

Vitalism, which postulated mysterious
"vital" forces, and teleology, which
postulated a supernatural directing
agency, have long ago been abandoned
by experimental biologists. However,
teleology is admissible in a modified
sense that an organ or function fulfils
a purpose toward aiding the survival
of the organism as a whole or survival
of the species.
          *The Art of Scientific Investiga-
          tion,* Ch. X

----

[1] See Preface, p. ix.

TEMPERANCE

See also ABSTINENCE, ALCO-HOL, EATING, INTEMPER-ANCE

Cicero [106–43 B.C.]

Exercise and temperance can preserve something of our early strength even in old age.
> *On Old Age,* X.34 (tr. by James Logan)

Duc François de La Rochefoucauld [1613–1680]

Temperance is the love of health, or the inability to overindulge.
> *Maxims,* No. 583 (tr. by Constantine FitzGibbon)

Joseph Addison [1672–1719]

The preservative I am speaking of is temperance, which has those particular advantages above all other means of health, that it may be practised by all ranks and conditions, at any season, or in any place. It is a kind of regimen into which every man may put himself, without interruption to business, expence of money, or loss of time.
> *The Spectator,* Vol. III, No. 195 (October 13, 1711)

Benjamin Franklin [1706–1790]

Eat not to dullness; drink not to elevation.
> *Autobiography,* Ch. 5

Jean Jacques Rousseau [1712–1778]

Temperance and labor are the two real physicians of man: labor sharpens his appetite and temperance prevents his abusing it.
> *Émile,* Bk. I

Charles Lamb [1775–1834]

What have I gained by health? intol-erable dulness. What by early hours and moderate meals? — a total blank.
> Letter to William Wordsworth, January 22, 1830

The Bible: Apocrypha

A very little is sufficient for a man well nurtured, and he fetcheth not his wind short upon his bed.

Sound sleep cometh of moderate eating: he riseth early, and his wits are with him: but the pain of watching, and choler, and pangs of the belly, are with an unsatiable man.
> *Ecclesiasticus* 31:19

Anonymous [1]

Nothing in excess.

Proverbs

Moderation in all things.

Temperance is the best physic.

TEMPERATURE

See also CLIMATE

Thomas Jefferson [1743–1826]

The living body (not like the dead one, which assumes the temperature of the surrounding atmosphere) maintains within itself a steady heat of about 96°. of Farenheit's thermometer, varying little with the ordinary variations of the atmosphere. This heat is principally supplied by respiration. The vital air, or oxygen of the atmospheric fluid inhaled, is separated by the lungs from the azotic and carbonic parts, and is absorbed by them; the caloric is dis-

[1] Attributed to Thales [640?–546 B.C.], Solon [638–559? B.C.], Cleobulus [628?–558? B.C.], Anacharsis [fl. 600 B.C.], Euripides [484–406 B.C.], and Socrates [470?–399 B.C.].

engaged, diffused thro' the mass of the body, and absorbed from the skin by the external air coming into contact with it.

> *Notes on the State of Virginia* (University of North Carolina, 1955), MS. note by Thomas Jefferson to Query VII

If the external air is of a high temperature, it does not take up the superfluous heat of the body fast enough, and we complain of too much heat: if it is very cold, it absorbs the heat too fast and produces the sensation of cold. To remedy this, we interpose a covering, which acting as a strainer, lets less air come into contact with the body, and checks the escape of the vital heat. As the atmospheric air becomes colder, more heat is conducted from the body. As it would be inconvenient in the day to be burthened with a mass of clothing entirely equivalent to great degrees of cold, we have resort to fire and warm rooms to correct the state of the atmosphere, as a supplement to our clothing.

> *Idem*

Of the substances we use for covering, linen seems the openest strainer, for admission of air to the body, and the most copious conductor of heat from it; and is therefore considered as a cool clothing. Cotton obstructs still more the passage of both fluids; and wool more than cotton: it is called therefore a worse conductor of heat, and warmer clothing. Next to this are the furs, and the most impermeable of all for heat and air, are feathers and down, and especially the down of the Eider duck.

> *Idem*

The Bible

My skin is black upon me, and my bones are burned with heat.

> *Job* 30:30

TERMINOLOGY

See also COMMUNICATION, WRITING

Plato [427?–347 B.C.]

They do certainly give very strange and new-fangled names to diseases.

> *Republic,* III.405.D (tr. by Benjamin Jowett)

Galen [fl. 2nd Cent.]

The chief merit of language is clearness, and we know that nothing detracts so much from this as do unfamiliar terms.

> *On the Natural Faculties,* I.ii (tr. by Arthur J. Brock)

Sir Francis Bacon [1561–1626]

The ill and unfit choice of words wonderfully obstructs the understanding.

> *Novum Organum,* "Aphorisms," XLIII

Jonathan Swift [1667–1745]

These Papers are delivered to a Set of artists very dextrous in finding out the mysterious Meanings of Words, Syllables, and Letters. For Instance, they can decypher a Close-stool to signify a Privy-Council; a Flock of Geese, a Senate; a lame Dog, an Invader; the Plague, a standing Army; a Buzard, a Minister; the Gout, a High Priest; a Gibbet, a Secretary of State; a Chamber pot, a Committee of Grandees; a Sieve, a Court Lady; a Broom, a Revolution; a Mouse-trap, an Employment; a bottomless Pit, the Treasury; a Sink, a C———t; a Cap and Bells, a Favourite; a broken Reed, a Court of Justice; an empty Tun, a General; a running Sore, the Administration.

> *Gulliver's Travels,* Pt. III, Ch. 6

Percivall Pott [1714–1788]

Clear and precise definitions of diseases, and the application of such names to them as are expressive of their true and real nature, are of more consequence than they are generally imagined to be: Untrue or imperfect ones occasion false ideas; and false ideas are generally followed by erroneous practice.

> *Chirurgical Works*, Vol. III, "A Treatise on the Fistula in Ano"

Sydney Smith [1771–1845]

People of wealth and rank never use ugly names for ugly things. Apoplexy is an affection of the head; paralysis is nervousness; gangrene is pain and inconvenience in the extremities.

> Letter to Mrs. Holland, January 1844

Peter Mere Latham [1789–1875]

There are things which will not be defined, and Fever is one of them. Besides, when a word has passed into everyday use, it is too late to lay a logical trap for its meaning, and think to apprehend it by a definition.

> *General Remarks on the Practice of Medicine*, Ch. X, Pt. 1

It is the great mystery of life itself which is at the bottom of all the mysterious language we are obliged to employ concerning it.

> *Ibid.*, Ch. XVI

Jane Welsh Carlyle [1801–1866]

Medical men all over the world . . . merely entered into a tacit agreement to call all sorts of maladies people are liable to, in cold weather, by one name; so that one sort of treatment may serve for all, and their practice be thereby greatly simplified.

> Letter to John Welsh, March 4, 1837

Frederick Saunders [1807–1902]

The language of the men of medicine is a fearful concoction of sesquipedalian words, numbered by thousands.

Oliver Wendell Holmes [1809–1894]

I would never use a long word, even, where a short one would answer the purpose. I know there are professors in this country who "ligate" arteries. Other surgeons only tie them, and it stops the bleeding just as well.

> *Medical Essays*, "Scholastic and Bedside Teaching"

Remember that even the learned ignorance of a nomenclature is something to have mastered, and may furnish pegs to hang facts upon which would otherwise have strewed the floor of memory in loose disorder.

> *Ibid.*, "The Young Practitioner"

Sir William Withey Gull [1816–1890]

If facts be nature's words, our words should be true signs of nature's facts. A word rightly imposed is a landmark indicating so much recovered from the region of ignorance.

> *Published Writings*, Vol. 156, "Study of Medicine"

Herman Melville [1819–1891]

Upon the strength of their dealing in the dark, they [the sorcerers] affected even more mystery than belonged to them; when interrogated concerning their science, would confound the inquirer by answers couched in an extraordinary jargon, employing words almost as long as anacondas.

> *Mardi*, Ch. 144

There is no counting the names, that surgeons and anatomists give to the various parts of the human body. . . . I wonder whether mankind could not get along without all those names,

which keep increasing every day, and hour, and moment; till at last the very air will be full of them; and even in a great plain men will be breathing each other's breath, owing to the vast multitude of words they use that consume all the air. . . . But people seem to have a great love for names; for to know a great many names seems to look like knowing a good many things.
Redburn, Ch. XIII

A man of true science . . . uses but few hard words, and those only when none other will answer his purpose; whereas the smatterer in science . . . thinks, that by mouthing hard words, he proves that he understands hard things.
White Jacket, Ch. LXIII

Paul Broca [1824–1880]

Greedy for explanations, and rather than being satisfied with ignorance, the human mind treats itself to words devoid of meaning, like those American savages who in time of famine swallow clay to silence their empty stomachs.
Mémoires de l'Académie Nationale de Médecine 16:453, 1852

Thomas Huxley [1825–1895]

Many of the faults and mistakes of the ancient philosophers are traceable to the fact that they knew no language but their own, and were often led into confusing the symbol with the thought which it embodied.
Science and Education, "Science and Art and Education"

Sir Benjamin Ward Richardson [1828–1896]

Such vague terms, as hidden seizures, sympathies, irritations, revulsions, crises, antiphlogistics, nervous exhaustions, and others familiar to our mouths — what do they mean? What are they worth? Where are the two men who shall give to them the same

definition? What other science would foster, or even permit, such ragged phraseologies?
Glasgow Medical Journal 4:80, 1856

Henry Maudsley [1835–1918]

As no one can have perfect knowledge of all parts of medicine . . . a simplicity of nomenclature would seem not merely desirable but essential.

Sir William Osler [1849–1919]

In our precious cabbage patches the holometabolous insecta are the hosts of parasitic polyembryonic hymenoptera, upon the prevalence of which rests the psychic and somatic stamina of our fellow-countrymen.[1]
The Old Humanities and the New Science

Charles Nicolle [1866–1936]

Suppose the term to be newly created, and I should hope, well chosen, clear, precise, and philologically respectable. The work of the inventor of this word is by no means finished. The principal portion of the task remains to be accomplished. It is requisite in the first place to define the term to give it community status. To define is to specify as to character. To the same extent it is the foreseeing of the pernicious uses to which the term may be put. The newly born word offers no self-defense. It is needful to watch over it, to protect it from encroachment, from deformation. It is not sufficient to content oneself with employing it rigorously; it is further essential to demand of others that they use it in the same way.
Les Responsibilités de la médecine

George Horace Lorimer [1868–1937]

You can insult a person or praise him

---

[1] Osler is illustrating the profusion of Greek derivatives in scientific terminology.

by the way in which you express your-self. For example: if a young man tells a young lady that her face could stop a clock, she is insulted: but if he tells her that when he gazes upon her face time stands still, she is flattered. They both mean the same thing.

> *Letters of a Self-Made Merchant to His Son*

Martin H. Fischer [1879–1962]

Idiopathic epilepsy is idiopathic ignorance on the part of the doctor.

> Quoted by Howard Fabing and Ray Marr in *Fischerisms*

When there is no explanation, they give it a name, which immediately explains everything.
> *Idem*

Whenever ideas fail, men invent words.
> *Idem*

You must learn to talk clearly. The jargon of scientific terminology which rolls off your tongues is mental garbage.
> *Idem*

Sir Ernest Gowers [1880–1966]

Some seventy years ago a promising young neurologist made a discovery that necessitated the addition of a new word to the English vocabulary. He insisted that this should be *knee-jerk*, and *knee-jerk* it has remained, in spite of the efforts of *patellar reflex* to dislodge it. He was my father;[1] so perhaps I have inherited a prejudice in favour of home-made words.
> *Plain Words*, Ch. 5

Sir Thomas Lewis [1881–1945]

Diagnosis is a system of more or less accurate guessing in which the end-point achieved is a name. These names applied to disease come to assume the importance of specific entities, whereas

[1] Sir William Richard Gowers [1845–1915].

they are for the most part no more than insecure and therefore temporary conceptions.
> *Lancet* 1:619, 1944

Hanns Sachs [1881–1947]

While I was listening eagerly to Freud's lectures I studied assiduously his technique of exposition with a view of modelling my own after him. I wondered how he succeeded in producing something unexpected and stupendous while his talk moved in simple terms, dispensing with the fireworks of baffling profundity or of glittering paradoxes. I found that he made use of Schopenhauer's recipe for a good style: "Say extraordinary things by using ordinary words."
> *Great Teachers* (ed. by H. Peterson), Ch. 17

James Murphy [1884–1950]

The sociologists and financial experts have a jargon that is all their own and it keeps them from being found out. The majesty of the law is upheld in like manner and the medical craft could not survive if it prescribed its medicines and described its diseases in the vernacular.
> Epilogue to Max Planck's *Where Is Science Going?*

Siegfried J. Thannhauser [1885–1962]

Dr. D———, don't you think a father should be allowed to name his own child?[1]
> Comment on medical grand rounds, New England Center Hospital, ca. 1958

John Punnett Peters [1887–1955]

The attachment of polysyllabic labels has throughout medical history created

[1] Referring to Dr. D———'s reclassification of several diseases which Dr. Thannhauser had originally described and named many years before.

such mental and spiritual satisfaction that it has tended to stifle curiosity.
> *Yale Journal of Biology and Medicine* 26:179, 1953

Horace B. and Ava C. English [1892–1961]   [20th Cent.]

Ad-i-ad-o-cho-kin-e-sis
Is a term that will bolster my thesis
That 'tis idle to seek
Such precision in Greek
When confusion it only increases.
> *A Comprehensive Dictionary of Psychological and Psychoanalytical Terms*

James Thurber [1894–1961]

[During an operation:] "Coreopsis has set in," said Renshaw nervously. "If you would take over, Mitty?"[1]
> *My World and Welcome to It,* "The Secret Life of Walter Mitty"

Homer W. Smith [1895–1962]

Though we name the things we know, we do not necessarily know them because we name them.
> *Circulation of the Blood* (ed. by A. P. Fishman and D. W. Richards), Ch. 9

David Harley [1904–   ]

It seems likely that the term allergy would itself have been dropped long since had it not been for the strong general feeling that a word so beautiful must mean something. The term allergy has been invested with such an all-embracing meaning that the word itself conveys but little, or rather

---

[1] Thurber later wrote to Edward Newhouse of *The New Yorker,* "It is my firm but sad conviction that ninety percent of Americans would figure coreopsis is a disease and I can only hope that the women's eyes do not brighten with the hope of flowers when a man says, 'I've brought you syphilis.'" (Quoted by Harold Stevens in *Journal of the American Medical Association* 190:1114, 1964.)

its vastness prevents any attempt at a precise definition.
> *Modern Practice of Dermatology*

Theodore C. Ruch [1906–   ]

In a world where splinter disciplines stake claims on words as though they were gold mines (which they are), perhaps our meaning of the word "biophysics" is not evident to all.
> *Physiology and Biophysics,* Preface

Richard Asher [1912–   ]

The modern haematologist, instead of describing in English what he can see, prefers to describe in Greek what he can't.[1]
> *Lancet* 2:359, 1959

Well I ask you? When you take your family on holiday, do you say "I am taking my gregarious egalitarian sibling group with me"?
> *Idem*

Of course some of the changes in illnesses between the centuries are due to a genuine biological change, better drains mean less typhoid and so on; yet a lot of it does depend on fashion and if it is all right to have "choreopsis," then choreopsis will occur.[2]
> *Twentieth Century,* Autumn 1962, "Fashions in Disease"

C. F. Consolazio [1913–   ], R. E. Johnson [1911–   ], and L. J. Pecora [1910–   ]

There is no more reason to retain the inch, the pound, and the quart than there is to retain the ell, the stone, and the pottle. All belong in the British Museum, Division of Antiquities. Nevertheless, American environmental physiologists still persist in describing a male subject, 160 lbs in weight (but

---

[1] Cf. Voltaire, p. 62b.
[2] Cf. James Thurber, p. 612a.

of surface area of 1.61 meters), who walks at 4 mph (but with a caloric expenditure of 300 Kcal/hr), with a fluid intake of 1 pint/hr (but a sweat rate of 0.8 liters/hr), at a dry bulb temperature of 86°F (24.4° C).
Physiological Measurements of Metabolic Functions in Man, Sect. 13

Anonymous

Nouns of multitude (e.g., a pair of shoes, a gaggle of geese, a pride of lions) . . . : a rash of dermatologists, a hive of allergists, a scrub of interns, a chest of phthisiologists; or, a giggle of nurses, a flood of urologists, a pile of proctologists, an eyeful of ophthalmologists; or, a whiff of anesthesiologists, a staff of bacteriologists, a cast of orthopedic rheumatologists, a gargle of laryngologists.
Journal of the American Medical Association 190:392, 1964

TEXTBOOKS

Theodor Billroth [1829–1894]

It is a most gratifying sign of the rapid progress of our time that our best text-books become antiquated so quickly.
The Medical Sciences in the German Universities, Pt. II

Wilder Penfield [1891–   ]

The Egyptians made a fatal mistake. They wrote textbooks, the hermetic books. They made another and more serious mistake, and that was to believe that the textbooks were correct. So they forbade physicians, at peril of their lives, to depart in any way from the treatment prescribed in the hermetic books. It was a remarkable experiment. . . . The experiment demonstrated that standardization can halt

advance but that it does not in any way hinder retrogression.
The Second Career, "Neurosurgery — Yesterday, Today and Tomorrow"

THEORY

See also HYPOTHESIS, RESEARCH, SCIENTIFIC METHOD, THEORY AND PRACTICE

Thomas Jefferson [1743–1826]

I have lived myself to see the disciples of Hoffmann, Boerhaave, Stahl, Cullen, Brown, succeed one another like the shifting figures of a magic lantern, & their fancies, like the dresses of the annual doll-babies from Paris, becoming, from their novelty, the vogue of the day, and yielding to the next novelty their ephemeral favor.
Letter to Dr. Caspar Wistar, June 21, 1807

Elisha Bartlett [1804–1855]

The old saying, so constantly and so blindly repeated, that the exception proves the rule, is as destitute of truth, as it is of meaning. Such an exception can prove only one thing, and that is, that the rule is not fully understood, or completely ascertained.
Philosophy of Medical Science, Pt. I, Ch. 3

Claude Bernard [1813–1878]

A scientific hypothesis is merely a scientific idea, preconceived or previsioned. A theory is merely a scientific idea controlled by experiment.
An Introduction to the Study of Experimental Medicine, Pt. I, Ch. 1, Sect. vi (tr. by H. C. Greene)

They [physiologists] should consequently have very little confidence in

the ultimate value of theories, but should still make use of them as intellectual tools necessary to the evolution of science and suitable for the discovery of new facts.
> *Ibid.*, Pt. III, Ch. 1, Sect. ii

Louis Pasteur [1822–1895]

Physicians are inclined to engage in hasty generalizations. Possessing a natural or acquired distinction, endowed with a quick intelligence, an elegant and facile conversation . . . the more eminent they are . . . the less leisure they have for investigative work. . . . Eager for knowledge . . . they are apt to accept too readily attractive but inadequately proven theories.
> *Études sur la bière*, Ch. III, Sect. ii (tr. by René J. Dubos)

Jean Martin Charcot [1825–1893]

In medicine . . . one never sees even the most stoic intellects limit themselves to stating the facts without looking for a way to relate them by some sort of theory: from the outset, one sees minds occupied more with the subjective relationships of things than with their reality itself; the empirical results of observation, scarcely acquired, are brought together, tested one against the other, to evolve theories or systems. There, one must recognize, is a necessity of the human mind.
> *Leçons sur les maladies des vieillards et les maladies chroniques*, Introduction

August Bier [1861–1949]

Medical theories are most of the time even more peculiar than the facts themselves.
> Aphorism

Nicholas Maurice Arthus [1862–1945]

Seek facts and classify them and you will be the workmen of science. Conceive or accept theories and you will be their politicians.
> *De l'Anaphylaxie a l'immunité*

J. Chalmers Da Costa [1863–1933]

A man who has a theory which he tries to fit to facts is like a drunkard who tries his key haphazard in door after door, hoping to find one it fits.
> *The Trials and Triumphs of the Surgeon*, Ch. 1

Béla Schick [1877–1967]

In making theories always keep a window open so that you can throw one out if necessary.
> Quoted by I. J. Wolf in *Aphorisms and Facetiae of Béla Schick*, "Early Years"

Martin H. Fischer [1879–1962]

Don't confuse *hypothesis* and *theory*. The former is a possible explanation; the latter, the correct one. The establishment of theory is the very purpose of science.
> Quoted by Howard Fabing and Ray Marr in *Fischerisms*

Henry E. Sigerist [1891–1957]

In glancing back over the history of medicine we realize that medical theories have always been the product of the contemporary "Weltanschauung," or world viewpoint.
> *Man and Medicine*, Ch. I (tr. by M. G. Boise)

W. F. Neuman [1919–   ] and C. M. Dowse [20th Cent.]

There is no irreversible damage to be incurred in developing a unifying concept, even a wrong one. After all, concepts, like automobiles, can be "traded in" every year or so, whenever they fail to serve as reliable conveyances for ideas and data or whenever new models become irresistibly attractive.
> *The Parathyroids*, Sect. 5

Stephen E. Toulmin [1922–   ]

The more we treat the theories of our predecessors as myths, the more inclined we shall be to treat our own theories as dogmas.[1]

Journal of the History of Ideas 18:206, 1957

THEORY AND PRACTICE

See also EMPIRICISM, PRACTICE, THEORY

Celsus [25 B.C.–A.D. 50]

In all theorizing over a subject it is possible to argue on either side, and so cleverness and fluency may get the best of it; it is not, however, by eloquence but by remedies that diseases are treated.

De Medicina, Prooemium (tr. by W. G. Spencer)

Leonardo da Vinci [1452–1519]

Those who are enamoured of practice without science are like a pilot who goes into a ship without rudder or compass and never has any certainty where he is going.

Practice should always be based upon a sound knowledge of theory.

Manuscript G, Library of the Institut de France (tr. by Edward MacCurdy in *The Notebooks of Leonardo da Vinci,* Vol. II, Ch. XXIX)

Thomas Sydenham [1624–1689]

I have ever held that any accession whatever to the art of healing, even if it went no further than the cutting of corns, or the curing of toothaches, was of far higher value than all the knowledge of fine points, and all the

---

[1] Toulmin notes, "This way of putting the point I owe to Dr. J. B. Thornton of the New South Wales University of Technology."

pomp of subtle speculations; matters which are as useful to physicians in driving away diseases, as music is to masons in laying bricks.

Medical Observations, Sect. II, Ch. 2 (tr. by R. G. Latham in *Works,* Vol. I)

Thomas Jefferson [1743–1826]

Perhaps I should concur with you in excluding the *theory* (not the *practice*) of medicine. This is the charlatanerie of the body, as the other [abstruse theology] is of the mind.

Letter to Dr. Thomas Cooper, October 7, 1814

Karl F. H. Marx [1796–1877]

In actual life, pious churchgoers may show up as deceitful tricksters and theorizing physicians as blind empirics.

Quoted by F. H. Garrison in *Bulletin of the New York Academy of Medicine* 4:1001, 1928

Elisha Bartlett [1804–1855]

The *inference* is not to be relied upon any farther than as an indication of an experiment or trial; the only foundation of our therapeutical knowledge consists in the results of the experiment or trial itself.

Philosophy of Medical Science, Pt. II, Ch. 8

Therapeutics is not founded upon pathology. The former cannot be deduced from the latter. It rests wholly upon experience. It is, absolutely and exclusively, an empirical art.

Idem

There is but one philosophical, or intelligible, indication; and that is to remove disease, to mitigate its severity, or to abridge its duration; and this indication never grows out of any *à priori* reasoning, but reposes solely upon the basis of experience.

Idem

Our ability to apply these principles successfully has nothing, whatever, to do with the soundness of the principles themselves. This ability will depend upon the knowledge, the sagacity, and the skill of the individual observer. The existence of individual diseases is one thing; the power of ascertaining this existence is another.

> *Ibid.,* Ch. 10

Rudolf Virchow [1821–1902]

There are circumstances in which the split between scientific and practical medicine is so great that the learned physician can do nothing, while the practical physician knows nothing. Lord Bacon has said, *scientia est potentia.* Knowledge which is unable to support action is not genuine — and how unsure is activity without understanding! This split between science and practice is rather new; our century and our country have brought it into being.

> *Disease, Life, and Man,* "Standpoints in Scientific Medicine" (tr. by L. J. Rather)

Abraham Jacobi [1830–1919]

While thus admitting the claims of the practitioner as paramount, I was ever of opinion that a careful physician and therapeutist required the very latest and soundest results of exact scientific investigations as the foundation and safeguard of his practice.

> *A Treatise on Diphtheria,* Preface

Abraham Flexner [1866–1959]

The fact that disease is only in part accurately known does not invalidate the scientific method in practice. In the twilight region probabilities are substituted for certainties. There the physician may indeed only surmise, but, most important of all, he knows that he surmises. His procedure is tentative, observant, heedful, respon-

sive. Meanwhile the logic of the process has not changed. The scientific physician still keeps his advantage over the empiric. He studies the actual situation with keener attention; he is freer of prejudiced prepossession; he is more conscious of liability to error. Whatever the patient may have to endure from a baffling disease, he is not further handicapped by reckless medication. In the end the scientist alone draws the line accurately between the known, the partly known, and the unknown. The empiricist fares forth with an indiscriminate confidence which sharp lines do not disturb. Investigation and practice are thus one in spirit, method, and object.

> *Medical Education, A Comparative Study*

Harvey Cushing [1869–1939]

In these days when science is clearly in the saddle and when our knowledge of disease is consequently advancing at a breathless pace, we are apt to forget that not all can ride and that he also serves who waits and who applies what the horseman discovers.

> *Consecratio Medici,* Ch. 1

Wilfred Trotter [1872–1939]

The history of medicine teaches us that when reason took a hand *there* it was not only truth that suffered. The rational system of a Stahl, a Brown, a Rush, or a Broussais unfortunately did not exist in a mere metaphysical vacuum but at the bedside — and armed with opium, antimony, alcohol, mercury, the lancet, and the purge. Thus the consequences of the confident use of reason in medicine have been gloomy enough.

> *Collected Papers,* "Has the Intellect a Function?"

Warfield T. Longcope [1877–1953]

If you find that you resent having to look after the patients on your wards and want to get back to the laboratory,

it probably means you'll be happier there. If on the contrary you find you are concerned all the time you are in the laboratory with what is going on in your patients, then that may indicate that you will be better off dealing with people.
> Statement to Dr. Lawrence A. Kohn

Martin H. Fischer [1879–1962]

In the sick room, ten cents' worth of human understanding equals ten dollars' worth of medical science.
> Quoted by Howard Fabing and Ray Marr in *Fischerisms*

THINKING

See also BRAIN, MIND, REASON

Confucius [551–478 B.C.]

Learning without thinking is useless. Thinking without learning is dangerous.
> *Analects*, Bk. II, Ch. XV (tr. by William E. Soothill)

Thomas Sydenham [1624–1689]

It is my nature to think where others read.
> *Works*, "A Treatise on Gout and Dropsy" (tr. by R. G. Latham)

Anton van Leeuwenhoek [1632–1723]

A man has always to be busy with his thoughts if anything is to be accomplished.

Oliver Wendell Holmes [1809–1894]

A thought is often original, though you have uttered it a hundred times.
> *The Autocrat of the Breakfast Table*, Sect. I

John Ruskin [1819–1900]

One of the worst diseases to which the human creature is liable is its disease of thinking.
> *"A Joy For Ever"*: *The Political Economy of Art,* Note 6

Oscar Wilde [1854–1900]

Thinking is the most unhealthy thing in the world, and people die of it just as they die of any other disease.
> *The Decay of Lying*

William J. Mayo [1861–1939]

It is better to think and sometimes think wrong than not to think at all.
> *Collected Papers of the Mayo Clinic and Mayo Foundation* 27:1212, 1935

Georg Groddeck [1866–1934]

It would not be at all a bad thing if the elite of the medical world would be a little less clever, and would adopt a more primitive method of thinking, and reason more as children do.
> *The Book of the It,* Letter XIII (tr. by V. M. E. Collins)

Martin H. Fischer [1879–1962]

You can't go out and teach a community to think clearly if you can't think clearly yourself.
> Quoted by Howard Fabing and Ray Marr in *Fischerisms*

THIRST

See also DROPSY, WATER

Horace [65–8 B.C.]

Tantalus, ever thirsty, catches at the streams that fly from his lips.
> *Satires*, I.i.68 (tr. by E. C. Wickham)

Ovid [43 B.C.–A.D. 17?]

Tantalus seeks for water in the midst of waters.
> *The Amores,* II.ii.43 (tr. by G. Showerman)

Sick men long most to drink, who know they mayn't.
> *Ibid.,* III.iv.18 (tr. by Sir Charles Sedley)

Petronius [fl. 1st Cent.]

There, with water everywhere, dry thirst burns the throat.
> *Poems,* 14 (tr. by M. Heseltine)

François Rabelais [1494?–1553]

'Appetite comes as you eat,' said Bishop Hangest of Le Mans; but thirst vanishes as you drink!
> *Gargantua,* Bk. I, Ch. 5 (tr. by Jacques Le Clercq)

William Shakespeare [1564–1616]

When they are thirsty, fools would fain have drink.
> *Love's Labour's Lost,* V, ii, 372

Benjamin Rush [1745?–1813]

In the beginning of a battle, I have observed *thirst* to be a very common sensation among both officers and soldiers.
> *An Account of the Influence of the Military and Political Events of the American Revolution upon the Human Body*

Anthelme Brillat-Savarin [1755–1826]

Thirst is the inner consciousness of the need to drink.
> *La Physiologie du Goût*

George Gordon, Lord Byron [1788–1824]

> Till taught by pain,
Men really know not what good water's worth.
> *Don Juan,* Canto II, Stanza 84

Eliza Cook [1818–1889]

Hunger is bitter, but the worst
Of human pangs, the most accursed
Of Want's fell scorpions, is Thirst.
> *Melaia*

Traverse the desert, and then ye can tell
What treasures exist in the cold deep well;
Sink in despair on the red parched earth,
And then ye may reckon what Water is worth.
> *Water*

Edna St. Vincent Millay [1892–1950]

I drank at every vine.
The last was like the first.
I came upon no wine
So wonderful as thirst.
> *The Harp-Weaver and Other Poems,* "Feast"

The Bible

Ho, every one that thirsteth, come ye to the waters.
> *Isaiah* 55:1

In that day shall the fair virgins and young men faint for thirst.
> *Amos* 8:13

I was thirsty, and ye gave me drink.
> *Matthew* 25:35

Anonymous

How dry I am! How dry I am!
Nobody knows how dry I am!
> American popular song

There it o'ertook me that I fell down for thirst, I was parched, my throat burned, and I said: "This is the taste of death."
> *The Story of Sinuhe* (German tr. by Adolf Erman in *The Literature of the Ancient Egyptians,* English tr. by A. M. Blackman)

Proverb

The wine in the bottle doth not quench thirst.

English Proverb

He that goes to bed thirsty rises healthy.

French Proverbs

He who is master of his thirst is master of his health.

They that are thirsty drink silently.

TIME

See also OLD AGE

Sophocles [496?–406 B.C.]

To the gods alone comes never old age or death, but all else is confounded by all-mastering time.

> *Oedipus at Colonus*, 607 (tr. by R. C. Jebb)

Virgil [70–19 B.C.]

Times carries all things, even our wits, away.

> *Eclogues*, IX.51 (tr. by J. Rhoades)

Ovid [43 B.C.–A.D. 17?]

Helen also weeps when she sees her aged wrinkles in the looking-glass, and tearfully asks herself why she should twice have been a lover's prey. O Time, thou great devourer, and thou, envious Age, together you destroy all things; and, slowly gnawing with your teeth, you finally consume all things in lingering death!

> *Metamorphoses*, XV.232 (tr. by F. J. Miller)

Seneca [4? B.C.–A.D. 65]

Time heals what reason cannot.

> *Agamemnon*, 130

Leonardo da Vinci [1452–1519]

Wrongfully do men lament the flight of time, accusing it of being too swift, and not perceiving that its period is yet sufficient; but good memory wherewith Nature has endowed us causes everything long past to seem present.

> *Codice Atlantico*, 76 (tr. by Edward MacCurdy in *The Notebooks of Leonardo da Vinci*, Vol. I, Ch. I)

Paracelsus [1493?–1541]

Just as time can bring rain, roses, flowers, and shape all things from their beginnings to their end, and no one can stop it, so can it also make diseases break out at will. The physician must never forget that time can do this, or he will be unable to discover what is possible and what is impossible, and to understand what he can nevertheless undertake to inspire people with respect for the medical art that God has created, and to prevent the disease from getting worse, for this cannot be the intention of God. Time is a brisk wind, for each hour it brings something new. . . . but who can understand and measure its sharp breath, its mystery and its design? Therefore the physician must not think himself too important; for over him there is a master — time — which plays with him as the cat with the mouse.

> *Hohenheim's German Commentary on the Aphorisms of Hippocrates*, Ch. I, Sect. 3 (tr. by Norbert Guterman in *Selected Writings*)

Geronimo Cardano (Jerome Cardan) [1501–1576]

I prefer solitude to companions, since there are few men who are trustworthy, and almost none who are truly learned. I do not say this because I demand scholarship in all men — although the sum total of men's learning is small

enough; but I question whether we should allow anyone to waste our time.
>   *The Book of My Life,* Ch. 18

Hester Lynch Piozzi (Mrs. Henry Thrale) [1741–1821]

A physician can sometimes parry the scythe of death, but has no power over the sand in the hourglass.
>   Letter to Fanny Burney, November 22, 1781

Benjamin Disraeli, Lord Beaconsfield [1804–1881]

Time is the great physician.
>   *Henrietta Temple,* Bk. VI, Ch. 9

Moses Gunn [1822–1887]

Gentlemen, I'm sorry I'm late. I feel as though there had been lost not two minutes of my time but two minutes' time of each one of you three hundred men. That makes a loss of 600 minutes, or ten hours. It is inexcusable.[1]
>   Quoted by James B. Herrick in *Memories of Eighty Years*

Sir William Osler [1849–1919]

Save the fleeting minute; do not stop by the way. Learn gracefully to dodge the bore.
>   *Bulletin of the Johns Hopkins Hospital* 30:198, 1919

Sir John Bland-Sutton [1855–1936]

In reflecting on my early aspirations, I am satisfied that *TIME* has arranged things for me better than I could have managed them for myself.
>   *The Story of a Surgeon,* Preface

Béla Schick [1877–1967]

The physician's best remedy is *Tincture of Time!*
>   Quoted by I. J. Wolf in *Aphorisms and Facetiae of Béla Schick,* "Early Years"

---

[1] Comment on being late to deliver a lecture.

Spanish Proverb

Time cures the sick man, not the ointment.

TOBACCO

Edmund Spenser [1552?–1599]

Divine Tobacco.
>   *The Faerie Queene,* Bk. III

James I of England [1566–1625]

Is it not both great vanitie and uncleannesse, that at the table, a place of respect, of cleanlinesse, of modestie, men should not be ashamed, to sit tossing of *Tobacco pipes,* and puffing of the smoke of *Tobacco* one to another, making the filthie smoke and stinke thereof, to exhale athwart the dishes and infect the air, when, very often, men that abhorre it are at their repast? Surely Smoke becomes a kitchen far better than a Dining chamber, and yet it makes a kitchen also oftentimes in the inward parts of men, soiling and infecting them, with an unctuous and oily kind of Soote, as hath bene found in some great *Tobacco* takers, that after death were opened.
>   *A Counter-Blaste to Tobacco,* Ch. 4

The publicke use whereof, at all times, and in all places, hath now so farre prevailed, as divers men very sound both in judgment, and complexion, have bene at last forced to take it also without desire, partly because they were ashamed to seeme singular. . . . Now it is become in place of a cure, a point of good fellowship, and he that will refuse to take a pipe of *Tobacco* among his fellowes . . . is accounted peevish and no good company.
>   *Idem*

Moreover, which is a great iniquitie, and against all humanite, the husband shall not bee ashamed, to reduce thereby his delicate, wholesome, and cleane complexioned wife, to that extremitie, that either shee must also corrupt her sweete breath therewith, or else resolute to live in a perpetual stinking torment.

> *Idem*

A custome lothsome to the eye, hatefull to the Nose, harmefull to the braine, dangerous to the Lungs, and the blacke stinking fume thereof, neerest resembling the horrible Stigian smoke of the pit that is bottomlesse.

> *Idem*

Ben Jonson [1573?–1637]

Neither doe thou lust after that tawney weede, tabacco.

> *Bartholomew Fair,* Act II, Sc. vi

I have my three sorts of tabacco in my pocket, my light by me, and thus I beginne.

> *Cynthia's Revels,* Induction

By gods deynes: I marle what pleasure or felicitie they have in taking this rogish tabacco: it's good for nothing but to choake a man, and fill him full of smoake, and imbers.

> *Every Man in His Humour,* Act III, Sc. ii

By *Hercules* I doe holde it, and will affirme it before any Prince in Europe to be the most soveraigne, and pretious herbe that ever the earth tendred to the use of man.

> *Idem*

Robert Burton [1577–1640]

Tobacco, divine, rare, superexcellent *Tobacco,* which goes far beyond all their Panaceas, potable gold, and Philosophers stones, a soveraign remedy to all diseases. A good vomit, I confesse, a virtuous herb, if it be well qualified, opportunely taken, and medicinally used, but as it is commonly abused by

most men, which take it as Tinkers do ale, 'tis a plague, a mischief, a violent purger of goods, lands, health, hellish, divelish and damned *Tobacco,* the ruine and overthrow of body and soul.

> *The Anatomy of Melancholy,* Pt. 2, Sect. 2, Memb. 2, Subsect. 2

Tobias Venner [1577–1660]

Tobacco drieth the brain, dimmeth the sight, vitiateth the smell, hurteth the stomach, destroyeth the concoction, disturbeth the humors and spirits, corrupteth the breath, induceth a trembling of the limbs, exsiccateth the windpipe, lungs, and liver, annoyeth the milt, scorcheth the heart, and causeth the blood to be adusted.

> *Via recta ad vitam longam*

Sir John Beaumont [1582–1628]

Me let the sound of great *Tabaccoes* praise
A pitch above those love-sicke Poets raise:
Let me adore with my thrice-happie pen
The sweete and sole delight of mortall men.

> *Metamorphosis of Tabacco*

Barten Holyday [1593–1661]

Earth ne're did breed
Such a joviall weed.

> *Technogamia,* Act II, Sc. iii

Molière [1622–1673]

No matter what Aristotle and all philosophy may say, there's nothing like tobacco. 'T is the passion of decent folk; and he who lives without tobacco isn't worthy of living.

> *Don Juan, or Le Festin de Pierre,* Act I, Sc. i (tr. by Katharine Prescott Wormeley)

Samuel Johnson [1709–1784]

Smoking . . . is a shocking thing, blowing smoke out of our mouths into

other people's mouths, eyes and noses, and having the same thing done to us.
> Quoted by James Boswell in *Tour to the Hebrides*, August 19, 1773

William Cowper [1731–1800]

Pernicious weed! whose scent the fair annoys,
Unfriendly to society's chief joys,
Thy worst effect is banishing for hours
The sex whose presence civilizes ours.
Conversation

Philip Freneau [1752–1832]

Tobacco surely was designed
To poison, and destroy mankind.
> *Poems,* "Tobacco"

Charles Lamb [1775–1834]

Tobacco has been my evening comfort and my morning curse for these five years.
> Letter to William Wordsworth, September 28, 1805

For thy sake, TOBACCO, I
Would do any thing but die.
> *Ibid.,* "A Farewell to Tobacco"

To do this [1] it will be necessary to leave off Tobacco. But I had some thoughts of doing that before, for I sometimes think it does not agree with me.
> *Ibid.,* June 26, 1806

This very night I am going to *leave off tobacco!* Surely there must be some other world in which this unconquerable purpose shall be realised.
> Letter to Thomas Manning, December 25, 1815

Jesse Torrey [1787–1834]

We shall not refuse tobacco the credit of being sometimes medical, when used

[1] To help his sister Mary with the version of *All's Well That Ends Well* which she was preparing for their *Tales from Shakespeare* and in which she was "stuck fast."

temperately, though an acknowledged poison.
> *The Moral Instructor,* Pt. IV, Sect. II, Ch. 17

George Gordon, Lord Byron [1788–1824]

Sublime tobacco! which from east to west
Cheers the tar's labour or the Turkman's rest; . . .
Divine in hookas, glorious in a pipe, . . .
Yet thy true lovers more admire by far
Thy naked beauties — Give me a cigar!
> *The Island,* Canto II, Sect. 19

Charles Sprague [1791–1875]

Thy clouds all other clouds dispel,
And lap me in delight.
> *To My Cigar*

Thomas Hood [1799–1845]

Some sigh for this and that;
My wishes don't go far;
The world may wag at will,
So I have my cigar.
> *The Cigar*

Edward Bulwer-Lytton [1803–1873]

The man who smokes, thinks like a sage and acts like a Samaritan!
> *Night and Morning,* Bk. I, Ch. VI

Charles Kingsley [1819–1875]

When all things were made none was made better than [tobacco]; to be a lone man's companion, a bachelor's friend, a hungry man's food, a sad man's cordial, a wakeful man's sleep, and a chilly man's fire, Sir; while for stanching of wounds, purging of rheum, and settling of the stomach, there's no herb like unto it under the canopy of heaven.
> *Westward Ho!,* Ch. 7

Charles Stuart Calverley
[1831–1884]

I have a liking old
For thee, though manifold
Stories, I know, are told,
    Not to thy credit;
How one (or two at most)
Drops make a cat a ghost —
Useless, except to roast —
    Doctors have said it.
        Ode to Tobacco

Mark Twain (Samuel L. Clemens)
[1835–1910]

I have made it a rule never to smoke
more than one cigar at a time. . . . As
an example to others, and not that I
care for moderation myself, it has always been my rule never to smoke
when asleep, and never to refrain when
awake.
        Mark Twain's Speeches, "Sev-
        entieth Birthday"

Elizabeth Amy Dillwyn
[1845–1935]

Cigarette-smoking is like drinking beer
out of a thimble.
        Aphorism

Eugene Field [1850–1895]

What smells so? Has somebody been
burning a Rag, or is there a Dead Mule
in the Back yard? No, the Man is
Smoking a Five-Cent Cigar.
        The Tribune Primer, "The
        Five-Cent Cigar"

Thomas Riley Marshall
[1854–1925]

What this country needs is a really
good five-cent cigar.
        Remark to Chief Clerk of the
        U.S. Senate (Quoted by C. M.
        Thomas in *Thomas Riley Mar-
        shall,* Ch. VII)

Oscar Wilde [1854–1900]

A cigarette is the perfect type of a
perfect pleasure. It is exquisite, and it

leaves one unsatisfied. What more can
one want?
        Picture of Dorian Gray, Ch. 6

Sir James M. Barrie [1860–1937]

The Elizabethan age might be better
named the beginning of the smoking
era.
        My Lady Nicotine, Ch. 13

Rudyard Kipling [1865–1936]

And a woman is only a woman, but a
    good cigar is a Smoke.
        The Betrothed

Richard Clarke Cabot [1868–1939]

In a smoker, probably the earliest
known indication of disease is that he
begins to give up tobacco.
        *New England Journal of Med-
        icine* 205:740, 1931

James Joyce [1882–1941]

Rarely smoke, dear. Cigar now and
then. Childish device. (*Lewdly.*) The
mouth can be better engaged than with
a cylinder of rank weed. . . . Sir Walter Raleigh brought from the new
world that potato and that weed, the
one a killer of pestilence by absorption,
the other a poisoner of the ear, eye,
heart, memory, will, understanding, all.
That is to say, he brought the poison
a hundred years before another person
whose name I forget brought the food.
        Ulysses, Bk. II

Graham Lee Hemminger
[1896–1949]

Tobacco is a dirty weed. I like it.
It satisfies no normal need. I like it.
It makes you thin, it makes you lean,
It takes the hair right off your bean.
It's the worst darn stuff I've ever seen.
I like it.
        Penn State Froth, November
        1915

Anonymous

May never lady press his lips, his
    proffer'd love returning,

Who makes a furnace of his mouth,
　and keeps his chimney burning;
May each true woman shun his sight,
　for fear his fumes should choke
　her,
And none but those who smoke them-
　selves have kisses for a smoker.

Caution: Cigarette Smoking May Be
Hazardous to Your Health.
　　　Statement required on cigarette
　　　packages and cartons by the
　　　89th U.S. Congress, 1st Session

Tobacco's an outlandish weed,
Doth in the land strange wonders
　breed;
It taints the breath, the blood it dries,
It burns the head, it blinds the eyes;
It dries the lungs, scourgeth the lights,
It 'numbs the soul, it dulls the sprite.
　　　Quoted by F. W. Fairholt in
　　　Tobacco: Its History and Asso-
　　　ciations, Ch. 3

English Proverbs

Tobacco hic,
If a man be well it will make him sick.

Tobacco hic,
Will make a man well if he be sick.

Estonian Proverb

It is better to be without a wife for a
bit than without tobacco for an hour.

Persian Proverb

Coffee without tobacco is meat without salt.

TONSILS

Plautus [254?–184 B.C.]

O that I now were changed into a
　quinsy,
To seize her throat, and strangle the
　evil jade.
　　　Mostellaria, I.iii.218

Lyman G. Richards [1893–　]

Never in the history of medicine have
so many physicians owed so much economic security to a single operation as
to tonsillectomy.
　　　Quoted in *The New York Times*
　　　Magazine, May 31, 1953

TRANSFUSIONS

Anonymous

Blood-transfusion is neither a panacea
nor a last rite.
　　　Lancet 1:288, 1951

TRANSPLANTATION

Sir Harold Gillies [1882–1960]
and
D. Ralph Millard, Jr. [1919–　]

It is frightening to contemplate what
will follow the solution of the crossgrafting mystery, for it may be as
revolutionary as fission of the atom.
Anyone could then drop in at the local
organ bank and, for a reasonable down
payment, trade in a weak heart and a
feeble brain for more vigorous ones, a
cirrhotic liver for a softer one. Death
vacancies on this planet would soon
be limited to civil accidents, war casualties and cosmic travel.
　　　The Principles and Art of Plas-
　　　tic Surgery, Vol. II, Ch. 32

TREATMENT

See also BLOODLETTING, DIAG-
NOSIS, DRUGS, HYDROTHER-
APY, PSYCHOTHERAPY, REM-
EDIES

Huang Ti (The Yellow Emperor)
[2697–2597 B.C.]

The people of these regions [the West]
. . . become robust and energetic. . . .

Hence evil cannot injure their external bodies, and if they get diseases they strike at the inner body. These diseases are most successfully cured with poison medicines.

> *Nei Ching Su Wên*, Bk. 4, Sect. 12 (tr. by Ilza Veith as *The Yellow Emperor's Classic of Internal Medicine*)

The treatment with poison medicines comes from the West.

> *Idem*

Confucius [551–478 B.C.]

Because the newer methods of treatment are good, it does not follow that the old ones were bad: for if our honorable and worshipful ancestors had not recovered from their ailments, you and I would not be here to-day.

Sushruta [5th Cent.? B.C.]

The physician, the patient, the medicine, and the attendants (nurses) are the four essential factors of a course of medical treatment. Even a dangerous disease is readily cured, or it may be expected to run a speedy course in the event of the preceding four factors being respectively found to be qualified, self-controlled, genuine and intelligently watchful.

> *Sushruta-Samhitá*, "Sutrasthánam," Ch. 34 (tr. by K. K. L. Bhishagratna)

Hippocrates [460?–377? B.C.]

For extreme diseases, extreme strictness of treatment is most efficacious.

> *Aphorisms*, I.6 (tr. by W. H. S. Jones)

As to diseases, make a habit of two things — to help, or at least to do no harm.

> *Epidemics*, Bk. I, Sect. XI (tr. by W. H. S. Jones)

People rather admire what is new, although they do not know whether it be proper or not, than what they are accustomed to, and know already to be proper; and what is strange, they prefer to what is obvious.

> *On Fractures*, I (tr. by Francis Adams)

What you should put first in all the practice of our art is how to make the patient well; and if he can be made well in many ways, one should choose the least troublesome.

> *On Joints*, 78 (tr. by E. T. Withington)

Plato [427?–347 B.C.]

And what would you say of the physician? In prescribing meats and drinks would he wish to go beyond another physician or beyond the practice of medicine? He would not. But would he wish to go beyond the non-physician? Yes.

> *Republic*, I.350.A (tr. by Benjamin Jowett)

When a carpenter is ill he asks the physician for a rough and ready cure; an emetic or a purge or a cautery or the knife — these are his remedies. And if someone prescribes for him a course of dietetics, and tells him that he must swathe and swaddle his head, and all that sort of thing, he replies at once that he has no time to be ill, and that he sees no good in a life which is spent in nursing his disease to the neglect of his customary employment; and therefore bidding good-bye to this sort of physician, he resumes his ordinary habits, and either gets well and lives and does his business, or, if his constitution fails, he dies and has no more trouble.

> *Ibid.*, III.406.D

Aristotle [384–322 B.C.]

To have a judgement that when Callias was suffering from this or that disease this or that benefited him, and similarly with Socrates and various other individuals, is a matter of experience; but to judge that it benefits all persons of a certain type, considered as a class, who suffer from this or that disease (e.g. the phlegmatic or bilious when suffering from burning fever) is a matter of art.

> *Metaphysics,* I.i (tr. by H. Tredennick)

Even in medicine, though it is easy to know what honey, wine and hellebore, cautery and surgery are, to know how and to whom and when to apply them so as to effect a cure is no less an undertaking than to be a physician.

> *Nicomachean Ethics,* V.ix (tr. by H. Rackham)

Herophilus [fl. 300 B.C.]

Medicines are nothing in themselves, if not properly used, but the very hands of the gods, if employed with reason and prudence.

Cicero [106–43 B.C.]

A careful physician . . . , before he attempts to administer a remedy to his patient, must investigate not only the malady of the man he wishes to cure, but also his habits when in health, and his physical constitution.

> *On the Orator,* II.xliv.186 (tr. by E. W. Sutton)

Ovid [43 B.C.–A.D. 17?]

Too late is the medicine prepared, when the disease has gained strength by long delay.

> *The Remedies of Love,* 91 (tr. by J. H. Mozley)

Medicine sometimes removes, sometimes bestows safety, showing what plant is healthful, what harmful.

> *Tristia,* II.269 (tr. by A. L. Wheeler)

Celsus [25 B.C.–A.D. 50]

During the same times the Art of Medicine was divided into three parts:

one being that which cures through diet, another through medicaments, and the third by the hand. The Greeks termed the first *dietetics,* the second *pharmaceutics,* the third *chirurgics.*

> *De Medicina,* Prooemium (tr. by W. G. Spencer)

Treatment is to be always directed to the part [of the body] which is mostly in trouble.

> *Ibid.,* I.iii.14

Seneca [4? B.C.–A.D. 65]

The physician cannot prescribe by letter the proper time for eating or bathing; he must feel the pulse.

> *Moral Epistles to Lucilius,* XXII (tr. by Richard M. Gummere)

Rhazes [850–923]

In treating a patient, let your first thought be to strengthen his natural vitality.

Arnold of Villanova [13th Cent.]

A wise Physician will not give Physic but upon necessity, & first try medicinal diet, before he proceed to medicinal cure.

> Quoted by Robert Burton in *The Anatomy of Melancholy,* Pt. 2, Sect. 1, Memb. 4, Subsect. 1

Amerigo Vespucci [1451–1512]

They [1] use in their sicknesses various forms of medicines, so different from ours that we marvelled how any one escaped: for many times I saw that with a man sick of fever, when it heightened upon him, they bathed him from head to foot with a large quantity of cold water: then they lit a great fire around him, making him turn and turn again every two hours, until they tired him and left him to sleep, and many were (thus) cured: with

[1] The Indians encountered by Vespucci on his first voyage to the Caribbean in 1497.

this they make use of dieting, for they remain three days without eating, and also of blood-letting, but not from the arm, only from the thighs and the loins and the calf of the leg: also they provoke vomiting with their herbs which are put into the mouth: and they use many other remedies which it would be long to relate.

> Letter to Pier Soderini, Gonfalonier of the Republic of Florence, 1497 (in *The First Four Voyages of Amerigo Vespucci,* tr. by M. K.)

Leonardo da Vinci [1452–1519]

You know that medicines when well used restore health to the sick: they will be well used when the doctor together with his understanding of their nature shall understand also what man is, what life is, and what constitution and health are. Know these well and you will know their opposites; and when this is the case you will know well how to devise a remedy.

> *Codice Atlantico,* 270 (tr. by Edward MacCurdy in *The Notebooks of Leonardo da Vinci,* Vol. I, Ch. VII)

Sir Thomas More [1478–1535]

The sycke (as I sayde) they see to with great affection, and lette nothing at al passe concerninge either Phisycke or good diete, whereby they may be restored againe to their health.

> *Utopia,* Bk. II, Ch. 7 (tr. by R. Robinson)

Henry VIII of England [1491–1547]

By which ye leve the often takyng of medicines that ye were wont to use and while ye so do, ye shall not faile of helthe, which our Lord long preserve.

> Quoted by Sir Thomas More in a letter written to Cardinal Wolsey at the command of Henry VIII, July 5, 1519

Ambroise Paré [1517?–1590]

I dressed him and God healed him.[1]

> *The Apologie and Treatise of Ambroise Paré,* Pt. I

Michel de Montaigne [1533–1592]

Of medicine I believe all the bad or the good you like, for we have, thank God, no dealings whatever. . . . I despise it always, but when I am sick, instead of making peace overtures, I begin also to hate and fear it; and I reply to those who urge me to take medicine that they should wait at least until I am restored to my strength and health, so that I may have more resources to withstand the impact and the hazards of their potion.

> *Essays,* Bk. I, Ch. 24, "Various Outcomes of the Same Plan" (tr. by Donald M. Frame)

The ordinary course of a cure is carried on at the expense of life: they incise us, they cauterize us, they amputate our limbs, they deprive us of food and blood. One step further, and we are completely cured.

> *Ibid.,* Bk. II, Ch. 3, "A Custom of the Island of Cea"

Both in health and in sickness I have readily let myself follow my urgent appetites. I give great authority to my desires and inclinations. I do not like to cure trouble by trouble; I hate remedies that are more nuisance than the disease. To be subjected to the stone and subjected to abstaining from the pleasure of eating oysters, those are two troubles for one. The disease pinches us on one side, the rule on the other. Since there is a risk of making a mistake, let us risk it rather in pursuit of pleasure. The world does the opposite, and thinks nothing beneficial that is not painful; it is suspicious of ease.

> *Ibid.,* Bk. III, Ch. 13, "Of Experience"

[1] Je le pensay, et Dieu le guarit.

Doctors . . . keep prescribing for sick men a way of life not only new, but contrary: a change that a healthy man could not endure. . . . If they do no other good, they do at least this, that they prepare their patients early for death, undermining little by little and cutting off their enjoyment of life.
Idem

The art of medicine is not so fixed that we are without authority, no matter what we do; it changes according to the climates and according to the moons, according to Fernel and according to L'Escale. If your doctor does not think it good for you to sleep, to drink wine, or to eat such-and-such a food, don't worry: I'll find you another who will not agree with him.
Idem

We should give free passage to diseases; and I find that they do not stay so long with me, who let them go ahead; and some of those that are considered most stubborn and tenacious, I have shaken off by their own decadence, without help and without art, and against the rules of medicine. Let us give Nature a chance; she knows her business better than we do. "But so-and-so died of it." So will you, if not of that disease, of some other. And how many have not failed to die of it, with three doctors at their backsides?
Idem

Sir Walter Raleigh [1552?–1618]

If we condemn natural *Magick,* or the wisdom of Nature, because the Devil (who knoweth more than any man) doth also teach Witches and Poisoners the harmful parts of Herbs, Drugs, Minerals and Excrements: then may we, by the same rule, condemn the *Physician,* and the Art of Healing.
History of the World, Bk. I, Ch. xi, Sect. 3

William Shakespeare [1564–1616]
Plutus himself,
That knows the tinct and multiplying med'cine,
Hath not in nature's mystery more science
Than I have in this ring.
All's Well That Ends Well, V, iii, 101

I will not cast away my physic but on those that are sick.
As You Like It, III, ii, 376

SICINIUS: He's a disease that must be cut away.
MENENIUS: O, he's a limb that has but a disease:
Mortal, to cut it off; to cure it, easy.
Coriolanus, III, i, 295

It is but as a body yet distempered,
Which to his former strength may be restor'd
With good advice and little medicine.
Henry IV, Part II, III, i, 41

Preserving life in med'cine potable.
Ibid., IV, v, 163

Thou speak'st like a physician, Helicanus,
That ministers a potion unto me
That thou wouldst tremble to receive thyself.
Pericles, I, ii, 66

'Tis known, I ever
Have studied physic, through which secret art,
By turning o'er authorities, I have,
Together with my practice, made familiar
To me and to my aid the blest infusions
That dwell in vegetives, in metals, stones;
And I can speak of the disturbances
That nature works, and of her cures; which doth give me

A more content in course of true de-
light
Than to be thirsty after tottering
honour,
Or tie my treasure up in silken bags,
To please the fool and death.
Ibid., III, ii, 31

Ben Jonson [1573?–1637]

We will be brave, *Puffe*, now we ha'
the *med'cine*.
The Alchemist, Act II, Sc. ii

John Milton [1608–1674]

In Physic, things of melancholic hue
and quality are used against melancholy, sour against sour, salt to remove
salt humours.
Samson Agonistes, Preface

Molière [1622–1673]

DOCTOR: The patient is a fool. In the
disease that he has it is not in the head
but according to Galen in the spleen
that he should have pain. . . . How
many times has he been bled?
COUNTRY GIRL: Fifteen times, sir,
within twenty days. . . .
DOCTOR: That proves that the disease is not in the blood. We will then
purge him an equal number of times
to find out whether it may be in the
humours and if that does not help, we
will send him to the baths.
Don Juan

Thomas Sydenham [1624–1689]

We are overwhelmed as it is, with an
infinite abundance of vaunted medicaments, and here they add a new one.
Medical Observations (3rd ed.),
Preface (tr. by R. G. Latham
in *Works*, Vol. I)

How I can make a patient vomit, and
how I can purge or sweat him, are
matters which a druggist's shopboy
can tell me offhand. When, however,
I must use one sort of medicine in
preference to another, requires an in-
formant of a different kind — a man
who has no little practice in the arena
of his profession.

It is a great mistake to suppose that
Nature always stands in need of the
assistance of Art . . . nor do I think
it below me to acknowledge that, when
no manifest indication pointed out to
me what was to be done, I have consulted the safety of my patient and
my own reputation effectually by doing nothing at all.

Increase Mather [1639–1723]

As it is unlawful to entreat witches to
heal bewitched persons, because they
cannot do this but by Satan, so is it
very sinful by scratching, or burnings,
or detention of urine, &c. to endeavour
to constrain them to unbewitch any;
for this is to put them upon seeking
to the devil.
Remarkable Providences, Ch. 8

Cotton Mather [1663–1728]

Let this advice for the *sick* be principally attended to: *Don't kill 'em!*
That is to say, with mischievous kindness. Indeed, if we stopt here, and
said no more, this were enough to save
more *lives* than our *wars* have destroyed.

Alain René Lesage [1668–1747]

Remember, my friend, that bleeding
and drinking warm water are the two
grand principles; the true secret of
curing all the distempers incident to
humanity.
Gil Blas de Santillana, Bk. II,
Ch. 3 (tr. by Tobias Smollett)

Alexander Pope [1688–1744]

Be not the first by whom the new are
tried,
Nor yet the last to lay the old aside.
An Essay on Criticism, Pt. II

Lady Mary Wortley Montagu [1689–1762]

I hope you will no more suffer the physicians to try experiments with so good a constitution as yours.
> Letter to Mr. Wortley Montagu, November 12, 1757

John Armstrong [1709–1779]

For want of timely care Millions have died of medicable wounds.
> *The Art of Preserving Health,* Bk. III

William Heberden [1710–1801]

Lastly, where there is no room for anything else, there it is the duty of a physician to exert himself as much as possible in supporting the powers of life, by strengthening the appetite and digestion, and by providing that the stools, and sleep, and every other article of health, shall approach as nearly as may be to its natural state.
> *Commentaries on the History and Cure of Diseases,* Ch. 2

New medicines, and new methods of cure, always work miracles for a while.[1]
> *Ibid.,* Ch. 9

Jean Jacques Rousseau [1712–1778]

However useful well-administered medicine may be to us, it is still certain that if the sick savage, left to himself, has nothing to hope for except from nature, on the other hand he has nothing to fear except from his disease; a circumstance which often renders his situation preferable to ours.
> *A Discourse Upon the Origin and the Foundation of the Inequality Among Mankind,* Pt. I

[1] Cf. Sir William Withey Gull, p. 495b.

With so few sources of sickness, man in his natural state hardly needs any medicines, and needs doctors even less; in that respect the human species is in no worse condition than any other, and it is easy to find out from hunters if in their travels they find many sick animals. Several have found animals whose extensive wounds have healed very well, who have had bones and even limbs broken and mended without any surgeon but time, without any regimen but their ordinary life, and who are no less perfectly cured for not having been tormented with incisions, poisoned with drugs, and exhausted with fasts.
> *Idem*

I shall always ask what real good the art of medicine has done to men. Some of those whom it cures would die, to be sure, but millions whom it kills would live. Sensible reader, do not invest in that lottery where the chances are so heavily against you. Suffer, die, or get well, but in any case *live* to your last hour.
> *Émile,* Bk. II

James Townley [1714–1778]

Wonderful is the skill of a physician; for a rich man he prescribeth various admixtures and compounds, by which the patient is brought to health in many days at an expense of fifty pounds; while for a poor man for the same disease he giveth a more common name, and prescribeth a dose of oil, which worketh a cure in a single night charging fourpence therefor.

Thomas Jefferson [1743–1826]

I would wish the young practitioner, especially, to have deeply impressed on his mind, the real limits of his art, & that when the state of his patient gets beyond these, his office is to be a watchful, but quiet spectator of the operations of nature, giving them fair play by a well-regulated regimen, & by all the aid they can derive from the excitement of good spirits and hope in the patient.

> Letter to Dr. Caspar Wistar, June 21, 1807

The patient, treated on the fashionable theory, sometimes gets well in spite of the medicine. The medicine therefore restored him, & the young doctor receives new courage to proceed in his bold experiments on the lives of his fellow creatures.

> *Idem*

To an unknown disease, there cannot be a known remedy. Here then, the judicious, the moral, the humane physician should stop. Having been so often a witness to the salutary efforts which nature makes to re-establish the disordered functions, he should rather trust to their action, than hazard the interruption of that, and a greater derangement of the system, by conjectural experiments on a machine so complicated & so unknown as the human body, & a subject so sacred as human life.

> *Idem*

I have been long sensible that while I was endeavoring to render our country the greatest of all services, that of regenerating the public education, . . . I was discharging the odious function of a Physician pouring medicine down the throat of a patient, insensible of needing it.

> Letter to Joseph C. Cabell, February 7, 1826

John Coakley Lettsom
[1744–1815]

When people's ill, they comes to I,
I physics, bleeds, and sweats 'em;
Sometimes they live, sometimes they die.
What's that to I? I lets 'em.

> *On Dr. Lettsom, by Himself*

George Colman, the Younger
[1762–1836]

But, when ill indeed,
E'en dismissing the Doctor don't *always* succeed.

> *Broad Grins,* "Lodgings for Single Gentlemen"

Christoph Wilhelm Hufeland
[1762–1836]

After thirty years' practice, I am fully convinced that two-thirds of all my patients would have recovered without the use of physic, or the attendance of a physician.

Napoleon Bonaparte [1769–1821]

Medicines are only fit for old people.

> Quoted by Barry O'Meara in *Napoleon in Exile,* August 19, 1816

Take a dose of medicine once, and in all probability you will be obliged to take an additional hundred afterwards.

> *Ibid.,* September 26, 1817

Our body is a watch that is designed to go for a given time. The watchmaker cannot open it, and must in handling it, grope his way blindfold and at random. For once that he assists and relieves it, by dint of tormenting it with his crooked instruments, he injures it ten times, and at last destroys it.

> Quoted by Dr. F. Antommarchi in *The Last Days of the Emperor Napoleon,* October 14, 1820

Sydney Smith [1771–1845]

Mrs. Sydney has eight distinct illnesses, and I have nine. We take something every hour, and pass the mixture from one to the other.

> Letter to R. Murchison, 1840

James Jackson [1777–1867]

A physician need not always declare his prognosis, but he should always try to make one for himself — it decides the treatment — the greater the danger, the bolder may be the treatment, if any reliance is to be placed on treatment.

Letter to James Jackson, Jr., August 28, 1831

Shall we ever have fixed laws? Shall we ever know, or must we ever be doomed to suspect or presume? Is *perhaps* to be our qualifying word forever? Do we know, for example, in how many cases such a treatment fails for the one time that it succeeds?

Quoted in *Vital Magnetic Cure*, "Contrast Between Medicine and Magnetism"

François Magendie [1783–1855]

I hesitate not to declare, no matter how sorely I shall wound our vanity, that so gross is our ignorance of the real nature of the physiological disorders called diseases, that it would perhaps be better to do nothing, and resign the complaint we are called upon to treat to the resources of *nature*, than to act as we are frequently compelled to do, without knowing the why and the wherefore of our conduct, and at obvious risk of hastening the end of the patient.

Quoted in *Vital Magnetic Cure*

Jacob Bigelow [1786–1879]

A man who falls sick at home or abroad is liable to get heroic treatment, or nominal treatment, random treatment, or no treatment at all, according to the hands into which he may happen to fall.

Address to the Massachusetts Medical Society, 1835

George Gordon, Lord Byron [1788–1824]

'Tis written in the Hebrew Chronicle,
How the physicians, leaving pill and potion,

Prescribed, by way of blister, a young belle,
When old King David's blood grew dull in motion,
And that the medicine answer'd very well.

Don Juan, Canto I, Stanza 168

Peter Mere Latham [1789–1875]

There is no such thing as calculating the results of medical treatment with certainty. Success and failure run contrary to expectation sometimes in every disease.

Diseases of the Heart, Lect. XI

There is such a thing as sober conjecture, as well as sober certainty. And diseases are treated, and cures are achieved, and lives are saved, as often under the guidance of one as the other.

Ibid., Lect. XX

Among the perils of disease we must not refuse to reckon the errors of physicians. . . . Nor among the perils of disease must we refuse to reckon the interference of friends with its treatment.

General Remarks on the Practice of Medicine, "The Heart and Its Affections," Ch. IV

David Craigie [1793–1866]

When the physician is at a loss, it is wiser to do nothing than to recommend what may be injurious.

Quoted in *St. Bartholomew's Hospital Reports* 52:47, 1916

Francis Hopkins Ramadge [1793–1867]

It cannot be denied that the present system of medicine is a burning reproach to its professors; if, indeed, a series of vague and uncertain incongruities deserve to be called by that name. How rarely do our medicines do good! How often do they make our patients really worse! I fearlessly assert that in most cases the sufferer would be safer without a physician than with one. I have seen enough of the mal-practice of my professional brethren to warrant the strong language I employ.

> Quoted in *Vital Magnetic Cure*

Robert James Graves [1796–1853]

This [the healthy appearance of convalescents from typhus at Meath Hospital, Dublin] is all the effect of our good feeding; and lest, when I am gone, you may be at a loss for an epitaph for me, let me give you one, in three words: — He Fed Fevers.

> Quoted in *A Memorial of Graves,* "The Life and Labours of Graves"

Edward Kentish [fl. 1797]

I presume one of the great causes of error is the assigning to various applications the cure of slight burns, some of which no doubt would have got well without any, and perhaps much sooner than with those which were used. This mistake frequently happens from good motives, and by the best intentioned people; for if we have seen a person recover from any complaint during the use of any particular means we naturally imagine such beneficial effect to have arisen from that cause, although upon further investigation, it may be found to have been inadequate.

> *Essay on Burns*

It falls to the lot of few men to appreciate properly the effect of various modes of treatment in a particular disease; for if a patient recovers, whatever was the treatment, whether good or bad, we flatter ourselves it was the effect of our superior merit in conducting the disease; but future experience may convince us that the recovery, of which we so vainly boasted, was a victory of Nature over the malpractice of art.

> *Idem*

Ralph Waldo Emerson [1803–1882]

The physician prescribes hesitatingly out of his few resources. . . . If the patient mends, he is glad and surprised.

> *The Conduct of Life,* Ch. VII

Elisha Bartlett [1804–1855]

Difficult as it may be to cure, it is always easy to poison and to kill.

> *Philosophy of Medical Science,* Pt. II, Ch. 16

John Y. Bassett [1805–1851]

I doubt, however, if, in the present state of medicine, a thorough physician is ever, in any stage of any disease, so completely without rational education as to be thus non-plussed, and driven to the necessity of dealing a blow in the dark. Where there are no intelligible indications, it is clear there should be no action.

> *Southern Medical Reports,* Vol. 2, 1850–51, "Reports from Alabama"

Josef Skoda [1805–1881]

Ach, das ist ja alles Eins! [1]
[Oh, that is all one!]

> Quoted by F. H. Garrison in *An Introduction to the History of Medicine,* Ch. XI

Frederick Saunders [1807–1902]

The best practitioners give to their patients the least medicine.

Oliver Wendell Holmes [1809–1894]

Nature, in medical language, as opposed to Art, means trust in the reactions of the living system against ordinary normal impressions.
Art, in the same language, as opposed to Nature, means an intentional resort

[1] Comment when, after having established a diagnosis, he was asked about the treatment of the patient.

to extraordinary abnormal impressions for the relief of disease.

> *Medical Essays*, "Currents and Counter-Currents in Medical Science"

There is nothing men will not do, there is nothing they have not done, to recover their health and save their lives. They have submitted to be half-drowned in water, and half-choked with gases, to be buried up to their chins in earth, to be seared with hot irons like galley-slaves, to be crimped with knives, like cod-fish, to have needles thrust into their flesh, and bonfires kindled on their skin, to swallow all sorts of abominations, and to pay for all this, as if blisters were a blessing, and leeches were a luxury. What more can be asked to prove their honesty and sincerity?

> *Ibid.*, "The Young Practitioner"

Claude Bernard [1813–1878]

When we begin to base our opinions on medical tact, on inspiration or on more or less vague intuitions about things, we are outside of science and offer an example of that fanciful method which may involve the greatest dangers, by surrendering the health and life of the sick to the whims of an inspired ignoramus. True science teaches us to doubt and, in ignorance, to refrain.

> *An Introduction to the Study of Experimental Medicine*, Pt. I, Ch. 2, Sect. vii (tr. by H. C. Greene)

J. Marion Sims [1813–1883]

Let man learn to be honest and do the right thing or do nothing.

Alfred Stillé [1813–1900]

It is quite as necessary for the physician to know when to abstain from the use of medicine as it is for him to prescribe when medication is neces-

sary; . . . he must, as far as possible, see the end of a disease from its beginning; . . . he must never forget that medical art has a far higher range and aim than the prescription of drugs or even of food and hygienic means, and that when neither of these avails to ward off the fatal ending, it is still no small portion of his art to rid his patient's path of thorns if he cannot make it bloom with roses.

> *Medical News* 44:433, 1884

Prince Otto von Bismarck [1815–1898]

Laws are like medicine; they generally cure an evil by a lesser or a passing evil.

> Speech in the Prussian Chamber of Deputies, March 6, 1872

Sir William Withey Gull [1816–1890]

Never forget that it is not a pneumonia, but a pneumonic man who is your patient. Not a typhoid fever, but a typhoid man.

> *Published Writings* (ed. by T. D. Acland), Memoir II

Rudolf Virchow [1821–1902]

What is dark and incomprehensible attracts some minds more than what is clear and understandable.

> Quoted by F. H. Garrison in *Bulletin of the New York Academy of Medicine* 4:994, 1928

Henrik Ibsen [1828–1906]

Many a wound must be probed till it bleeds before you are cured of your sickness.

> *Brand*, Act IV

Abraham Jacobi [1830–1919]

Treat the man who is sick and not a Greek name.

> Quoted by F. H. Garrison in *Bulletin of the New York Academy of Medicine* 4:1003, 1928

Samuel Butler [1835–1902]

These people say further, that the greater part of the illness which exists in their country is brought about by the insane manner in which it is treated.

Erewhon, Ch. XII

Sir Thomas Lauder Brunton [1844–1916]

There are various recommendations which a doctor gives to his patients, and which are very hard to get carried out. One of those is work for those who will not take it; another, rest for those who cannot get it; yet another is restraint of the appetites.

Lectures on the Action of Medicines, Lect. 1

Sir William Osler [1849–1919]

The physician without physiology and chemistry flounders along in an aimless fashion, never able to gain any accurate conception of disease, practicing a sort of popgun pharmacy, hitting now the malady and again the patient, he himself not knowing which.

Aequanimitas, with Other Addresses, "Teaching and Thinking"

From Hippocrates to Hunter the treatment of disease was one long traffic in hypotheses.

British Medical Journal 2:185, 1909

Robert Tuttle Morris [1857–1945]

It is the patient rather than the case which requires treatment.

Doctors Versus Folks, Ch. 2

Frederick Peterson [1859–1938]

Whatever will help the patient to get well, I'm in favor of, whether Osteopathy, New Thought, Hindu Yoga or Christian Science. We need catholicity of mind in the treatment of nervous disorders. We must treat the soul as well as the body.

Quoted by Mary Lou Mc-Donough in *Poet Physicians*

Sir Andrew MacPhail [1864–1938]

For a perfect sight of the old medicine, let me conduct you to the bedside of Charles II: With a cry he fell. Dr. King, who, fortunately, happened to be present, bled him with a pocket knife. Fourteen physicians were quickly in attendance. They bled him more thoroughly; they scarified and cupped him; they shaved and blistered his head; they gave him an emetic, a clyster, and two pills. During the next eight days they "threw in" fifty-seven separate drugs; and towards the end, a cordial containing forty more. This availing nothing, they tried Goa stone, which was a calculus obtained from a species of Indian goat; and as a final remedy, the distillate of human skull. In the case report it is recorded that the emetic and the purge worked so mightily well that it was a wonder the patient died.

British Medical Journal 1:445, 1933

Alfred Cox [1866–1954]

You'll often find yourself puzzled about the nature of a complaint and about what you ought to prescribe for the patient. I find it is a good thing in such cases to find out what the patient likes most and firmly *knock him off it.*[1]

Among the Doctors

Stephen B. Leacock [1869–1944]

In the old-fashioned days when a man got sick he went to the family doctor and said he was sick. The doctor gave him a bottle of medicine. He took it home and drank it and got well.

On the bottle was written, "Three times a day in water." The man drank it three times a day the first day,

[1] Advice given to him by the older doctor with whom he served his apprenticeship

twice the second day, and once the third day. On the fourth day he forgot it. But that didn't matter. He was well by that time. . . .

Such medicine was, of course, hopelessly unscientific, hopelessly limited. Death could beat it round every corner. But it was human, gracious, kindly.

> *The Leacock Roundabout,* "The Doctor and the Contraption," Sect. I

Hugh Cabot [1872–1945]

It is better to shoot the patient than to shoot the works.

> Lecture

Russell John Howard [1875–1942]

Diagnosis precedes treatment.

> Quoted by F. G. St. Clair Strange in *The Hip,* Ch. 7

Reduce the deformity, maintain the reduction, restore the function.

> *Ibid.,* Ch. 10

Thomas Mann [1875–1955]

We are aware that the intercalation of periods of change and novelty is the only means by which we can refresh our sense of time, strengthen, retard, and rejuvenate it, and therewith renew our perception of life itself. Such is the purpose of our changes of air and scene, of all our sojourns at cures and bathing resorts; it is the secret of the healing power of change and incident.

> *The Magic Mountain,* Ch. IV, "Excursus on the Sense of Time" (tr. by H. T. Lowe-Porter)

Martin H. Fischer [1879–1962]

I feel sorry for you, Boys! We used to learn our therapy from a professor. Now he disparages the subject and you learn it from the drug house or a radio.

> Quoted by Howard Fabing and Ray Marr in *Fischerisms*

Some day, when you have time, look into the business of prayer, amulets, baths and poultices, and discover for yourself how much valuable therapy the profession has cast on the dump.

> *Idem*

You have allowed the drug hawkers, the cosmeticians, the masseurs and the colon flushers to run off with the major portion of your practice — treatment.

> *Idem*

Thomas Addis [1881–1949]

Practice is entirely concerned with the individual, whereas classification abstracts from the individual and considers the group. Classification is, therefore, at first disowned even while implicitly it is continuously in operation. But as time passes and decisions are reached on the treatment of each of these unique individuals, we begin to think of them less as people and more as instances of a series of general rules. Ultimately the detachment from individual considerations is complete, for disease in individuals has an end — they recover or they die. When all the facts are in and there is nothing more to do we can afford to be "scientific."

> *Glomerular Nephritis, Diagnosis and Treatment,* Ch. 5

Albert R. Lamb [1881–]

The physician has two sleeves, one containing a diagnostic and the other a therapeutic armamentarium; these sleeves should rarely be emptied in one move; keep some techniques in reserve; time your maneuvers to best serve the status and special needs of your patient.

> Quoted by David Seegal in *Journal of Chronic Diseases* 16:443, 1963

Arthur L. Bloomfield [1888–1962]

Every hospital should have a plaque in the physicians' and students' entrances: "There are some patients whom we cannot help; there are none whom we cannot harm."

> Personal communication after iatrogenic tragedy (ca. 1930–1936)

William Faulkner [1897–1962]

What do doctors know? They make their livings advising people to do whatever they are not doing at the time, which is the extent of anyone's knowledge of the degenerate ape.

> *The Sound and the Fury,* "April Sixth 1928"

Alfred Blalock [1899–1964]

It usually requires a considerable time to determine with certainty the virtues of a new method of treatment and usually still longer to ascertain the harmful effects.

> *Principles of Surgical Care*

Sir Theodore Fox [1899–   ]

We shall have to learn to refrain from doing things merely because we know how to do them.

> *Lancet* 2:801, 1965

David Seegal [1899–   ]

The young physician today is so generously provided with a kit of diagnostic and therapeutic tools, his attention might be wisely directed to the question of "what not to do" as well as "what to do."

> *Journal of Chronic Diseases* 17:299, 1964

Fuller Albright [1900–   ]

One cannot possibly practice good medicine and not understand the fundamentals underlying therapy. Few if any rules for therapy are more than 90 per cent correct. If one does not understand the fundamentals, one does more harm in the 10 per cent of instances to which the rules do not apply than one does good in the 90 per cent to which they do apply.

> *Textbook of Medicine* (9th ed. by Russell L. Cecil and Robert F. Loeb), "Diseases of the Ductless Glands," Introduction

George H. Day [1900–   ]

Apart from poisoning by stealth there is no form of therapy from which the effects of suggestion can be entirely eliminated.

> *British Journal of Physical Medicine* 18:15, 1955

Ogden Nash [1902–   ]

I haven't the slightest idea where fashions in pathology are born. . . .

Possibly some of my older readers dimly recollect the days when modish scientists declared that the only dependable method of relieving a toothache was a clean, conclusive appendectomy. Then the whistle blew for the quarter, the two teams changed goals, and it developed that if you had a pain in your side it was high time your teeth came out. Late in the second half, tonsils got into the game and broke away for a long run; two plays later, colitis recovered a fumble and kicked out of danger, and the issue has been terribly confused ever since. Only one point is clear: it's better to be dead, or even perfectly well, than to suffer from the wrong affliction. The man who owns up to arthritis in a beriberi year is as lonely as a woman in a last month's dress.

> *Saturday Evening Post,* October 14, 1933, "How's Your Sacro-iliac?"

Sir George W. Pickering [1904–   ]

Medicine is not yet liberated from the medieval idea that disease is the result of sin and must be expiated by mortification of the flesh.

> *Resident Physician* 11 (No. 9): 71, 1965

David Littmann [1906–   ]

It came to me, in times gone by,
That nature often helped the cure,
That doctors tried but not to hurt
And drugs were mercifully weak.
It's little help, these modern days,
To urge restraint, to watch and wait.
To stay the hot and eager hand
With sharpened blade and two-edged
    drug.
The patient's come with a disease,
He must be healed tomorrow. . . .
And now to thwart what might oc-
    cur —
Thrombosis is an ugly thought;
Dicumarol and heparin,
Statistics show, prevent most ills
Like thrombus of the coronary,
Infarction of the heart and baldness,
Angina pectoris and heartburn,
Flatulence and morning nausea.
And tests are made so many times
That arms turn blue and blood runs
    thin.

When my time comes, no matter how,
I plan to hide, deny and lie.
I'll not complain, divulge a symptom,
Betray a sign, confess a hurt.
I'll not accept my brother's kidney,
Or wear a heart of chimpanzee;
I'll not be joined to wires and tubing,
I'll not be tracheostomized.
If this seems strange from a physician,
It must be I'm not ready yet.
> *New England Journal of Medi-
> cine* 273:1201, 1965, "The
> Good Old Days"

Stanley O. Hoerr [1909–   ]

It is difficult to make the asymp-
tomatic patient feel better.
> *American Journal of Surgery*
> 103:411, 1962

C. Stuart Welch [1909–   ]

Enemas are enemies.
> Aphorism

Alexander Lenard [1910–   ]

Everything depends, as in all human
relations, upon dosage.
> *The Valley of the Latin Bear,*
> Ch. 10

Thomas F. Main [1911–   ]

The sufferer who frustrates a keen
therapist by failing to improve is always in danger of meeting primitive
human behavior disguised as treatment.
> *British Journal of Medical Psy-
> chology* 30:129, 1957

James M. Hunter [1924–   ]

Treat the patient, not the x-ray.
> Address, American Fracture As-
> sociation, October 1964

Alvan R. Feinstein [1925–   ]

Before the changes of the past century,
the practice of medicine could be illustrated by a single, traditional picture
. . . a physician seated at a bedside,
studying a sick patient and administering the most effective available treatment: compassion.
> *Annals of Internal Medicine*
> 61:757, 1964

Anonymous

Even where medicine cannot heal, it
obtains one of its greatest triumphs in
palliating disorder.

Modern therapy, particularly of malignancy, makes good use of the Borgia
effect — two poisons are more efficacious than one.

Of old when folk lay sick and sorely
    tried
The doctors gave them physic, and
    they died.
But here's a happier age: for now we
    know
Both how to make men sick and keep
    them so.
> *On Hygiene*

Where there is no treatment, there are many treatments.

Proverbs

He's the best physician that knows the worthlessness of the most medicines.

Many medicines, few cures.

African (Nupe) Proverb

If you intend to give a sick man medicine, let him get very ill first, so that he may see the benefit of your medicine.

Danish Proverbs

Good advice is no better than bad advice unless it is taken at the right time.

Nothing kills like doing nothing.

French Proverb

The presence of the doctor is the beginning of the cure.

Hindu Proverb

If you have a toothache, cut off your tongue; if you have a sore eye, cut off your hand.

Indian (Tamil) Proverb

Hospitality and medicine must be confined to three days.

Spanish Proverb

Bleed him and purge him; if he dies, bury him.

TRICHINOSIS

Ambrose Bierce [1842–1914?]

TRICHINOSIS, n. The pig's reply to proponents of porcophagy.
The Devil's Dictionary

TRUTH

See also PATIENT–PHYSICIAN RELATIONSHIP

Plato [427?–347 B.C.]

Truth should be highly valued; if, as we were saying, a lie is useless to the gods, and useful only as a medicine to men, then the use of such medicines should be restricted to physicians.
Republic, III.389.B (tr. by Benjamin Jowett)

Sir Francis Bacon [1561–1626]

What is Truth? said jesting Pilate; and would not stay for an answer.
Essays, "Of Truth"

Truth is to be sought for not in the felicity of any age, which is an unstable thing, but in the light of nature and experience, which is eternal.
Novum Organum, "Aphorisms," LVI

Sir Thomas Browne [1605–1682]

A Man may come unto the *Pericardium,* but not the Heart of Truth.
Christian Morals, Pt. II, Sect. 3

William Heberden [1710–1801]

No aphorism of Hippocrates holds truer to this day, than that in which he laments the length of time necessary to establish medical truths, and the danger, unless the utmost caution be used, of our being misled even by experience.
Commentaries on the History and Cure of Diseases, Ch. 13

John Morgan [1735–1789]

As the most precious metals in a state of ore are mixed with dross, so the choice truths of Medicine are frequently blended with a heap of rubbish.

> *A Discourse upon the Institution of Medical Schools in America*

Johann Kaspar Lavater
[1741–1801]

Let me repeat it: if you cannot bear to be told by your bosom friend that you have a strong breath, you deserve not to have a friend.

> *Aphorisms on Man,* CCCLVII (tr. by Henry Fuseli)

Peter Mere Latham [1789–1875]

Truths without exception are not the truths most commonly met with in medicine.

> *Diseases of the Heart,* Lect. III

Truth in all its kinds is most difficult to win; and truth in medicine is the most difficult of all.

> *Ibid.,* Lect. V

Next to knowing the truth itself, is to know the direction in which it lies. And this is the peculiar praise of a sound conjecture.

> *Ibid.,* Lect. XX

How is it that in medicine Truth is thus measured out to us in fragments, and we are never put in trust of it *as a whole?*

> *General Remarks on the Practice of Medicine,* Ch. XIII

Robert Browning [1812–1889]

Truth is within ourselves; it takes no rise
From outward things, whate'er you may believe.
There is an inmost centre in us all,
Where truth abides in fullness; and around,
Wall upon wall, the gross flesh hems it in,
This perfect, clear perception — which is truth.

A baffling and perverting carnal mesh
Binds it, and makes all error: and, "to know"
Rather consists in opening out a way
Whence the imprisoned splendour may escape,
Than in effecting entry for a light
Supposed to be without.

> *Paracelsus,* Pt. I

Herbert Spencer [1820–1903]

Scientific truths, of whatever order, are reached by eliminating perturbing or conflicting factors, and recognizing only fundamental factors.

> *The Data of Ethics,* Ch. XV

Thomas Huxley [1825–1895]

Irrationally held truths may be more harmful than reasoned errors.

> *Darwiniana,* "The Coming of Age of the *Origin of Species*"

It is the customary fate of new truths to begin as heresies and to end as superstitions.

> *Idem*

Theodor Billroth [1829–1894]

He who cannot quote his therapeutic experiences in numbers is a charlatan; be truthful for clarity's sake, do not hesitate to admit failures, as they must show the mode and places of improvement.

Santiago Ramón y Cajal
[1852–1934]

To be right before the right time is heresy, which is sometimes paid for by martyrdom.

> *Charlas de Café*

Willem Einthoven [1860–1927]

The truth is all that matters; what you or I may think is inconsequential.

> Remark to C. J. Wiggers

William J. Mayo [1861–1939]

Scientific truth which I formerly thought of as fixed, as though it could be weighed and measured, is change-able. Add a fact, change the outlook, and you have a new truth. Truth is a constant variable. We seek it, we find it, our viewpoint changes, and the truth changes to meet it.

> *Annals of Surgery* 94:799, 1931

J. Chalmers Da Costa [1863–1933]

Sometimes a man tells the truth out of pure meanness.

> *The Trials and Triumphs of the Surgeon*, Ch. 1

Rudyard Kipling [1865–1936]

At a time when few things are called by their right names — when it is against the Spirit of the Time even to hint that an act may entail conse-quences — you are going to join a profession in which you will be paid for telling a man the truth, and every departure you may make from the truth you will make as a concession to man's bodily weakness, and not to your own mental weakness.

> *A Doctor's Work,* address to students at London's Middlesex Hospital, October 1, 1908

Richard Clarke Cabot [1868–1939]

Before you tell the "truth" to the pa-tient, be sure you know the "truth," and that the patient wants to hear it.

> Quoted by David Seegal in *Journal of Chronic Diseases* 16:443, 1963

I have never known a man or woman made worse by telling them the truth.

Burton J. Hendrick [1870–1949]

The great glory of modern medicine is that it regards nothing as essential but the truth.

Martin H. Fischer [1879–1962]

Truth is rarely writ in ink; it lives in nature.

> Quoted by Howard Fabing and Ray Marr in *Fischerisms*

William Sharpe [1882–   ]

Yes, to fear something and *not* have it — that frequently seems to have more serious effects upon the patient than having the condition itself. So why not tell the patient the truth if he wants to know it.

> *Brain Surgeon,* Ch. XXVII

Alan Gregg [1890–1957]

The truth will always be found, in some curious and interesting way, to differ from assumption and opinion.

> Aphorism (Quoted by Wilder Penfield in *The Difficult Art of Giving,* Appendix A)

Chauncey D. Leake [1896–   ]

Let us remember always that whatever truth we may get by scientific study about ourselves and our environment is always relative, tentative, subject to change and correction, and that there are no final answers.

> *New York State Journal of Medicine* 60:1496, 1960

TUBERCULOSIS

Aretaeus of Cappadocia [1st–2nd Cent.]

This is a mighty wonder: in the dis-charge from the lungs alone, which is particularly dangerous, the patients do not despair of themselves, even al-though near the last.

> *On the Causes and Symptoms of Acute Diseases,* II.ii.18 (tr. by Francis Adams)

Niccolò Machiavelli [1469–1527]

In its beginning the malady [tubercu-losis] is easier to cure but difficult to detect, but later it becomes easy to detect but difficult to cure.

William Shakespeare [1564–1616]

Thy food is such
As has been belch'd on by infected
lungs.
Pericles, IV, vi, 178

Consumption catch thee!
Timon of Athens, IV, iii, 201

Sir Thomas Browne [1605–1682]

The common Fallacy of consumptive
Persons, who feel not themselves dy-
ing, and therefore still hope to live.
A Letter to a Friend

John Milton [1608–1674]

O Fairest flower no sooner blown but
blasted.
*On the Death of a Fair Infant
Dying of a Cough*

John Bunyan [1628–1688]

The captain of all these men of death
that came against him to take him
away, was the consumption; for it was
that that brought him down to the
grave.[1]
*The Life and Death of Mr.
Badman*, "Of Badman's disease, death, etc. etc."

William Heberden [1710–1801]

Consumptive women readily conceive,
and during their pregnancy the progress of the consumption seems to be
suspended; but as soon as they are
delivered, it begins to attack them
with redoubled strength; the usual
symptoms come on, or increase with
great rapidity, and they very soon
sink under their distemper.
*Commentaries on the History
and Cure of Diseases*, Ch. 43

Dissections of those who have died
of pulmonary consumptions, have acquainted me, that their lungs are full

[1] Cf. Sir William Osler, p. 432a.

of little glandular swellings, many of
which are in a state of suppuration.
Ibid., Ch. 72

In England we have very little apprehensions of the contagious nature of
consumptions; of which in other
countries they are fully persuaded. I
have not seen proof enough to say,
that the breath of a consumptive person is infectious; and yet I have seen
too much appearance of it, to be sure
that it is not; for I have observed
several die of consumptions, in whom
infection seemed to be the most probable origin of their illness, from their
having been the constant companions,
or bed-fellows, of consumptive persons.
Idem

The phthisis pulmonum usually begins with a dry cough, so slight and
inconsiderable, that little or no notice
is taken of it, till its continuance, and
gradual increase, begin to make it regarded. Such a cough has lasted for
a few years without bringing on other
complaints. It has sometimes wholly
ceased, and after a truce of a very
uncertain length it has returned, and
after frequent recoveries and relapses
the patient begins at last to find an
accession of other symptoms, which in
bad cases will very soon follow the
appearance of the first cough. These
are shortness of breath, hoarseness,
loss of appetite, wasting of the flesh
and strength, pains in the breast, pro-
fuse sweats during sleep, spitting of
blood and matter, shiverings succeeded
by hot fits, with flushings of the face,
and burning of the hands and feet, and
a pulse constantly above ninety, a
swelling of the legs, and an obstruction of the menstrua in women; a very
small stone has sometimes been
coughed up, and in the last stages
of this illness a diarrhoea helps to
waste the little remainder of flesh and
strength.
Idem

George Colman, the Younger [1762–1836]

And why should this be thought so
   odd?
   Can't men have taste who cure a
      phthisic?
         Broad Grins, "The Newcastle
         Apothecary"

Thomas Moore [1779–1852]

Described Byron after his illness at
Patras looking in the glass and saying,
"I look pale; I should like to die of
consumption." "Why?" "Because the
ladies would all say, 'Look at that
poor Byron, how interesting he looks
in dying.' "
         Diary, February 19, 1828

William Cullen Bryant [1794–1878]

Ay, thou art for the grave; thy
   glances shine
Too bright to shine long; . . .
And they who love thee wait in anxious
   grief
Till the slow plague shall bring the
   fatal hour.
Glide softly to thy rest, then; Death
   should come
Gently, to one of gentle mould like
   thee,
As light winds wandering through
   groves of bloom
Detach the delicate blossom from the
   tree.
Close thy sweet eyes, calmly and without pain.
         Consumption

Alexandre Dumas père [1802–1870]

[In 1823 and 1824] it was all the
fashion to suffer from chest complaint;
everybody was consumptive, poets especially; it was good form to spit
blood after each emotion that was at
all inclined to be sensational, and to
die before reaching the age of thirty.
         Memoirs, Vol. III, Bk. I, Ch. I
         (tr. by E. M. Waller)

Charles Dickens [1812–1870]

There is a dread disease which so pre-
pares its victim, as it were, for death;
which so refines it of its grosser aspect, and throws around familiar looks,
unearthly indications of the coming
change — a dread disease, in which the
struggle between soul and body is so
gradual, quiet, and solemn, and the
result so sure, that day by day, and
grain by grain, the mortal part wastes
and withers away, so that the spirit
grows light and sanguine with its
lightening load, and, feeling immortality at hand, deems it but a new term
of mortal life — a disease in which
death and life are so strangely blended,
that death takes the glow and hue of
life, and life the gaunt and grisly form
of death — a disease which medicine
never cured, wealth warded off, or
poverty could boast exemption from
— which sometimes moves in giant
strides, and sometimes at a tardy
sluggish pace, but, slow or quick, is
ever sure and certain.
         Nicholas Nickleby, Ch. 49

Henry David Thoreau [1817–1862]

Decay and disease are often beautiful,
like the pearly tear of the shellfish and
the hectic glow of consumption.
         Journal, June 11, 1852

Henri Amiel [1821–1881]

Autumn landscape. Sky draped in
gray, pleated by subtle shading, mists
trailing on the distant mountains; nature melancholy, leaves falling on all
sides like the lost illusions of youth
under the tears of incurable grief. . . .
The earth strewn with brown, yellow
and reddish leaves, the trees half bare.
. . . The fir tree, alone in its vigor,
green, stoical in the midst of this
universal phthisis.
         Journal Intime, October 31,
         1852

Henri Murger [1822–1861]

[Mimi was] pale like the angel of phthisis.
> *Scènes de la vie de Bohême*, Ch. XIV

If only I had a diseased lung, long hair, and a black suit, I would now be as famous as the sun.
> *Ibid.*, Ch. XVII

Robert Koch [1843–1910]

If we are continually guided in this enterprise by the spirit of genuine preventive medical science; if we utilise the experience gained in conflict with other pestilences, and aim, with clear recognition of the purpose and resolute avoidance of wrong roads, at striking the evil at its roots, then the battle against tuberculosis cannot fail to have a victorious issue.
> *The Fight Against Tuberculosis*

Marie Bashkirtsev [1860–1884]

I cough continually! but for a wonder, far from making me look ugly, this gives me an air of languor that is very becoming.
> *Journal*, January 3, 1880

Katherine Mansfield [1888–1923]

Almighty Father of All and Most Celestial Giver;
Who has granted to us thy children a heart and lungs and a liver;
If upon me should descend thy beautiful gift of tongues
Incline not thine Omnipotent ear to my remarks on lungs.
> *Journal*, 1918, "Verses Writ in a Foreign Bed"

Norman Bethune [1890–1939]

I believe in Trudeau,
the mighty father of the American Sanatorium,
maker of a heaven on earth for the tuberculous;
and in Artificial Pneumothorax;
which was conceived by Carson;
born of the Labors of Forlanini;
suffered under Pompous Pride and Prejudice;
was criticized by the Cranks whose patients are dead and buried;
thousands now well,
even in the third stage,
rose again from their bed;
ascending into the Heaven of Medicine's Immortals,
they sit on the right hand of Hippocrates our Father,
from thence they do judge those phthisiotherapists
quick to collapse cavities or dead on their job.
I believe in Bodington, Brehmer, Koch and Brauer,
in Murphy, Friedrich, Wilms, Sauerbruch, Stuertz and Jacobeus,
in the unforgiveness of the sins of omission in Collapse Therapy,
in the resurrection of a healthy body from a diseased one
and long life for the tuberculous with care everlasting.
Amen.
> *A Compressionist's Creed*

Arthur M. Walker [1896–1955]

I would like to remind those responsible for the treatment of tuberculosis that Keats wrote his best poems while dying of this disease. In my opinion he would never have done so under the influence of modern chemotherapy.
> Quoted by Julius L. Wilson in *Walkerisms*

René and Jean Dubos [1901–   ] [1918–   ]

Melancholy meditations over the death of a youth or a maiden, tombs, abandoned ruins, and weeping willows became popular themes over much of Europe around 1750, as if some new circumstance had made more obvious the ephemeral character of human life.
> *The White Plague*, Ch. V

Throughout medical history there runs this suggestion — that the intellectually gifted are the most likely to contract the disease, and furthermore that the same fire which wastes the body in consumption also makes the mind shine with a brighter light.
Idem

It is probable that every consumptive became, in some measure, an opium addict, and it may be wondered whether the drug did not contribute to the mental effervescence that expressed itself in poetry and artistic creation.
Idem

There is no evidence that tuberculosis breeds genius. The probability is, rather, that eagerness for achievement often leads to a way of life that renders the body less resistant to infection.
Idem

But disease was rarely presented [in the Victorian novel] as something loathsome, unless it affected the villain. Rather, it was used as a device to enlist the sympathies of the reader.
Idem

Edgar Allan Poe . . . looked on his wife's illness as the source of a strange additional charm, which rendered more ethereal her chalky pallor and her haunted, liquid eyes.
Idem

Indian (Tamil) Proverb

If fresh-drawn milk unboiled be drunk, consumption may be cured.

TWINS

William Shakespeare [1564–1616]

By her he had two children at one birth.
Henry VI, Part II, IV, ii, 147

Henry Wheeler Shaw ("Josh Billings") [1818–1885]

There iz 2 things in this life for which we are never fully prepared, and that iz twins.
Josh Billings: His Sayings, Ch. VIII

Henry S. Leigh [1837–1883]

In form and feature, face and limb,
  I grew so like my brother,
That folks got taking me for him,
  And each for one another. . . .
For one of us was born a twin;
  And not a soul knew which.
    Carols of Cockayne, "The Twins"

TYPHUS

Samuel Butler [1835–1902]

They made a clean sweep of all machinery that had not been in use for more than two hundred and seventy-one years (which period was arrived at after a series of compromises), and strictly forbade all further improvements and inventions under pain of being considered in the eye of the law to be labouring under typhus fever, which they regard as one of the worst of all crimes.
Erewhon, Ch. IX

ULCER

Sushruta [5th Cent.? B.C.]

A wise physician, with any regard to his own reputation, should abandon a patient laid up with an ulcer which appears to have been dusted over with a sort of pulverised crust, or who has been suffering from one accompanied by loss of flesh and strength, cough, difficult respiration and aversion to food. An ulcer, which occurring at any of the vital parts of the body

secretes a copious quantity of pus and blood, and refuses to be healed even after a course of proper and persistent medical treatment, is sure to have a fatal termination.
> *Sushruta-Samhitá,* "Sutrasthá-nam," Ch. 28 (tr. by K. K. L. Bhishagratna)

William Shakespeare [1564–1616]

It will but skin and film the ulcerous place,
Whiles rank corruption, mining all within,
Infects unseen.
> *Hamlet,* III, iv, 147

Victor Hugo [1802–1885]

A foreign war is like a scratch on the elbow; a civil war is an ulcer which eats away your liver.
> *Ninety-Three,* Pt. II, Bk. II, Ch. 2 (tr. by A. Delano)

William J. Mayo [1861–1939]

Unfortunately, only a small number of patients with peptic ulcer are financially able to make a pet of an ulcer.
> *Journal of the American Medical Association* 79:19, 1922

J. A. D. Anderson [1926–   ]

The view that a peptic ulcer may be the hole in a man's stomach through which he crawls to escape from his wife has fairly wide acceptance.
> *A New Look at Social Medicine*

URINARY STONE

Michel de Montaigne [1533–1592]

Oh, why have I not the faculty of that dreamer in Cicero who, dreaming he was embracing a wench, found that he had discharged his stone in the sheets! Mine extraordinarily diswench me.
> *Essays,* Bk. II, Ch. 37, "Of the Resemblance of Children to Fathers" (tr. by Donald M. Frame)

People . . . see you sweat in agony, turn pale, turn red, tremble, vomit your very blood, suffer strange contractions and convulsions, sometimes shed great tears from your eyes, discharge thick, black, and frightful urine, or have it stopped up by some sharp rough stone that cruelly pricks and flays the neck of your penis.[1]
> *Ibid.,* Bk. III, Ch. 13, "Of Experience"

Thomas Sydenham [1624–1689]

Gout produces calculus in the kidney. . . . the patient has frequently to entertain the painful speculation as to whether gout or stone be the worst disease. Sometimes the stone, in passing . . . , kills the patient, without waiting for the gout.
> *A Treatise on Gout and Dropsy* (tr. by R. G. Latham in *Works,* Vol. II)

Samuel Pepys [1633–1703]

This day it is two years since it pleased God that I was cut for the stone at Mrs. Turner's in Salisbury Court. And did resolve while I live to keep it a festival, as I did the last year at my house.
> *Diary,* March 26, 1659

William Heberden [1710–1801]

The signs of a stone in the bladder are, great and frequent irritations to make water, a stoppage in the middle of making it, and a pain with heat just after it is made; a tenesmus, pain in the extremity of the urethra, incontinence or suppression of urine, to-

---

[1] Montaigne, who suffered from "the stone" for many years, thus describes an attack.

gether with a quiet pulse, and the health in no bad state.

> *Commentaries on the History and Cure of Diseases,* Ch. 16

URINE

See also BLADDER, KIDNEY, URINARY STONE

Christopher Marlowe [1564–1593]

I view'd your urine, and the hypostasis
Thick and obscure doth make your
    danger great,
Your vaines are full of accidentall
    heat,
Whereby the moisture of your blood
    is dried.

> *Tamburlaine the Great,* Act V, Sc. iii

William Shakespeare [1564–1616]

FALSTAFF: What says the doctor to my water?
PAGE: He said, sir, the water itself was a good healthy water; but, for the party that owed it, he might have moe diseases than he knew for.

> *Henry IV, Part II,* I, ii, 1

MACDUFF: What three things does drink especially provoke?
PORTER: Marry, sir, nose-painting, sleep and urine.

> *Macbeth,* II, iii, 29

            If thou could'st, doctor, cast
The water of my land, find her disease,
And purge it to a sound and pristine
    health,
I would applaud thee to the very
    echo,
That should applaud again.

> *Ibid.,* V, iii, 50

When he makes water, his urine is congeal'd ice.

> *Measure for Measure,* III, ii, 117

And others, when the bagpipe sings
    i' the nose,
Cannot contain their urine.

> *The Merchant of Venice,* IV, i, 49

HOST: A word, Mounseur Mock-water.
DR. CAIUS: Mock-vater? Vat is dat?

> *The Merry Wives of Windsor,* II, iii, 59

Carry his water to th' wise woman.

> *Twelfth Night,* III, iv, 114

Thomas Fuller [1608–1661]

He [the good physician] *trusteth not the single witnesse of the water if better testimony may be had.* For reasons drawn from the urine alone are as brittle as the urinall. Sometimes the water runneth in such posthast through the sick mans body, it can give no account of anything memorable in the passage, though the most judicious eye examine it.

> *The Holy State,* Bk. II, Ch. 2

Parson Swift [fl. 18th Cent.]

[If the urine is] Bright as Gold, [the diagnosis is] Lust or Desire to marry.[1]

If you see your face in her Water, if she hath not a Fever, she is with Child.

Davach de La Rivière [18th Cent.]

Their experience has taught them, as mine has me, that one must listen to reason and agree with Hippocrates, Avicenna, Galen and many others, ancient and modern, that there is no surer way to determine the temperaments and constitutions of people of either sex [than to look at the urine].

> *The Mirror of Urines*

William Heberden [1710–1801]

Very pale urine, unless the patient have drunk a great quantity of small

---

[1] His system of uroscopy provided forty-one means of diagnosis.

liquors, is a bad sign in fevers, and it is very desirable to see it become thick, and deposit a sediment.
> *Commentaries on the History and Cure of Diseases,* Ch. 37

A total suppression has lasted seven days, and yet the patient has recovered. It has been fatal so early as on the fourth day. But in general those patients, who could not be cured, have sunk under their malady on the sixth or seventh day.
> *Ibid.,* Ch. 55

Whatever probability there may be, that the bladder is empty, and that the disease is in the kidneys, it will still be advisable in every suppression to make the matter certain by the introduction of a catheter.
> *Idem*

Count Antoine François de Fourcroy [1755–1809]

The urine of man is one of the animal matters that have been the most examined by chemists, and of which the examination has at the same time furnished the most singular discoveries to chemistry, and the most useful application to physiology, as well as the art of healing. This liquid, which commonly inspires men only with contempt and disgust, which is generally ranked amongst vile and repulsive matters, has become, in the hands of the chemists, a source of important discoveries.
> *A General System of Chemical Knowledge, and Its Application to the Phenomena of Nature and Art,* Vol. X, Article 25 (tr. by W. Nicholson)

John Blackall [1771–1860]

Yet the experiment is the easiest possible; and every practitioner may shortly convince himself beyond the possibility of doubt, that in a considerable number of dropsical cases the urine coagulates [on the application

of heat] like diluted serum of the blood.
> *Observations on the Nature and Cure of Dropsies*

Herman L. Kretschmer [1879–1951]

Gentle, Doctor, it makes lots of difference which end of that thing you're on.
> Instruction to interns and residents on the use of a cystoscope

Thomas Addis [1881–1949]

When the patient dies the kidneys may go to the pathologist, but while he lives the urine is ours. It can provide us day by day, month by month, and year by year, with a serial story of the major events going on within the kidney. The examination of the urine is the most essential part of the physical examination of any patient with Bright's disease.
> *Glomerular Nephritis, Diagnosis and Treatment,* Ch. 1

UROSCOPY

See URINE

VACCINATION

See also SMALLPOX

Lady Mary Wortley Montagu [1689–1762]

I am Patriot enough to take pains to bring this usefull invention [vaccination] into fashion in England, and I should not fail to write to some of our Doctors very particularly about it if I knew any one of 'em that I thought had Virtue enough to destroy such a considerable branch of their Revenue for the good of Mankind, but that Distemper is too beneficial to them not to expose to all their Resentment the hardy wight that should undertake to put an end to it.

> Letter to Sarah Chiswell, April 1, 1717

Thomas Huxley [1825–1895]

If he [my next-door neighbor] is to be allowed to let his children go unvaccinated, he might as well be allowed to leave strychnine lozenges about in the way of mine.
> *Method and Results*, "Administrative Nihilism"

VARICOSE VEINS

Sir William Osler [1849–1919]

Varicose veins are the result of an improper selection of grandparents.
> Quoted by William B. Bean in *Sir William Osler: Aphorisms*, Ch. 5

VEGETARIANISM

See also DIET

William Cullen [1710–1790]

Persons living very entirely on vegetables are seldom of a plump and succulent habit.
> *First Lines of the Practice of Physic*, Pt. III, Bk. I

Percy Bysshe Shelley [1792–1822]

There is no disease, bodily or mental, which adoption of vegetable diet and pure water has not infallibly mitigated, wherever the experiment has been fairly tried.
> *Queen Mab*, Notes

Sir Robert Hutchison [1871–1960]

Don't scrape your insides with much roughage as it is more likely to do harm than good. Vegetarianism is harmless enough though it is apt to fill a man with wind and self-righteousness.
> Address, Session of the British Medical Association, Winnipeg, 1930

VENEREAL DISEASE

Girolamo Fracastoro [1483–1553]

To begin with, there was this strange fact; though the infection was there, the moon had often four times circled the earth before clear symptoms of the disease appeared. For when it has once been received into the body it does not immediately declare itself; rather it lies dormant for a certain time and gradually gains strength as it feeds. Meanwhile, however, the sufferers, weighed down by strange heaviness and irresistible langour, are going through life with increasing weakness, moving sluggishly in every limb. Their eyes, too, have lost their natural keenness; the colour is driven from their faces and deserts their unhappy brows.
> *Syphilis or the French Disease*, Bk. I (tr. by Wynne-Finch)

And first among them all, Syphilus, who had established the worship of the King with blood-sacrifices, and raised altars to him among the mountains, manifested the foul sores in his own body. . . . And from him, first to suffer it, the disease took its name, and was called Syphilis by the native race.
> *Ibid.*, Bk. III

Benvenuto Cellini [1500–1571]

It was true indeed that I had got the sickness; but I believe I caught it from that fine young servant-girl whom I was keeping when my house was robbed. The French disease,[1] for it was

[1] Syphilis was referred to as the "French disease" because it was brought to Italy and disseminated among the people by the soldiers of Charles VIII of France.

that, remained in me more than four months dormant before it showed itself, and then it broke out over my whole body at one instant. It was not like what one commonly observes, but covered my flesh with certain blisters, of the size of six-pence, and rose-colored. The doctors would not call it the French disease, albeit I told them why I thought it was that.

> *The Life of Benvenuto Cellini Written by Himself*, Bk. I, Ch. 59 (tr. by John Addington Symonds)

I went on treating myself according to their [the doctors'] methods, but derived no benefit. At last, then, I resolved on taking the wood,[1] against the advice of the first physicians in Rome; and I took it with the most scrupulous discipline and rules of abstinence that could be thought of; and after a few days, I perceived in me a great amendment. The result was that at the end of fifty days I was cured and as sound as a fish in water.

> *Idem*

Johann Fernelii Ambiani [1506–1558]

The cause of Lues venerea is obscure. Apparently, it is a dangerous and toxic disease contracted by contact or contamination. The poison seems to be without structure — at any rate, it cannot be seen — , does not exist, free, in nature, but vegetates in the secretions of the body which, so to speak, serve as carriers. Since it has no sharp edge, it can only enter through apertures, and be transmitted only by smearing secretions on the denuded parts.

> *Therapeutics*, Vol. VII (tr. by Max Samter)

[1] "Taking the wood" refers to guaiac, derived from the heartwood of certain flowering trees of tropical America, introduced as a treatment for syphilis, gout, and other diseases around 1500.

William Shakespeare [1564–1616]

A man can no more separate age and covetousness than 'a can part young limbs and lechery; but the gout galls the one, and the pox pinches the other.

> *Henry IV, Part II*, I, ii, 256

FALSTAFF: You make fat rascals, Mistress Doll.
DOLL: I make them? Gluttony and diseases make them. I make them not.
FALSTAFF: If the cook help to make the gluttony, you help to make the diseases, Doll. We catch of you, Doll; we catch of you.

> *Ibid.*, II, iv, 45

> To the spital go,
> And from the powd'ring tub of infamy
> Fetch forth the lazar kite of Cressid's kind.
> *Henry V*, II, i, 78

> News have I, that my Nell is dead i' th' spital
> Of malady of France.
> *Ibid.*, V, i, 86

I have purchas'd as many diseases under her roof as come to . . . three thousand dolours a year.

> *Measure for Measure*, I, ii, 46

BOULT: Do you know the French knight that cow'rs i' the hams?
BAWD: . . . As for him, he brought his disease hither: here he does but repair it.

> *Pericles*, IV, ii, 112

Have you that a man may deal withal and defy the surgeon?

> *Ibid.*, IV, vi, 28

> Most ungentle fortune
> Have plac'd me in this sty, where, since I came,
> Diseases have been sold dearer than physic.
> *Ibid.*, IV, vi, 103

She whom the spital-house and ulcerous sores
Would cast the gorge at, this [gold]
embalms and spices
To th' April day again.
Timon of Athens, IV, iii, 39

Be a whore still. They love thee not
that use thee.
Give them diseases, leaving with thee
their lust.
Make use of thy salt hours. Season the
slaves
For tubs and baths; bring down rose-
cheeked youth
To the tub-fast and the diet.
Ibid., IV, iii, 83

Consumptions sow
In hollow bones of man; strike their
sharp shins,
And mar men's spurring. Crack the
lawyer's voice,
That he may never more false title
plead
Nor sound his quillets shrilly. Hoar
the flamen,
That scolds against the quality of flesh
And not believes himself. Down with
the nose —
Down with it flat; take the bridge
quite away —
Of him that, his particular to foresee,
Smells from the general weal. Make
curl'd-pate ruffians bald,
And let the unscarr'd braggarts of the
war
Derive some pain from you.
Ibid., IV, iii, 151

Sir Thomas Browne [1605–1682]

He that is Chast and Continent not to
impair his strength, or honest for fear
of Contagion, will hardly be Heroically
virtuous.
Christian Morals, Pt. I, Sect. 3

Alexander Pope [1688–1744]

Pox'd by her love.
Satires and Epistles Imitated,
"The First Satire of the Second
Book of Horace"

Abraham Colles [1773–1843]

I may be told by some that men may
contract syphilis by sitting in a public
privy; to this I can only answer that I
have never witnessed a single instance;
nor did the late Mr. Obre, who had
been for many years most extensively
engaged in treating the venereal disease; for on asking him if he believed
that the disease was propagated in this
manner, he shrewdly answered, that it
sometimes was the manner in which
married men contracted it, but unmarried men never caught it in this manner.

George Gordon, Lord Byron
[1788–1824]

I said the small pox has gone out of
late;
Perhaps it may be follow'd by the
great.
Don Juan, Canto I, Stanza 130

Sir William Osler [1849–1919]

Know syphilis in all its manifestations
and relations, and all things clinical
will be added unto you.
*Aequanimitas, with Other Ad-
dresses*, "Internal Medicine as
a Vocation"

John H. Stokes [1885–1961]

There are instances in which one positive Wassermann test will convict a la-
borer over his own denial, two will make
a case against a banker or a railroad
president, but three successive posi-
tives will scarcely convince the medical advisor of the guilt of a clergyman.

J. Earle Moore [1892–1957]

Two minutes with Venus, two years
with mercury.
Aphorism

René J. Dubos [1901–   ]

The epidemic of syphilis which spread
through all of Europe in the late fifteenth and early sixteenth century

gave many physicians frequent occasions to observe, often in the form of a personal experience, that a given disease can pass from one individual to another.

> *Louis Pasteur, Free Lance of Science*, Ch. IX

W. I. B. Beveridge [1908–]

John Hunter deliberately infected himself with gonorrhoea to find out if it was a distinct disease from syphilis. Unfortunately the material he used to inoculate himself contained also the syphilis organism, with the result that he contracted both diseases and so established for a long time the false belief that both were manifestations of the same disease.

> *The Art of Scientific Investigation*, Ch. II

VIRGINITY

See also SEX

Soranus of Ephesus [2nd Cent.]

It is advisable that menstruation begin before the individual ceases to be a virgin.

> *Text on Diseases of Women*, V (tr. by François J. Herrgott)

Christopher Marlowe [1564–1593]

Virginitie, albeit some highly prise it,
Compar'd with marriage, had you tried them both,
Differs as much as wine and water doth.

> *Hero and Leander*, Sestiad I

William Shakespeare [1564–1616]

Virginity breeds mites, much like a cheese; consumes itself to the very paring, and so dies with feeding his own stomach. Besides, virginity is peevish, proud, idle, made of self-love, which

is the most inhibited sin in the canon.

> *All's Well That Ends Well*, I, i, 154

Andrew Marvell [1621–1678]

Had we but World enough, and Time,
This coyness Lady were no crime. . . .
But at my back I alwaies hear
Times winged Charriot hurrying near:
And yonder all before us lye
Desarts of vast Eternity.
Thy Beauty shall no more be found:
Nor, in thy marble Vault, shall sound
My ecchoing Song: then Worms shall try
That long preserved Virginity:
And your quaint Honour turn to dust;
And into ashes all my Lust.
The Grave's a fine and private place,
But none I think do there embrace.

> *To His Coy Mistress*

Maxwell Anderson [1888–1959]

Virginity is rather a state of mind.

> *Elizabeth the Queen*, Act II, Sc. iii

VISION

See BLINDNESS, EYE, SIGHT

VITALISM

See also REDUCTIONISM

William Harvey [1578–1657]

Persons of limited information, when they are at a loss to assign a cause for anything, very commonly reply that it is done by the spirits. . . . Some speak of corporeal, others of incorporeal spirits; and they who advocate the corporeal spirits will have the blood, or the thinner portion of the blood, to be the bond of union with the soul, the spirit being contained in the blood as the flame is in the smoke of a lamp or candle, and held admixed by the incessant motion of the fluid. . . . There is nothing more uncertain and questionable, then, than the doctrine of the spirits.

> *On the Circulation of the Blood,* "Second Essay to Jean Riolan" (tr. by Robert Willis)

Rudolf Virchow [1821–1902]

As long as vitalism and spiritualism are open questions so long will the gateway of science be open to mysticism.

> Quoted by F. H. Garrison in *Bulletin of the New York Academy of Medicine* 4:994, 1928

Merkel H. Jacobs [1884–   ]

To many persons in those days an explanation of cellular behavior, to be scientific, had to be of a very simple physicochemical character. The possibility that the plasma membrane might be a part — even a complex part — of the cell itself seems to have been disregarded, possibly because such a belief was thought to be too vitalistic.

> *Circulation* 26:1013, 1962

René J. Dubos [1901–   ]

Scientists . . . may assume on faith that life is the expression of some divine vital spirit, or accept — *also* on faith — that living processes are but the expression of the activities of a kind of chemical molecule which happens to be fashionable at the time.

> *The Dreams of Reason,* Ch. I

Francis H. C. Crick [1916–   ]

I also suspect that many workers in this field [molecular biology] and related fields have been strongly motivated by the desire, rarely actually expressed, to refute vitalism.

> *British Medical Bulletin* 21: 183, 1965

VITAMINS

See also DIET, NUTRITION

Richard Mead [1673–1754]

That experienced and brave admiral, Sir Charles Wager, once told me . . . his sailors were terribly afflicted with the Scurvy. . . . Recollecting, from what he had often heard, how effectual these fruits [oranges and lemons] were in the cure of this distemper, he ordered a chest of each to be brought upon deck, and opened every day. The men, besides eating what they would, mixed the juice in their beer. It was also their constant diversion to pelt one another with the rinds; so that the deck was always strewed and wet with the fragrant liquor. The happy effect was, that he brought his sailors home in good health.

> *Medical Works,* "A Discourse on the Scurvy"

John Blackall [1771–1860]

Towards the conclusion of the voyage, the sailors had been attacked with dropsical symptoms. . . . This disorder was attributed, no doubt with great reason, to the use of damaged rice, upon which, circumstances not necessary to detail, had reduced them in great measure to subsist. On their arrival in port, the principal improvement in their diet was well-fermented bread, which operated as a very active diuretic within twenty-four hours after they had begun its use; and no doubt remained in the minds of many of the sick, what it was that performed the cure.

> *Observations on the Nature and Cure of Dropsies*

WASTING

Ovid [43 B.C.–A.D. 17?]

Whether the contagion of a sick mind

affects my limbs or the cause of my ills
is this region, since I reached the Pont-
us, I am harassed by sleeplessness,
scarce does the lean flesh cover my
bones, food pleases not my lips.
> *Tristia,* III.viii.25 (tr. by A. L.
> Wheeler)

Guillaume de Salluste, Seigneur du Bartas [1544–1590]

Weakened and wasted even to skin and
bone.
> *Devine Weekes and Workes,*
> Week II, Day IV, "The Decay"
> (tr. by Joshua Sylvester)

WATER

See also THIRST

I. GENERAL

Clement of Alexandria [150?–220?]

The natural, temperate and necessary
beverage, therefore, for the thirsty is
water.
> *The Instructor,* Bk. II, Ch. II
> (tr. by William Wilson in *The
> Anti-Nicene Christian Library*)

St. Francis of Assisi [1182–1226]

Praised be my Lord for sister water
the which is greatly helpful and humble and precious and pure.
> *Praises of the Creatures,* "The
> Canticle of the Sun"

Tobias Venner [1577–1660]

Water . . . doth very greatly deject
their appetite, destroy the naturall
heat, and overthrow the strength of the
stomacke, and consequently, confounding the concoction, is the cause of
crudities, fluctuations, and windinesse
in the bodie.
> *Via recta ad vitam longam,*
> Sect. III

Tobias Smollett [1721–1771]

Pure water is certainly of all others
the most salutary beverage. . . . These
admirable qualities inherent in simple
water are clearly evinced by the uninterrupted health, good spirits and longevity of those who use nothing else
for their ordinary drink.
> *Essay on the External Use of
> Water*

Edmund Burke [1729–1797]

Water, when simple, is insipid, inodor-
ous, colorless, and smooth; it is found,
when *not cold,* to be a great resolver
of spasms, and lubricator of the fibres;
this power it probably owes to its
smoothness.
> *On the Sublime and Beautiful,*
> Pt. IV, Sect. XXI

Napoleon Bonaparte [1769–1821]

The greatest necessity of the soldier is
water.
> Quoted by Barry O'Meara in
> *Napoleon in Exile,* February
> 17, 1817

Samuel Taylor Coleridge [1772–1834]

Water, water, every where,
Nor any drop to drink.
> *The Rime of the Ancient Mari-
> ner,* Pt. II

Oliver Herford [1863–1935]

Here's to old Adam's crystal ale,
    Clear-sparkling and divine,
Fair H_2O, long may you flow,
    We drink your health (in wine).
> *Toast: Adam's Crystal Ale*

Anonymous

Full many a man, both young and old,
    Is brought to his sarcophagus
By pouring water, icy cold,
    Adown his warm esophagus.

Proverbs

Drinking water neither makes a man sick, nor in debt, nor his wife a widow.

We never miss the water till the well runs dry.

Slovakian Proverb

Pure water is the world's first and foremost medicine.

II. WATER POLLUTION

Plato [427?–347 B.C.]

And let this be the law: If anyone intentionally pollutes the water of another, whether the water of a spring, or collected in reservoirs, either by poisonous substances, or by digging, or by theft, let the injured party bring the cause before the warden of the city.
> *Laws*, VIII.845 (tr. by Benjamin Jowett)

William Clowes [1544–1604]

That fish which is bred in the dirt will always taste of the mud.
> *Treatise on Struma* (ed. by F. N. L. Poynter in *Selected Writings*, Ch. 5)

William Blake [1757–1827]

Expect poison from the standing water.
> *The Marriage of Heaven and Hell*, "Proverbs of Hell"

Sydney Smith [1771–1845]

He who drinks a tumbler of London water has literally in his stomach more animated beings than there are men, women, and children on the face of the globe.
> Letter to the Countess Grey, November 19, 1834

West African Proverb

Filthy water cannot be washed.

WILLS

William Shakespeare [1564–1616]

Bid a sick man in sadness make his will.
Ah, word ill urg'd to one that is so ill!
> *Romeo and Juliet*, I, i, 209

John Donne [1573–1631]

To Schoolemen I bequeath my doubtfulnesse;
My sicknesse to Physitians, or excesse.
> *The Will*

To him for whom the passing bell next tolls,
I give my physick bookes.
> *Idem*

Alexander Pope [1688–1744]

But thousands die, without or this or that,
Die, and endow a College, or a Cat.
> *Moral Essays*, Epistle III

Spanish Proverb

More people have died because they made their wills than because they were sick.

WISDOM

See also KNOWLEDGE, LEARNING

Moses ben Maimon (Maimonides) [1135–1204]

Teach thy tongue to say "I do not know."

Laurence Sterne [1713–1768]

Sciences may be learned by rote, but Wisdom not.
> *Tristram Shandy*, Bk. V, Ch. 32

Oliver Wendell Holmes
[1809-1894]

It is the folly of the world, constantly, which confounds its wisdom.
> *The Professor at the Breakfast Table,* Sect. 1

William J. Mayo [1861-1939]

Knowledge is static; wisdom is active and moves knowledge, making it effective.
> *Minnesota Medicine* 19:468, 1936

Frederic J. Cotton [1869-1938]

Wisdom did not begin with this generation, but we have had an unusual opportunity to learn.
> *Dislocation and Joint-Fractures,* Introduction

Harry Allen Overstreet
[1875-   ]

The psychological growth of man must keep pace with his physical powers; every increase in power must be matched by an increase in understanding.
> *The Mature Mind,* Ch. 4, Sect. 10

Martin H. Fischer [1879-1962]

Knowledge is a process of piling up facts; wisdom lies in their simplification.
> Quoted by Howard Fabing and Ray Marr in *Fischerisms*

Alan Gregg [1890-1957]

The essence of wisdom is the ability to make the right decision on the basis of inadequate evidence.

The Bible

Who hath put wisdom in the inward parts? or who hath given understanding to the heart?
> *Job* 38:36

Anonymous

He who remains silent, has often said all he knows.

WIVES

See also MARRIAGE

Euripides [484-406 B.C.]

In the hour of sorrow or sickness, a wife is a man's greatest blessing.
> *Antigone,* Fragment 164

John Abernethy [1764-1831]

[To the daughter of a widowed patient:] I have witnessed your devotion and kindness to your mother. I am in need of a wife, and I think you are the very person that would suit me. My time is incessantly occupied, and I have therefore no leisure for courting. Reflect upon this matter until Monday.[1]
> Quoted by Samuel D. Gross in *Autobiography*

Sir James Paget [1814-1899]

In May 1844, I married, and began to enjoy that happiness of domestic life which has already lasted without a break, without a cloud, for 39 years. From this time, the "being alone" was the being alone with one who never failed in love, in wise counsel, in prudence and in gentle care of me. With her it was easy to work and be undisturbed by anything going-on around me; a habit I can advise everyone to learn. . . . she wrote for me, copying for the press my roughly written manuscripts, sitting with me till midnight or far into the morning.
> *Memoirs and Letters,* Pt. I, Ch. VII

[1] She did, and subsequently became Mrs. Abernethy.

Louis Pasteur [1822–1895]

I prepare my lectures easily, and often have five whole days a week that I can devote to the laboratory. I am often scolded by Madame Pasteur, whom I console by telling her that I shall lead her to posterity.

> Letter to Charles Chappuis, December 12, 1851

Alfred Cox [1866–1954]

Osler's *Aequanimitas* is a favorite and oft quoted book of mine. But I remember Lady Osler's remark that it was all very well for William to preach Aequanimitas, but she had noted that every time they had to move (and this was frequently) he always had a good excuse for *not being there*, leaving her if possible to cultivate Aequanimitas in the uncomfortable circumstances.

> Letter, 1946

W. Sampson Handley [1872–1962]

People were known to have consulted Mr. Hunter [1] professionally in the hope of being invited to Mrs. Hunter's assemblies.

> *Lancet* 1:369, 1939

Eleanor (Mrs. Alan) Gregg [1889–   ]

As Alan would say — Don't answer until you've passed through the negative stage!

> Letter to Wilder Penfield, May 1959 (Quoted by Penfield in *The Second Career,* "The Epic of Alan Gregg")

Wilder Penfield [1891–   ]

Don't always be a physician! . . . The help you need is the help a wife could give you. Through her you would learn the other half of life. Without her you may live to be only half a man. . . . "Nothing in excess."

[1] John Hunter [1728–1793].

Too much medicine, too much work, even too much kindly service may be excessive.

> *The Torch,* Ch. 5

You physicians are a group apart. You are a strange race. The wife of a physician should be as different from other women as her husband is different from other men.

She needs more than beauty and poetry to support her through the years of medical practice. She must know how to work. She must have patience. She must be able to understand and to suggest. She must love you, but more than that, she must love your work. Otherwise she will not be happy, nor you. Otherwise you can never do all that you want to do for the sick.

> *Ibid.,* Ch. 8

It may be that physicians need a woman's guidance and companionship more than other men. Happiness comes to them as a reward, secondarily. There are other urges than the pursuit of happiness that keep them going. But what can a physician do? No woman would marry him if she were in her right mind.

> *Ibid.,* Ch. 10

William B. Terhune [1893–   ]

Fatigue . . . is a doctor's greatest personal enemy. . . . His wife's greatest opportunity is to prevent, ameliorate and cure this fatigue . . . by standing between him and the unthinking public, as well as by bringing him love and understanding, both in almost superhuman amounts.

> *Connecticut State Medical Journal* 11:576, 1947

The watchful public expects the doctor's wife to set a good example by having an efficiently run house, well-trained children, a sensibly organized personal life, and marital felicity.

> *Idem*

Being a doctor's wife carries a certain amount of occupational hazard, largely due to the realization that you are not first in your husband's interests (Medicine, you know, is his great love).
> *Idem*

Ellen M. Firebaugh [fl. 1894]

And now I would like to ask physicians' wives, Do your husbands ever get sick? Then, angels and ministers of grace defend you! A doctor is so accustomed to being director in a sick-room that he wants to be director at the same time that he is a patient, when he is not himself and not capable of directing things.
> *The Physician's Wife and the Things That Pertain to Her Life*

James B. McClinton [1897–   ]

The doctor's children have 50% more chances of being failures than others of their kind because there is only one to teach them. She must take them hurriedly to the toilet, slowly to the Sunday School, and proudly to the graduation, all alone. The doctor is often busy.
> *Canadian Medical Association Journal* 47:472, 1942

Joyce Dennys [20th Cent.]

The only person to whom a Doctor can say exactly what he thinks about another Doctor is his Wife. That is why practically all Doctors are married.
> *The Over-Dose*

Cyril Connolly [1903–   ]

The true index of a man's character is the health of his wife.
> *The Unquiet Grave*, Pt. II

Samuel Zelman [1912–   ]

[The physician's] wife proved a better diagnostician. Her medical education, obtained from long reading of popular magazines, although deficient in basic sciences, was remarkably current.
> *New England Journal of Medicine* 265:1203, 1961

Anonymous

Said she, "My medulla, O light of my life
  And pith of my skeleton's ossa!"
And she buried her head, like a dutiful wife,
  In her husband's subclavian fossa.[1]

WOMAN

See also MATERNITY, SEX, WIVES, WOMEN IN MEDICINE

Euripides [484–406 B.C.]

Strange that God hath given to men
Salves for the venom of all creeping pests,
But none hath ever yet devised a balm
For venomous woman, worse than fire or viper.
> *Andromache*, 269 (tr. by A. S. Way)

Aristotle [384–322 B.C.]

We must look upon the female character as being a sort of natural deficiency.

Menander [343?–291? B.C.]

Though many wild beasts on land and in the sea, the beastliest one of all is woman.
> *Fragments*, 488 (tr. by F. G. Allinson)

---

[1] This is the last stanza of an anatomical poem on the doctor's wife, the other stanzas of which have been lost. Dr. W. W. Francis of the Osler Library, McGill University, states that it was a favorite quotation of Sir William Osler's.

A woman is necessarily an evil, but he that gets the most tolerable one is lucky.
>   *Ibid.,* 532

Seneca [4? B.C.–A.D. 65]

The illustrious founder of the guild and profession of medicine [Hippocrates] remarked that women never lost their hair or suffered from pain in the feet; and yet nowadays they run short of hair and are afflicted with gout. . . . in rivalling male indulgences, they have also rivalled the ills to which men are heirs. They keep just as late hours, and drink just as much liquor; they challenge men in wrestling and carousing; they are no less given to vomiting from distended stomachs and to thus discharging all their wine again; nor are they behind men in gnawing ice, as a relief to their fevered digestions. And they even match the men in their passions, although they were created to feel love passively (may the gods and goddesses confound them!). They devise the most impossible varieties of unchastity, and in the company of men they play the part of men. What wonder, then, that we can trip up the statement of the greatest and most skilled physician, when so many women are gouty and bald! Because of their vices, women have ceased to deserve the privileges of their sex; they have put off their womanly nature and are therefore condemned to suffer the diseases of men.
>   *Moral Epistles to Lucilius,*
>   XCV (tr. by Richard M.
>   Gummere)

Favorinus [fl. 2nd Cent.]

Do you too perhaps think . . . that nature gave women nipples as a kind of beauty spot, not for the purpose of nourishing their children, but as an adornment of their breast?
>   Quoted by Aulus Gellius in
>   *Attic Nights,* XII.i.7 (tr. by
>   J. C. Rolfe)

Arnold of Villanova [1235–1311]

In this book I propose, with God's help, to consider diseases peculiar to women. And since women are, for the most part, poisonous creatures, I shall then proceed to treat of the bites of venomous beasts.
>   *Commentaries,* Bk. III

Geoffrey Chaucer [1340?–1400]

And bet than old boef is the tendre
>   veel.
I wol no womman thritty yeer of age.
>   *The Canterbury Tales,* "The
>   Merchant's Tale"

Heinrich Kramer and James Sprenger [ca. 15th Cent.]

And the tears of a woman are a deception, for they may spring from true grief, or they may be a snare. When a woman thinks alone she thinks evil.
>   *Malleus Maleficarum* (tr. by
>   M. Summers)

Francis Beaumont [1584–1616] and John Fletcher [1579–1625]

>   As men
Do walk a mile, women should talk
>   an hour
After supper: 'Tis their exercise.
>   *Philaster,* Act II, Sc. iv

Samuel Johnson [1709–1784]

Yet more remote from common conceptions are the numerous and restless anxieties, by which female happiness is particularly disturbed. A solitary philosopher would imagine ladies born with an exemption from care and sorrow, lulled in perpetual quiet, and feasted with unmingled pleasure; for what can interrupt the content of those, upon whom one age has laboured after another to confer honours, and accumulate immunities. . . . But experience will soon discover how easily those are disgusted who have been

made nice by plenty and tender by indulgence.
> *The Rambler,* No. 128 (June 8, 1751)

Edmund Burke [1729–1797]

A woman is but an animal, and an animal not of the highest order.
> *Reflections on the Revolution in France*

Hannah Cowley [1743–1809]

What is woman? — only one of Nature's agreeable blunders.
> *Who's the Dupe?,* Act II

Oliver Wendell Holmes [1809–1894]

A lady's portrait has been known to come out of the finishing-artist's room ten years younger than when it left the camera. But try to mend a stereograph and you will find the difference. Your marks and patches float above the picture and never identify themselves with it. No woman may be declared youthful on the strength of a single photograph; but if the stereoscopic twins say she is young, let her be so acknowledged.
> *Atlantic Monthly,* July 1861, "Sun-painting and Sun-sculpture"

A woman never forgets her sex. She would rather talk with a man than an angel, any day.
> *The Poet at the Breakfast Table,* Sect. IV

S. Weir Mitchell [1829–1914]

The moral world of the sick-bed explains in a measure some of the things that are strange in daily life, and the man who does not know sick women does not know women.
> *Doctor and Patient,* Introduction

Ambrose Bierce [1842–1914?]

You are not permitted to kill a woman who has wronged you, but nothing forbids you to reflect that she is growing older every minute. You are avenged fourteen hundred and forty times a day.
> *Epigrams*

Anatole France [1844–1924]

We have medicines to make women speak; we have none to make them keep silence.
> *The Man Who Married a Dumb Wife,* Act II, Sc. iv (tr. by Curtis H. Page)

Friedrich Nietzsche [1844–1900]

God created woman. And boredom did indeed cease from that moment — but many other things ceased as well! Woman was God's *second* mistake.
> *The Antichrist,* Sect. 48

When a woman has scholarly inclinations there is generally something wrong with her sexual nature.
> *Beyond Good and Evil,* Ch. IV, Sect. 144 (tr. by Helen Zimmern)

From a woman you can learn nothing of women.

Sir William Osler [1849–1919]

I do not know at what age one dare call a woman a spinster. I will put it, perhaps rashly, at twenty-five.
> *Aequanimitas, with Other Addresses,* "Nurse and Patient"

It is the prime duty of a woman of this terrestrial world to look well.
> *The Johns Hopkins Hospital Nurses Alumnae Magazine* 12: 72, 1913

The surgical cycle in woman: Appendix removed, right kidney hooked up, gall-bladder taken out, gastro-enterostomy, clean sweep of uterus and adnexa.
> Quoted by William B. Bean in *Sir William Osler: Aphorisms,* Ch. 5

Santiago Ramón y Cajal
[1852–1934]

A woman venerates her parents, esteems her husband, but adores only her sons.
Charlas de Café

Sir James M. Barrie [1860–1937]

You see, dear, it is not true that woman was made from man's rib; she was really made from his funny bone.

August Bier [1861–1949]

Medicine is like a woman who changes with the fashions.
Aphorism

Oliver Herford [1863–1935]

A woman's mind is cleaner than a man's — she changes it oftener.

W. Somerset Maugham
[1874–1965]

The Professor of Gynaecology. . . . began his course of lectures as follows: Gentlemen, woman is an animal that micturates once a day, defecates once a week, menstruates once a month, parturates once a year and copulates whenever she has the opportunity.
A Writer's Notebook, 1894

An acquaintance with the rudiments of physiology will teach you more about feminine character than all the philosophy and wise-saws in the world.
Ibid., 1896

Otto Weininger [1880–1903]

No one who is not female can be in a position to make accurate statements about women.
Sex and Character, Pt. II, Ch. 2

There have never been any great discoveries in the world of science made by women, because the facility for truth only proceeds from a desire for truth, and the former is always in proportion to the latter. Woman's sense of reality is much less than man's, in spite of much repetition of the contrary opinion.
Ibid., Ch. 9

Samuel Hoffenstein [1890–1947]

A woman, like the touted Sphinx,
Sits, and God knows what she thinks;
Hard-boiled men, who never fall,
Say she doesn't think at all.
Poems in Praise of Practically Nothing, "Love Songs, at Once Tender and Informative"

Henry E. Sigerist [1891–1957]

A determining point in the history of gynecology is to be found in the fact that sex plays a more important part in the life of woman than in that of man, and that she is more burdened by her sex.
American Journal of Obstetrics and Gynecology 42:714, 1941

Spanish Proverb

Six men give a doctor less to do than one woman.

WOMEN IN MEDICINE

William E. Gladstone [1809–1898]

Sir W. Jenner was good enough . . . to state what greatly confirmed all [my] previous impressions . . . with respect to the repulsive subject of any combination of men and women in the reception of some of the instruction absolutely necessary for the effective pursuit of the medical profession.[1]
Letter to Queen Victoria, May 11, 1870

[1] Queen Victoria had written to Gladstone on May 8 suggesting that Sir William Jenner could tell him "what an *awful* idea this is — of allowing *young girls* & young men to *enter* the dissecting room together."

Alfred Stillé [1813–1900]

Another disease has become epidemic. "The woman question" in relation to medicine is only one of the forms in which the *pestis muliebris* vexes the world. In other shapes it attacks the bar, wriggles into the jury box, and clearly means to mount upon the bench; it strives, thus far in vain, to serve at the altar and thunder from the pulpit; it raves at political meetings, harangues in the lecture-room, infects the masses with its poison, and even pierces the triple brass that surrounds the politician's heart.

To the vulgar apprehension, nothing seems more natural than that women should be physicians, for is not nursing the chief agent in the cure of disease, and who so fit a nurse as woman! The logic is worthy of its subject, and is of the sort in which Eve's daughters excel.

> *Transactions of the American Medical Association* 22:73, 1871

Mary Putnam Jacobi [1842–1906]

I have heard repeated on all sides, "a woman could not enter the amphitheatre in safety, so great would be the *tapage* among the students, so impossible the efforts of the professor to screen her from the insult and annoyance." Now I always knew this was humbug but I wanted to have it demonstrated.

> Letter to her mother, Mrs. G. P. Putnam, January 25, 1868

Day before yesterday, for the first time since its foundation several centuries ago a petticoat might be seen in the august amphitheatre of the *Ecole de Médecine*. That petticoat enrobed the form of your most obedient servant and dutiful daughter!

> *Idem*

Perrin H. Long [1899–1965]

We have never understood just why there are not more women in surgery.

We once heard Dr. Edward D. Churchill jokingly say, speaking of the difference between a surgeon and an internist, that the surgeon was the captain of the team, while an internist never had a team. Does this mean that women don't make good captains?

> *Resident Physician* 10:75, October 1964

Anonymous

A maiden at college, named Breeze,
Weighed down by B.A.'s and M.D.'s
    Collapsed from the strain.
    Said her doctor, "It's plain
You are killing yourself by degrees!"

> *The World's Best Limericks*

WORK

See also IDLENESS

Sophocles [496?–406 B.C.]

Who in season labors best,
His labors ended, has the sweetest rest.

> *Philoctetes*, 637 (tr. by F. Storr)

Galen [fl. 2nd Cent.]

Employment is nature's physician, and is essential to human happiness.

St. John Chrysostom [345?–407]

So powerful a medicine is labour, that . . . the servant is able to sleep.

> *Homilies on the Statutes*, Homily II (tr. by John H. Parker)

Bishop Richard Cumberland [1631–1718]

It is better to wear out than to rust out.

> Quoted by Bishop George Horne in *The Duty of Contending for the Faith*

Jean Jacques Rousseau [1712–1778]

Temperance and labor are the two real

physicians of man: labor sharpens his appetite and temperance prevents his abusing it.
> *Émile*, Bk. I

Thomas Young [1773–1829]

Leisure and application are the great requisites for improving the mind: leisure is useless without application; but application with a very little leisure may produce very material benefit. If you are careful of your vacant minutes, you may advance yourselves more than many do who have every convenience afforded them.
> Quoted in *Biographical Memoirs of the Most Celebrated Physicians and Surgeons*, Vol. IV

Thomas Carlyle [1795–1881]

Work is the grand cure of all the maladies and miseries that ever beset mankind.
> Inaugural address at Edinburgh University, 1866

Thomas Hood [1799–1845]

Work — work — work
Till the brain begins to swim;
Work — work — work
Till the eyes are heavy and dim!
> *The Song of the Shirt*

Oliver Wendell Holmes [1809–1894]

What have we to do with time but to fill it up with labor?

John Ruskin [1819–1900]

Now in order that people may be happy in their work, these three things are needed: They must be fit for it: They must not do too much of it: And they must have a sense of success in it.
> *Pre-Raphaelitism*

Wilhelm His [1831–1904]

For the progress and success of one's own intellectual labors it is more advantageous to be burdened with a moderate number of obligations than to possess absolute freedom. In particular I have often found that at the beginning of a desired vacation, simultaneously with the appearance of the ability to dispose freely of one's time, there is also a relaxation of intellectual tension which can only be overcome gradually and by compulsion.
> *Lebenserinnerungen*, "Abschlussder Studienzeit"

John Shaw Billings [1838–1913]

There's nothing really difficult if you only begin — some people contemplate a task until it looms so big, it seems impossible, but I just begin and it gets done somehow. There would be no coral islands if the first bug sat down and began to wonder how the job was to be done.
> Quoted by John Y. W. MacAlister in *British Medical Journal* 1:642, 1913

Sir William Osler [1849–1919]

Though a little one, the master-word looms large in meaning. It is the open sesame to every portal, the great equalizer in the world, the true philosopher's stone, which transmutes all the base metal of humanity into gold. . . . And the master-word is *Work*.
> *Aequanimitas, with Other Addresses*, "The Master-Word in Medicine"

William Stewart Halsted [1852–1922]

When oppressed by the seeming magnitude of one of my little anthills of work I have recalled the advice of Dr. [John Shaw] Billings: "Devote a small amount of time each day to it and the mountain will melt away with astonishing rapidity."
> *Bulletin of the Johns Hopkins Hospital* 25:244, 1914

George Bernard Shaw [1856–1950]

The secret of being miserable is to have leisure to bother about whether you are happy or not. The cure for it is occupation.

> *Misalliance,* Preface, "Parents and Children"

Sir Arthur Conan Doyle [1859–1930]

Work is the best antidote to sorrow, my dear Watson.

> *The Return of Sherlock Holmes,* "The Adventure of the Empty House"

Walter W. Palmer [1882–1950]

As the day's problems accumulate, I have three piles of work in front of me: first you tackle the one about which you can make immediate decisions, get it done and over with; then after appraising the second pile, containing insufficient data, arrange for the collection of the required missing information; finally there is the third pile of imponderables which should be filed or thrown into the basket; above all, don't waste any time on them.

> Quoted by David Seegal in *Journal of Chronic Diseases* 16:442, 1963

William E. Tanner [1889–   ]

Genius is the art of taking pains. Taking pains means work. . . .
    Work is effort directed to an end — the result of thought plus action.
    Work is also what is achieved — performance plus the result.

> *Sir W. Arbuthnot Lane,* Epilogue

Henry E. Sigerist [1891–1957]

Work is an essential factor of health. It balances and gives significance to our lives, ennobling them and permitting man to create those material and cultural values without which human existence would be meaningless.

> *Medicine and Human Welfare,* Ch. 3

C. Northcote Parkinson [1909–   ]

Work expands so as to fill the time available for its completion.

> *Parkinson's Law,* Ch. 1

Dutch Proverb

The labour we delight in physics pain.

WORRY

See also ANXIETY

John Wolcot ("Peter Pindar") [1738–1819]

Care to our coffin adds a nail, no doubt,
And every grin so merry draws one out.

> *Expostulatory Odes,* XV

J. Chalmers Da Costa [1863–1933]

A man who doesn't worry at all doesn't care a whole lot. I should not want a man who did not care a whole lot operating on me or mine. Perhaps worry is a device of nature to make us try to do our very best. If we knew we should not worry, we might be tempted at times to be careless. If a surgeon analyzes his worry he can get a line on what sort of man he is himself. If he worries only because he fears he may be sued, may lose a bill, or may hurt his reputation, then with him the voice of conscience is the fear of getting caught. If he worries because of the poor patient and the credit of surgery, then he is really a conscientious man.

> *The Trials and Triumphs of the Surgeon,* Ch. 1

Martin H. Fischer [1879–1962]

Stop telling men not to worry; all thinking men do; and such only do the world's work.
>> Quoted by Howard Fabing and Ray Marr in *Fischerisms*

English Proverb

It is not work that kills, but worry.

WOUNDS

See also SCARS

Horace [65–8 B.C.]

Fools, through false shame, hide the unhealed sore.
>> *Epistles,* I.xvi.24 (tr. by H. R. Fairclough)

Livy [59 B.C.–A.D. 17]

Wounds . . . unless handled and treated . . . cannot be healed.
>> *History,* XXVIII.xxvii.7 (tr. by G. F. Moore)

Ovid [43 B.C.–A.D.17?]

Perhaps in long time a scar will form; a raw wound quivers at the touch of a hand.
>> *Pontic Epistles,* I.iii.15 (tr. by A. L. Wheeler)

John Lyly [1554?–1606]

The wound that bleedeth inward is most dangerous.
>> *Euphues*

Sir Philip Sidney [1554–1586]

None can speak of a wound with skill, if he hath not a wound felt.
>> *Arcadia,* Bk. I

Sir Francis Bacon [1561–1626]

Wounds cannot be cured without searching.
>> *Essays,* "Of Expense"

William Shakespeare [1564–1616]

Here is a letter, lady —
The paper as the body of my friend,
And every word in it a gaping wound
Issuing lifeblood.
>> *The Merchant of Venice,* III, ii, 263

Have by some surgeon . . .
To stop his wounds, lest he do bleed to death.
>> *Ibid.,* IV, i, 257

What wound did ever heal but by degrees?
>> *Othello,* II, iii, 377

Dead Henry's wounds
Open their congeal'd mouths and bleed afresh!
Blush, blush, thou lump of foul deformity;
For 'tis thy presence that exhales this blood
From cold and empty veins where no blood dwells.
>> *Richard III,* I, ii, 55

The new-heal'd wound of malice should break out,
Which would be so much the more dangerous.
>> *Ibid.,* II, ii, 125

He jests at scars that never felt a wound.
>> *Romeo and Juliet,* II, ii, 1

MERCUTIO: Go, villain, fetch a surgeon.
ROMEO: Courage, man. The hurt cannot be much.
MERCUTIO: No, 'tis not so deep as a well, nor so wide as a church door; but 'tis enough, 'twill serve. Ask for me to-

morrow, and you shall find me a grave man.
Ibid., III, i, 97

Samuel Butler [1612–1680]
    H' had got a hurt
O' th' inside of a deadlier sort.
Hudibras, Pt. I, Canto III

John Oldham [1653–1683]
A wound, tho' cured, yet leaves behind a scar.
Satires Upon the Jesuits, No. 3

John Hunter [1728–1793]
Many wounds ought to be allowed to scab in which this process is now prevented; and this arises, I believe, from the conceit of surgeons who think themselves possessed of powers superior to nature and therefore have introduced the practice of making sores of all wounds. The mode of assisting the cure of wounds by permitting a scab to form is likewise applicable, in some cases, to that species of accident where the parts have not only been lacerated but deprived of life. . . . This practice is the very best for burns and scalds.
Lectures on the Principles of Surgery

George Gordon, Lord Byron
[1788–1824]
What deep wounds ever closed without a scar?
Childe Harold's Pilgrimage, Canto III, Stanza 84

Sir William S. Gilbert [1836–1911]
Bind up their wounds — but look the other way.
Princess Ida, Act III

The Bible
But a certain Samaritan . . . went to him, and bound up his wounds, pouring in oil and wine.
Luke 10:33

English Proverbs
A green wound is soon healed.

A wound heals but the scar remains.

WRITING

See also COMMUNICATION, LITERATURE, TERMINOLOGY

Horace [65–8 B.C.]
Doctors undertake a doctor's work; carpenters handle carpenters' tools: but, skilled or unskilled, we scribble poetry, all alike.
Epistles, I.i.114 (tr. by H. R. Fairclough)

Juvenal [60?–140?]
The itch for writing and making a name holds you fast as with a noose.
Satires, VII.50 (tr. by G. G. Ramsay)

Pliny the Younger [62–113]
Too much polishing weakens rather than improves a work.
Epistles, IX.xxxv

Su Shih ("Su Tung-p'o")
[1036–1101]
To be a writer requires the wasting of paper: to be a doctor requires the sacrificing of lives.
Quoted by F. H. Garrison in *Bulletin of the New York Academy of Medicine* 5:148, 1929

John of Mirfield [1362–1407]
I protest, however, at the finish of this little work, just as I also did at the beginning thereof, that with regard to all the things which are contained in this little tract, I myself have added nothing of my own to the matter at hand, for the reason that I have not discovered anything of my very own to add. I have simply collected the

words of authoritative philosophers and scientists, as well as the opinions of practical men, and having collected them together, have written them all down in one little summary: so that poor and unlearned men who do not possess a plenty of books at hand may here be able to find, at least in a superficial degree, not a few remedies for very many diseases.

> *Breviarum Bartholomei,* Epilogue (tr. by H. R. Aldridge)

William Clowes [1544–1604]

Thus much I have thought good to write briefly against that vain cavill of publishing books in English, seeing that herein I deserve no more blame than those excellent men who, by their famous writings in their own language, have purchased themselves immortal thanks of all men that succeed them.

> *A Profitable and Necessarie Booke of Observations* (ed. by F. N. L. Poynter in *Selected Writings,* Ch. 21)

Miguel de Cervantes [1547–1616]

And for the Citation of so many Authors, 'tis the easiest Thing in Nature. Find out one of these Books with an alphabetical Index, and without any farther Ceremony, remove it *verbatim* into your own: And tho' the World won't believe you have Occasion for such Lumber, yet there are Fools enough to be thus drawn into an Opinion of the Work; at least, such a flourishing Train of Attendants will give your Book a fashionable Air, and recommend it to Sale.

> *Don Quixote,* "The Author's Preface to the Reader" (tr. by P. A. Motteux)

Sir Thomas Browne [1605–1682]

Some men have written more than others have spoken. Pineda quotes more authors, in a work, than are necessary in a whole world.

> *Religio Medici,* Pt. I, Sect. 24

Blaise Pascal [1623–1662]

The present letter is a very long one, simply because I had no leisure to make it shorter.

> *Provincial Letters,* Ch. XVI (tr. by Thomas M'Crie)

Thomas Sydenham [1624–1689]

In writing the history of a disease, every philosophical hypothesis whatsoever, that has previously occupied the mind of the author, should lie in abeyance. This being done, the clear and natural phenomena of the disease should be noted — these, and these only. They should be noted accurately, and in all their minuteness; in imitation of the exquisite industry of those painters who represent in their portraits the smallest moles and faintest spots.

> *Medical Observations* (3rd ed.), Preface (tr. by R. G. Latham in *Works,* Vol. I)

John Mayow [1640–1679]

As a rule disease can scarcely keep pace with the itch to scribble about it.

> *De Rachitide,* Pt. V

Hermann Boerhaave [1668–1738]

To offset all these inconveniences of the profession there remains the necessity of writing all singularity of disease and indeed of each disease observable. For such a task it is required that the case history be so clear that when it is read the Reader will immediately see the evident correspondence, so that he will learn of the present disease from that previously described. Everything pertaining to the case must be listed; nor that least thing neglected which a critical Reader might rightly seek to understand the malady.

> *Atrocis, nec Descripti Prius, Morbi Historia*

Narration must be done carefully so that the order of events be unchanged;

there must be arrangement according to the surging change of events, and each event must be recorded in its proper place.
Idem

Benjamin Franklin [1706–1790]

If you wou'd not be forgotten
As soon as you are dead and rotten,
Either write things worth reading,
Or do things worth the writing.
Poor Richard's Almanack, 1738

John Mitchell [d. 1768]

You seem to request of me, concerning the yellow fever . . . , to publish my Account of it. That I cannot by any means do, at least at this time, & am uncertain if ever I shall. But that I may not seem to you to act without Reason, . . . my office & business in the world is to know & understand as much of those things as I can, in order to apply them, & not to teach them; Enough, shall I say, or too much, for any one Man to do! at least I have found it too much for me; when joyned to the fatigues of such a slavish Practice, as you know ours is.
Letter to Dr. Cadwallader Colden, September 10, 1745

Charles Churchill [1731–1764]

Little do such men know the toil, the pains,
The daily, nightly racking of the brains,
To range the thoughts, the matter to digest,
To cull fit phrases, and reject the rest.
Gotham, Bk. II

John Wolcot ("Peter Pindar") [1738–1819]

Astronomers should treat of stars and comets;
Doctors of *assa faetida* and vomits,
And apoplexies, those light troops of Death,

That use no ceremony with our breath;
Ague and dropsy, jaundice and catarrh,
The grim-look tyrant's heavy horse of war.

Farriers should write on farcys and the glanders;
Bug-doctors, only upon bed-disorders;
Farmers on land, ploughs, pigs, ducks, geese and ganders;
Nightmen alone, on aromatic ordures.
The artists should on painting solely write;
Like David, then they may "good things indite."
But when the mob of *gentlemen*
Desert their province, and take up the pen,
The Lord have mercy on the art!
Their crow-quills can no light impart.
Farewell Odes for 1786, Ode V

Richard Brinsley Sheridan [1751–1816]

You write with *ease,* to shew your breeding;
But *easy writing's* vile *hard reading.*
Clio's Protest

Samuel Hahnemann [1755–1843]

I beg you to publish only the most accurate and careful experiment.

Martin J. Routh [1755–1854]

You will find it a very good practice *always to verify your references,* sir!
Quoted in *Quarterly Review,* July 1878

John Abernethy [1764–1831]

Various advantages result even from the publication of opinions; for though we are very liable to error in forming them, yet their promulgation, by exciting investigation, and pointing out the deficiencies of our information, cannot be otherwise than useful in the promotion of science.
Surgical and Physiological Works, Vol. I, Preface

Sydney Smith [1771–1845]

In composing, as a general rule, run your pen through every other word you have written; you have no idea what vigor it will give your style.

> Quoted by Lady Holland in *A Memoir of the Rev. Sydney Smith,* Ch. 11

Samuel Lover [1797–1868]

When once the itch of litherature[1] comes over a man, nothing can cure it but the scratching of a pen.
Handy Andy, Ch. 36

Oliver Wendell Holmes [1809–1894]

I never saw an author in my life — saving, perhaps, one — that did not purr as audibly as a full-grown domestic cat . . . on having his fur smoothed in the right way by a skilful hand.

> *The Autocrat of the Breakfast Table,* Sect. III

Should you become authors, express your opinions freely; defend them rarely. It is not often that an opinion is worth expressing, which cannot take care of itself. Opposition is the best *mordant* to fix the color of your thought in the general belief.

> *Medical Essays,* "Border Lines of Knowledge in Some Provinces of Medical Science"

There is no form of lead-poisoning which more rapidly and thoroughly pervades the blood and bones and marrow than that which reaches the young author through mental contact with type-metal. . . . So the man or woman who has tasted type is sure to return to his old indulgence sooner or later.

> *Ibid.,* "Some of My Early Teachers"

[1] This dialogue is written in an Irish dialect.

John Brown [1810–1882]

Men who rejoiced in making clear things obscure, and plain things the reverse, he could not abide, and spoke with some contempt of those who were original merely from their standing on their heads, and tall from walking upon stilts.

> *Horae Subsecivae,* Series II, "Letter to John Cairns"

Rudolf Virchow [1821–1902]

Brevity in writing is the best insurance for its perusal.

> Quoted by F. H. Garrison in *Bulletin of the New York Academy of Medicine* 4:994, 1928

The conjunction "and" commonly serves to indicate that the writer's mind still functions even when no signs of the phenomenon are noticeable.

> *Idem*

In my journal, anyone can make a fool of himself.[1]

Jean Martin Charcot [1825–1893]

There is, in any well executed description of disease, a remarkable power of transmission. If made at the right time, it will penetrate even the least prepared minds. What had hitherto remained in the womb of nothingness has begun to live. A description of a hitherto unknown species of disease is an event, a very great event, in pathology.

> Quoted by F. H. Garrison in *Bulletin of the New York Academy of Medicine* 4:1000, 1928

Walter Bagehot [1826–1877]

Writers, like teeth, are divided into incisors and grinders.

> *Literary Studies,* "The First Edinburgh Reviewers"

[1] Cf. W. I. B. Beveridge, p. 251b.

Theodor Billroth [1829–1894]

Become familiar not only with teaching but also with writing.

> Quoted by James B. Herrick in *Memories of Eighty Years*

Sir Clifford Allbutt [1836–1925]

Slovenly writing reflects slovenly thinking and obscure writing usually confused thinking.

John Shaw Billings [1838–1913]

First have something to say, 2nd say it, 3rd stop when you have said it, and finally give it an accurate title.

> Prescription for writing a medical paper

Mary Putnam Jacobi [1842–1906]

I . . . have a real dread of becoming a "literary physician," like (though a *long* way after), Holmes. Such men are never worth anything for medicine or science.

> Letter to her father, G. P. Putnam, September 12, 1867

Anatole France [1844–1924]

When a thing has been said and well said, have no scruple: take it and copy it. Give references? Why should you? Either your readers know where you have taken the passage and the precaution is needless, or they do not know and you humiliate them.

Sir William Osler [1849–1919]

The young physician should be careful what and how he writes. Let him take heed to his education, and his reputation will take care of itself.

> *Aequanimitas, with Other Addresses,* "Internal Medicine as a Vocation"

There is no more difficult art to acquire than the art of observation, and for some men it is quite as difficult to record an observation in brief and plain language.

> *Ibid.,* "On the Educational Value of the Medical Society"

Always note and record the unusual. Keep and compare your observations. Communicate or publish short notes on anything that is striking or new.

> *Bulletin of the Johns Hopkins Hospital* 30:198, 1919

It is often harder to boil down than to write.

> Quoted by Harvey Cushing in *Life of Sir William Osler*

Sir John Bland-Sutton [1855–1936]

I always read carefully reviews of my own books in order to amend faults of style, correct errors and false references. Often I have been pleased with a review written by a friend and gained much from the criticisms of an adversary.

> *The Story of a Surgeon,* Ch. XIV

Stephen Paget [1855–1926]

Has everybody got something to say worth saying? Are not they the nicest people who say nothing? Indeed, that may be true; and if ever, like Prospero, I recover my dukedom, I will drown my book: but there comes a time, even to people who might otherwise be nice, when they find pleasure in writing. They are tired of their own company; they have lived inside their hearts till they know every stick of the furniture: they desire now, before it is too late, to leave that narrow lodging, to say what they think, and to proclaim what they have learned. Silence is golden; but gold is for circulation.

> *Confessio Medici,* Preface

A. E. Housman [1859–1936]

I have seldom written poetry unless I was rather out of health, and the

experience, though pleasurable, was generally agitating and exhausting.
> *The Name and Nature of Poetry*

Sir James M. Barrie [1860–1937]

The scientific man is the only person who has anything new to say and who does not know how to say it.

James B. Herrick [1861–1954]

I recall . . . the thrill of excitement . . . as I was looking through the high-toned Virchow and Hirsch's *Jahresbericht* and saw my name . . . and the title of a recent article of mine. The thrill changed to a jolt as I read this terse, clear, yet comprehensive epitome: "Nichts neues." [Nothing new.]
> *Memories of Eighty Years*, Ch. XI

J. Chalmers Da Costa [1863–1933]

To write an article of any sort is, to some extent, to reveal ourselves. Hence, even a medical article is, in a sense, something of an autobiography.
> *The Trials and Triumphs of the Surgeon*, Ch. 1

Benjamin N. Cardozo [1870–1938]

There is an accuracy that defeats itself by the overemphasis of details. I often say that one must permit oneself, and quite advisedly and deliberately, a certain margin of misstatement.

Marcel Proust [1871–1922]

Each of us finds lucidity only in those ideas which are in the same state of confusion as his own. Many simply do not have the will power to resist writing a book when they have reached a point of "understanding" this abstract subject.

Wilfred Trotter [1872–1939]

At no time has the astringent tonic

of critical writing been more necessary for the health of medicine and the medical sciences.
> *Collected Papers*, "Has the Intellect a Function?"

W. Somerset Maugham [1874–1965]

If you could write lucidly, simply, euphoniously and yet with liveliness you would write perfectly: you would write like Voltaire.
> *The Summing Up*, Sect. xiii

I have seen men since as I saw them then [as a medical student], and thus have I drawn them.
> *Ibid.*, Sect. xx

Martin H. Fischer [1879–1962]

You must acquire the ability to describe your observations and your experiences in such language that whoever observes or experiences similarly will be forced to the same conclusions.
> Quoted by Howard Fabing and Ray Marr in *Fischerisms*

Stanley Cobb [1887–1968]

If the ladies of the Record Room will prepare for me a list of the words they wish deleted from the records, I shall be happy to give it my attention.[1]

Archibald Malloch [1887–   ]

The greatest men I have ever known have written their own papers.
> Quoted by F. H. Garrison in *An Introduction to the History of Medicine* (4th ed.)

Sir F. M. R. Walshe [1888–   ]

Good God! This is a dreadful record. You can't tell anything about the pa-

---

[1] Comment when ladies of the Record Room at Massachusetts General Hospital objected to many of the words being quoted verbatim in psychiatric histories.

tient. You can't tell whether he's married, single, or Australian!

Comment on a case record written by an Australian clinical clerk, National Hospital, London, 1930

I see you have an interesting paper in the latest number of *Brain*. When is the English translation coming out? [1]

Remark to Dr. Derek Denny-Brown, National Hospital, London

Morris Fishbein [1889–   ]

Increasing organization in the field of medicine, as in every other field of human endeavor, has raised the level of contributions to medical literature. Far too often, however, physicians still prepare their contributions with a striving and agony and delay comparable to the delivery of human progeny by one untutored in the refinements of obstetrics.

Medical Writing (3rd ed.), Introduction

John A. Ryle [1889–1950]

Although our instruction, as well as our destruction, now comes from the air, the written word still has its little part to play.

Fears May Be Liars, Foreword

Percival Bailey [1892–   ]

I am not one of those who believe that prefaces are written but not read. Sometimes the preface suffices.

American Journal of Psychiatry 113:387, 1956

Richard M. Hewitt [1892–   ]

I do not know two people who agree about [hyphenation], although I know a number who have bowed to authority in order to eat. . . . Hyphenation is

[1] Dr. Denny-Brown explained, "After a long and rather obscure paper of mine had appeared in *Brain*."

strictly a family affair, to be fought over behind closed doors. It never should be mentioned when guests are present or when members of the family are out in company.

The Physician-Writer's Book, Ch. 34

Joseph Garland [1] [1893–   ]

There is no good medical writing — just good rewriting.

Arthur M. Walker [1896–1955]

A life-long aversion to publishing single case reports.

Quoted by Julius L. Wilson in *Walkerisms*

Walter Modell [1907–   ]

Time was when symposium was not a portentous word for a ragbag of second rate papers artfully salted with a few "names."

Clinical Pharmacology and Therapeutics 1:689, 1960

W. I. B. Beveridge [1908–   ]

He is a bold man who submits his paper for publication without it having first been put under the microscope of friendly criticism by colleagues.

The Art of Scientific Investigation, Ch. IX

William B. Bean [1909–   ]

The vapidity of medical *writing* which reflects very little logical or rigorous thought indicates that the cultural potential of physicians, instead of leading, has fallen below the average. Anyone forced by editorial obligations to read critically many medical papers is struck by the singular and consistent absence of form, a vast desert of data with the rare oases of prose, all too often the dried up water holes of the alkali plains.

Archives of Internal Medicine 92:153, 1953

[1] Attributed to Joseph Garland.

The pseudo prestige of long and difficult words transcends the useful scientific term and diffuses widely through our papers. Simple things are made complicated, and the complex is made incomprehensible. Chaos reigns. The so-called medical literature is stuffed to bursting with junk, written in a hopscotch style characterised by a Brownian movement of uncontrolled parts of speech which seethe in restless unintelligibility.
> *Journal of Laboratory and Clinical Medicine* 39:3, 1952

Stanley Gilder [1909–   ]

Last year Sir George Pickering castigated examiners, teachers and editors for allowing medical students and doctors to get away with an abominably low standard of composition. He was immediately assailed with the counter-argument that an illiterate doctor was not necessarily a bad doctor; but he would no doubt have retorted that muddled writing means muddled thinking and muddled thinking is not conducive to good diagnosis.
> *Medical Journal of Australia* 1:957, 1962

The cardinal sin in medical writing is not grammatical error but obscurity.
> *Idem*

Richard Asher [1912–   ]

Quote what you guess, and do not fight
To trace its source or get it right.[1]
> *Archives of Internal Medicine* 113:612, 1964, "Tough on Clough"

Robertson Davies [1913–   ]

[Of Sir Thomas Browne's style:] Every sentence is a stately torchlight procession from subject to predicate.
> *Bulletin of the Academy of Medicine of Toronto* 36:7, 1962

[1] Cf. Arthur Hugh Clough, p. 159b.

M. Therese Southgate [1928–   ]

Unfortunately, too many authors write as though they will never have another chance — and they are correct.
> *Journal of the American Medical Association* 181:1124, 1962

The Bible

My tongue is the pen of a ready writer.
> *Psalms* 45:1

Anonymous

Saving only the doctors, there are none more stupid than the grammarians.

No one but the author is interested in a long list of references stuck onto the end of an article like barnacles on a ship's bottom. . . . The publication of a long list of authors' names after the title is a little like having all a vessel's ballast hanging from the masthead, as if to counterbalance the barnacles.
> *New England Journal of Medicine* 271:1068, 1964

X-RAY

William Shakespeare [1564–1616]

Come, come, and sit you down. You
    shall not budge!
You go not till I set you up a glass
Where you may see the inmost part of
    you.
> *Hamlet*, III, iv, 18

Samuel Butler [1835–1902]

X-RAYS: Their moral is this — that a right way of looking at things will see through almost anything.
> *Note-Books*, Vol. V (*Further Extracts*, ed. by A. T. Bartholomew)

Wilhelm Conrad Roentgen [1845–1923]

If the hand be held between the discharge-tube and the [fluorescent] screen, the darker shadow of the bones is seen within the slightly dark shadow-image of the hand itself. . . . For brevity's sake I shall use the expression "rays" and to distinguish them from others of this name, I shall call them "x-rays."

> *On a New Kind of Rays* (tr. by Otto Glasser in *Wilhelm Conrad Röntgen and the Early History of the Roentgen Rays,* Ch. 2)

Merrill C. Sosman [1890–1959]

One look is worth a thousand listens.[1]
Aphorism

Anonymous

O Röntgen, then the news is true,
  And not a trick of idle rumor,
That bids us each beware of you,
  And of your grim and graveyard humor.

We do not want, like Dr. SWIFT,
  To take our flesh off and to pose in
Our bones, or show each little rift
  And joint for you to poke your nose in.

> *Punch,* January 25, 1896, "The New Photography"

YAWNING

Ashley Montagu [1905–   ]

Yawning warns one of the reduction in critical consciousness and, as in sleepiness or weariness, suggests that one ought to sleep or rest or, as in boredom, that one ought to do something about the boredom.

> *Journal of the American Medical Association* 182:732, 1962

[1] A radiologist's opinion of the stethoscope.

YELLOW FEVER

Mathew Carey [1760–1839]

Many never walked on the foot path, but went into the middle of the streets, to avoid being infected in passing by houses wherein people had died. Acquaintances and friends avoided each other in the streets, and only signified their regard by a cold nod. The old custom of shaking hands fell into such general disuse, that many were affronted at even the offer of the hand.

> *A Short Account of the Malignant Fever* [1] *Lately Prevalent in Philadelphia* (1793)

YOUTH

> *See also* ADOLESCENCE, AGE, CHILDREN

Homer [ca. 850 B.C.]

He hath the flower of youth, wherein is the fulness of strength.

> *Iliad,* XIII. 484 (tr. by A. T. Murray)

Leonardo da Vinci [1452–1519]

In youth acquire that which may requite you for the deprivations of old age; and if you are mindful that old age has wisdom for its food, you will so exert yourself in youth, that your old age will not lack sustenance.

> *Codice Atlantico,* 112 (tr. by Edward MacCurdy in *The Notebooks of Leonardo da Vinci,* Vol. I, Ch. I)

Michel de Montaigne [1533–1592]

If I were to enumerate all the beautiful human actions, of whatever kind, that have come to my knowledge, I should think I would find that the greater part were performed, both in ancient times

[1] This Malignant Fever was yellow fever.

and in our own, before the age of thirty, rather than after. Yes, often even in the lives of the same men.
> *Essays*, Bk. I, Ch. 57, "Of Age" (tr. by Donald M. Frame)

Sir Francis Bacon [1561–1626]

A man that is young in years may be old in hours, if he have lost no time.
> *Essays*, "Of Youth and Age"

Robert Southey [1774–1843]

Live as long as you may, the first twenty years are the longest half of your life.
> *The Doctor*, Ch. 130

William Hazlitt [1778–1830]

No young man believes he shall ever die.
> *The Monthly Magazine*, March 1827, "On the Feeling of Immortality in Youth"

Alexandre Dumas père [1802–1870]

Youth seems a sad mistake — when one is no longer young.
> *Twenty Years After*

W. Somerset Maugham [1874–1965]

The world of my twenties was a middle-aged world and youth was something to be got through as quickly as possible so that maturity might be reached.
> *The Summing Up*, Sect. lxxiii

Gertrude Stein [1874–1946]

We, living now, are always to ourselves young men and women.
> *The Making of Americans*, Introduction

Alan Gregg [1890–1957]

We are young when we expect variety, and indeed anything that promises variety or seeks change has youth. It is a curious paradox that we desire stability for our plans and require change for our souls' sake.
> Aphorism (Quoted by Wilder Penfield in *The Difficult Art of Giving*, Appendix A)

The Bible

The glory of young men is their strength.
> *Proverbs* 20:29

Index of Authors

Index of Authors

AN ASTERISK following the name of an author indicates that he is quoted more than fifty times. For these few authors no page numbers are given, since it is believed that an overabundance of page numbers (in Shakespeare's case, over 400) would be of little help.

Names containing connective elements (da, de, de la, du, la, le, van, von) are alphabetized according to usage. American and British names appear under these connectives (Da Costa, La Guardia, van Dyke). Names in the Romance languages follow no set pattern of alphabetization, but cross-references are given to aid the reader (Rochefoucauld, Duc François de La. *See* La Rochefoucauld, Duc François de).

A

Abbas, Haly, 134
Abell, Irvin, 302
Abernethy, John, 44, 50, 136, 195, 292, 354, 395, 656, 668
Acuna, Manuel, 265
Adams, Franklin P. (F.P.A.), 119, 207, 557
Adams, John Quincy, 259, 543
Adams, Samuel Hopkins, 228, 301, 321, 444, 458
Adams, Thomas, 450
Addis, Thomas, 60, 98, 116, 636, 648
Addison, Joseph, 21, 23, 37, 51, 78, 122, 165, 203, 211, 229, 244, 258, 269, 394, 548, 553, 607
Addison, Thomas, 422
Ade, George, 10, 274
Adler, Francis Heed, 507
Aeschylus, 37, 110, 414, 491
Aesop, 570

Aetios, 4, 188
Agathias Scholasticus, 87
Aikin, John, 296, 465
Akenside, Mark, 498, 517
Albright, Fuller, 236, 385, 637
Aldrich, Henry, 7
Aldrich, Thomas Bailey, 555
Alexander of Tralles, 442
Alexander the Great, 257
Ali ibn-Hazm, 21
Allbutt, Sir Clifford, 115, 152, 156, 206, 230, 233, 277, 286, 330, 411, 423, 520, 537, 564, 587, 670
Alpinus, Prosper, 549
Amberson, J. Burns, 98
Ambiani, Johann Fernelii, 650
Ames, Adelbert, 548
Amidon, Elsworth, 569
Amiel, Henri, 84, 92, 96, 119, 205, 339, 401, 545, 643
Ammianus Marcellinus, 188
Anderson, J. A. D., 646
Anderson, Maxwell, 340, 652
André, Major John, 258

B

C

D

G

K

M

Salluste, Guillaume de. *See* Bartas, Seigneur du

Salter, William T., 248

Sand, René, 302

Santayana, George, 30, 165, 266, 332, 343, 528, 539

Sarton, George, 484

Sauerbruch, Ernst Ferdinand, 133

Saul, Leon J., 288

Saunders, Frederick, 481, 609, 633

Savonarola, 399

Saxe, John Godfrey, 339

Sayers, Dorothy L., 2

Scarlett, Earle P., 157, 215, 334

Schatzki, Richard, 336

Schauffler, Robert Haven, 403

Schick, Béla, 38, 53, 57, 168, 275, 305, 374, 445, 513, 614, 620

Schiller, Friedrich von, 37, 40, 354

Schopenhauer, Arthur, 229, 290, 309, 431

Schulberg, Budd, 385

Schweitzer, Albert, 56–57, 220, 267, 332, 356, 361, 459

Scott, Sir Walter, 183, 184, 204, 309, 346, 379, 460, 543, 553

Sedley, Sir Charles, 326

Seegal, Beatrice, 109, 508

Seegal, David, 33, 76, 99, 109, 117, 164, 207, 212, 216, 248, 251, 261, 320, 349–350, 357, 413, 417, 461, 507–508, 576–577, 601, 603, 637

Selden, John, 130, 585

Semmelweis, Ignaz, 54

Seneca, 5, 36, 73, 77, 110–111, 175, 186, 200, 237, 238, 268, 278, 284, 344, 353, 405, 492, 548, 579, 598, 619, 626, 659

Senn, Nicholas, 300

Servetus, Michael (Villanovanus), 73, 378

"Seuss, Dr." *See* Geisel, Theodor S.

Sévigné, Marie, Marquise de, 354

Shakespeare, William*

Shands, Harley C., 468, 473

Shao Tze, 450

Sharp, William ("Fiona Macleod"), 555

Sharpe, William, 174, 641

Shattuck, Lemuel, 450

Shaw, George Bernard, 31, 41, 69, 132, 167, 177, 206, 241, 245, 266, 280, 300, 309, 320, 350, 382, 415, 431, 458, 475, 520, 527, 555, 578, 606, 664

Shaw, Henry Wheeler ("Josh Billings"), 44, 177, 196, 230, 282, 291, 533, 581, 645

Shaw, Irwin, 557

Shelley, Percy Bysshe, 84, 252, 307, 347, 355, 429, 559, 649

Shenstone, William, 203

Sheppard, Eugenia, 430

Sheridan, Richard Brinsley, 92, 153, 668

Sherrington, Sir Charles, 20, 46, 140

Shippen, William, Jr., 166, 462, 573

Sidney, Sir Philip, 174, 552, 665

Sieffert, Aloysius, 465

Sigerist, Henry E., 49, 109, 184, 215, 221, 303, 337, 384, 445, 452, 476–477, 484, 506, 522, 562, 566, 614, 661, 664

Silius Italicus, 184

Simonides of Ceos, 201

Simpson, Sir James Young, 410–411

Sims, J. Marion, 17, 634

Singer, Sir Charles, 86, 521

Skelton, John, 31

Skoda, Josef, 633

Smellie, William, 316

Smith, Adam, 354, 517

Smith, Alexander, 90, 290

Smith, Homer W., 147, 253, 267, 287, 486, 507, 531, 612

Smith, Jackson A., 567–568

Smith, Joseph, 488

Y

Z

Index

Index

IN THIS ALPHABETICAL INDEX of key words, hyphenated words are indexed as one word. Singular possessives, plurals, and plural possessives of identical spelling are arranged in the following sequence:

> Medicine, ready money ready m., 134a
> useless because uncertain, 295a
> Medicine-men, no medicine only m., 397a
> Medicine's, heaven of m. immortals, 644b
> Medicines, need of new m., 220a
> Medicines' worthlessness, 639a

Archaic, dialect, and other variant spellings have for the most part been modernized; very familiar variants, however, appear in both modern and original forms. Modern British variants have been changed to the preferred American spellings.

Application, dealing in laboratories with a. of science, 506b
for benefit of human being, 222a
leisure useless without a., 663a
of scientific medicine, 299a
requisites for improving mind, 663a
Applications, assigning to a. cure of burns, 633a
joy when studies find practical a., 502a
of sciences human, 517a
science and a. of science, 519a
worn me out with a., 378a
Applied, no category of a. sciences, 519a
Apply it I don't know where, 496b
understand in order to a. not teach, 668a
Appointments weeks in advance, 371b
Appreciation of relative values of ideas, 234a
Apprehension, not avert danger of which no a., 229a
roll-tobacco took away a., 429a
Apprehensions to terrify objects of spleen, 191b
Apprehensive, becomes newly a., 230a
Apprentice not permitted advancement until tested, 576b
Apprentices, attended with train of a., 390b
Apprenticeship, advice by doctor with whom served a., 635b
life a. to truth, 463a
system not satisfactory, 577b
Approach, wits to find right a., 501b
Apricot, determined whether currant or a., 212a
April, gold embalms to A. day again, 651a
in A. refrain from horseradish, 188a
Aptitude, led to medicine through a., 382b
Aqua vitae, I have bought a., 6a
recovered with a., 122b
Arabian, diseases A. Nights' entertainment, 115b
dysentery of A. coast, 128a
Arbuthnot, Dr. John, 419b
removed from kind A.'s aid, 419b
Arcadias, utopias memories of A., 257a
Archetype, nature has a. in human imagination, 231a
Architect, point of view of a., 219b
unaware of engineering, 303b
Architects allow for bidet, 228a
Arctic loneliness of age, 347b
Arduous, no road to health a., 202a
Are, what you a. stands over you, 454a
Argue against new idea before completely stated, 234a
in theorizing a. on either side, 615a
Argument, heard great a., 277a
single fact worth shipload of a., 171a

Arguments for as well as against, 251b
physicians engage in heated a., 453a
Arise, lie down say when shall I a., 557b
Aristocracy of enlightened public opinion, 141b
Aristocratic, culture a. thing, 457b
Aristocratical, in circles a. scientific ideas in contempt, 520a
Aristotle discovered all half-truths, 256a
Galen and A. unanimous, 153a
Hunter in same rank as A., 422b
Latin quotations from A., 378a
more secrets discover'd than from A. to us, 516b
no matter what A. say, 621b
why quote A. in Greek, 62b
Arithmetic, knowledge and skill controlled by a., 299b
physician ought to know a., 399b
Arm, bloodletting not from a., 627a
can honour set an a., 594a
hand instrument at end of a., 199a
shrink a. like shrub, 70b
something the matter with this a., 354b
the a. our soldier, 15a
this a. of mine now prisoner to palsy, 357b
tied up with ribbon, 35b
wounded in shoulder and left a., 515b
young are a.-achy, 58a
Armchair medicine used in disparaging way, 304a
Armed with antiseptic chloroform and healing hands, 385b
Armies lose more by sickness than sword, 533a
Armpits, bad odor from mouth and a., 538a
Arms, breaks out of keeper's a., 180a
clasped about neck, 179b
face aslant upon a., 179b
legs and a. and heads chopp'd off, 81b
pains in a., 190b, 514a
severed by frost, 184a
swing a. about with weight in hand, 165b
take a. against sea of troubles, 580a
turn blue blood runs thin, 698a
Armstrong, Dr. P. M., 43a
Army, homesickness frequent disease in a., 217a
medical men detailed by A., 207a
plague signify standing a., 608b
professions for gentleman A., 459a
save a. by frugal means, 134b
travels on stomach, 131a
Arnold, as Matthew A. said of religion, 444b
Arnoldus Villanova, 419b
Around, lot of it going a., 99b
Arquebusade, clean teeth with a. water, 604b
Arrangements, surgeon destroy natural a., 596a

Arrested, man expects to be a., 346b
Arrogance, inhibit presumptuous a., 157b
Arrow, appearance of disease swift as a., 547b
Arrows, blunted a. of death, 298b
fame pierced with a. of malignancy, 328b
leech worth many for cutting a., 387a
poisoned a. of Iroquois, 185a
slings and a. of outrageous fortune, 580a
Arrowsmith, psychiatry in *A.* called plot against medicine, 385a
Ars longa vita brevis, 150b
Arsenic and Old Lace, 440b
Art, absence of a. absence of correctness, 150b
as a. surgery incomparable in medium, 596a
at times disease stronger than a., 236b
bears ideal of a., 490b
course of nature is a. of God, 316b
cultivate science and exercise a., 297b
delicate a. of handling ideas, 234a
distinguish between medical science and physician's a., 299b
exercises a. with caution, 400a
generosity possible to those who practise a., 389b
has three factors, 293a
him who taught A. equally dear as parents, 325b
human achievement in a., 290b
immeasurably too long, 380b
impart knowledge of A. to own sons, 325b
important part of a. of medicine, 272a
impressed on mind limits of a., 630b
in medical language opposed to Nature, 633b
in this a. of medicine consists, 293b
increment of power of hand, 524a
itself is nature, 158b
judge that benefits all matter of a., 626a
justified for sake of a., 596b
knows his a. not the trade, 419b
life short the a. long, 292b
long life short, 297a
lose health renders a. inglorious, 541b
love of man love of the a., 50a
luck no less than a. claim influence, 315a
many require of a. what a. can not bestow, 400b
mark of effort upon a., 333b
mean when lack control, 266a
medicine a. of probability, 300b
medicine both science and a., 303a
medicine for Hippocrates the a. of arts, 141a
medicine is a. has principles, 293b
medicine like all great a., 303b

Body, invigorator of b. is exercise, 165b
jump b. with dangerous physic, 122a
knows human b. as whole, 588b
knows properties of human b., 400a
less resistant to infection, 645a
life imprison'd in b. dead, 81b
light of b. is eye, 170a
like a bakery, 38b
like a ship, 38a
long as b. affected through mind, 171b
loves and desires of b., 293b
machine so complicated as human b., 631a
mad receipts into sick man's b., 400a
magazine of inventions, 37b
maintains steady heat, 607b
maketh man whole in b., 128b
man's b. from lower animal form, 161a
material in which artist works, 589b
meats that nourish man's b., 324b
medicine regards to b., 296a
medicine task powers of b. and mind, 457a
medicine unites laws which apply to b. and mind, 561a
melancholy not indisposition of b., 305b
members of b. rebelled, 570b
members of b. revolted against belly, 571a
members refused assistance to b., 571a
men of lean habit of b., 259b
microorganisms in b. of animals, 241a
milk causeth b. to waxe grosse, 102b
mind and b. are one, 41b
mind and b. develop in harmonious proportions, 166a
mind begotten with b., 39b
mind dependent on b., 40a
mind like b. healed, 311b
mind may affect b., 41a
mind with separate existence in b., 469a
money for health of soul now for health of b., 479b
monstrous multiplicity of individuals, 352b
more than if own b. at stake, 408a
more wisdom in b. than philosophy, 38a
most abhorrent b. without mind, 536a
most extremely compounded, 36b
moving in every part of b., 318b
must be separated from spirit, 91a
nature commands mind suffer with b., 243b
neither tamper with integrity of b., 570a
neither too stout nor lean, 36a
newborn child not realise b. part of self, 356b
no better in mind than b., 39b

Body, no counting names to parts of b., 609b
no riches above sound b., 207b
no spare parts for b., 38a
nonnatural things not parts of b., 279a
not all food for b., 6a
not carriage but omnibus, 38a
not ignorant of idiosyncrasy b. has, 201b
not merely cure b. but whole man, 387a
not permanent dwelling, 36a
not proven that b. only machine, 486a
not viewed as chemical laboratory, 485b
nourishment of other parts of b., 324b
observations of b. in health and disease, 334b
of Benjamin Franklin printer, 149a
of woman heart of king, 36b
old in b. but old in spirit never, 341b
once disease entered b., 111a
organs and tissues of b., 358b
pain of mind worse than of b., 314a
pain wastes b., 431a
pains in legs because carried b. so long, 513b
paper as b. of my friend, 665b
penance and fasting waste b., 173b
physic ministred to b., 472b
physic too strange for b., 121b
physician ruler having b. as subject, 362b
physician torments b., 456a
physician unacquainted with your b., 370b
physician who confines attention to b., 370b
physicians find diseases of b., 94b
physicians ignorant of parts of b., 405b
pictures depicted by mind on b., 181b
plan of human b., 14a
pleasures which b. enjoy, 431a
power of b. to resist disease, 413a
powers and actions of b., 6b
prettinesses of the b., 82b
psyche in union with b., 470a
psychology of individual sick in b., 367b
quest into mysteries of human b., 303b
remain healthy all life, 226b
repaired and supported, 39b
resurrection of healthy b. from diseased, 644b
secrets of structure of b., 92a
semen emitted to excess b. consumed, 538a
sick mind worse, 39b
sicker in b. and mind for present, 544a
sickly b. sickly mind, 42b
skin regarded as part of b., 550b
sleep not support my impoverished b., 551b
slow to grow quick to decay, 73a

Body, solids of our b., 45a
soul and b. have arts corresponding, 293b
soul oppressed so is b., 39b
soul subject to health and disease as b., 529a
sound b. product of sound mind, 41b
sound mind in sound b., 39b
spasm may carry off weakened b., 483a
strength of b., 40a
strength of mind greater than b., 39a
strong b. above wealth, 207b
strong b. makes mind strong, 40b
struggle between soul and b. gradual, 643b
study nature of b., 36a
syphilis broke out over whole b., 650a
system of tubes and glands, 37a
tetter bark'd about my smooth b., 438b
think another twenty years left in b., 337b
tobacco not for b., 488b
tobacco ruine of b. and soul, 621b
torments in effect on b., 431a
transform food into elements of b., 555b
treat soul as well as b., 635b
tune harp of man's b., 295a
ulcer at vital parts of b., 645b
uneasy sensations anywhere in b., 204b
uninformed mind with healthy b., 40b
unless b. defective from creation, 226b
watch designed to go given time, 631b
water cause of windinesse in b., 654a
water post-hast through sick b., 647b
well in b. sick in mind, 39b
what concerns b. and health, 488a
what food best for b., 100a
what may be wrought upon b. of man, 497b
will be lightsome, 130b
will master of b., 41a
winds own springs, 37b
wine reduces firmness of b., 5b
with what b. nourished, 106a
without sickness b. and soul part, 342b
without superfluous flesh on b., 424a
woman without man b. without head, 541b
wound of b. like sensitive plant, 588b
wrong operation on b. of patient, 405a
you who restore health to b., 378a
Body snatcher robber of worms, 42b
Body's, end of physicke is b. health, 378a
members rebell'd against belly, 571a

Conduct, in London professional c. so nice, 454b

no power to compel necessary c., 409a

obliquity of c. not actual crime, 380a

one rule of professional c., 456b

progress based on integrity in professional c., 215b

regulate c. at outset of career, 401a

rule of c. "More light," 68a

Confessed, if Nihilist I should have c. all, 259a

Confession, psychoanalysis c. without absolution, 467b

suicide is c., 581a

Confessional, doctor's office c., 367a

Confessor, deceive not c., 460a

Confidence and hope more good than physic, 217b

breach of c. of eminent physicians, 241b

cannot have c. in doctors, 395a

change in c. of friends, 415b

conferred by endowment, 510b

men have c. to intrust selves to physician, 460a

people will have c. in him, 134b

required in patient c., 373a

restore c. to patient, 404b

roots of character in public c., 365a

shorn of c. of professional brethren, 63a

useful in emergency, 222a

winning patients' c., 366a

Confined, patients not too c. unto beds, 249a

person does enjoy any sort of outing, 350b

Confirm, advice sought to c. position, 331a

Conflagration, shun presence as c., 405a

Conflict between desire and desire, 13a

broadest range to c. of medical views, 321b

life c. with evil, 265b

pain resultant of c., 356b

Conflicts, analysis not only way to resolve c., 468a

psychic health not absence of c., 470b

Conformity of technique of language, 507a

Confused, keep c. until right answer forces solution, 529a

Confusion as to meaning of pulse, 94b

greater c. in compound medicine, 121b

in vulgar mind, 255a

lucidity in ideas in same c. as own, 671a

make think c. own fault, 566b

perfection of means c. of goals, 333a

Congenital weak-mindedness, 158b

Congress, program for consideration of C., 221a

Congresses, talks worst in International C., 304b

Congressional, warrant prompt c. action, 246b

Congressional Record, rather read *C.* than see bishop hanged, 333a

Conjectural, medicine c. art, 294a, 297a

war like medicine c., 456a

Conjecture, existence of atoms c., 231b

fail experience as well, 294a

no correct idea from c., 136a

praise of sound c., 640a

sober c. as well as certainty, 632b

Conjectures, medicine supported by mere c., 295a

out of trifling investment of fact, 520a

Conjuror, man ideot before pretend to be c., 395a

Connection, experiment discovers c. between phenomena, 503a

Conquering, idea of c. nation, 458a

so sharp the c., 294b

Conscience always inestimable, 401a

born of custom, 64b

defiance to c., 61b

digestion depends upon good c., 107a

disease of evil c., 64b

fear of getting caught, 664b

hint impiety of warfare against Providence, 394a

important in physician, 590a

is cancer that eats self, 64b

keen c. on part of surgeon, 590a

my c. is clear, 324a

not c. diseased, 64b

quiet compunctions of c., 370b

science without c. death of soul, 516a

senses have advantage over c., 537a

surgeon answerable to c., 586b

surgeons of c., 591b

those who take up burdens without c., 587b

time in c. he should die, 338a

value health next to c., 203a

with good c. work in surgery, 594a

Consciences, when alumni have c. pricked pockets picked, 292b

Conscientious, physician generally c., 388b

physicians allocate causes, 48b

then really c. man, 664b

Conscious, makes us c. of our being, 264a

memory dies with death, 172b

mind as organ of c. thought, 366b

rays of sense focus in c. pattern, 287b

thinking primer for brain, 109b

Consciousness, ebb and flow on shore of c., 537b

forces not recognize personal c., 366b

if c. in Nature, 317a

pain ushers us into c., 355a

symbols in c., 41b

without c. every muscle in action, 534b

yawning warns of reduction in c., 674a

Consecutive, error that things c. have cause and effect, 276b

Consensus, denying entry into scientific c., 154b

Consent, advice and c. of such as are skillful, 157b

Consequences, hint act may entail c., 641a

rules absolute c. variable, 294a

science knowledge of c., 516a

Conservative functions of kidneys, 253a

healthy stomach c., 107a

jealousy of rank due profession, 457a

neglect of kidney's c. services, 253b

Consolation, thought of suicide c., 581b

Consonants, language abound in c., 59b

Constipated, he whose intestines c., 65a

heal intestines slightly c., 65a

mind grows c. as grows old, 344b

Constituents, actions between ultimate c. of matter, 316b

Constitution, attends to c. of patient, 293b

causes independent of c., 115a

diagnosis include c. of patient, 96a

doctor understand c. and health, 627a

doctor who knows her c., 360b

error not attributed to c. of patient, 593b

for amending dry c., 102b

gets well or if c. fails dies, 625b

herbs for c. of man, 488b

how much of c. from progenitor, 212a

ignorance of c. of matter, 231b

injure c. without result, 499b

investigate malady habits c., 626a

know of own c., 65b

laws of life developed by c., 450b

length of life not so much good c., 279a

liquors pernicious to c., 8a

mastery through natural c., 236b

more stress upon man's c., 182a

no more experiments with c. as yours, 630a

of mind capable of growth, 260a

over which no initial control, 212a

people of same c. same illness, 391a

reconcile hostile elements in c., 293b

some defend c. some destroy it, 459b

strength of Marquesans' c., 554b

such men possess vigorous c., 189b

survived illness and remedy, 36a

tinkering with human c. four thousand years, 495a

unwilling to allow c. breaking, 346a

Constitutional, neglect c. factor in neuroses, 319a

remained alive on account of c. slowness, 461a

Credit, originator gets most c. if idea correct, 233a
others get c. for enterprises they initiated, 502b
physician get more c. than entitled to, 380a
preferring regard for me before c., 419b
suffers reward same, 393b
to man who convinces world, 502b
when maladies end happily, 392b
when recover doctor gets c., 382b
Credulity, course of mind from c. to scepticism, 549a
doctors infect with c., 394b
doctors work on c. of patient, 370a
homeopathy mass of imbecile c., 71b
mind rising above c., 136a
of men is such, 479a
relating to disease, 115b
Credulous hope market for proprietary remedies, 321b
not so c. of cure, 74a
Creed, found c. in biliary duct, 490a
mute obedience to outworn c., 464a
science suicide when adopts c., 519b
Creep cry out for thee, 408a
little bug c. behind you some day, 308a
Cressid, lazar kite of C.'s kind, 650b
Cries, as if c. of pain cause no emotion, 582c
Crime, absolves guilty of responsibility for c., 330a
best country has fewest laws c., 474a
insanity during c. required irrational behaviour, 245a
needless ignorance a c., 463a
obliquity of conduct not actual c., 380a
Crimean, since C. war nurses into novels, 322b
Crimes, authority on c. connected with poisons, 419b
subdivisions of illnesses into c. and misdemeanours, 545a
typhus fever one of worst c., 645b
Criminal, challenge to ideas of c. responsibility, 470b
expose newborn to infection c., 53a
illness in Erewhon c., 545a
more easily appeale than from c. decree, 460b
nearer person killed greater c., 579b
Cripple does not irritate us, 244a
Earth has more need of c., 191a
recognizes we go straight, 244b
restore c. to legs, 70b
sciatica c. senators, 515b
Crippled, majority of children c. can be restored, 489b
mind irritate us, 244a
spirit says we limp, 244b
Crippling, war against c., 489b

Crises, hygienic law supersedes rights in c., 228a
vague terms as c., 610a
Crisis, bring distemper to c. and cure, 370b
Critical, astringent tonic of c. writing, 671a
but beware lest ideas rejected, 251b
doctrines repay c. examination, 256b
method dominate teaching, 504a
people usually c. of hypothesis, 233a
Criticising, when c. may discourage him, 233a
Criticism, be sparing of c., 69a
creation and c. equal, 68b
dead in fields not advancing, 68b
desire c. on contributions, 68a
discovery tacit c., 109a
education constantly under c., 142b
homeopathy c. on medical practice, 71b
ignorant c. doubts on principle, 68a
of sources of cognition important, 214a
people ask c. want praise, 332b
submits paper for publication without c., 672b
work which excites c., 68b
Criticisms, gained from c. of adversary, 670a
Crito I owe cock to Aesculapius, 257a
Croaking, sit c. idly by stream, 266a
Crocodile, longevity of c., 280a
same if lived three hundred years of c., 340a
Crocus, mummy preferred to c., 280b
Crookback, valiant c. prodigy, 70b
Crooked, if thou wert c., 70b
two midwives baby's head c., 310b
were I c., 345a
Crookedness effect of cloths that pinch, 227a
Crops, life like c. harvested, 284a
Cross, house marked with red c., 429a
over river and rest under trees, 259a
Crossgrafting, what follow solution of c. mystery, 624b
Crotchets, hypothetical c. in brain, 232a
Croup, careful not to get c., 53a
child suffocating with c., 411b
Crow, die like c. with king birds, 457a
Crowd device for temporary insanity, 470a
individual one of active c., 469b
physician not rush with c., 413b
Crowds keep one another in countenance, 329a
Crown, iron of c. more valuable than gold, 167a
Jack fell down broke c., 496b
of experience like c. of Lombardy, 167a
true heir to th' English c., 447b
Crucible, cannot test faith in c., 172a

Crucible, chemist putting entire animal in c., 502b
Crudity, know how to manage a c., 134b
Cruel, canst not c. prove, 281b
subconscious self c., 469b
Cruelty, death hath drawn together c., 77b
deprive of death merely c., 581b
that anye in nede of comforte forsaken, 344a
Crusade, problem demands c., 489a
Crusoe, like dissipated Robinson C., 574a
Crust, ulcer over which pulverised c., 645b
Crusts, investigator may live on c., 504a
Crutches are forgot, 193a
seaman offer self upon c., 191a
Cry and go that is death, 271b
come and c. that is life, 271b
first c. of pain call for physician, 303a
infants not c. without cause, 55b
mankind's eternal c. for release, 367a
not to be born, 29b
symptoms c. from suffering organs, 599b
those that c. by night, 54a
Crying, goes out c., 57a
went on c. with satisfaction, 57a
Crystal, older personality like c., 349b
Crystals, uric acid c. spin, 198a
Cubas, emitted odour of C., 574a
Cubs, bears lick c. into shape, 523a
Cucumber I've eat and can't digest, 239b
Cuds, youth prepare savory c., 339a
Cullen, disciples of C., 613b
Culprit, increasing understanding of c., 470b
Cult accepts ruthless egotism, 330a
Cultist, leave reassurance to c., 230b
Cultivation, study like c. of fields, 134b
what potency has c. of illness, 187a
Cultural, plead for more c. side in medicine, 331b
potential of physicians below average, 672b
Culture aristocratic thing, 457b
general c. of mind best aid, 137a
in no profession c. count so much as medicine, 184b
phallic fallacies of import to c., 541a
science not more obvious for lack of literary c., 395b
Cunning, diseases affecting c. man, 236a
to restore cripple, 70b
Cup, before handing c. of knowledge to young, 603b
life's c. sparkles near brim, 347a
thirst not justify draining c., 100b
Cupid cast away quiver, 541a

Cupped, scarified and c. him, 635b

Cups that cheer not inebriate, 600a

Curable, appearing in c. form at outset, 236b
deafness c. and not c., 76b
patient with c. disease, 372a
presume disease c., 114a
what is less c. seventy-five, 346a

Curative, barriers between preventive and c. medicine, 452b
cease to regard function as c., 185b
consider not poison but its c. virtue, 438a
doctor's work more educational less c., 452a
in c. particular thinking physician has advantage, 379a
statements as to c. properties falsehoods, 321b

Cure, accede to requests if not interfere with c., 583a
all feel ill shun c., 542b
amuses patients while Nature effects c., 400a
anthology for prevention as c., 473b
as much business of physician as to c. diseases, 408a
assigning to applications c. of burns, 633a
assisting c. of wounds by permitting scab, 666a
at expense of life, 627b
at loss in c. of patient, 135a
bad physicians themselves cannot c., 414b
bath against maladies sovereign c., 224b
be eternized for wondrous c., 378a
before c. one kill ten, 398a
best c. upon own purse, 176a
better have recourse to quack if can c., 480b
bring distemper to crisis and c., 370b
broken senses stand in hard c., 552b
by tried methods, 157a
carpenter ill asks for ready c., 625b
contributed all in power towards c., 371a
death c. of all diseases, 88a
desperate c. for desperate ills, 75a
die of diseases they profess to c., 382b
difficult to c. easy to kill, 633b
disease kill patient, 370b
disorder called fever set of remedies to c. it, 480a
doctor doing best to c., 366a
doctor effects trumpery c., 578a
doctors not c. own complaints, 414b
doctors prescribe no c., 98b
effected avarice sets in, 179a
evil by lesser evil, 634b
faces ask can we not c., 283b
false promises of c., 370a
first water c. the Flood, 225a
for being miserable occupation, 664a
for everything but stark dead, 93b

Cure, for extreme diseases extreme c., 72b
for one disorder doctors c. produce dozen, 472a
for poor worketh c. in night, 630b
forbear advice not necessary to promote c., 364b
four things needful to c., 73b
frequent change of medicine hinders c., 73a
give ill he cannot c. a name, 238a
good leech himself can c., 399b
have no patients to c., 494b
her of that, 243b
herbs and rootes to c. thee, 387b
how effectual fruits in c. of scurvy, 532b, 653b
if c. elephant could c. anything, 75a
if kill or c. please c., 447a
if not c. quickly kill, 392a
if ye will c., 15a
impossible duty to lighten affliction, 238a
in minds of sick what was that performed, 653b
investigate man he wishes to c., 626a
is too easy price too dear, 176b
know cause before he can c., 48b
know how to effect c. no less than to be physician, 626a
knowledge by which c. diseases, 586a
learn by experience method of c., 230b
life ill whose c. death, 260b
manage c. best who foreseen what to happen, 460a
means care of sick, 367a
mission to c. incurable diseases, 481a
more important to c. than diagnose, 97a
more slowly than disease, 73a
mortal to cut off to c. easy, 628b
must answer to disease, 74a
nature often helped c., 638a
never forgive guarantee of c. that failed, 461b
never say c. due to medicine, 593b
new methods of c. work miracles for while, 630a
no c. discovered for epilepsy, 534b
no c. for birth and death, 30a
no c. for lucre only, 584b
no c. for this disease, 238a
no herb will c. death, 93b
no hope of c. one saves medicine, 238b
not always in physician's power to c., 236b
not c. unless caste in other syckeness, 406a
not cut off but c., 585b
not like to c. trouble by trouble, 627b
not merely c. body but whole man, 387a

Cure, not promise to c. physician, 460b
not prostitute past-c. malady to empirics, 237a
not same to feel and c. disease, 110b
not so credulous of c., 74a
not take much pains to c. disease, 229a
not worth pain, 72b
nursing chief in c. of disease, 662a
of disease more grievous than endurance, 447a
of gout depends upon two things, 194a
of many diseases unknown, 39a
old age disease we cannot c., 344a
only c. for seasickness, 533a
only things for which man not found c., 238a
part of c. to wish health, 373a
part of c. to wish to be cured, 73a
past c. past care, 237a
past c. still past care, 237b
patience c. of incurable, 359b
patient believes in c., 172a
patients I failed to c., 152a
patients when want c., 176a
perceive c. too grate for thee, 65b
perform something extraordinary like c. gout, 189a
physic more harm than evils it professes to c., 394b
physician dies of disease he claimed to c., 386a
physician thought good for c., 370b
physicians kill more than c., 393b
plying means of c., 50b
presence of doctor beginning of c., 639a
prevention better than c., 452b
prevention better than c. also cheaper, 452a
psychoanalysis disease it purports to c., 467b
purse of patient protracts c., 179a
radical c. for gout, 190a
rather c. patient and lose fee, 401b
removing teeth c. belief that c. everything, 605a
ridiculous that one undertake to c. another, 393a
science madness if good sense not c., 523a
second office c. of diseases, 278b
shall win thee wealth, 196a
sick man with c. up sleeve, 73b
sickness almost past c., 111a
sometimes relieve often comfort always, 410a
spend many times amount to c., 452b
sure c. for complaints, 495b
Sydenham humanely preoccupied with c., 528a
teaching men c. of all diseases, 418b
think more of doctors if they c. cold, 61b
three parts of c. without surgeon's power, 73b

Customs, obsessed with sex and romance in c., 540b
Cut, any fool can c. off leg, 587b
 burn torture every part, 281b
 disease that must be c. away, 628b
 diseased part, 17a
 eyes like calf that had throat c., 258a
 finger make bold with cobweb, 493b
 foot c. off for sake of body, 284a
 good surgeon medical man who can c., 590a
 have sore eye c. off hand, 639a
 have toothache c. off tongue, 639a
 I am c. to th' brains, 585a
 if surgeon tell him leg must be c. off, 585b
 incurable c. off the rest reforme, 594a
 many c. out of womb, 54b
 mortal to c. off to cure easy, 628b
 not c. off but cure, 585b
 not moved by cries to c. less, 582b
 not slightest pain although c., 187b
 off to c. cure-lesse limbe, 585a
 two years since c. for stone, 646b
Cuts, in good hand every sword c. well, 598a
Cutting, give surgeon pecuniary interest in c. off leg, 177b
 leech worth many for c. arrows, 387a
 like babe c. teeth, 193b
 use prescription without c. out something, 453a
Cymbal, charity like tinkling c., 50b
Cynic, touch of c. gives physician authority, 379b
Cynical, felt c. but hopeful, 275a
Cynics among philosophers, 67b
Cyrano de Cognac nose, 321a
Cystic, surgeons to give me c. examination, 240b
Cystoscope, instruction on use of c., 648b
Czech, every C. musician, 386b

D

Da Costa, Jacob M., 273b
Daily, how d. life is, 266a
 moral world of sick-bed explains d., 66oa
Dainty, hunger not d., 224a
 to be sick if leisure for it, 544a
Daisies, feel d. growing over me, 259a
Damned, better d. than not nam'd, 172b
 go earn d. guinea, 176b
Damocles, gout hangs like sword of D., 194b
Damp, course along d. walks, 474a
 like old man's mouth, 349a
Dampness of the atmosphere, 12a
Damsel, if man come near d., 1a

Damsel, what chance hath d. at pink tea, 324a
Dance, wench could sing and d., 305b
Danger, adore on brink of d., 370a
 agreed as to d. of innovations, 462a
 fixed person in future public d., 463b
 forego customary employment may be d., 512b
 free from disease's d. and thee, 176a
 greater d. bolder treatment, 632a
 hatch and disclose be some d., 243a
 hypostasis make your d. great, 647a
 in no fraud greater d., 391b
 in rewards of success, 578b
 industry created new sources of d., 337a
 like ague taints, 181a
 more d. in steamboat or railroad, 83b
 more d. of rusting than wearing out, 340a
 never operation without d., 350b
 not avert d. of which no apprehension, 229a
 not dangerous operations until lessening d., 583a
 on side of not retiring soon enough, 512a
 past same dull life, 271b
 sick greatest d. for healthy, 545b
 so much knowledge as to be out of d., 255b
 spice of d., 301b
 that we will do nothing, 262b
 what effect telling him he in d., 370b
Dangerous age, 309b
 ailments more annoying than d., 535a
 committees d. things, 505b
 if little knowledge d., 255b
 immoral to experiment on man when d., 168a
 in medicine to be too clever, 407b
 little trained nurse d. thing, 324b
 most d. physicians, 407a
 most d. thing to go to bed, 83b
 nowhere untruth more d., 377b
 pitiful surgeon makes d. sore, 585b
 such men are d., 259b
 thinking without learning d., 260a, 617a
 thirty-eighth year d., 308b
 to be sentenced by physician as judge, 460b
 to take a cold, 61a
 waiting for practice d., 409b
 when d. to apply remedies, 494a
 when men d. disease did 'scape, 176a
 wound of malice break out more d., 665b
 wound that bleedeth inward most d., 665a

Dangers, exaggerate real d., 94b
 happy man whom d. make cautious, 158a
 physicians acquire knowledge from our d., 390b
 possession threaten present d., 342b
 relative d. of treatment, 383a
Dark amid blaze of noon, 32a
 fear death as children in d., 90b
 great leap in d., 257b
 necessity of dealing blow in d., 633b
 not suffered me to die in d. Tower, 257b
 spirit of death so d., 89b
 spots float before eyes, 199b
Darkness, better light candle than drink beer in d., 334a
 death shrouded in d., 86a
 land of d., 80a
 restful and agreeable, 169a
Darrow, Clarence, 55a
Dart, with one stroke of d., 90b
Darwin as much emancipator as Lincoln, 162a
 Charles D. Abraham of scientific men, 421a
 impelled by appetite for discovery, 425a
Darwinian fitness mutual relationship, 163a
 Man only monkey shaved, 161b
 theory support to spiritual nature, 161a
Data, brain analyse incredible number of d., 143b
 check d. of confreres and instructors, 577a
 desert of d. with oases of prose, 672b
 entities based on inferences from observed d., 471a
 fail as conveyances for d., 614b
 no programming make salad of garbage when d. processed, 509b
 not mousetrapped by tangential d., 99a
 outlaw d. from other schools, 466b
 publication of d. exclude ideas, 483a, 522b
 skeptical toward d. of profession, 402b
 theories founded on uncertain d., 450b
 work containing insufficient d., 664a
Date, lengthen life beyond appointed d., 281a
Daughter and a goodly babe, 449a
 as mother so d., 213a
 behold d. I have parted from appendix, 324a
 died like Duke-and-Duchess's d., 581a
 Jukes fifty-four when married d., 310a
 of Bacchus and Aphrodite gout, 186b
 of widowed patient, 656b
 petticoat enrobed most dutiful d., 662a
Daughters, healthy sons with healthy d. pair, 211a

David died in good old age, 281a
King D.'s blood dull in motion, 632b
like D. good things indite, 668b
span of life same as when D. played before Saul, 343b
Davis, inscription on statue of W. E. B. D., 421a
Day, as morning shews d., 56a
each d. a life, 559a
every d. in every way better, 473a
give me health and a d., 205a
I have had d., 434b
incidents which most occupied thoughts during d., 117b
insurmountable d. mare, 61a
life in d.-tight compartments, 266a
life like winter's d., 150a
life sultry d., 270a
much sleep not medicinal in d., 552a
not sleep during d., 552a
others have dimmer sight in d., 548a
ready to answer alarm d. and night, 403a
riseth late trot all d., 128b
what dwelt on by d., 118a
Daybreak, begin day from d., 129a
Daydreams, night dreams wish-fulfillment as d., 119b
Daylight, not waste d. listening, 484a
rising before d. recommended, 128b
Days, few golden d. spend with you, 340b
grow short when reach September, 340b
hours are like d., 181a
hurried away from unamusing d., 346b
my salad d., 2b
of childhood d. of woe, 56a
of years threescore and ten, 349a
travel toward death, 81a
Dazzle, their ideal of surgery to d., 589b
DDT more toward eradication of malariologists, 283b
Dead, all d. before them, 345b
are hopeless, 217a
as a doornail, 77b
as a herring, 78b
as living to us as living, 271a
assumes temperature of atmosphere, 607b
atoms return to earth when he d., 384a
await medical student, 42b
before man wise half d., 345b
being d. raise to life, 378a
better d. than suffer wrong affliction, 637b
bodies when d. lie quietly, 78b
book of ye d., 149a
break jests on d., 587a
carts began to go about, 429b
cure for everything but stark d., 93b
discover me fifteen years after d., 173a
doctor enters d. man leaves, 395a
doubt whether person d., 95a

Dead, dread to die but not being d., 80b
early to bed wish you were d., 129a
Egyptian had nine hours lien d., 74a
examination of d., 499a
examination of d. source of knowledge, 136a
fault of fellow who's d., 393a
fetch one to life that was d., 74b
grievest for d., 29a
hand of medical tradition, 153b
Henry's wounds open congeal'd mouths, 665b
how many physicians d., 77b
invaluable when alive forgotten after d., 401a
is d. mule in yard, 623a
is for long time, 80b
leaves d. are driven, 429b
life imprison'd in body d., 81b
life-weary taker fall d. violently, 439b
living distinguished from d. by changes, 265a
maid not d. but sleepeth, 559b
male healthy wealthy and d., 129a
man haven for d., 28a
man not born until d., 29b
man's as good as d., 66b
Marley was d. as doornail, 79a
master d. ere you return, 237b
medical literature and live, 272b
medicine sailed by d. reckoning, 146a
men's fingers call them, 183a
Nell d. of malady of France, 650b
no longer young already d., 340b
no medicine for life when man d., 77a
not be forgotten soon as d., 668a
not deserve to be called d. because inorganic, 266b
now with multitude of d., 148b
one that's d. is quick, 447b
preference for d. or live patient, 466b
relatives of d. man, 42b
reputation on foundation of d. bodies, 382b
rest is for d., 511a
say I'm sick I'm d., 174a
she feels young one kick, 447b
sick dying and d. crammed together, 218b
tired of having people say thought you were d., 417a
twenty years been d. and buried, 79a
Tyrawley and I d. two years, 338b
unable to understand that alive, 271a
useless to physic d., 341a
vertigo never leave till d., 535b
we are the d., 436a
we become lumber, 78b
well at night d. in morning, 150a
what matter if make d. walk, 394b
woke up d., 87a

Dead, you're a lang time d., 271b
Deadlier, hurt inside of d. sort, 666a
Deadly, give no d. medicine to any one, 325b
sleep does good is not d., 551b
though slow d., 438a
Deadness, total d. and distaste, 61a
Deaf, advantages that are d. man's, 76b
always hear better, 77a
as a doore, 76a
dumb and d. as post, 75b
ears more d. than adders, 76a
giddy helpless, 76a
husband blind wife happy, 288b
live in world divorced from sound, 76b
men distrustful, 77a
nearly blind totally d., 347a
rendered all he taught less d., 602a
scientists d. to argument that not fit, 532a
shalt not curse d., 33a
speak louder for I am d., 76a
tenant in own body, 201b
to all those motives, 285b
why for d. irritable bind, 33a, 76b
Deafens, too much sound d., 536b
Deafness, apoplexy kind of d., 572a
it is a kind of d., 76a
none complaining of d., 76b
two kinds of d., 76b
Dean, see how D. begins to break, 535b
Dear as ruddy drops that visit heart, 58b
man to all country d., 418a
want to be d. old lady, 340b
Dearth, disease and d. sweep superfluous from earth, 441a
Death, absence and d. the same, 78b
advertizes doctor, 578a
affair of being more frightened than hurt, 271a
afflictions to which d. about to put end, 342b
after d. joy and pleasure none, 432a
after d. the doctor, 80b
after life greatly please, 552b
against d. no medicine, 91b
against d. no remedy, 93b
all that makes d. hideous show, 84b
all there is in life, 270b
all things swallowed in d., 91a
analysis unappetizing as d., 467a
Angel of D. behind physician, 397b
Angel of D. throughout land, 79a
any man's d. diminishes me, 78a
apoplexies light troops of d., 668a
ashamed besides d. diseases incurable, 363b
at last not unwelcome, 343b
aught seen but ghastly views of d., 429b

Dislike, inveterate d. of interruption, 339a
save me from doing anything I d., 193b
Dislocated, man has d. shoulder, 376b
Dislocation, pain like that of d., 189b
Disorder, better a quack if can cure d., 480b
by heating of blood, 112a
called fever set of remedies to cure it, 480a
catches any d. tried before jury, 545a
chronic d. places among majority, 320a
conceptual d. by no means always bad, 528b
correlate symptoms with overall mental d., 468a
doctor intuitively divining d., 401b
for one d. doctors cure produce dozen, 472a
has thousand prescriptions not single remedy, 495a
her last d. mortal, 83a
little things of functional d., 115a
medicine triumphs in palliating d., 638b
never same in two patients, 26a
scarcely d. incident to humanity, 321a
why this d., 404b
Disordered understanding with quiet pulse, 244b
Disorders, anthology medicine for mental d., 473b
classes of d. which springs relieve, 225a
in disease normal, 427b
of animal body, 113a
offspring stigmatized by heredital d., 212b
province to remove d., 371a
separates d. of chest from d. of bowels, 99b
tinkering four thousand years to cure d., 495a
uprooted several contagious d., 329a
wisdom to recognize d., 446a
Disparagingly, talk d. of best things, 329b
Dispatch, physicians give quick d., 377a
Dispensary, The D. by Samuel Garth, 50b
Dispersal, catalytic d. called death, 287a
Disperse, meetings of Trustees disburse and d., 510b
Displaced, restore things d., 594a
Disposition, natural d. like soil, 134a
of this disease from parents to children, 189a
possessed of natural d., 134a
surgeon have temperate d., 583b
Dispositions, possess virtues and d., 210b
secret d. of men revealed, 467b
Disproportion in every part, 70b
Disputations, not d. before those who not know medicine, 583a

Dispute, like doctors when d. past, 67b
no scientific d. with respect to faith, 171b
Disputes, dividing efforts by personal d., 454a
Dissect, butcher can d. joint well, 26a
the dead, 15b
through creatures you d., 15b
Dissected, body d. by fiendish men, 42b
friend died I d. him, 25a
no man marry until d. woman, 288b
those who d. learn'd to doubt, 15b
Dissecting, discussing cadaver while d., 332b
girls and men enter d. room together, 661b
influences of d. room and laboratory, 566a
Dissection, Galen leader of professors of d., 14b
repugnance to d., 14a
statistical analysis delicate d., 56gb
Dissections, beasts and birds for d., 497b
no discovery by d., 20a
of those died of consumptions, 642a
Dissector, could d. have revealed power, 485b
Dissembling, clever at d., 69b
Dissipate, afflicted are those who d., 248b
Dissipated, sleep of d. profound as of innocence, 554b
Dissipation, accompanying d. of motion, 161a
in d. little dreams of gout, 194b
lead life of d., 236b
of ill-directed industry, 270a
Dissolute indulgence of appetites, 190b
of such d. habits, 190a
Dissolution, anguish not often in d., 84a
death by natural d., 278b
has begun, 318a
Dissymmetry of natural products, 27b
Distance, doctor from d. blind eye, 408a
holding page to see clearly bothered by d., 548b
too great d. hinders views, 536b
Distemper, body easy to d., 36b
bring d. to crisis and cure, 370b
epidemical d. l'influenza, 241b
of no d. he dy'd, 279a
often fatal, 560a
rich foods source of d., 195a
soon sink under d., 642a
they dug pits when d. spread, 429b
too beneficial to doctors, 648b
Distempered, as body yet d., 628b
Distempers, alone capable of curing d., 398a
God visited people with d., 371a
have fashion on their side, 192a
in blood never security, 192a
man hold in abeyance these foul d., 424b
must be propagated, 5a

Distempers, one d. within other blisters without, 585b
secret of curing all d., 629b
topic forbidden to well-bred mortals their d., 544a
Distended stomach swill barrel, 132a
vomiting from d. stomachs, 659a
Distinction between us and other animals, 288a
Distinguish diseases from one another, 96a
Distinguished think rules for young, 156b
Distortions, making d. with gout not unpleasant, 355a
Distracted, sight mortifying as d. person, 244b
without risk of being d., 250b
Distraction, gout hardly tolerates d., 196b
Distress, feel d. at futile struggle, 411b
in spite of dire d., 223b
leave prolonging thy d., 81b
lunacy refuge of weak nature against d., 246a
Distressed, patience sanctuary to d., 359b
Distresses, I take pleasure in d., 431b
Distributions, favorable d. in this world, 222b
without which body not subsist, 165a
Distrust, intolerance conceived in d., 331a
laboratory in which d., 454a
not for awing human mind to d. own vision, 517a
seek simplicity and d. it, 550a
Distrustful, deaf men d., 77a
Disturbances in healthy body, 115b
knowledge of internal d., 94b
remedy for d. let them run course, 493b
Disturbed, in d. mind as body sanity not, 242a
Disuse, iron rusts from d., 234a
use strengthens d. debilitates, 489a
Diswench, stones extraordinarily d. me, 646b
Diuretic, bread operated as d., 653b
Diver poised in albumen, 179b
Diversity, science discovery of identity amidst d., 520a
Dividing efforts by personal disputes, 454a
Divine, against self-slaughter prohibition d., 579b
diagnosis of things human and d., 376b
doctor's life d. vocation, 382a
eat is human digest d., 107a
guides human discourse to d., 169a
life expression of d. vital spirit, 653a
medicine not lucrative d., 296b
more needs d. than physician, 243b
nurse given d. touch, 323a
regard suicide breaks d. law, 582a
secrets just as inexplicable, 161a

Doctor, wonder where is d., 368a
work eighteen hours seven days a week, 409b
work without having to talk, 459a
worth many another man, 389a
writes prescriptions till patient dies or cured, 394a
young country d. anxious over chance, 282a
young d. receives new courage, 631a
Doctoral cap upon my head, 326a
Doctoring is like logic, 278a
killed all by d. them, 181a
unwise when represent d. as art or science, 277b
Doctor's, always read d. bill niver purscription, 449a
anatomical poem on d. wife, 658b
ape wears d. cape, 163b
apothecaries taught to play d. part, 121a
apples every day takes d. bread away, 452b
being d. wife occupational hazard, 658a
brow crowned with camomile, 124a
character should be square, 404b
chief end of d. existence, 408b
children more chances of being failures, 658a
error will of God, 153a
errors covered with earth, 153a
expects d. wife set good example, 657b
fatigue d. greatest enemy, 657b
ill jesting with joiner's tools worse with d., 534b
intemperance is d. wet-nurse, 248b
life divine vocation, 382a
office confessional, 367a
offices admirable in dwelling of poor, 388b
patient longs for d. visit, 366a
patients perplexed, 66a
prone to spite d. mission, 371a
qualified to pass examinations for d. degree, 573a
role as orderer, 350a
slam door on d. nose, 227a
some out-liv'd d. pill, 122b
task to undiagnose, 99a
work more educational less curative, 452a
Doctors, acquire wealth to give to d., 175b
advertising d. possessed with antidote, 321a
advise one another, 175b
agreed he ought to die, 461a
always changing opinions, 396b
always trusting folk, 153b
American d. in war experience, 310b
amongst finest men, 389b
antipathy for d. hereditary, 278b
are frightful race, 396b
are our friends, 392b
believe in sorcerers instead of d., 236b
best d. sign most death certificates, 407b
best of d. go to hell, 397a

Doctors best-natured except when fighting, 454a
better appreciated, 277b
bug-d. write upon bed-disorders, 668b
bungling d., 152a
call three d. and play bridge, 62a
called to be d. when not yet babies, 382a
cannot do without d., 395a
city whose d. have gouty feet, 198b
clinicians in danger of becoming poor d., 60b
come in ails delighting, 131a
confuse color with chemistry, 104b
consult d. about children, 52b
consult patient dies, 67a
death terminus d. stokers, 271b
die of diseases they profess to cure, 382b
differ, 453b
dignity in dying d. should not deny, 87a
dismiss your d., 394b
do good without prospect of reward, 388b
don't see enough, 335a
dreamed about d. and bills, 411a
each generation of d. upon shoulders of predecessors, 464b
eat melon, 102a
either good or bad, 385a
endless train of d. on march, 384b
evils from d. and imagination, 229b
exposed to attacks, 20b
exposed to contempt of gifted amateur, 383a
families of d. take little medicine, 124a
felt as d. about medicines, 275a
felt her all over, 289b
first last and all the time, 60b
folks want d. mouldy, 416a
for one disorder d. cure produce dozen, 472a
found her last disorder mortal, 83a
gave them physic they died, 638b
generally dull dogs, 396a
get away with low standard of composition, 673a
give what they would take, 457a
good d. rather cure patient lose fee, 401b
got education off dirt pavements, 142b
greatest deceivers d., 370b
had more Christianity, 72a, 323a
half under d. half to Nature, 391a
have failed, 112b
have front row seat, 412b
have said it, 623a
have sense for complications unstated, 389b
have serious responsibility, 389a
honor d. for love of themselves, 387b
hospitals will attract d., 221a

Doctors, how get d. to submit patients to treatment, 454b
how many die with three d. at backsides, 628a
if d. destroy revenue for good of mankind, 648b
if d. had not caps and robes, 393a
ill do everything forbidden, 414b
imagine diseases, 372b
in dangerous illness call three d., 67a
in London d. never contradict each other, 454b
in natural state needs d. less, 630b
indeed called to be d., 382a
infect with fear of death, 394b
is all swabs, 396b
jests against d. uttered thousand years ago, 396b
kill patients and paid for it, 449a
king gains freedom from d., 395a
like d. can't let pity into it, 407b
like d. when dispute past, 67b
like diet prescribed by d., 100a
love d. hate their medicine, 389a
made point of mistrusting d., 458a
make bad seem worse, 461b
make health itself sick, 391b
make worst patients, 415b
medicine for people not d., 153b
meet to discuss case, 66a
men neither born d. nor love science, 381b
moral disorder of young d., 322b, 402a
more d. more diseases, 398a
more old drunkards than d., 12a
more stupid moment one in their hands, 396b
most generous of men, 277b
most learned d. leave, 74a
most sensible men, 457a
mostly imposters, 416b
music can be made with other d., 217a
must die too, 93a
never forget sincerities, 157b
never say anything unkind about each other, 455a
nobody supposes d. less virtuous than judges, 458a
not cure own complaints, 414b
not fault of d. that medical service absurdity, 177b
not more stupid than other people, 396b
not one of d. that make market of patients, 393a
not train enough d., 142b
not uncommon in young d., 416b
one object of most d., 85b
order strict regime, 414b
our d. don't know gout, 196b
overpopulated professions d. fools advisers, 459b
oxydable products, 380b
passed on from generation of d. to next, 369a

Doctors pray for fever, 181b
prescribe medicine of which know little, 394a
prescribe no cure, 98b
prescribing way of life contrary, 628a
procession of four or five d., 67a
pronounce attack rheumatism, 196b
pronounced insane by smart d., 246a
public find out skilled d., 457b
recover as soon as d. give over, 392b
rob and kill you, 458a
same as lawyers, 458a
saving d. none more stupid than grammarians, 673b
say eight hourse of slepe in sommer, 552a
scoundrels less among d., 178a
secrecy highly developed among d., 384b
see human race naked, 361b
social cement, 381b
some called to be d., 382a
talk Latin name diseases in Greek, 393a
teaching hospital to train d., 221a
think more of d. if they cure cold, 61b
thought it good you hear a play, 305a
to praise of d. let us say, 388b
torture sick then demand fee, 175a
training rising generation of d., 603a
treat assa faetida and vomits, 668a
tried not to hurt, 638a
trouble with us d., 459a
two classes of mankind d. and patients, 374b, 383a
two d. left leg and right, 166a
two sorts of d., 381b
two Swiss d. can't dispatch him, 191a
undertake doctor's work, 666b
urged by d. to give up salt meats, 188b
vegetate in dependence upon d., 249b
very brave about it, 362a
what d. know taught by sick, 361a
what do d. know, 637a
whatever speciality never forget to be d., 566a
where sunshine no d., 60a
who decide when d. disagree, 453b
why d. often make mistakes, 96a
why practically all d. married, 658a
William Mayo approached meeting of d., 382b
winter brings d. cheer, 60a
work on credulity of patient, 370a
working to preserve health, 203b
worry over remedies, 110b, 492a
would not call it French disease, 650a

Doctors, young d. make humpy cemeteries, 397b
Doctors', more filthy d. fees, 176b
Doctrinal, object distorted by d. medium, 232a
Doctrine, commit selves to d., 65a
Harvey established new d., 422a
influences men, 58b
investigation of neglected d., 500a
lack of rational d., 301b
unlike any in annals of medicine, 549b
Doctrines and techniques tools, 424b
continual reexamination of d., 503b
repay critical examination, 256b
resist fascination of d., 573b
speculative d. in regard to disease, 425b
Dodo-diseases of middle age, 310a
Doers, America land of d., 592a
Does, who d. well drinks well, 11b
Dog, as d. to person who gives bone, 254a, 281a
becomes like superintendent's d. orgulous, 384a
Chief of Service should have pet d., 513a
hair of d. that bit me, 12a
injecting as Mr. Wren into veins of d., 494a
lame d. signify invader, 608b
man recovered of bite d. died, 483b
not allowed to fall into grave like old d., 288a
not even d.-killer learn trade from books, 166b
only one who recognize him his d., 513a
sick as a d., 542a
that I were a d., 453b
to kill d. in Broadway, 125a
went mad and bit man, 483b
Dogdays, where escape d., 240b
Dogfish, nourished inside fish as d. are, 160a
Dogma, shackles of d. removed, 520b
Dogmas, misled by d. of schools, 443a
treat own theories as d., 615a
Dogmatic system requires standstill, 255b
Dogmatical, apothecaries and priests d., 121a
Dogmatism, greater the ignorance greater d., 235a
Dogmatist, surgeon disciple of Galen who was d., 386a, 592b
Dogmatize on practice invite controversy, 444b
Dog's, learning mitral stenosis as know d. bark, 209b
more deadly than mad d. tooth, 483b
Dogs bark and vomit, 67b
bark at me as I halt, 71a
delight more in d. than children, 20a
doctors generally dull d., 396a
live miserably like d., 388b
physicians upon whom set d. when well, 381b
practice operation upon d., 588a

Dogs, take away salt throw flesh to d., 515a
throw physic to d., 244a
traveled science in manner of d. for walk, 529b
Doing, joy of research in d., 504a
Doleful, more d. than procession of doctors, 67a
Doll, we catch of you D., 650b
Dollars lure men into research, 510a
Dolls, cut out paper d., 48a
Dolors, diseases come to three thousand d., 650b
Dolphinese, no human learned d., 261b
Dolphins learned English, 261b
Dolts, members of medical profession ordinary d., 396b
Domestic, happiness of d. life, 656b
medicine preferable to physician, 535a
Domiciliary, first charter for d. care, 373b
Don Quixote, Sydenham replied D., 273b
Done, so little d. so much to do, 259b
things never yet d. by means never yet tried, 524b
Donne jump into river, 541a
Dooley, said Mr. D., 72a, 323a
Doom, feeling of impending d., 21a
Door, came out by same d., 277a
deaf as a d., 76a
drunkard who tries key in d. after d., 614b
extort money from those at death's d., 175a
go from d. to d., 331b
iron d. yielded, 267a
keep physician from d., 391a
nor so wide as church d., 665b
shut out sun from window doctor in at d., 397b
slam d. on doctor's nose, 227a
tell what happens inside house by d., 306b
Doornail, dead as a d., 77b
Marley was dead as d., 79a
Doors, considering thousand d. to death, 542b
death hath so many d., 82a
death hath ten thousand d., 81b
searchers sealed up d., 429a
Dope, despair treated with hope not d., 306b
Doris hates having doctor, 397a
Dormitive, in opium a d. virtue, 351a
Dosage, everything depends upon d., 638b
Dose of opium every morning, 351b
one d. make boy willing to go to school for month, 496a
take d. of medicine once, 631b
worse the scrawl d. the better, 449a
Doses, digitalis in dangerous d., 125a
remedies less effect d. increased, 496a
world of filthy d., 176b
Dotage differ from melancholy, 305b

Drink, neither healing food nor d., 491b
nor any drop to d., 654b
nor d. unless thirsty, 225b
not d. wine whenever feel like it, 487a
not the third glass, 6b
not to elevation, 607a
on day of phlebotomy d. less, 35a
one another's health, 9b
one man's poison another's d., 439b
potion or two of good d., 305b
sick men long most to d., 618a
sleep is d. for thirsty, 552a
smaller d. clearer head, 7a
strong d. is raging, 11a
strong or not at all, 11b
takes the man, 12b
tea or wine and water, 494b
that may follow strong d., 11b
thin d. doth over-cool blood, 16b
third of stomach with d., 105a
thirst consciousness of need to d., 618a
thirst vanishes as you d., 22a, 618a
thirsty and ye gave me d., 618b
thirsty d. silently, 619a
this distilled liquor d., 122a
to improve understanding d. coffee, 60b
victuals and d. illusion of senses, 558a
well, 226b
what does d. provoke, 6a, 647a
what you don't like, 206a
when thirsty fools fain have d., 618a
which feaverish men desire, 281b
while of d. they take fill, 90a
wine and have gout, 188b
wine by measure, 103a
with him that wears hood, 106a
without being thirsty, 288a
women d. as much liquor, 659a
your health in wine, 654b
Drinkers candidates for chalk-stones, 195b
Drinketh, he that d. well sleepeth well, 102b
Drinking and sweating life of dyspeptic, 238b
appetite measure of d., 22a
as qualification for gentleman, 7b
at someone else's expense, 9a
bleeding and d. warm water grand principles, 629b
cut out d. , 48a
I naturally hated d., 7b
ill with eating and d. too much, 239a
life consists of d., 130a
men more given to intemperate d., 276a
Miniver kept on d., 10a
more general than card-playing, 9b
not d. blamed but excess, 130b
poison would waste it, 440a
rather heat liver with d., 275b
ruins health by d., 115a
scandalous habit of d., 8a
since leaving d. of wine, 7a
started day by d., 130a

Drinking takes away stomach, 23a
temperance in eating and d., 225a
water neither makes sick, 655a
without being thirsty, 539a
Drinks, choleric d., 49b
from cooling stream, 204a
he that sips often d. it up, 8a
holds nose and d., 123b
hot d. not for body, 488b
more he d. thirstier he grows, 120a
push under so d. fill against will, 483a
strong d. not for belly, 488b
tumbler of London water, 655a
who d. one bowl, 8b
who d. well sleeps well, 11b
Drive, men very hard to d., 286a
Drivelling, like old man's mouth d., 349a
Drivelry, dealing delusions d. despair, 347b
Drives, fundamental d. back to first life, 287a
Drones drive from marriage hive, 211a
Drop, draw out old age d. by d., 337b
nor any d. to drink, 654b
Drops, count d. that make lakeful, 557b
let patients die with colored d., 428a
one of physicians used d. of colored water, 428a
ruddy d. that visit heart, 58b
Dropsical, in d. cases urine coagulates, 648a
sailors attacked with d. symptoms, 653b
Dropsied, it is d. honour, 120b
patients died, 253b
Dropsies of ventricles of brain, 244b
swollen parcel of d., 120b
wherein were laid d., 218a
Dropsy, ague and d., 668b
belly swells with d., 120a
body of patient dying with d., 253a
diseases asthma d. and seventy-five, 346a
drown this fool, 120b
healing art helps not d., 237a
puffed his lips, 120a
pursues with thirst, 120a
rears bloated form, 120b
swelling increase to d., 120b
Drosophila, genetic study of D., 186a
Dross, metals in ore mixed with d., 639b
that man is heir to, 89a
Drought, plague of pestilence or d., 226b
Drown, dropsy d. this fool, 120b
Drowned, Bacchus d. more than Neptune, 12a
man virtually d. and revived, 86b
more d. in goblet than sea, 12a
submitted to be half-d., 634a
taken with cramp and d., 70a
Drowsiness in hollows of gridiron, 193b
senescence with comforting d., 343b

Drowsy, few relevant stimuli we become d., 340b
syrups of world, 122a
through veins run d. humour, 122a
when old age d. death nigh, 77b
Drudgery, innure self to d. in science, 575b
Drug agent with specimens, 412b
cannot have d. for every malady, 125a
contribute to mental effervescence, 645a
hawkers run off with treatment, 636b
injected into rat produces paper, 127b
learn therapy from d. house, 636a
merit of d. measured by use, 127a
murderous to senses, 122a
of such damn'd nature, 438b
patients believe every symptom benefited by d., 125b
self-analysis subtle as d.-taking, 469b
sharpened blade and two-edged d., 638a
treat with new d. while has power, 125a
what purgative d. would scour English, 122a
Drugging, humanity delivered from d., 124a
imperative d. no longer, 125a
rescue practice of medicine from d., 272b
Druggist questions it ask him to call, 121a
Druggist's, matters d. shopboy tell, 629a
Drugs, apothecary thy d. are quick, 439b
appropriately called wonder d., 127a
are kind of alchemy, 202a
by d. churchyard fills, 392a
cause cramp, 582b
clown more beneficial than d., 494a
devil teach harmful parts of d., 628a
did me no good, 150a
educated physician gives d. as placebos, 428a
effects known to follow d., 146a
for one disorder doctors cure with d., 472a
half modern d. thrown out window, 125b
higher aim than prescription of d., 634b
Holmes said no use in d., 181a
illusion that diseases conquered by d., 233a
knowledge of how to use d., 256b
less confidence in d., 488b
medical men don't know d., 391a
mercifully weak, 638a
no really safe d., 127a
nor sending to East Indies for d., 400a
not a man for d., 124b
not poisoned with d., 630b

Embrace, shun soft e. emasculant, 539a

Embryo, illnesses transmitted to e., 210a

seed of mother has power in e., 185b

Embryologist, assume spectacles of e., 318a

Emergency, confidence useful in e., 222a

good health until e., 374a

incapable of judgment in e., 586b

instruments ready for e. operations, 376b

makes e. of almost every case, 178a

Emeritus quit making fuss, 417a

Emetic, carpenter asks for e., 625b

gave him e. clyster two pills, 635b

worked so well wonder patient died, 635b

Emigrant best understood by native land, 299b

Eminent, more e. less investigative work, 614a

very few become e., 576a

Emoluments bestowed for deception, 380a

Emotion, as if cries of pain cause no e., 582b

contagious, 116a, 206b

data tinted in e., 143b

ebb and flow of e., 537b

good to spit blood after e., 643a

practice science touched with e., 444b

religion morality touched with e., 444b

see without e. child with croup, 411b

suppression of e. injurious, 145a

Emotional, disease affected by e. life, 116b

poisons by e. excess, 472a

preference for dead or live patient, 466a

sickness produces e. state, 42a

side to behavior, 145a

tensions mount, 104b

therapist's e. maturity, 473a

well attributed to sick own e. equipment, 250a

Emotions, able to rule our e., 279a

balance of forces in which e., 287a

influence of passions and e., 471b

judgment when e. engaged, 425b

no idea about man's e., 140a

physician on whom e. played continuously, 414a

undisciplined e., 20b

Emperors, make pomp of e. ridiculous, 205a

Empiric, don't despise e. truth, 146a

let not e. peepe in window, 387b

practitioner without sciences an e., 26a

scientific physician advantage over e., 616b

Empirical generalizations in rational generalization, 526b

Empirical, human nature inferred from e. study, 471a

medicine was e., 146a

results of observation, 614a

therapeutics become e., 550b

therapeutics e. art, 615b

Empirici accept evident causes, 145a

Empiricism, effort to narrow range of e., 301a

foundation laid for e., 573b

has done more than universities, 145a

medicine blend of superstition e. observation, 301a

Empiricisms, surgery seeded with e., 597b

Empiricist and theorist called other quack, 455a

with indiscriminate confidence, 616b

Empiric's, from powerful causes spring e. gains, 480a

Empirics excrescences of medical profession, 481a

happy many times in cures, 145b

not prostitute past-cure malady to e., 237a

suppositors to doctor, 479a

theorizing physicians may show as e., 615b

Employed, never e. you as my physician, 337a

Employers, many humane benevolent e., 336b

Employment divert lunatics from morbid, 472b

great preserver of health, 227a

mousetrap signify e., 608b

nature's physician, 662b

no length of life want e., 270a

not lightly forego customary e., 512b

nursing disease to neglect of e., 625b

retirement not due to lack of e. opportunities, 513a

Emptied, distended stomach e. occasionally, 132a

Empty, full bellies e. skulls, 132b

imagination takes possession of mind when e., 234b

never purpose e. of meaning, 225b

no man patriot on e. stomach, 224a

rest of stomach left e., 105a

thin people never exercise on e. stomach, 164b

to e. stomach food is God, 224a

Encyclopedia, in science I am e. behind, 517b

Encyclopedias, statistics in e., 255b

Encysted part ceases general life, 168b

End, afflictions to which death about to put e., 342b

attempt e. never stand to doubt, 498a

difference which e. you're on, 648b

ere e. work of noble note, 343a

flows from beginning, 29a

happy physician called at e. of illness, 386b

no e. to our researches, 497b

End, see e. of disease from beginning, 634b

so near mine e., 338a

think every illness beginning of e., 346b

Endearment, mutual anxiety begets mutual e., 363b

Endocrine, patient with e. insufficiency, 236a

Endocrines, pathologist venturing on sea of e., 146b

Endomorph with gentle hands, 404a

Endow college or cat, 655b

Endowing, importance of e. few big things, 510b

Endowment, agitation for e. of science, 510a

medical education worthy of e., 503a

soundest way to secure results, 510b

Endure, happiness motive of all willing to e., 286b

no skill to grow old trick to e. it, 338b

strong man wretched and e., 263b

Endured, can't be cured best e., 237a

life much e. little enjoyed, 264a

Endureth all things, 51a

Enema, give e. bleed purge, 494a

Enemas are enemies, 638a

physicians smelled of e., 392a

Enemies, disease entities recognized as e., 116a

doctor fights e. to life, 387b

enemas are e., 638a

forged letters describing death of e., 472b

health and sickness double e., 207b

humanity has three great e., 181b

insensible to pinpricks of e., 280a

mankind at large for e., 58b

physician in league with e., 155a

say out of conceit with own systems, 418a

Enemy, drive off e. at throats, 387b

fatigue doctor's greatest e., 657b

feed on war at expense of e., 131a

formula-worship real e., 521b

friend who is physician send to e., 398a

from e. reconciled liberate us, 397b

gout only e. not wish at feet, 195b

last e. destroyed is death, 91a

little trusted as general in pay of e., 458a

must get by man of ninety, 343a

old e. the gout, 196a

reason can become e., 485b

scurvy more destructive e. than French and Spanish, 533a

world small if would avoid e., 332a

Energetic, people of West e., 201a, 624b

Energies, directing e. with useful purpose, 489a

F

Glass, drunk my last g., 338a
get thee eye. eyes, 169b
letters large through g. filled
with water, 548a
not live running of one g., 275b
of fashion mould of form, 243a
some have urine-g. in hands,
384b
where see inmost part of you,
673b
Glasses, how find g. if not have
them on, 549a
pair with double g. not get to
fit eye, 548b
received spectacles and g. you
send, 548b
seldom make passes at girls who
wear g., 549a
Glassware, background of complicated g., 251a
Glaucoma, distinguish cataract
from g., 169a
Glister only way to help, 73a
Globe, hysteric g. in throat, 319a
more animated beings than on
face of g., 655a
Globule, trace ancestry to atomic
g., 161b
Gloom, ceremonious air of g., 84b
lost in g. of uninspired research, 499a
Gloomy, who would in g. state remain, 553b
Glorious, many g. men cut out of
womb, 54b
so death be but g., 84a
Glory, craves sympathy for sickness as portion of g., 543b
hallelujah I am with the Lord,
259b
heedless of g., 121b
is oblivion postponed, 173a
matter immortal as g., 265b
of surgeons like actors, 587a
of young men is strength, 675b
physician achieves g., 410a
ready go, 259b
there the sun outshines, 432b
Gloves, rubber g. to prevent infecting, 451b
Glow, hectic g. of consumption,
643b
Glutton committing dyspepsia,
131b
craves whole boars, 129b
digs grave with teeth, 133a
Gluttons tumble victuals in, 132a
Gluttony, belly full of g., 133a
cook make g. you make diseases
Doll, 650b
in g. must be eating, 130b
kills multitudes, 132b
no sin if doesn't injure, 132b
preacher of avoiding g. doctor,
387a
suffer not so much g. as starvation, 327b
those given to g., 22b
Gnaw, only seems to g. itself,
605b
Go, cry and g. that is death, 271b
Goa, they tried G. stone, 635b
Goal, healing ultimate g. of efforts, 381a
health for all is continuing g.,
477b
many run that few reach g.,
508b
physicians seek same g., 384b

Goal, prevention of disease g. of
every physician, 452b
Soley drove self to reach g.,
426a
Goals, able to abandon competitive g., 473b
perfection of means confusion
of g., 333a
Goat, calculus from Indian g.,
635b
in midst of illness promise g.,
179a
Goats careful in selecting foods,
311b
Gobble, don't g. as much as can,
129b
Goblet, more drowned in g. than
sea, 12a
Goblins, charge g. grind joints,
70a
God and doctor we alike adore,
370a
and recuperating power of nature restore, 175b
big bellyache heap G., 239b
brought me into light to die,
257b
caused deep sleep, 18b
chemistry G. has given cow,
104a
could have made better berry,
420b
course of nature is art of G.,
316b
cursed Eve, 55a
dealt well with midwives, 310b
doctor the g., 362a
doctor's error will of G., 153a
doth G. exact day-labour, 32a
doubt G. given unwholesome
refreshment, 307b
feel love of G. in work, 401b
few physicians rise to G., 43a
forbids us go hence, 579b
forgive sins nervous system
won't, 318b
forgotten doctor slighted, 370a
gave him no children, 235b
gave navels altogether useless,
318a
granted him easy death, 86b
guide not hand of G., 222b
happy he who bears a g. within,
490b
have them of His Grace, 149b
he seems to be, 176a
heals doctor takes fee, 179a
hear words and make them
true, 206b
herbs G. ordained for man,
488b
how little know of nature of
G., 235a
human pun made by G., 287b
I dressed him G. healed him,
627b
indigestion charged by G. with
enforcing morality, 239b
indignation directed to G., 371a
indulged Devil to create one
thing, 191a
is in her child, 290a
law of G. allows no man touch
life, 157b
live as long as G. wills,
388b
lost fear of G., 308b
lover of wisdom equal of a g.,
399a

God make known power of anger,
190b
man in image of G., 286a
medicine from G. no man despise it, 387a
more faith than in affirmative
statements about G., 491b
nature art of G., 316a
never made work for man to
mend, 165a
no one so mindful of G., 188a
not alter faulty incision, 598a
not exhaust power in making
Galen, 421b
not intention of G., 619b
not take life until G. summons,
579b
O G. O Kinsey O Jehoshaphat,
541b
of contemporary man's idolatry,
522b
of physic and sender of diseases,
296a
on side of best digestion, 107a
only one of arts which produced a g., 294b
or something very like Him,
490b
ordered motion but no rest,
285a
pleased G. to take to mercy,
73b
prefer to die by decree of G.,
83b
prefer to die by hand of G., 81a
put physic in mere muck,
492b
receives small honour from vulgar, 498a
relenting G. placed within my
hand, 283b
render soul to G. unclouded,
83a
reveal million-murdering cause,
283b
sick served for honour of G.,
372a
some call it evolution others G.,
162a
study of anatomy lifted to G.,
15a
temptation to imagine self a g.,
384a
thanks to G. it's them not me,
198b
theories not dangerous to G. or
capital, 530b
think motion of heart only
comprehended by G., 209b
this g. did shake, 180a
to empty stomach food is G.,
224a
to G. belongeth chiefest part,
73b
waiting for me, 258b
we owe G. a death, 91b
what G. did when saw free one,
471a
who rules within us, 579b
who understands quicksilver a
g., 386b
wipe nose and not blame G.,
320b
work upon temple of G., 593b
Goddess, fair g. as companion,
203b
who hatest poor, 187b
Goddesses, swear by all gods and
g., 325b

Hair, harsh red h. big merciless hands, 587a
head without h. an eyesore, 25a
heads whose h. falls, 25b
horrid image unfix my h., 174a
if had diseased lung long h., 644a
in a bag, 32b
in head worth two in brush, 25b
let barber shave off h., 25a
mats of h. betray character, 49b
no time to recover h., 25b
of dog that bit me, 12a
on sheets his h. sticking, 314b
painted upon skull, 179b
plenteous lack of h., 416a
sent h. to editors of medical journals, 374b
should loosen h., 128a
sweet Alice whose h. was so brown, 434a
takes h. right off bean, 623b
those dim of vision like number of h., 547b
time when necessarily loses h., 345a
upreared, 314b
with long wig cover h., 397a
women short of h., 659a
women never lost h., 659a
Haircut, lies h. and shave, 25b
Hairdresser, no need to have h., 25a
Hairs, animals that have h., 13a
bedded h. stand on end, 243b
collect straggling h., 25a
palsy shakes last gray h., 347a
trouble brung grey h., 25b
Half doctor near better, 390a
first twenty years longest h. of life, 675a
knowledge dreads whole knowledge, 255a
loquacity of h. knowledge, 25a
of objects appear, 199b
of what you are taught wrong, 143a
pain of one h. of head, 199b
scarce h. made up, 70b
too bad cannot cut patient in h., 168b
under doctors h. to Nature, 391a
what it h. knows, 25a
without wife only h. man, 657a
Half-truths, Aristotle discovered all h., 256a
Half-witted, money for health of body by h. men, 479b
Hall, science of life lighted h., 500b
Hallelujah, glory h. I am with the Lord, 259b
Hallucination, pity result of h., 249b
Hallucinations, hatters developed h., 247a
tranquilizers eliminate h., 126a
Hallucinoses, how to get rid of h., 473a
Halo, glorifieth her as h., 324a
Halt and the blind, 33a, 71a
cry out for thee, 408a
Ham, cursing h., 188b
Hamlet, story of H. without Ghost, 352a
walked softly as ghost in H., 418b

Hamlet with doublet unbrac'd, 242b
without Prince of Denmark, 359a
Hammer, dysentery fall like h., 128a
Hampshire, sleeps in peace H. Grenadier, 11b
Hams, together with most weak h., 345a
Hamsters, teacher paid not to sacrifice h., 604a
Hand, affronted at offer of h., 674b
art increment of power of h., 524a
between discharge-tube and screen, 674a
dead h. of medical tradition, 153b
Death's h. warmer than my own, 349a
dying bless h. that gave blow, 82b
finger of each h. pouring chalk, 193b
gout in h., 187a
have sore eye cut off h., 639a
have you not dry h., 345a
holds out h. to physician ridiculous, 337b
in good h. every sword cuts well, 598a
instrument at end of arm, 199a
last grasp of h. precious by touch of gold, 177b
lay h. on heart that's sore, 331b
mother spared rod used h., 57b
old age lays jewelled h. in mine, 343a
operates with h. not heart, 587a
others attend to disorders of h., 563b
raw wound quivers at touch of h., 665a
relenting God placed within my h., 283b
scratching ready at h. as any, 532b
such sanctity given his h., 74a
surgeon with strong and steady h., 582b
surgeons of future not divorce h. from brain, 597b
that which cures by h., 626b
through h. line of gout, 193b
tongue do more good and evil than h., 62b
unison of h. and head, 588b
unskilled h. into divine mechanism, 587a
walked with death in h., 349a
where man feels pain he lays his h., 357b
wipe face with handkerchief not h., 598b
Handicaps, better grave h. than trifling, 71a
to practice of medicine, 445b
Handicraft, surgery h. with elaborate techniques, 597b
surgery of future not merely h., 597b
true test of h., 430b
Handiwork, G.P. live with results of h., 185a
Handkerchief, knit my h. about brows, 199b

Handerchief, wipe face with h., 598b
Hands abroad display'd, 314b
and feet distorted, 197a
appointed surgeon who had no h., 512b, 596b
armed with healing h., 385b
asked why shook h. with patient, 368b
burning of h. and feet, 642b
chirurgien have h. of woman, 584b
distance between fingers of h., 13b
eats bread without washing h., 228a
feet and h. may slow down, 216b
folding of h. to sleep, 555b
frosted pawed me, 390b
harsh red hair big merciless h., 587a
in need of eating have no h., 197a
many h. needed for discovery, 109a
message h. bear to patient, 385a
nursing hard work for h., 322a
repented of folly, 571a
shakes h. with relish, 66b
shaking h. fell into disuse, 674b
surgery motion of steady experienced h., 593a
take fever'd h., 283b
wash h. before sitting down to table, 227a
wash h. often, 228b
washing h. between patients, 228a
when tormented h. ready, 197a
whose h. are four, 163a
with wrist bones like shank of ham, 424a
Handsaw, know hawk from h., 243a
Hang, one more reason to h. him, 245a
Hanged, make diagnosis and get h., 98a
man knows be h. in fortnight, 312b
rather read *Congressional Record* than see bishop h., 333a
Hangest, Bishop H. of Le Mans, 22a, 618a
Hanging, as h. advertizes barrister, 578a
Hangman, difference only from h., 392a
Hangover became part of day, 10b
Hannibal knew how to subdue Romans, 327b
Happenings of yore occurred day before, 347b
Happiness, anxieties by which female h. disturbed, 659b
comes secondarily, 657b
credit to my lady H., 437a
diseases disturbing our h., 263b
duty of physician to bring h., 238a
employment essential to h., 662b
essential to good citizenship, 475a
found by wayside, 206b
gives energy, 205b

Hues, paint everything with lurid h., 252b
Hufeland, Christoph Wilhelm, 146b
Hugo, Victor H. in exile, 489a
Human, abnormalities of h. behaviour, 470b
abominations down throats of h. beings, 124b
application of scientific discipline to h. problem, 303b
as in all h. relations, 638b
beautiful h. actions before thirty, 674a
behold in suffering only h. being, 447a
being and terrible thing happening, 288a
being ingenious portable plumbing, 287b
beings of which know nothing, 394a
care of h. mind most noble branch of medicine, 465b
contribution of psychoanalysis to h. progress, 468a
control of h. evolution, 185b
course of h. mind from credulity to scepticism, 549a
death privilege of h. nature, 269b
death proclaims how small our h. bodies, 77a
diagnosis of things h. and divine, 376b
difficulties from h. condition, 320a
discount h. achievement as naught, 298a
divine mechanism as h. body, 587a
doctor sees h. nature bare, 361b
doctors see h. race naked, 361b
doctrine vouched for by feelings of h. beings, 527b
eat is h. digest divine, 107a
experience of h. nature, 53a
experimental science relation to h. welfare, 508a
face novel situations, 463b
fellow sufferers from h. condition, 517a
forgetting claims of h. brotherhood, 331a
fraud to call sciences h. invention, 517a
great concern h. being, 287a
greeting another h. being, 368b
guides h. discourse to divine, 169a
hear aloof h. tempest beat, 342b
how guileless h. nature, 324b
how h. body improved, 186a
increases total of h. ignorance, 274b
influenced conception of h. nature, 470a
intimate knowledge of h. body, 296b
invalid is all body, 249b
joy one of greatest felt by h., 502a
judgment founded on knowledge of h. nature, 409a
knowledge of h. reactions, 451b
laws of h. nature, 286a
lessons practice teaches, 603b
life much endured little enjoyed, 264a

Human life mutual service, 582a
link between apes and h. beings, 163a
little knowledge of h. nature, 312b
love majesty of h. suffering, 578b
machine so complicated as h. body, 631a
medicine concerned with entire h. organism, 297a
medicine humane as well as h., 298b
medicine old as h. race, 298b
most sudden change h. race known, 287b
mystical qualities of h. nature, 9a
nature has archetype in h. imagination, 231a
nature never observed as such, 471a
nature would lose h. species, 538b
no h. learned dolphinese, 261b
not integrated complex systems, 404a
nothing h. foreign, 284a
nurse given h. touch, 323a
one of heaviest loads on h., 322b
one of most advanced types of h., 402b
one of worst diseases to which h. liable is thinking, 617b
passions of h. heart unchanged, 265b
precision of h. organism, 123a
prerogative of h. species, 169b
psyche in union with body, 470a
psychology of h. relationships, 601b
purposes unworthy h. nature, 229a
pursuit of development of h. mind, 214a
quest into mysteries of h. body, 303b
race cancer of planet, 287b
relationship in which observer teaches observed, 468a
roads to h. power and knowledge close, 524b
science exists only in h. beings, 519a
science not encompass h. factors, 256b
scientific scholar of h. biology, 403b
seat in front row of h. drama, 413b
see another h. with understanding, 466a
semi-deliverance from h. prison, 119a
sense horses have never to bet on h. beings, 333b
setting at naught strongest instinct of h., 582a
sleep perverse as h. nature, 555b
so vast art so narrow h. wit, 523a
species in no worse condition than other, 630b
study of h. mind, 465a
subtlety makes inventions, 315a
sum of h. achievement, 290b

Human, surgery take into account nature peculiar to h., 597b
to professional skill join h. warmth, 367b
touch counts for most, 366b
touch that counts, 435b
traits specialized as appropriate of one sex, 540b
units are to h. whole, 85a
varying conditions of h. life, 301a
wish to ascertain laws of h. life, 450b
worst of h. pangs thirst, 618b
you who restore health to h. body, 378a
Humane, in good health devote to h. activities, 201b
medicine h. as well as human, 298b
sense in which knowledge employed, 156a
study fear in h. regard, 174b
triumph of h. civilization, 142b
Humanism neither atheistic nor pantheistic, 255b
science serving mankind h., 368a
without h. medicine must degenerate, 157a
Humanist, clinician possess qualities of h., 367b
practices profession as h., 403b
Humanistic faculty of medicine, 286b
Humanitarian, school carries on aims of h. accomplishments, 292a
Humanities, neglect of h. general, 139a
of four or five generations, 212a
sciences encouraged to neglect of h., 142a
surgery one of h., 597a
Humanity, benefit to h. of such heritage, 589a
cause of h. my own, 363b
children escape into h., 58a
cry of h. that life too short, 561b
curing all distempers incident to h., 629b
delivered from drugging, 124a
despair of political h., 177b
doctor without sense of h., 155b
doing good to h. with skill, 410a
each of us accident in history of h., 545a
fear casts out h., 174b
future belong to who done most for h., 463a
gout delights in assaulting h., 197b
has three great enemies, 181b
history of medicine history of h., 214b
idea of h. degenerated, 116b
indiscreet zeal for h., 328b
interests of h. ennoble disgusting, 328b
knowledge belongs to h., 519a
listen to still sad music of h., 380b
love hope fear faith make h., 265b
lover of h. or either sex of it, 464a

Indigestion enforcing morality on stomach, 239b
excellent common-place, 239a
for first time troubled with i., 239a
gout referred to i., 189b
know how to manage i., 134b
makes Styx through liver flow, 239b
patient mistake for religious conviction, 239b
sows hurry reaps i., 239b
Indignation directed to Cot Almighty, 371a
of reformer, 178a
reaction spurred by moral i., 330a
Indiscretions, diseases of young pardonable i., 291b
Indispensable, no one more i. than doctor, 387a
Indisposition, late occasion of i., 204b
melancholy not i. of body, 305b
remedies harm thanks to lasting i., 496b
to do anything, 61a
Individual, anxiety of the i., 21b
avoid examination of i. symptoms, 468a
conflict between stimulus and whole i., 356b
contribute under sense of responsibility, 273b
difference between i. and fellows, 3b
doctor needs to know i., 368a
doctor subordinates i. to society, 157a
every i. derived from lowest forms, 161b
experiences by which i. unique, 49b
genius strictly i., 186b, 212b
government never replace i. responsibility, 478a
human i. with personality of own, 404a
leaves little to i. excellence, 525a
obsession that its responsibility is to the i., 186a
practice concerned with i., 636b
provision for needs which no i. can, 475b
realistic concept of i., 330a
right of i. to be sick, 475b
studies patient as i., 404a
thus become i., 409b
Individualism turn into egotism, 330a
Individualist, in future i. by roadside, 597b
Individuality, letting own i. interact with i. of patient, 361b
subconscious self lacks i., 469b
Individualized physician man of world, 380a
Individualizing disease as well as patient, 446a
Individuals best fitted survive, 160b
body monstrous multiplicity of i., 352b
disease in i. has end, 636b
feel sharply, 329a
insanity in i. rare, 245b
management same for i. of all ages, 445b

Individuals, men not i. but components, 85a
no two i. alike, 115b
sick people not numbered i., 323a
Indolence in fashion diseases multiplied, 195a
not destroy i. by awakening effort, 376a
require help of medicine by i., 110b
Indolent, gout attacks eunuchs who lead i. life, 192a
maladies which afflict i., 204a
medical student too i. to exercise, 575a
question of i. citizen, 195a
Induction, false i. from genuine facts, 277b
only hope in true i., 276b
sciences need i. which analyse experience, 524b
Inductions, legitimate i., 136b
Inductive, no process of i. reasoning used by Newton, 525b
reasoning experimentally obtained, 525b
Indulgence, dropsy by i. nursed, 120a
in pleasures of youth capital offence, 345b
of sensual appetites, 190b
patient abstain from i., 177a
Indulgences, rivalling male i. rivalled ills, 569a
Industrial, health centers in i. center, 445b
Industrialists, doctor needs more brains than i., 185a
not recall help from organized i., 336b
Industries, solemnest of i. on earth, 79a
Industry contributes to good stomach, 106b
created new sources of danger, 337a
dissipation of ill-directed i., 270a
fundamental to success in medicine, 402b
ingenuity in mechanical beneficial in i., 592a
make good use of i., 135b
rather excite i. than inflame vanity, 594b
success depends upon i., 578a
to quote poets feeble i., 261b
Inebriate, cups that cheer not i., 600a
Ineffable, mystic sees i., 466a
Inefficacy, at Aix long enough to prove i., 224b
Inevitable, poor to fear what is i., 91b
Inexperienced, any i. man finds it possible to be physician, 359b
Inexplicable, divine secrets just as i., 161a
Infallible, none of us i., 152b
Infamy, eternal i. his name surround, 539a
Infancy, bring up from i. and diet him, 279a
idiocy of i., 56b
importance of experiences of i., 470b
nerves in i. again, 318b

Infancy, stage between i. and adultery, 3b
tetchy and wayward thy i., 55b
Infant all gut and squall, 56a
birth painful to i., 29b
diseases affecting i., 236a
is disagreeable, 56a
mother seldom in hospital to attend i., 52b
newborn i. upon bosom, 289b
Infants, American i. not rosy, 16b
hospital for deserted i., 289a
not cry without cause, 55b
savor of person by whom suckled, 55b
Infarction of heart, 638a
Infect, flowery speakers i. one another, 304b
one i. other against wind, 428b
Infected, food belch'd on by i. lungs, 642a
in thee nature i., 305b
minds to pillows discharge secrets, 243b
one i. pig stock destroys, 147a
they are i., 429a
to save whole sawes off i. part, 585a
went into streets to avoid being i., 674b
wife's liver i. as her life, 275b
Infecting, rubber gloves to prevent i., 451b
Infection, body less resistant to i., 645a
expose newborn to i. criminal, 53a
lest his i. spread further, 240a
not by geniality recognize i., 184b
origin of consumptions, 642b
Pasteur attacked for views on i., 240b
plague come by i., 240a
there before symptoms appeared, 649b
will be banished, 54b
with germs of haughty contempt, 563b
without disease rule, 241b
Infections, forces help survive i., 48a
secondary or terminal i. cause of death, 85b
that sun sucks up, 240b
Infectious agents must be bacteria, 241a
disease one of few adventures left, 505a
germ doctrine of i. diseases, 108b
horror ran face to face, 429a
house where i. pestilence did reign, 429a
learn what relation i. agents bear, 451a
nature of childbirth fever, 54b
not proof that breath of consumptive i., 642b
old age i. chronic disease, 348a
patients whose pulses felt with tongs, 240b
Infective material independently alive, 307b
Infects, rank corruption i. unseen, 646a
Inference *per enumerationem simplicem*, 277a
science matter of i., 528a

Insatiable, pangs of belly with i. man, 607b
Inscription, bell with i. asking to ring it, 320b
for University of Pennsylvania Hospital, 218a
gloomy i. on monuments, 149b
house of physician adorned with i., 387b
Insecta, holometabolous i., 610b
Insecurity, growing feeling of i., 21b
Insensibility, measure of i. advantage, 402a
oysterlike i., 61b
Insensible, at forty far from cold and i., 309a
death leaves outward parts i., 93b
Inside, he who cuts your i. out, 177b
hurt i. of deadlier sort, 666a
tender state of i., 43b
Insides, don't scrape i. with roughage, 649a
neurotic less addicted to listening to i., 319b
Insidious, traditionalism more i., 154a
Insight into humours of mankind, 177a
moment's i. worth life's experience, 330a
Insignificant, nothing in medicine i., 334b
Insomnia, every man's i. different, 557b
troubles those who can sleep any time, 557a
Inspection, discover from actual i., 209a
Inspiration, genius one per cent i., 186a
grandeur of acts measured by i., 490b
greater than himself in i., 154b
ideas come like i., 501b
in glorious past, 214a
secret of i. in literature, 265b
Instability, warmth generated by i., 266b
Instant obsolescence in medical knowledge, 257b
Instep, ankle and i. tortured, 195a
pain more rarely in i., 189b
wine mine its way through i., 197b
Instinct, brutes by i. produced discoveries, 107b
for being unhappy highly developed, 306b
for self-determination, 268a
pathologic development of amorous i., 273b
setting at naught strongest i. of human, 582a
sexual i. always active in woman, 540a
Instincts, endeavors to satisfy i., 117b
Institute, make fools of selves at i., 251b
Royal College of Physicians not research i., 508a
Institution, dual standards within i., 577b
good practice and public i. besides, 418b

Institution, priesthood not question of i., 154a
Institutions, clinicians in variety of i., 601b
for research worthy of endowment, 503a
mentally disabled in i., 246b
provided hospitals sanitaria and i., 489a
senior citizens in obsolete mental i., 349a
sin tends to beset all i., 323a
Instructed those not yet ill, 449b
Instruction comes from air, 672a
essential i. at bedside, 137a
from evident causes, 48b
in medicine like culture of earth, 134a
in the art takes place, 134a
like planting seed, 134a
medical i. to make possible protection of health, 474b
men and women in i. for medical profession, 661b
mind hardly sees anything without i., 313a
talk with purpose of i. about common, 602b
throughout educational life, 227b
wards great book of i., 602a
Instructions, nurse follows i. of physician, 322a
Instructor, best i. may have no conception of higher work, 600b
perform examination under i., 144a
Instructors, low scholastic ratings from i., 577a
medical students have faith in i., 573b
wise infidelity against i., 136a
Instrument, body i. easy to distemper, 36b
fever Nature's i., 181a
most important i. in research mind, 509a
of death fly on wall, 241a
to take away one of greatest calamities, 328b
worship of i. leads to enslavement, 248a
Instruments, equipped with surgical i., 398b
give student power to use i., 199b
ideas intellectual i., 233b
need of new i., 220a
physicians keep i. ready, 376b
polish rust from my i., 437a
save from confusion of i., 447a
silver case with i. at girdle, 585a
tormenting with crooked i., 631b
Insufficiency, conditions due to i., 49a
patient with endocrine i., 236a
Insulin, led to discovery of i., 109b
Insult, efforts of professor to screen her from i., 662a
or praise by way in which express self, 610b
Insulted, profession i. from without, 71b
Insurance companies not charge different, 373b

Insurance, confuse provisions of national health i., 476a
life i. agent, 412b
only genuine medical i., 562b
Insure, to i. self from hurt to i. self from growth, 356a
Integration, accompanying i. of matter, 161a
phenomena investigated at different levels of i., 508b
Integrity fundamental to success in medicine, 402b
health i. of functions, 264b
in profession paramount, 157b
neither tamper with i. of body, 570a
progress based on i. in professional conduct, 215b
quality of good teacher i., 602a
success depends upon i., 578a
therapist's personal i., 473a
Integument regarded as part of body, 550b
Intellect, any knowledge useful to i., 254a
drains large water-shed of i., 330a
has i. a function, 313b
higher order of i. for observation, 334b
in addition to three-story i., 426b
means of strengthening i., 313a
nature fixed so i. learn it, 317a
not by magic of great i., 525b
ordained to excellence, 24a
sciences in which truth discoverable by i., 250b
side to behavior not of i., 145a
sorry share of i., 309b
suppression of emotion injurious to i., 145a
too much pride of i., 490b
uses not i. but memory, 485a
Intellects, never i. limit to stating facts, 614a
suppose old man decayed in i., 536a
Intellectual, backbone of i. training in education, 142a
by superior i. qualifications, 331b
combined i. with nobility of character, 389a
counterpart in i. life, 508b
courage necessary to i. honesty, 591a
doctor near patient in i. capacity, 366b
emulate in i. endowments, 296a
faculties had another origin, 161a
greater i. freedom greater suicides, 582b
harmony between men and women, 539b
high i. ferment, 68b
home in which I grew up, 299a
hypothesis i. instrument of discovery, 231a
ideas i. instruments, 233b
Lydgate felt growth of i. passion, 419a
never allowing i. powers interfered with, 398b
occupation allow i. freedom, 301b
occupation for which training i., 457b

Inventions, remembered not as age of technical i., 476a

three great i. from Ireland, 332b

Inventiveness smothered by poor method, 526a

Inventor, many an i. sounder philosopher, 470a

work of i. of word, 610b

Inverse, common sense in i. ratio to education, 331a

Investigate, necessary to i. to prevent depravity, 465a

Investigated, phenomena i. at different levels, 508b

Investigates, prefer scholar who i. limited field, 501b

Investigation and practice one, 616b

difficulties by i. of natural phenomena, 454a

fallacy elude other species of i., 525b

means of i. now hidden, 462b

motives, 506b

no i. true science without mathematical tests, 482a

of neglected doctrine, 500a

of rarer forms of disease, 498a

promulgation exciting i., 668b

removing hindrance to immediate i., 576a

until forty, 348a

Investigations, ascertain what i. already done, 509a

follow workings of mind through i., 500a

goal of i. recognition of truth, 502b

imagination needed at beginning of i., 526b

latest i. safeguard of practice, 616b

of problem in all directions, 501b

Investigative, difficult to keep abreast of i. reports, 595a

more eminent less i. work, 614a

Investigator, discovery not monopoly of i., 109b

every physician clinical i., 251a

greatness of scientific i., 251a

may dwell in garret, 504b

neglects control, 116b

nor practitioner blinded by prejudice, 528a

observes experiments judges, 528a

reported that rat got away, 569a

should be independent, 250b

surgical i. bridgetender, 592a

worth of i. pursuing what did not seek, 501b

Investigator's obligation to make fact known, 63b

Investigators, few recount labours of i., 503b

how many brilliant i. wretched teachers, 600b

in search for truth, 528a

make you great, 223a

motive attracting i., 108a

personal characteristics of i., 250b

settled for what measurable, 509b

Investment, headache at sharpest seems bad i., 200a

Investment, no finer i. for community, 53a

Investments, more than capitalist over i., 204b

Invigorator of body is exercise, 165b

Invited, consulted Hunter in hope of i. to assemblies, 657a

Involuntary, muscles actions of which i., 318b

voluntary and i. movement, 46b

Inward, who put wisdom in i. parts, 656a

wound that bleedeth i. most dangerous, 665a

Ions, peering through maze of hydrogen i., 303b

Ipecac, rhubarb scarce i. high, 434a

I.Q.'s combining so beautifully, 213a

Irascible, man of i. temperament, 236a

Ireland, diseases of I. many, 111a

three great inventions from I., 332b

Irish, dialogue in I. dialect, 669a

over head and ears in I. claret, 193b

throw spirits into I. Channel, 9a

Irishman, give I. lager for month, 9a

lined with copper, 9a

said I. if I take stone to Heaven, 395b

Iron, band of i. in band of gold, 167a

of crown more valuable than gold, 167a

rusts from disuse, 234a

Iron Virgin, mercy from I., 198a

Ironing, patients assist in i., 222a

Irons, merit in multiplicity of hot i., 594a

seared with hot i., 634a

Iroquois, poisoned arrows of I., 185a

Irrational, insanity during crime required i. behaviour, 245a

side to behavior, 145a

subconscious self i., 469b

surgery seeded with i. beliefs, 597b

Irrationally held truths more harmful, 151b, 640b

Irregular, nature contriving i. parts, 316a

Irremediable, amount of i. disease enormous, 237b

Irritability, decrease i. of patient, 367b

sickness adds to i., 364a

theory of i., 231a

Irritable nerves of invalid, 249a

Irritation, another man's disappointment allays i., 282a

reducing i. of antiseptic, 20a

with things of present, 229b

Irritations, vague terms as i., 610a

Isaac old eyes dim, 33a

Ischia, tuberosities of the i., 16a

Ischuria, most dangerous i., 253a

Island, no man i., 284b

Islands, no coral i. if first bug wonder how, 663b

Isolation, aura of i. in childbirth, 55a

Israel, of stock of I., 59b

Issue, children bury and sow fresh i., 284a

following i. full-term, 449a

Italian, belladonna in I. lady, 124b

draughts of I. wine, 187b

every I. doctor, 386b

woman preparing frogs' legs, 109a

Italy, lascivious friars in I., 102b

syphilis brought to I. by soldiers, 649b

Itch, difficult to stand i., 252a

disease scarcely keep pace with i. to scribble, 667b

faith in Lord but sulphur for i., 252a

for writing and making name, 666b

more intolerable than smart, 252a

not to be concealed, 70a

of litterature comes over man, 66ga

old as the i., 252a

pleasing to touch, 251b

rubbing i. of your opinion, 252a

unguent to take away i., 126a

would thou didst i. from head to foot, 252a

Itched, elbow i. thought scab follow, 252a

Itches, better than riches to scratch when i., 252a, 532b

sow Athenian bosoms, 262b

Itching, good for physician to have i. piles, 403b

violent i. without eruption, 252b

J

Jack and Jill, 496b

Jack Sprat loved no fat, 105a

Jackass, doctor j. when no longer on terms, 381a

Jackson, Andrew, 543b

Jackson, Samuel J. said rest panacea, 181b

Jacobeus, I believe in J., 644b

Jade, pulse like string of red j., 208b

Jahresbericht, looking through J., 671a

Jails, society pay greater bill by j., 476b

James I laughs at medicine, 295a

Janitor, mentally sick lucky if j. comes, 246a

January, in J. glass of wine, 188a

Jar of person walking in room, 189b

Jargon, answers couched in extraordinary j., 609b

murders with j. where med'cine fails, 393b

of scientific terminology, 611a

sociologists and financial experts have j., 611b

Jastrow, Joseph, 262a

Jaundice and catarrh, 668b

disease your friends diagnose. 252a

grief set j. o'er cheeks, 252a

itching without eruption familiar to j., 252b

Killing, Sicilians ended by k. patient, 152b

yourself by degrees, 662b

Kills, amusing patient until nature k. or cures, 295b

bad doctor k. you no appeal, 379b

doctor k. earth hides, 386b

doctor k. more than general, 393b

first insults victim he k., 480b

gout k. more rich than poor, 189b

if he operates and k. patient, 578a

millions medicine k. would live, 630b

near relative, 579b

not work k. but worry, 665a

nothing k. like doing nothing, 639a

physician k. us priest sings, 456a

quartan ague k. old, 181b

rat or only child, 183b

self to avoid misery, 580a

who k. thousand half a doctor, ·398a

worse is he who k. self, 579b

Kimmelstiel-Wilson lesion, 417a

Kin, mole above chin never beholden to k., 551a

one of k. has weak pia mater, 244a

Kind, cannot be clever always be k., 403a

heart always inestimable, 401a

prefer k. doctor to efficient, 369a

Kindest man ever known medical, 389a

Kindliness, losing finer edge of k., 330b

Kindly, age frosty but k., 342a

as many k. old specialists, 369b

scientific spirit make modest and k., 454a

Kindness, don't kill sick with k., 629b

follow objects of profession in k., 410b

for k. they remain in debt, 175b

here you will find human k., 220b

our work's unembarrassed k., 412a

to k. promises only, 356a

King, Dr. K. bled him with pocket knife, 635b

King, ague in spring physic for k., 181b

among blind one-eyed k., 33a

body of woman heart of k., 36b

care for K. better than poor, 327b

diseases affecting k., 236a

gains freedom from doctors, 395a

God bless the k., 433a

hath heavy reckoning, 81a

he shall receive honour of K., 390a

he that is drunk great as k., 11b

health to Englands K., 487a

healthy man k., 208a

languishes of fistula, 182a

King, miraculous work in good k., 74a

of topics operations, 350b

open medical career with permission of k., 398b

touch many attacked by ailment, 73b

King's, caught cold ringing in K. affairs, 61a

death of K. disease, 417b

Kings, care for poor as for k., 327b

Kinsey, O God O K. O Jehoshaphat, 541b

Kinship, by likeness k. show, 210a

Kirk, physic not work prepare for k., 238b

Kiss, coffee sweet like k., 60b

definition of k., 314a

place to make well, 495a

Kisses, straight on k. dream, 182a

those who smoke have k. for smoker, 624a

Kissing, saw her k. last lover, 149a

understanding between men and women k. in dark, 540a

Kitchen, chief physic comes from k., 101b

good apothecary's shop, 102a

in inward parts of men, 620b

lighted hall reached through ghastly k., 500b

physic best, 103a

relinquish flirting with sirens of k., 198a

smoke becomes k. better than dining chamber, 620b

Kitchens, in k. reformation must be, 103b

Knee a joint not entertainment, 16a

by painefull k. guesse what weather be, 513b

facts on wise man's k., 171a

got water on k., 310a

sing to child on thy k., 79b

Knee jerk remained in spite of *patellar reflex*, 611a

Knee jerks, examine his k., 207a

Knees, his k. knocking each other, 242b

wine mine its way through k., 197b

Knell of thirtieth year sounded, 291a

ring out doleful k., 88a

Knew, if youth only k., 417a

what once k. little consequence, 255a

Knife, Brutus drew murd'rous k., 34a

by k. churchyard fills, 392a

carpenter asks for the k., 625b

Death's indifferent hand drives home, 436b

dip k. in it, 438b

diseases cured by k., 110b

happier using k. than trying to save limb, 587a

in patients arme, 35b

malady needs the k., 593a

not always have fields for conquest, 595a

patients would not allow k., 567b

people which contrived Bowie k., 443b

Knife, surgeon uses k. physician prescribes medicines, 385b, 592b

use k. to cure moral necrosis, 152a

waiting for the k., 17b

Knight, French k. that cow'rs i' hams, 650b

what can ail thee k. at arms, 433b

Knights, blistered k. of Middle Ages, 185a

Knits, sleep that k. sleave of care, 552b

Knitting, medical practice not k. and weaving, 442a

Knives, crimped with k., 634a

Knobs size of pea upon fingers, 198b

Knock, every k. at door is alarm, 346b

find what patient likes most k. him off it, 635b

Knocker, tie up k., 174a

Know, all answers except I do not k., 531b

be sure you k. truth and patient wants to hear, 641a

divest of everything we suppose k., 254b

express selves upon sciences about which k. nothing, 529a

few k. how to be old, 338a

formula I do not k., 255b

Galen well patient not at all, 406b

grey hair makes appear k. more, 403b

healthy are sick who don't k. it, 207a

I do not k. stick in physician's throat, 235a

man of seventy assume to k. all, 347b

many things ye k. sires knew not, 463a

more than able to wield, 254b

never pretend to k. what cannot be known, 400b

nor physician work cures on who k. him, 370a

not k. them because name them, 612a

not that doctors don't k. enough, 335a

not to guess but to k., 408a

nothing but itself to k. itself, 313a

occupy minds with what continue to k., 255a

older doctor is more pretend to k. everything, 416b

papers tell what we k. in complicated manner, 275a

poetry for those who k., 523b

really k. very little, 454a

refrain from doing things because k. how, 637a

say to fellow students I do not k., 600b

teach tongue to say I do not k., 655b

that we k. hindrance to learning, 255b

to k. consists in opening way, 640b

what don't k. won't hurt poor principle, 228a

where not k. be cautious, 65a

Man, only One M. upon earth, 85a
passage for food, 28a
passes seed into womb, 64a
pattern of neural activity, 287b
physician must view m. in world, 361a
possesses sexual organs, 540a
prisoner has no right to run away, 579a
proper study of mankind m., 285a
protagonists m. and nature, 503b
put m. in circle with skunk, 162b
rather talk with m. than angel, 660a
reasoning animal, 284a
recovered of bite dog died, 483b
reveal figure of m. in words, 13b
science bestowed immense powers on m., 521b
science of m. no different from other sciences, 471a
scientist pontificate about M., 531a
sex more important in woman than m., 661b
show me m. who needs Medicare, 292b
six hours' sleep for m., 556a
still Faustus and a m., 378a
strength of sexual impulse in m., 540a
such as m. made of, 286a
suicide best gift to m., 579b
support to spiritual nature of m., 161a
task of science never end till m. ceases, 520b
that is born of woman, 92a
that is m. which is going to be one, 1b
that which distinguishes m. from beast, 539a
theory that denies Creation of m. as in Bible, 163b
thinking and feeling in opposition in m., 145a
this is m. doctor should know and treat, 366b
three events concern m., 29b, 269b
thus become real m., 409b
to whom death of fellow-creatures amusing, 314b
took medicine like m., 286a
true study of m. is m., 284a
unlawful to teach that m. descended from lower animals, 163b
victim of blood sugar, 94b
viewless beings live like m., 307b
wants little here below, 285a
what a m. gout makes, 188a
what are you a m., 284a
what incomprehensible machine is m., 285b
what may be wrought upon body of m., 497b
wheel in machine of civilisation, 93a
where m. who out of danger, 255b
why has m. not microscopic eye, 169b

Man without woman head without body, 541b
woman's desire for desire of m., 539b
you detached no longer m., 284b
Managers, felt as m. about plays, 275a
Mandamus of death binds all, 92b
Mandible, brimstone and gunpowder with butter rub m., 605b
Mandragora, give me m., 121b
not poppy nor m., 122a
Mange of pig destroys herd, 240a
Manhood is struggle, 4a
period of life, 4a
poisons genial love and m. stains, 539a
sickness breaks down pride of m., 544b
sins of m., 56b
Manipulative, correction by m. measures, 72b
Manipulator, thank God not dextrous m., 107b
Mankind advancing man always same, 265b
arrive at decisions that benefit m., 455a
ask but folly of m., 84b
at large for enemies, 58b
best interests of m., 71b
better for m. worse for fishes, 124b
contempt profession must give of m., 388b
distempers among m. living close, 5a
eats twice as much, 130b
enable to relieve burden of m., 504b
encompass aspirations of m., 288a
establish permanent mating relationship, 288b
future of m. depends upon better minds, 186a
get along without all those names, 609b
greater blessing to m. than medicine, 295a
I am involved in m., 78a
if doctors destroy revenue for good of m., 648b
immense importance to welfare of m., 503a
in original perus'd m., 135a
insight into humours of m., 177a
insist on pouring draught down throats of m., 321b
medicine greatest boon to m., 304a
medicine second of benefit to m., 296a
misery of m. want of control over conditions, 450b
mistake indigestion for concern for salvation of m., 239b
more fatal than useful to m., 124a
outlook of m. immeasurably larger, 464a
problems whose solution important to m., 499a
profit from gifted it produces, 234a
promote health of m., 521b

Mankind, proper study of m. is man, 285a
science serving m. humanism, 368a
sorry intellect endowed five-sixths of m., 309b
two classes of m. doctors and patients, 374b, 383a
under pain and pleasure, 431a
united aims of noblest of m., 298a
we fail m., 414a
wine pernicious to m., 5a
work cure of all maladies that beset m., 663a
Manly, brings m. mind from heights, 538a
not m. to fear sweat, 598a
voice toward childish treble, 344b
Manner, pray for quiet m., 402b
sympathizing should be m., 365a
Manners, limbs halt lamely as m., 515b
physicians had courtly m., 27a
plain manly fashion in m., 400a
scientists have odious m., 530a
truth in spight of m. told, 338a
Man's bane or benison, 183b
body from lower animal form, 161a
desire for woman, 539b
dignity to value ideals above life, 287b
dung heals wounds, 492b
might understand m. destiny, 235a
new system to compose, 211a
nothing so difficult as m. experience, 167a
speculation concerning m. fate, 469b
tune harp of m. body, 295a
woman's mind cleaner than m., 661a
woman's sense of reality less than m., 661b
Mansion, divinely built m. as body, 37a
Mansions, medicine house of many m., 304a
Manslaughter, rational yet commit m., 245a
Manuscript, nature universal and publik m., 316a
Manuscripts, American mind reflected in m., 274a
she copying my m., 656b
Map, I their m. lie on this bed, 360a
Marasmus, wherein were laid m., 218a
March, in M. mix sweets, 188a
mad as M. hare, 247a
Marcus, physician M. laid hand on stone Zeus, 390b
Marines, post M. to guard him, 207a
Marital, doctor's wife have m. felicity, 657b
Mark, come into world with m. of descent, 211a
physicians themselves bear disease's m., 415a
try shot frequently hit m., 506b
Market, fell down in m. place, 534a
science comes from m., 523b

Medicine, not that good in organized m., 154a
nothing in m. insignificant, 334b
now separates bacillus, 308a
obligation of m. sacred, 301b
obligations to m. beyond measurement, 298a
observation nowhere more difficult than m., 335b
occupation for slaves, 296b
of m. believe bad or good, 627b
of which know little, 394a
old as human race, 298b
old student scarcely recognizes Dame M., 299a
older in m. more chary about prognoses, 461a
oldest learned profession, 464b
one experiment in m. to convince self, 505b
one m. cure various kinds, 478b
one of greatest follies, 392a
one of nine low trades, 304b
only m. for foot is rest, 189a
only world-wide profession, 300b
ought to be rational, 48b
Pantagruel thought of studying m., 392a
part of m. little attended to, 471b
particularly true of clinical m., 577a
patience best m., 359a, 359b
patient has no right to all m., 365a
patients would not allow m., 567b
perfect sight of old m., 635b
philosophic minds tend to experimental m., 589a
physician concerned with science of m., 369b
physician patient m. nurses factors of treatment, 625a
physician unversed in science of m., 303b
physician versed in science of m., 398b
physicians loathe m., 414b
physiology stepchild of m., 427b
place of m. in stream of life, 302a
played with cards under table, 156a
plead for more cultural side in m., 331b
pleasure which has no equal from m., 296b
Plutus knows multiplying m., 628b
poisons and m. often same, 124a, 440a
practical m. application of scientific m., 299a
practice of m. all or none, 445a
practice of m. art not trade, 444a
practice of m. become ineffective, 444b
practice of m. lonely road, 444a
practice of m. often choleric business, 444a
practice of m. perpetual compromise, 443b
practice of m. thinker's art, 596b

Medicine, practice of m. would win benefits, 174b
praised in physition of experience, 399b
preached principles of scientific work, 518b
prepared for study of m., 135b
present m. reproach to professors, 632b
present system of m. educate diseases, 110b
preserving life in m. potable, 628b
pressed to verge of destroying life, 264b
priesthood in m., 154a
profession for social service, 561b
professions for gentleman added m., 459a
professor of clinical m. or pathology, 250b
progress in m., 20b
progress of m. wonderful, 464a
promise health to sick, 294a
proper m. produces similar symptoms, 71b
prophylactic meaning precautionary m., 451b
psychiatry called plot against m., 385a
psychiatry shown tendencies to devour m., 466a
purposefully acting science, 168b
quacks in m. religion politics, 480b
qualities of good teacher of m., 602a
reaches highest ideal in m., 402a
reading of men in m., 577a
ready money ready m., 134a
real satisfaction in practice of m., 445a
reasons for m. perpetual, 296a
regards nothing essential but truth, 641a
regimen superior to m., 488a
removes bestows safety, 626a
render student of m. discriminating, 275a
require help of m. disgrace, 110b
rescue practice of m. from drugging, 272b
restored with advice and m., 628b
rules as expounded in books on m., 226b
sacred calling, 300b
safest for patient in hands of man teaching m., 601a
said master word of m. work, 302b
scene of disunited effort, 301b
scheme of things drags along m., 315b
science and art of m. little understood, 589b
science important to practice of m., 303b
science in the making, 297b
science must accompany modern m., 300b
science of agencies healthful and harmful, 294a
science of m. based on assumption, 317a

Medicine science of uncertainty art of probability, 300b
scientific specialized costly, 303a
scientists go to m. for principles, 48b
second of benefit to mankind, 296a
secrets of m. revealed, 143b
sensitive to outside influences, 298b
shall m. thee to sleep, 122a
should enable to live out lives, 86a
should not be in clinical m., 603b
sighing no m., 563b
skill in m. in timing remedies, 194a
sleep better than m., 556a
sleep only m. that gives ease, 551a
so emaciated as not able to swallow m., 236b
so powerful m. labour, 662b
social science, 561b
socialized m. used to confuse, 476a
some shapen in m., 382a
sought admission to study of m., 403b
sovereign m. and sheet-anchor, 165b
specialisms bad for soul of m., 566b
specialized and access uneven, 566b
split between scientific and practical m., 616a
state of m. worse than total ignorance, 254b
sterile unproductive heath, 300b
stick to m. for good, 393a
still ineffectual speculation, 297b
stone flung down Bowery, 125a
student forever excluded from art of m., 141a
study and practice m. in proper manner, 297a
studying m. never through, 261a
success in m. selfish, 578b
such m. hopelessly unscientific, 636a
such men never worth anything for m., 670a
superstition and m. incompatible, 300a
sure foundations of m., 296b
surgeon know m. philosophy logic, 583b
surgeon know principles of m., 584a
surgeon nothing if ignorant of m., 583b
surgery most important of science of m., 593a
surgery salvation of inner m., 587b
surgery superior to m., 593a
surprise to patients I know m., 360b
take dose of m. once, 631b
takes m. and neglects diet, 105b
task of m., 562a
task of m. to promote health, 452b
teach disciples bound according to law of m., 325b
teachers of m. in Paris, 144a

Melancholy, what charm can soothe her m., 433b
  wherein were laid moaping m., 218a
  wine taketh away hurt of m., 6b
Mellhorn, Doc M. asked what like first, 419b
Mellon, give Andy M. part of revenues, 333a
Melon, doctors eat m., 102a
Melt, too solid flesh m., 579b
Member, nature of evrye m., 15a
Members, body's m. rebell'd against belly, 571a
  heart most noble of m., 209a
  refused assistance to body, 571a
  revolted against belly, 571a
Membrane is so irritable, 13a
  nutriment reaches to m., 324b
  possibility plasma m. part of cell, 653a
Membranes, if nose m. feel irritation hold breath, 560b
Memoirs which fill libraries, 503b
Memories, balance of forces in which m., 287a
  balsam of our m., 172b
  burden of one's m., 348b
  utopias m. of Arcadias, 257a
Memory, begot in ventricle of m., 243b
  causes everything past seem present, 619b
  everyone complains of m., 151a
  exercised by nerves, 318b
  facts strewed floor of m., 609b
  fails vigour fled, 342b
  his m. decays, 535b
  inaccessible in lumber-room of m., 334b
  is fair and bright, 78a
  lends light no more, 346b
  oblivion deals with m. of men, 172b
  of man dies with death, 172b
  of man float to posterity, 172b
  pluck from m. rooted sorrow, 244a
  poetry strays into m., 41b
  pray for good m., 402b
  save from lapses of m., 447a
  shrug and say his m. going, 536a
  spanking penetrated to m., 57b
  thou fond deceiver, 433a
  to record and recall, 96b
  too much attention to m., 140b
  unconscious m. of nature, 172b
  unforeseen indelibly in m., 137a
  uses not intellect but m., 485a
  weed poisoner of m., 623b
  written something which escaped m., 273a
Men about me that are fat, 326a
  above common herd, 389a
  all women mothers of great m., 290a
  always to selves young m. and women, 675b
  American m. at thirty, 16b
  and women agree only in conclusions, 539b
  and women in instruction for medical profession, 661b
  aspect of m. widely different, 59b
  at thirty lost vivacity, 290b
  before thirty m. seek diseases, 117a

Men born of woman have navel, 318a
  born with indelible character, 211b
  children of larger growth, 285a
  Christ of m. most perfect, 448a
  doctor sees m. as they are, 459b
  drunkenness unmans m., 7a
  engendered inside fish, 160a
  girls and m. enter dissecting room together, 661b
  God give us m., 434b
  great m. not discovered for fifty years, 173a
  happiness for most m. motive, 286b
  have broad chests narrow hips, 538b
  helpers of m. they're call'd, 379b
  how many m. die, 64b
  husband different from other m., 657b
  hypochondriac affection in m., 229b
  hysteric globe scarcely among m., 319a
  in company of m. play part of m., 659a
  in m. nine of ten tumours malignant, 47b, 448a
  lose minds look less lost than women, 246b
  many m. cut out of womb, 54b
  match m. in passions, 659a
  melancholy made for m., 305a
  more affected with scirrhous livers, 276a
  more than war's destroyer of m., 235a
  more things to admire in m. than to despise, 430a
  narrow twisted m., 537b
  Nature includes m. and ways, 137b
  neither m. nor times out of temper, 328a
  nine of ten m. have piles, 428a
  not individuals but components, 85a
  not treat women unless m. present, 325a
  observations of no more worth than of m., 469a
  of science want fair day's wages, 133a
  old m. look alike, 337b
  ordinary m. experience no fear of death, 79b
  pampered race of m., 165a
  possession of gods, 579a
  prefer to believe they are degenerated angels, 162a
  principles which have guided great m., 422b
  say she doesn't think at all, 661b
  scheme of things takes care of m., 315b
  seen m. as medical student, 671b
  seldom make passes, 549a
  should keep close, 29b
  six m. give doctor less to do than woman, 661b
  smooth and nicely rounded m., 537b
  some m. called to be doctors, 382a

Men, sorry for m. their dull way of dressing, 246b
  suffer diseases of m., 659a
  suffering made less than m., 579a
  take diseases one of another, 240a
  talk at random, 62b
  they fail to give us m., 394b
  think all mortal but themselves, 78b
  thus m. and know not how, 285a
  very queer animals, 286a
  vitalizing principle in university m., 139a
  walk women talk after supper, 659b
  wealth accumulates m. decay, 433a
  what m. in women require, 539a
  wise in proportion to capacity for experience, 167a
  women as afraid of death as m., 80a
  worry over diseases, 110b, 492a
Menace, man becomes public m., 167b
Mending, need no m., 263b
Menenius concluded with fable, 571a
Mens sana in corpore sano, 41b
Menses, after m. subject to piles, 428a
  not take gout unless m. stopped, 186b
Menstrua, obstruction of m. in women, 642b
Menstrual, history of missed m. period, 64a
Menstruates once a month, 661a
Menstruation begin before ceases to be virgin, 652a
Mental, adapt knowledge as part of m. organization, 484a
  advancement of knowledge of m. disease, 469a
  anthology medicine for m. disorders, 473b
  apprehension in dying, 85b
  attitude antagonistic to foreign, 331a
  cause and effect m., 72a
  characteristics of women, 468b
  concession to bodily weakness not m., 641a
  conditions symbols, 41b
  contact with type-metal, 669a
  correlate symptoms with overall m. disorder, 468a
  drug contribute to m. effervescence, 645a
  energy into m. state, 42a
  evaluate thinking about m. illness, 246b
  experience leaves m. scars, 167b
  exposing unconscious basis of m. attitudes, 470b
  failing of faculties m. and physical, 348b
  great source of m. day, 517a
  habits independent of initial m. force, 212a
  incapacity matters of national concern, 477b
  influence of m. on corporeal, 471b

Mental, lacks m. balance in and without pneumonia, 246a

manifestations, 45a

more difficult case if m. effect, 297b

national m. health program, 246b

national program to combat m. retardation, 246b

no disease bodily or m. vegetable diet not mitigated, 649a

not accompanied by advance in m. faculties, 464b

not best for wide m. vision, 381b

obesity m. state, 327a

open about flagrant m. diseases, 545b

opium contribute to m. effervescence, 352b

part of m. disease, 115a

patient in need of m. comfort, 230b

penetrating into patient's m. life, 366b

physical fitness goes with m., 182b

powers exercised by nerves, 318b

probable descendants suffer m. defect, 570a

reading often m. dissipation, 484a

reversal in approach to m. affliction, 246b

Rush's ideas about m. health, 425b

sacrifice m. independence, 184b

science has being in m. restlessness, 522a

senior citizens in obsolete m. institutions, 349a

sharpening of m. edge, 31b

tranquilizers affect m. patients, 126a

understanding m. state of patient, 368a

Mentality of teaching profession, 565b

Mentally, prohibit marriage of m. unfit, 158b

shabby treatment of m. disabled, 246b

sick lucky if janitor comes, 246a

Mentor, physician take up position as m., 465b

Merchant, every German m., 386b

loses power to enjoy, 137a

on conquering ship stood m., 458a

Merchants, doctors begun to act like m., 385b

Mercies have their commissions, 222b

Merciful, life taken in most m. manner, 159a

Mercuric, hatters exposed to m. nitrate, 247a

Mercury, hot spring raises m. to 112 degrees, 225a

in theory of m. I opposed Rush, 425a

rational system armed with m., 616b

repletion by m., 231a

two minutes with Venus two years with m., 651b

Mercy from Iron Virgin, 198a

pity for others styled m., 563a

Mercy, trained nurse seeketh him at her m., 324a

transient claim for m., 289b

Merit, oblivion deals without distinction to m., 172b

spurns patient merit takes, 580a

Merits, examine suggestions on m., 251b

Merry, grin so m. draws nail out of coffin, 51b, 664b

heart doeth good, 52a

to bedwarde be you m., 552a

Merryman, best physicians Diet Quiet M., 386b

use three physicians Quiet M. Dyet, 487a

Mescaline, give me m., 126b

Message hands bear to patient, 385a

Messenger, pain m. of harm, 357a

Met, indigestion common-place for people that never m., 239a

part of all I m., 286a

Metabolic, derangements of m. processes, 307a

woe, 198a

Metabolism, complexities of m., 267b

continuous movement, 307a

intermediate processes of m., 307a

intermediate products in m., 307a

intermediate steps of m., 307a

Metal, dentist putting m. in mouth pulls coins out of pocket, 605a

lead-poisoning through type-m., 669a

Metals, infusions in vegetives m. stones, 628b

precious m. mixed with dross, 639b

Metaphysical concept prevalent among medical scientists, 486b

no progress until shaken off m., 469a

rational system not in m. vacuum, 616b

Metaphysicians usually not polite, 67b

Metaphysics, for philosophers pain problem of m., 357a

may have use, 26b

science not exist without m., 521a

Meteorological phenomena exert influence, 146b

Meteors, cannot explain m., 146b

Method, all m. imperfect, 152b

believe belief replaced by scientific m., 528b

determine virtues of new m., 637a

discovered m. of treating, 48b

experimental m. living philosophy, 424b

first comes improved m., 463b

influences of physical and chemical m., 566a

inventiveness smothered by poor m., 526a

lack of interest in m., 301b

madness yet m. in't, 243a

never strayed from your m. never saved patient, 417b

no conception of scientific m., 528a

Method of research invariably same, 527a

of teaching art of healing, 462a

progress of experimental m., 462b

scientific m. in practice, 616a

take m. and try it, 168b

virtue of m. make successful, 223a

watched what m. Nature take, 316a

with which unconscious studied, 467b

Methodical, developmental research by m. scientist, 509a

Methodists, therapeutics of m. from pathology, 232a

Methodology, problems for which m. not existent, 531b

Methods, achievers using established m., 531b

change from age to age, 384b

common to medical profession, 457b

cure by tried m., 157a

distinguished in practice not reject m., 400a

following everywhere same m., 300b

give student good m., 138a

give student power to use m., 139b

good m. teach to develop faculties, 526a

ignorant of surgeon's m., 586b

Lister altered m., 20a

more happy and successful m., 67b

must find right m., 251a

new m. work miracles for while, 630a

no art change m. oftener than medicine, 294a

not ashamed to change m., 520b

not content to imitate m., 463b

of which not know all secrets, 574b

results of new m., 477b

Methuselah, days of M. nine hundred sixty and nine, 280b

sees M. ahead of him, 337b

slept in open air, 279b

Methuselites, must we be M., 280b

Metropolis, responsibility diminished in m., 360b

Metropolitan, Great M. Fallacy, 361a

Michaelmas, forty times M. pass, 309b

Microbe, inoculation of m. in guinea pig, 20b

keeps m. in box, 397a

so very small, 308a

two to make disease m. and host, 241a

Microbes, acquired fear of m., 308b

doubt unwholesome refreshment except m., 307b

more virulent than m. idea that one is ill, 472a

watch m. and nurses, 447a

Microcosm, I am m. or little world, 328a

meeting with salt of our m., 429b

Mind, flashed upon m. unforeseen, 267a
follow workings of m. through investigations, 500a
free from maladies of m., 295b
functions of m. dependent upon body, 469a
functions when no phenomenon, 669b
general culture of m. best aid, 137a
Goldsmith asked if m. at rest, 258b
greatest derangement of m., 502a
greatness of m. ability to examine honestly, 497a
grows constipated as grows old, 344b
growth of American m. in medicine, 274a
habits of m. independent, 212a
hard work give peace to m., 511a
hardly sees anything without instruction, 313a
has mountains, 313a
health condition of m., 41a
health lightens efforts of m., 204b
how little know of m., 235a
hypothesis that occupied m. of author, 667b
ideal prototype has open m., 403b
ideas presented to m., 44b
ill health of m. defeat, 205a
illness from affliction of m., 471b
ills more severe in m. than body, 39a
imagination takes possession of m. unoccupied, 234b
in disease wandering m. often found, 93b
in diseases of m., 123b
in disturbed m. sanity can not be, 242a
in his right m., 314a
in right m. unable to cope, 246a
in sickness m. reflects upon self, 541b
in theory bear it in m., 319b
inability to comprehend state of m., 256a
inaction sap vigour of m., 234b
incompetence of m. to observe without prejudice, 445a
insanity logic of m. overtasked, 245a
instrument by which ideas presented to m., 312b
intellectual and moral qualities of m., 285b
keep m. free to give up hypothesis, 232a
last infirmity of noble m., 172b
learning disposeth m. capable of growth, 260a
lectures temptation to contemplative m., 261b
libraries cradles and sepulchres of m., 263a
life use of m., 264a
like body healed, 311b
like physicke ministred to m., 472b
likes strange idea little, 234a

Mind, long as body affected through m., 171b
make *tabula rasa* of m., 335b
make up m. about nothing, 313a
making up m. not believe what you want, 485b
man above all m. of man, 366b
man with slightest power of m., 309b
many supposed to have sound m., 40b
master surgeon man of m., 588a
matter secreted by brain, 313a
may affect body, 41a
medicine in development of m., 214a
medicine task powers of body and m., 457a
medicine unites laws which apply to body and m., 561a
melancholy commotion of m., 305b
members trained to fulfillment of wishes of m., 583b
minister to m. diseas'd, 243b
more thing knows own m. more living, 313a
most abhorrent body without m., 536a
most important instrument in research m., 509a
movement of m. toward discovery, 108a
muddleheadedness proper state of m., 529a
narrowness of student's m., 564b
nature commands m. suffer with body, 243b
nature of the m., 39b
necessary weakness of m., 501a
necessity of human m., 614a
never know how m. acts on matter, 312b
no better in m. than body, 39a
no method of controlling m., 313a
noble m. here o'erthrown, 243a
nobler in m. to suffer slings, 580a
not enough attention to m., 140b
not for awing human m. to distrust own vision, 517a
not m. diseased, 64b
not of sound m., 247a
nursing vexation of m., 322a
object to rouse m., 136b
observation of nature requires purity of m., 334b
of man working at best, 222a
of Sydenham not operate differently from Galileo, 528a
only knowledge which satisfies m., 255a
pain of m. worse than of body, 314a
passions of m. exercised by nerves, 318b
passions of m. nonnatural things, 279a
philosophers find diseases of m., 95a
philosophy regards to m., 296a
physician heal his m., 410a
pictures depicted by m. on body, 181b
piercing searchlight, 314a

Mind prepared before study of surgery, 585b
preserved in vigour, 39b
priesthood state of m., 154a
prolong youth of m., 339b
proud and intolerant m., 501a
psychiatrist obstetrician of m., 467a
pursuit of development of m., 214a
quickened by pain, 354a
rather accurate than exalted, 388b
rational society informs m., 264a
requisites for improving m., 663a
research state of m., 503b, 505a
research worker keep m. malleable, 251b
saneness of m. has for basis tranquillity, 242a
scintillate in brilliant fashion, 262a
searching into Nature inlarges m., 316b
seem occupied with transitory, 312a
sensation connection of m. with world, 41b
separates vulgar from superior m., 255a
sick in m. rendered more so, 245a
sick m. affects limbs, 653b
sicker in body and m. for present, 544a
sickly body sickly m., 42b
siege of death against m., 93b
skepticism opposed to progress of m., 549b
slave of preconceived ideas, 423a
soothe troubled m., 370b
sorrows of m. breed corrupt humours, 189a
sound body product of sound m., 41b
sound m. in sound body, 39b
start from nature with open m., 315b
state of m. philosophers term insanity, 242a
strength of m., 40a
strength of m. greater than body, 39a
strong body makes m. strong, 40b
structure of Sydenham's m., 426a
student's m. must be strong, 136a
study of human m., 465a
stuff for disorderliness of m., 473a
stupid substitutes for divine M., 495b
stupor, 61b
sudden epilepsies seize m., 211a
taints by long sitting, 313a
that which enters m. through reason, 172a, 485a
that which treats diseases of m., 471b
theater for interplay of forces, 366b
theology charlatanerie of m., 615b

North Pole, still look like N., 430b

Northern lights, cannot explain n., 146b

Nose, between n. and eyes strange contest, 548b
custom hateful to n., 621a
Cyrano de Cognac n., 321a
down with the n., 651a
drink provokes n. painting, 6a, 647a
fell a-bleeding Black Monday, 320b
holds n. and drinks, 123b
if alive will scratch n., 95a
if n. membranes feel irritation hold breath, 560b
linen by which n. held fast, 598a
make and remake n., 276a
of Mrs. Gamp red and swollen, 310a
Panacea turned head holding n., 182b
pray that mucus in n. not run, 320b
pug-n. betrays character, 49b
slam door on doctor's n., 227a
spectacles on n. pouch on side, 344b
treatment for broken n., 598a
uterus like n. on one side, 230a
venerable man with purple n., 321a
who gave thee jolly red n., 321a
wipe n. and not blame God, 320b
wringing of n. bringeth blood, 321a

Noses blossom as lobster, 321a
blowing smoke into other people's n., 621b
rubicund n., 224b

Nosographer not always clinician, 96b

Nosography description of regular phenomena, 96b

Nosologically, effects of treatment upon disease n., 168a

Nosology, class sick man in n., 96a

Nostalgia frequent disease in army, 217a

Nostrils, apply onion to n., 95a
old men suffer watery discharge from n., 344a
plugs of linen inside n., 598a
solution of opium to n., 13a
stretched with struggling, 314b

Nostrum, ignorant physician believes n. vendor, 428a
placebo giving fosters n. evil, 428b

Nostrums, presentations of educational n., 142a

Note and record unusual, 670b
down all I see, 283b

Notebook, student-practitioner requires n., 138b

Notes, never miss death n. in papers, 340a
publish short n. on new, 670b
read several times and make n., 484b

Nothing, better know n. than keep fixed ideas, 500b
better to do n., 632a
clinician knows n. about everything, 60b

Nothing, consulted safety of patient by doing n., 629b
did n. because thought n. could be done, 262b
die of things we know n. about, 86b
do right thing or n., 634a
good remedy sometimes to use n., 492a
in excess, 607b
kills like doing n., 639a
nicest people say n., 670b
on six days decided to do n., 62a
physician at loss do n., 632b
physician heals for n. worth n., 178b
researcher knows everything about n., 60b
sometimes give services for n., 49b
working for n. half tam' mebbe, 412a

Nothingness, it will never pass into n., 433b

Notice, if n. out of work when I am gone, 259b

Notions, words symbols of n., 276b

Notoriety, Andrew Jackson ravenous of n., 543b

Nouns of multitude, 613a

Nourish, starve measles n. smallpox, 291b, 560b
stomach receive meats that n., 324b
way of dealing with breasts that n., 56a

Nourished, men n. inside fish, 160a
with what body n., 106a

Nourisher, chief n. in life's feast, 552b

Nourishes, what one relishes n., 105b

Nourishing, nipples not for n. children, 659a

Nourishment, agriculture promises n., 294a
belly send n. back again, 571a
call for n. in body, 571b
fault of n., 124b
of other parts of body, 324b
sleep n. of sucking child, 52a
to children in womb, 318a
what organism takes in as n., 306b

Novel, admitted truth of n. without scrutiny, 549b
disease in Victorian n., 645a

Novels, majority of bad n., 348b
since Crimean war nurses into n., 322b

Novelty, periods of n. refresh sense of time, 636a

November, in N. bathing prohibited, 188a

Now, health makes you feel n. best, 207a

Noxious, vegetable kingdom robbed of n. growths, 124b

Nuclear, first threat n. war, 441b

Numb soporifical goodfornothingness, 61a

Number, way to get insight must be to n., 482a

Number Six, never forget effects of N., 496a

Numbered, sick people not n. individuals, 323b

Numbers, cannot express in n. scarcely to stage of science, 482b

Numbness pains my sense, 434a

Nurse, better be sick than n. sick, 322a
came with bedpan, 259a
consider n. proof of sympathy of women, 323a
disease support patient n. doctor, 333a
enlightened put them out to n., 290a
falling in love with patient, 322b
fear three things third trained n., 324a
foster n. of nature repose, 556b
given divine touch, 323a
head n. swept place clean with look, 323b
head of every department mature n., 323a
if we obey dying n., 491a
if ye had a good n., 72a, 323a
learns moments better to leave patient alone, 323b
little trained n. dangerous thing, 324b
man make very bad n., 323b
mother no parent but n., 358a
Mrs. Gamp monthly n., 310a
one of great blessings of humanity, 323a
patient falling in love with n., 322b
point of view of n., 219b
practical n. marries rich patient, 324b
she must not herself n., 289b
sleep nature's soft n., 556b
sleeps sweetly, 322a
take sick child from n., 52b
talk of patience of Job said n., 323a
that person alone is fit to n., 321b
to each child, 52b
turn woman into good n., 322b
who so fit n. as woman, 662a

Nursed, famished must be slowly n., 224a

Nursemaid, which every n. knows, 119a

Nurses, children have two important n., 397a
condemned to bed favorite remedy with n., 250a
examining board for registration of n., 322b
giggle of n., 613a
health no better than n., 477b
ignorant old n., 52b
isolated in home under watch of n., 465b
moral disorder of young n., 322b, 402a
oldster insists on changing n., 350a
physician patient medicine n. factors of treatment, 625a
since Crimean war n. into novels, 322b
smile at what patients say under ether, 323b
watch microbes and n., 447a

Nursing chief in cure of disease, 662a
going to bed in n. home, 375a
home architects allow for bidet, 228a
meant as stay, 30b
mystery of n., 139b
nature and n. save greater proportion, 218b
nurse given n. divine touch, 323a
patients assist n. others, 222a
sisters sweetness in presence of death, 323b
vexation and hard work, 322a
Nurture, fish as one with us in n., 160a
Nurtured in wretched place, 147a
little sufficient for man well n., 607b
Nutriment reaches to all parts, 324b
Nutrition, mind as organ of bodily n., 366b
natural function of n., 72b
wine helpeth n., 6b
Nuts, bed before eleven n. before seven, 129a
that's n. to crack, 604b

O

Oak, plant me beneath big o. tree, 436a
Oars, two physicians like pair of o., 66a
Oases, desert of data with o. of prose, 672b
Oath, Gallic idea of Hippocratic o., 326a
Hippocratic o. enjoins secrecy, 156a
keep this O. and stipulation, 325b
men took o. of Hippocrates seriously, 384a
should I violate this O., 326a
while I keep O. unviolated, 325b
Oats, measles like sowing wild o., 291b
Obedience, tradition kept alive not by mute o., 464a
Oberlin, liver to O. College, 24b
Obesity mental state, 327a
Obey, pain we o., 355a
Object, men of age o. too much, 344b
Objectionable people numerous, 412a
Objective, health of whole race practical o., 476a
Objectives, medical detectives with powerful o., 307b
Objects, doctor has to learn serve two o., 361b
of perception seem to vary, 537a
Obligation, consultant's o. to patient, 361a
to make fact known, 63b
Obligations, moderate number of o., 663b
to medicine beyond measurement, 298a
Obligatory, experiments that do good o., 168a

Oblivion, glory is o. postponed, 173a
lie in dead o., 553b
scattereth poppy, 172b
second childishness and mere o., 344b, 535b
Obre treating venereal disease, 651b
Obscure, rejoiced in making clear o., 669b
Obscurities, light of discovery dispels o., 108a
Obscurity, cardinal sin in medical writing o., 673a
too deep for reason, 222b
Observable, entities not directly o., 471a
Observation after serious illness, 362a
determine from o. sources of health, 450b
difficult art, 335b
difficult to record o. in plain language, 670b
discloses numerous phenomena, 503a
disqualification of mind for o., 232a
effort to systematize o., 301a
empirical results of o., 614a
experiment induced o., 168a
facts of general o., 336a
false induction from facts of o., 277b
first step in research, 527a
further from truth than clinical o., 508a
growth of o., 336a
higher intellect to elicit truths by o., 334b
hypothesis based on accurate o., 383b
if only material for o., 250b
in plenty on gout, 193b
insight into creation within our o., 482a
key to learning by episode is o., 576b
know by experience as well as o., 328b
know by o. of effects, 335b
knowledge dependent upon o. increasing, 462a
knowledge gained by own o., 602a
learn by o. diagnostics, 230b
makes the physician, 403a
medical practice must be equipped with o., 442a
medicine blend of superstition empiricism o., 301a
medicine professedly founded on o., 298b
mistakes from lack of o., 152b
naturalist school based on o., 566b
no more difficult art than o., 670a
of causes themselves, 335b
of effects of medicinal substances, 296b
of living subject, 499a
of nature requires purity of mind, 334b
of patient as he is, 116b
own o. best physic, 202b
patient born with o., 365a
reason o. experience trinity of science, 527a

Observation, recent medical knowledge based on o., 336a
science matter of o., 528a
sciences single out for o., 75b
search for concept to explain o., 509b
search for truth by experiment and o., 525b
seed of important o., 508a
skilful doctor knows by o., 95a
skin calls for close o., 550b
statement supported by o., 190a
study o. and experience united, 564a
surgeon taught o. by physician, 590b
that what happens in bodies useful, 606b
truths by o. and practice, 398b
unless we teach o., 140a
use of o. disappearing, 164a
value set on clinical o., 231a
waste when piecemeal, 335a
Observations, ability to describe o., 671b
after death, 24a
correlation of o. into laws, 528b
few o. much reasoning error, 336a, 485b
in direction of ideas, 501a
in experimental laboratory, 506a
incapable of simple truth as to o., 273a
interpret facts from o., 526b
keep and compare o., 670b
long series of o., 108b
make very poor o., 500b
many o. little reasoning truth, 336a, 485b
miracles from ordinary o., 498a
of body in health and disease, 334b
omitted distinctive o., 334b
on diseased source of knowledge, 136a
science begins by o., 526b
women's o. of no more worth than of men, 468b
Observe, above all must o., 526a
doctor trained to o. critically, 404a
incompetence of mind to o. without prejudice, 445b
let what you o. penetrate soul, 336a
man interrogate as well as o. nature, 261a
observer who learned to o. self, 468a
physician as hee disease, 360a
practice of many physicians, 335a
waiting for practice learn to o., 409b
Observed, entities based on inferences from o. data, 471a
of all observers, 243a
teaches o. to become self-observant, 468a
Observer, clinician as o., 335b
delineate likeness, 494b
experiments leaving no place to imagination of o., 526b
Hippocrates o. and doer, 507a
ideal doctor judicial o. 403a
listens to Nature, 499a
only competent o. yourself, 336a

Physician productive if intends to heal, 400b
  protect patient as child, 362b
  quack p. of fools, 482a
  reason p. to love, 485a
  recognize individual diseases, 96a
  required latest investigations, 616a
  research of p. emanates from bedside, 508a
  respect to gout p. lout, 198b
  revive springtime of life, 390a
  reviving exhausted women, 491a
  ruler having body as subject, 362b
  safer with p. naturally wise, 404a
  said to leg of mutton go, 105a
  says he not need it, 375a
  scholar of human biology, 403b
  scientific p. advantage over empiric, 616b
  seek out good p., 363a
  self-conceit of p. hot from studies, 394b
  servant of nature, 315b
  should be the patient, 414b
  should consider, 155a
  should look healthy, 399a
  shun p. eminent for speech, 406a
  sick person who lies to p., 370a
  sickness comes call for p., 377a
  skill of p. lift up his head, 390a
  skillful p. distinguishes symptoms, 480a
  small difference between good p. and no p., 379b
  social p. protecting people, 562b
  something greater a p., 421a
  sometimes blamed unjustly, 380a
  soothing hand of p., 279b
  speakest like p., 628b
  still unskillful p., 365b
  strives for good, 380a
  strongest impulse which moves p., 383b
  studied nature from youth, 400a
  study hygienic potentialities, 227b
  study of nature by p., 497b
  substitutes presumption for knowledge, 230b
  successful p. tempted by press, 63a
  sufferer safer without p., 633a
  superior p. helps before budding of disease, 449b
  supreme reward to p., 414a
  sure p. death, 188b
  surely forgets himself, 407a
  surgeon should be young p. old, 417a
  surgeon taught observation by p., 590b
  surgeon uses knife p. prescribes medicines, 385b, 592b
  surgeon who is own p., 591a
  sympathy of p. makes one of family, 363b
  take fee without thought, 177a
  take up position as mentor, 465b
  tasks assigned to p., 562b

Physician teacher should be best of city, 457b
  tell it to p., 360a
  tench p. of fishes, 363b
  testifies temporary insanity, 245a
  these are duties of p., 410a
  they that whole need not p., 547a
  thinking p. has advantage, 379a
  thinks his pills best, 127b
  this is business of p., 408b
  this is what p. has to do, 293b
  this seems strange from p., 638a
  thoroughly studied science of medicine, 398b
  three faces p. hath, 176a
  three factors disease patient p., 293a
  Tiberius jest at arts of p., 390b
  time great p., 620a
  time p. heals grief, 200b
  to himself and friends, 134b
  to p. humanity laid bare, 361a
  torments body, 456a
  touch of cynic gives p. authority, 379b
  trip up statement of greatest p., 659a
  true p. do own thinking, 399b
  trust not the p., 392a
  turned self over to trainer as to p., 487a
  twinkling of star between p. and man-slayer, 378b
  two-thirds of patients recovered without p., 631b
  unable to escape slovenliness unless he teaches, 220a
  unacquainted with your body, 370b
  understand meaning of health, 106a
  unknown beyond sick room, 137a
  until p. killed he not p., 398a
  unversed in science amateur, 303b
  upon whom set hopes when ill dogs when well, 381b
  versed in science of medicine, 398b
  versed in surgery experienced in practice, 398a
  walks Angel of Death behind, 397b
  warnings of p. forgotten, 194b
  wastes skill of p., 105b
  watchful against covetousness, 176b
  whatever p. prescribes is remedy, 497a
  when sick bawls for p., 371b
  where strength of p. lies, 381a
  whether practitioner or hospital p., 250b
  who become p. if foresee hardships, 413a
  who can do no good, 156b, 178a
  who confines attention to body, 370b
  who learned medicine a p., 455a
  who most perfect p., 399a
  who not admit reality of disease, 229a
  who pays p. does cure, 179a
  who practices with regard to facts, 236b

Physician who puts too much trust in what reads, 483b
  who treats self who has fool for patient, 535a
  who understands powers of herbs, 386a
  who worse than p. would report become, 91b
  whose remedies efficacious is p., 493a
  wide difference between good p. and bad, 379b
  wife of p. different, 657b
  wise p. abandon patient with ulcer, 645b
  wise p. do much for us, 388b
  wish to die soon make p. heir, 371b
  wish to go beyond non-p., 625b
  withholding or making acquainted opinion, 364b
  without physiology and chemistry, 635a
  wonderful is skill of p., 630b
  young p. careful what and how he writes, 670a
  young p. twenty remedies for every disease, 494b
  young p. with diagnostic and therapeutic tools, 637a
Physician's, apothecary p. accomplice, 121a
  best remedy Tincture of Time, 620a
  business to avert disease, 408b
  distinguish between medical science and p. art, 299b
  foot in chamber knife in arme, 35a
  I do not know stick in p. throat, 235a
  interest in survival of matter, 384a
  lodged in p. house, 122b
  medicine absorbs p. whole being, 297a
  name for rheumatism of rich, 197a
  no part of p. business, 369b
  not always in p. power to cure, 236b
  office to draw healing waters, 380b
  patient feel better after p. visit, 367a
  peace bringeth p. gain, 392a
  perform true p. part, 100b
  physiology has relation to healing, 427a
  proof of p. skill, 400a
  restored without p. effort, 175b
  rule of life, 384b
  surgeon's fingers stiff before p. cerebral vessels, 512b
  this is p. aphorism, 205a
  wife better diagnostician, 658a
  words received with more attention, 163b
Physicians, abandoned by skill and care of p., 217a
  abandoned operative procedures, 583b
  acquire knowledge from our dangers, 390b
  all conditions of famous p., 241a
  allocate causes to natural laws, 48b

Practical, America land of p. men, 592a

collected opinions of p. men, 667a

discovery and knowledge without p. purpose, 521a

good deal of mysterious in whatever p., 490a

joy when studies find p. applications, 502a

man practices mistakes, 152b

medicine application of scientific medicine, 299a

minds cannot help speculating, 231a

nurse marries rich patient, 324b

physician knows nothing, 616a

research untrammeled by reference to p., 504a

scarcely aware of until p., 151a

show p. man at what cost scientist conquers, 530a

split between scientific and p. medicine, 616a

student have mind upon p., 573b

systematic knowledge much not p., 255a

testing idea for p. utility, 222a

theory useful when p. results beneficial, 525b

whatever p. people say, 233b

Practice, abuses committed in p. of physic and surgery, 442b

advance proper p. of medicine, 498a

advantage p. of medicine has over surgery, 297a

all else in p. derives from consultation, 368b

all p. is theory, 593b

and marriage extinguishers of science, 519b

attended with privileges, 411a

based upon sound knowledge of theory, 615a

became vulgarity, 277b

beware of p., 444b

calls of p. of necessity, 297b

causal in theory rule in p., 561b

concerned with individual, 636b

daily life forecast of life in p., 574b

diagnosis beginning of p., 97b

diseases he must meet in p., 96a

distinguished in p. not reject methods, 400a

does it to poor person for p., 177b

dogmatize on p. invite controversy, 444b

dreamed of ups and downs of p., 411a

enjoy life and p. of art, 325b

errors must occur in p., 152b

essential unit of medical p., 368b

evil conscience beyond p. of physicians, 64b

excluding theory not p. of medicine, 615b

faith and knowledge in p. of medicine, 443a

false ideas followed by erroneous p., 609a

false philosophy of disease influence p., 425b

falsehoods as to results of p., 273a

Practice, fight way into p. and in p., 381b

first in p. make patient well, 625b

first law on medical p. in colonies, 158a

from discovery of principle to adoption in p., 445a

general p. as difficult as special, 185a

good advice for p., 445a

good p. to verify references, 668b

handicaps to p. of medicine, 445b

homeopathy criticism on medical p., 71b

how content with any but heroic p., 443b

human lessons p. teaches, 603b

illustrated by traditional picture, 638b

important rules of p. unknown in former ages, 462a

in p. difficult to single out dull day, 413b

in p. mistakes made, 152b

in stress of p., 184b

internal medicine and surgery separated in p., 294b

investigation and p. one, 616b

joined to fatigues of p., 668a

latest investigations safeguard of p., 616a

learn art properly or cease p., 151a

Lydgate gained excellent p., 419a

man of few words learns by p., 399a

man who has no little p., 629b

matter-of-fact influence of p., 137a

medical p. not knitting and weaving, 442a

medicine in clinical p., 507a

medicine learned from p., 295b

methods of p. improved within limit, 595a

misrepresentation mingled in p., 71b

most eligible mode of p., 176b

music requires little p., 217a

my p. never very absorbing, 444b

mystery about p. of medicine, 300a

neglect constitutional factor in p., 319a

no person shall p. in New York before examined, 443a

no punishment with p. of medicine, 293a

not p. good medicine and not understand therapy, 637a

not possible in private p. possible in hospital, 221a

obscure causes rejected from p., 48b

observe p. of many physicians, 335a

of medicine all or none, 445a

of medicine art not trade, 444a

of medicine become ineffective, 444b

of medicine lonely road, 444a

of medicine often choleric business, 444a

Practice of medicine perpetual compromise, 443b

of medicine thinker's art, 596b

of medicine undergone considerable changes, 297b

of osteopathy, 72b

of physic jostled by quacks and science, 480b

of physick undervalued with reason, 442a

of surgery glorious, 402a

operations kept down my p., 586a

physician experienced in p., 398a

physician throw self out of p., 443a

physician who commands decent p., 398b

preparation begun in p. end there, 444a

principle for guidance in p., 595a

pure science end in correct p., 444a

putting religion of love into p., 459a

raise sciences from relation to p., 524b

rare that one sets aside p. to study, 444a

real satisfaction in p. of medicine, 445a

rescue p. of medicine from drugging, 272b

result if p. upon dogs omitted, 588a

retired from p. of physic, 512a

review of p. of surgery, 590a

run off with major portion of p., 636b

satisfaction in p., 546a

science more important to p., 303b

science touched with emotion, 444a

scientific method in p., 616a

should be acquainted with real p., 442b

split between science and p. new, 616a

student removed from environment in which p., 577b

study and p. medicine in proper manner, 297a

support through years of p., 657b

surgeon reviewing years of p., 587b

surgeon's ideas put in p., 68b

tact valuable in gaining p., 367a

teaching hospital to set example of p., 221a

thereby simplified, 609a

things work in p. without proof, 146a

those p. with brains those with tongues, 381b

three fifths of p. common sense, 451b

together with my p., 628b

truths by observation and p., 398b

under sway of rationalized beliefs, 232b

unskillful p. in America, 573a

waiting for p. hard, 409b

Purity, observation of nature requires p. of mind, 334b
stagnant water loses p., 234a
Purples, garlands of long p., 182b
Purpose, by fidelity to p., 331b
directing energies with useful p., 489a
establishment of theory p. of science, 232b, 614b
life's p. to go on living, 267b
of life to serve, 267a
organ fulfills p. aiding survival, 606b
other world in which p. realized, 622a
physicians disagree of set p., 453a
practical p. in medical education, 141a
pray for simplicity of p., 402b
seeking p. in rain wind lightning, 267b
techniques devoid of moral p., 157a
to do something worthy recognition, 331b
why always seek p. in selves, 268a
Purr, author p. on having fur smoothed, 669a
Purse, best cure upon own p., 176a
diagnosis forecast by pulse and p., 96b
lawyer torments p., 456a
not knowledge but p. built renown, 417b
not niggardly of p., 373a
of patient protracts cure, 179a
restore man to health p. open to thee, 202b
shibboleth loosened p. strings of nation, 510b
sickness soaks p., 547a
would be right in p., 129a
Purses, not removing consumption out of bodies into p., 400a
Pursue, more you p. health more it flees, 206b
Pursuer, morbid condition flew at throat of p., 116a
Pursuit, progress based on p. of knowledge, 215b
Pus, ulcer secretes p. and blood, 646a
Push, function of muscle pull not p., 314b
make one brave p., 238a
Pushing, no muscle uses power p., 314b
Putrefaction, malignant salts cast us into p., 429b
Putrefactions in gummes bred, 604a
Putrefied, blood blushing at that so p., 34b
Putrid, poison with p. exhalations, 19a
Pycroft, dear old Doctor P., 320b
Pyemia, no instance of p., 19a
Pylorus, unhappiness from agitated p., 239a
Pythagoras, persuade to hold with P., 382a
Pythagorean as I subject to gout, 193b

Q

Quack, advertising q. who wearies, 481a
be a better q., 481b
beheld q. on public stage, 480a
better have recourse to q. if can cure, 480b
compelled to call self what is, 482a
don't cry out against q., 481b
empiricist and theorist called other q., 455a
essential to large class of society, 482a
imposter in common with physicians, 479b
lame and unhealthy duped by every q., 479b
leave reassurance to q., 230b
long versed in human ills, 480b
not bad if simply a q., 481b
strength of physician be he q., 381a
unable to distinguish particularities, 480a
who believed in self, 481b
Quacked self to death, 480a
Quackeries, vulgar q. drop off, 71b
Quackery all but immortal, 481a
beset by q., 304a
bewitching cup of self-q., 321b
consumers waste on medical q., 481b
disgusted with learned q., 145b
ever the same, 481a
followers of quacks causes of q., 482a
gives death to all, 480b
great outcry in journals against q., 482a
left to rude q., 52b
placebo giving is q., 428b
waste dollars on q., 127a
Quack's words heard but no one trusts him, 478b
Quacks, followers of q. causes of quackery, 482a
great outcry in journals against q., 482a
greatest liars except patients, 479b
impotence fills coffers of q., 236a
imprisoned q. replaced by new ones, 481a
in medicine religion politics, 480b
in religion physic law government, 479b
index to regular profession in locality, 481b
laws not against q. but superstition, 481a
modes of generating q., 573b
now q. gamesters, 480a
physic jostled by q. and science, 480b
Quacksalver, let not q. peepe in window, 387b
Quacksalvers suppositors to doctor, 479a
Quacksalving cheating mountebanks, 479a
Quadrangle of health, 488b
Quaffing, long q. maketh short life, 6a

Quain, Sir Richard, 259a
Quaker women of Nantucket taking opium, 351b
Qualification, first q. for physician hopefulness, 402a
Qualifications, prime q. of physician, 401b
Qualitative, approach to psychology q., 262a
quibbling over q. differences sophistry, 482b
results not attended quantitative effort, 510b
Quality, improving q. of life, 268a
increase in literature not improvement of q., 274b
of mind will help, 139a
of writings indication of intellectual state, 275a
Qualms, have no q. my dear, 334a
Quantitative aspects of desire, 541a
error most complete, 482b
qualitative results not attended q. effort, 510b
systems analysis q. common sense, 483a
truth most satisfying, 482b
vital distinctions q., 482b
Quarantine, best q. hygiene, 227b
to protect community, 147b
Quarantines that nourish yellow fever, 240b
Quarrel, ceased to q. with physicians, 371b
physicians in consultation not q., 65b
take up our q. with foe, 436a
takes two to make q., 241a
Quarrels, controversies without personal q., 68a, 454a
half q. of physicians fomented by patients, 454b
ignoble when sours temper in q., 407a
Quarry, go not like q. slave, 84a
Quart, no reason to retain q., 612b
Quartan ague kills old heals young, 181b
Queasily, before breakfast man feels q., 184a
Queen, Cinderella often turns out q., 427b
is dead, 91b
of Scotlandis leichter of sonne, 569b
will live, 74b
your mother rounds apace, 448a
Queen's in labour, 54a
Quest, not possession of knowledge but q. for truth, 532a
Question after right course presented, 156b
answer to leading q., 216b
experiments of light settle q., 525a
more knowledge more we q., 549b
not answer q. because not read chapter, 603a
that is the q., 580a
Questionable, least questioned assumptions most q., 232b
Questioned, least q. assumptions most questionable, 232b

Rest might have balm'd broken senses, 552b
more in need of r. than exercise, 166a, 511b
Nature oppress'd with care sinks to r., 553a
now cometh r., 270b
on day of phlebotomy, 35a
only medicine for foot is r., 189a
patients should have r., 488b
results in rust, 511b
sleep thou r. of all things, 551b
sleep three weeks to get rested from r., 511b
take now and then day's r., 488a
take r. greater than take cities, 511a
those living at r., 102b
vomit and shalt have r., 132b
who labors best has sweetest r., 511a, 662b
wild trash of sleep without r., 553a
with legs as high as seat, 511a
work play r. in proportion, 488b
Restaurant, if food in Vientiane r. safe, 334a
Rested, after sixtieth year best if men r., 348b
Restful, darkness r. and agreeable, 169a
Restless forms bound on sickbeds, 366a
Restlessness, science has being in mental r., 522a
Restoration, travelling means of r., 495a
Restorative, sleep gave nature r., 559a
Restore cripple to legs, 70b
Restored, hundreds by you r., 417b
without physician's effort, 175b
Restores, diet neither r., 100a
Restraint and neglect synonymous, 472b
unconfined r., 554b
Restriction, extreme cure as to r., 72b
Restrictions, little attention except r., 413a
novelty of r. upon life, 546a
Restrictive, happiness freedom from r. sensations, 51b
Result, reputation greater than r., 72a
work performance plus r., 664a
Results, books of science records of r., 503b
confused statements of r., 274b
endowment soundest way to secure r., 510b
highest r. produced, 186a
problem-solvers feel r. justify existence, 531b
qualitative r. not attended quantitative effort, 510b
talk about r. too soon, 531b
use r. of other departments, 380b
will be better, 588b
Resurrection of healthy body from diseased, 644b
Resuscitation, 74a, 74b
Retardation, national program to combat mental r., 246b

Retention and evacuation non-natural things, 279a
Retina, brain integrated with r., 508a
Retire all men at sixty, 348a
make competence and r., 85b
supper at five r. at nine, 489a
time to r. from labor has come, 512a
world sorry that you r., 512a
Retired, at sixty r. on double allowance, 348a
from practice of physic, 512a
Retirement, age of r. for surgeon and physician, 512b
cold wind across landscape that's r., 512b
fellows looking forward to r., 512b
few that court r. aware of toils, 512a
friend to life's decline, 512a
getting old and want r., 339a
through choice not compulsion, 513a
Retires, brother soon r. from case, 66b
Retiring, don't think of r. until world will be sorry, 512a
hours of r. regular, 225a
Retort, could r. of analyst have revealed power, 485b
Retreat, seek stillness of r., 342b
Return, time which can never r., 264a
Revenge, deformed persons take r., 70b
Revenue, appendicitis for r., 22a
if doctors destroy r. for good of mankind, 648b
Revenues, give such r. as can gouge out, 333a
Reverence for life, 267a
thinking being feels r. for life, 267a
Reverie, found self in kind of r., 328b
Review, pleased with r. by friend, 670b
Reviews, read r. of own books, 670b
Reviling vices no longer have enterprise to commit, 347b
Revised and corrected by Author, 149a
Revivals, takes place of normal personality in r., 469b
Revive, stop air by which he r., 171b
Revived, man virtually drowned and r., 86b
Revolt, quack furtively in r., 481b
Revolting, end life by death most r., 257a
Revolts, suppress r. already developed, 449b
Revolution, broom signify r., 608b
in medical science, 445b
medical r. extended life, 349a
people which has r. once in four years, 443b
Revolver, people which contrived r., 443b
Revolvers, statistics like r. in mining districts, 568b
Revulsions, vague terms as r., 610a

Reward according to means of patient, 584a
credit suffers r. same, 393b
doctors do good without prospect of r., 388b
earn least corruptible r., 413a
in gratitude of patients, 411a
no r. worthy faithful doctor, 176a
not becoming to regard r., 50b
Pasteur obtain r. of devotion, 424b
rarer is material r., 411b
science like virtue own r., 518b
supreme r. to physician, 414a
Rewards, in medicine r. immediate, 411b
nothing but pecuniary r. not desired, 411a
Rewriting, no good medical writing just r., 672b
Reynolds, Sir Joshua, 76a
Rhapsodies, condemn swarms of r., 272a
Rhetoric, persuaded to do what would not do by r., 567b
physician ought to know r., 399b
Rheum, curse r., 111b
for purging of r. no herb like tobacco, 622b
Rheumatic, coincidence of r. heart disease and r. fever, 513a
diseases abound, 513b
fever licks joints bites heart, 513a
raw r. day, 513a
were I r., 345a
Rheumatism distemper of coachman, 190b, 514a
doctors pronounce attack r., 196b
gout r. of rich patient, 197a
gout to arteries what r. to heart, 197a
has patrons, 113a
have r. thank Heaven aint gout, 196a
name for many pains, 514a
replaced by headaches, 282a
reputation for dignity because r. in neck, 514a
tax paid by grog drinker, 195b, 514a
vise tightly as possible r., 198b
why suffer from r. with rise in humidity, 514a
writhing in beds with r., 514a
Rheumatisms caught in nocturnal pastimes, 474a
Rheumatologists, cast of orthopedic r., 613a
Rheums, long sleepe at afternoones breeds r., 551b
very subject to r., 543a
wherein were laid r., 218a
Rhubarb, gives diarrhoea quicker than r., 240a
no one picks goes to seed, 511b
nor r. always purge, 123a
scarce ipecac high, 434a
what r. would scour English, 122a
Rhythm, neurosis produce broken r. of cardiac, 319b
Rib, not true woman from r. from funny bone, 661a

Sexual, woman devoted wholly to s. matters, 540a
woman scholarly something wrong with s., 660b
Seymour, I knew a Doctor S., 406b
Shade, rest under s. of trees, 259a
Shadow of bones seen within hand, 674a
of death, 80a
valley of s. of death, 80a
Shaêta, old woman brings S., 1a
Shake his sapient head, 238a
mark how he did s., 180a
Shaken, when taken to be well s., 123b
Shakes, developed hatter's s., 247a
Shakespeare, quality S. possessed enormously, 329b
Shaking hands fell into disuse, 674b
Shaky, got here s. in shoes, 152a
Shamans of primitive tribes, 384b
Shame, fixed the s. in himself, 305b
in decline of life s. short, 342b
released from all s., 117b
through false s. hide unhealed sore, 665a
Shames mother who does not resemble father, 213a
Shank, hose world too wide for s., 344b
Shape, contemplate my flaccid s., 163a
like lute, 120a
shocked at s. of fingers, 199a
Shapes, ring out s. of disease, 114b
way of making fine s., 227a
Shark, man like s. must have prey, 131b
Sharp remedy but sure one, 257b
so s. the converynge, 294b
stomach makes short devotion, 224a
things rot teeth, 604a
Sharp, such were S., 586a
Sharper than serpent's tooth, 55b
Sharpest, headache at s. seems bad investment, 200a
Shattered, doctor cured s. limb, 175a
Shave, lies haircut and s., 25b
Shaved and blistered his head, 635b
Darwinian Man only monkey s., 161b
physician should be well s., 398b
Shaven, bald head soon s., 25b
Sheep careful in selecting foods, 311b
death devours lambs as well as s., 93b
medicine not field in which s. safely graze, 304a
one scabby s. flock destroys, 147a
scab of s. destroys herd, 240a
Sheets, death's worse winding s., 348a
dreamer discharged stone in s., 646a
Shekels, take s. of silver, 175a
Shelf, ought to help clear s., 605b
Shellfish, pearly tear of s., 643b
Shells given to poor, 104a
Shelter gone when night o'er, 436a

Shepherd, above common herd the s., 389a
guides of whom Bunyan tells, 444a
Shepherds give grosser name, 183a
Sherrington found Pflüger superficial, 425a
portrait of Sir Charles S., 20b
Sherris, your excellent s. warms blood, 6a
Shibboleth, ancient s. that should be liquidated, 334a
Shield nobler than spear, 450b
Shift from side to side, 181a
Shin, plantain leaf for broken s., 493b
Shins, strike s. mar spurring, 651a
Ship, as select s. so choose death, 579b
body like a s., 38a
every s. spared one surgeon, 310b
fat man like s. stocked for last voyage, 327a
fool to put about s. entering harbour, 580b
handle body like sail of s., 225b
like s. in dock for repairs, 544b
not safe but with gouty master, 191a
on prow of conquering s., 458a
under sail and big-bellied woman, 448a
without rudder or compass, 615a
Shipload, single fact worth s. of argument, 171a
Ship's, references like barnacles on s. bottom, 673b
Ships, disregard on hospital s., 310b
Shiraz, turning wine of S. into urine, 287a
Shirt, find garment s. of Nessus, 601a
Shiverings succeeded by hot fits, 642b
Shivers, sweats and at same time s., 179b
Shock, like s. of corn in season, 86b
Shocks, thousand natural s. flesh is heir to, 558b
Shoe, could not wear s., 197a
no more than old s. become dancing slipper, 184b, 565a
Shoes, any crime sufficient for large s., 195a
be so good to bodies as to hosen and s., 363a
man may go over s. in grime of it, 598b
physician put on s., 398b
too short s. worn, 69a
Shoot, better s. patient than works, 636a
Shopboy, matters druggist's s. tell, 629a
Shops, two s. in three shut up, 429a
Shore, never saile more willing bent to s., 432b
Short, art long life s., 297a
but s. time to live, 92a
days grow s. when reach September, 340b
highest pain not consequently s., 187a

Short, leg s. opposite member longer, 317b
life far too s., 380b
life s. the art long, 292b
life so s. craft so long to lerne, 294b
men eat more than tall, 133a
never use long word where s. answer, 609b
sharp stomach makes s. devotion, 224a
too s. shoes worn, 69a
Shortcut, no s. to longevity, 280a
to knowledge, 136a
Shortens, desire to live increases as life s., 340a
Shorter, letter long because no leisure to make s., 667b
physicians make life s., 391b
Shortness, consistent with desires s. of life, 285b
of life generally forgotten, 270a
Short-winded, chest specialist long-winded about s., 47a
Shoulder, carrying away s. as came in, 376b
knot of scarlet ribbon on s., 326a
man has dislocated s., 376b
wounded in s. and left arm, 515b
Shoulders, each generation of doctors upon s. of predecessors, 464b
Shout for I am deaf, 76a
Show, all that makes death hideous s., 84b
medicine where s. stripped off, 361b
people put on tremendous s., 412b
revenues in return for s., 333a
ticket to greatest s. on earth, 413b
Shower, coming s. corns presage, 69a, 605b
with cold water two hours, 496b
Shrieks, keen s. day after day, 355a
Shrink, against fire I s. up, 180b
arm like shrub, 70b
Shrug, who notes s., 156a
Shut door good John, 173b
Shuttle, death busy with s., 302a
man is s., 285a
Sibling, gregarious egalitarian s. group, 612b
Sibyl sweet and mystic sense, 208a
Sicilians ended by killing patient, 152b
Sick, above all care had of s., 372a
advice for s. don't kill 'em, 629b
after contracting eyebrows over s., 77b
all become s. and die, 117a
appetite desires increase evil, 542a
are you s. or sullen, 40a
as a cat, 545a
as a dog, 542a
as a horse, 547a
ask physicians' wives do husbands get s., 658a
at fifty lost s. headaches, 200a
attended in own houses, 373b
avoid contact with s., 240a

Sleeps, who s. well thinks well, 11b

Sleepy, doctor may be s., 320b

Sleeve, sick man with cure up s., 73b
 sleep that knits s. of care, 552b

Sleeves, Angel of Death s. turned up, 397b
 physician has two s., 636b
 teach in gown with wide s., 326a

Slender, fat die earlier than s., 326a
 sleep which is food to s. frame, 551b
 way of making s. waists, 227a

Slept in caves and woods, 69b
 Methuselah s. in open air, 279b
 not s. one wink, 556b
 we thought her dying when she s., 559b

Slighted, in first case she is s., 230a

Slings and arrows of outrageous fortune, 580a

Slipper, no more than old shoe become dancing s., 184b, 565a

Sloane, Hans, 26a

Slop, uncourtly figure of Doctor S., 418a

Slops, doctors keep patient tied down to s., 102a

Sloth, be temperate in s., 192a
 emblems of s. and indigestion, 224b
 excess began s. sustains trade, 393b
 in slumber of s., 270a
 long sleepe at after-noones breeds s., 551b

Slow, difficult to s. down, 445a
 in s. motion outdone snail, 186b
 spirit of death so s., 89b

Slowly, eat s., 132a
 science moves s. s., 518b

Slowness, O your s. if I balk, 276a
 remained alive on account of constitutional s., 461a

Slows, Gen. McClellan got the s., 311b
 milk sick name of s., 311b

Sluggishness and activity equally surprised, 270a

Slumber, bringeth patient in sense-lesse s., 585a
 if my dear you seek to s., 557b
 never limbs affected s. more, 432b
 nor s. to mine eyelids, 555b
 not s. in calm repose, 544b
 to soothing s. seven, 488a
 yet a little sleep a little s., 555b

Slumbers not sleep, 556b
 sweet are s. of virtuous, 553a

Small, all things both great and s., 308b
 change of death pain, 92b
 children stamp on lap, 58a
 death proclaims how s. our bodies, 77a
 hurt in eye great one, 170a
 microbe so very s., 308a
 praise physician whose mistakes s., 150b
 rage for fame attends great and s., 172b

Smallness, greatness or s. determined at birth, 212a

Smallpox accompanied by fever, 35b
 blood ridding self of impurities, 560a
 cut claws and wings of s., 329a
 gone out follow'd by great, 560b, 651b
 know by history only s. existed, 560b
 likely to spread, 560a
 rash of s. spot after spot, 291a, 560a
 signs nearly same as s., 291a, 560a
 starve measles nourish s., 291b, 560b
 until over s. parents not count child own, 560b

Smart, can fool man by saying he s., 340a
 itch more intolerable than s., 252a
 too s. to pay doctor, 179a

Smatterer in science, 610a

Smelfungus, I'll tell it cried S., 360a

Smell, best s. is bread, 515a
 causes water to s. bad, 311a
 conscious of s. of spirits, 310b
 ill conception of my s., 429a
 tobacco vitiateth s., 621b
 warns against flavour, 123b
 who s. stench for sake of discovery, 498b

Smells, what s. so, 623a

Smile at what patients say under ether, 323b
 friends with whom seldom s., 379b
 greets with blandest s., 66b
 runneth over, 324a
 short s. of sunshine, 366b
 sweet with certainties, 423b
 wept with delight when gave her a s., 434b

Smith, Theobald S. built temples to nature, 426a

Smock, maid pleased wife and I in her s., 239a

Smoke appetite provoke, 447b
 at table men puffing s. of tobacco, 620b
 becomes kitchen better than dining chamber, 620b
 blowing s. out of mouths, 621b
 consume your own s., 63a
 gentlemen who s. in streets, 574a
 good cigar is a s., 623b
 never s. more than one cigar at time, 623a
 never s. when asleep refrain when awake, 623a
 rarely s. dear, 623b
 spirit in blood as flame in s., 653a
 stinking fume resembling Stigian s., 621a
 those who s. have kisses for smoker, 624a
 tobacco fill full of s., 621a

Smoker, in s. earliest indication of disease, 623b
 those who smoke have kisses for s., 624a

Smokes, who s. thinks like sage acts like Samaritan, 622b

Smoking, cigarette s. may be hazardous, 624a

Smoking, cigarette-s. drinking beer out of thimble, 623a
 cut out s., 48a
 Elizabethan age beginning of s. era, 623b
 is shocking thing, 621b
 man s. five-cent cigar, 623a

Smollett, Sterne's caricature of S., 360a

Smother, some freeze others s., 60a

Snail, in slow motion outdone s., 186b

Snake, as s. to pig, 131b

Snakeroot, farmer decided white s. caused milk sick, 311a
 milk sick caused by white s., 311b
 remind of Seneca s., 123a

Snare, tears of woman from grief or s., 659b

Sneer, though we s. in health, 371a

Sneeze, I recommend for dis-ease a s., 561b
 interrupt his sigh, 281b
 you must not s., 560b

Sneezed, he s. thrice turn out of hospital, 561a

Sneezes, beat him when he s., 560b
 with wheezes and s., 472a

Sneezing, anything sets me s., 13a
 before King and Queen, 560b
 removes hiccup, 213b

Sneezles, if s. turn into mumps, 241a

Snob value of rooms on chosen street, 153b

Snore, why can't hear self s., 555a

Snoring, whom s. she disturbs, 322a

Snow, Dr. John, 17b

Snow, children naked in s., 52b
 merely because s. coming, 319b
 when men asleep s. came flying, 435a

Snowballs, as well swallow s., 65b
 for pills, 27b

Snowy, let s. fountains flow, 289a

Snubbed if epidemic overlooks, 147b

Snuff, rather the worse for s., 310a
 shifted trumpet and took s., 76a

Soap best disinfectant, 19b
 try s. and water, 20a

Sober as a hymn, 381b
 ordinary meats relish s. man, 22b
 things narrow hope, 312a

Soberly, news bad tell it s., 461a

Sobriety, persistent preacher of s. doctor, 387a

Social and economic structure of society, 562b
 brain which made s. evolution possible, 235a
 comfort learnt in hospital, 219a
 cost of sickness incalculable, 452a
 disease has s. causes, 49b
 doctor near patient in s. background, 366b
 doctors s. cement, 381b
 forces deform trends, 287a
 forces that influenced medical history, 233a
 if physician s. animal, 304b

Social, investigator deprived of s. recognition, 504b
leave s. medicine department, 144a
measures of s. amelioration, 186a
medicine basically s. science, 562a
medicine involved in s. organization, 561b
medicine is s. science, 562b
medicine must enter s. life, 561a
medicine profession for s. service, 561b
physician protecting people, 562b
physicians know s. conditions best, 562b
physicians must play s. role, 562b
position varies, 384b
possibility in mental illness, 246b
practice psychosomatic also s. medicine, 562b
problems of medical care, 563a
problems of our race, 561b
problems should be solved by physicians, 561b
science leavens s. fabric, 520b
tranquilizers facilitate s. adjustment, 126a
truth in conflict with s. circumstances, 502b
Social science, medicine s., 561a
Social worker, we see physician as s., 562b
Socialized medicine used to confuse, 476a
Socially, occupational diseases s. different, 337a
Societies, fixed person in older s. godsend, 463b
have organization to fight disease, 477a
Society, among most valuable rational s., 264a
cannot afford what cannot be without, 51a
characteristic of affluent s., 132a
conflict and confusion within s., 464b
demonstrating benefits of free s., 477a
discouraging things they learn about s., 458b
doctor subordinates individual to s., 157a
drunk from delusions of freedom, 330a
for Preservation of Use of Five Senses, 164b
leave you at large, 391a
make collective provision for needs, 475b
Morrison's Pill for curing maladies of s., 321a
no members of s. listen more, 380b
not care if work useful to s., 531b
not escape responsibility for life, 280a
of scientists more important than discoveries, 532a
pathology of s. function of medical man, 561b

Society pay greater bill by hospitals and jails, 476b
physician key medical expert of s., 384b
physician must know history of s., 215b
progress based on service to s., 215b
quack essential to large class of s., 482a
responsibility to individual rather than s., 186a
sick man parasite of s., 249b
think of health of race as practical, 476a
think work useful to s., 531b
wise to support men for what might find, 505b
Society's, unfriendly to s. joys, 622a
Sociologic concept find support in fact, 540b
Sociologists have jargon, 611b
Sociology, conflict between biology and s., 287a
technology of medicine outrun s., 522a
Socrates asked all important questions, 143a
phenomena in sickness of S. of simpleton, 599b
similarly with S., 625b
Soda, invention of s. water, 332b
reads of American fortunes takes bicarbonate of s., 510a
Sofa suits gouty limb, 194a
Soil concerned with plants in it, 112b
ecology that involves s., 287a
fame no plant on mortal s., 172b
family doctor natural sprout from s., 185a
keep half knowledge under by enriching s., 255a
natural disposition like s., 134a
potassium of s. not sea, 514b
simples as our s. doth yeeld, 121b
Sold, diseases s. dearer than physic, 650b
Soldier, above common herd the s., 389a
as sleeping s. in alarm, 243a
greatest necessity of s. water, 654b
in hut, 266a
not a s. desires peace of country, 390a
Soldiers aim straight at my heart, 259a
bore operations after battle, 310b
epidemics more influential than s., 147b
homesickness among s. of New England, 217a
life fighting unarmed amongst thousand s., 264b
like s. equipped to fight last war, 477a
long for war, 375b
physicians commit more deaths than s., 394b
physicist and chemist s. without arms, 502b
syphilis brought by s. of France, 649b

Soldiers, thirst common among officers and s., 618a
Solemnity as a disease, 306a
Soley, Mayo Hamilton S. brings to mind Elizabethan, 426a
Solicitude, not frustrate self with s., 237b
Solidarity, fraternity and s., 457b
Solitary, I lead s. life, 239b
pain only experience by nature s., 357a
Solitude, death more welcome than s., 88b
if I with thee dwell, 183a
prefer s. to companions, 619b
regal s. is sick bed, 544a
Solomon places wisdom in proper times, 194a
say with S. medicine from God, 387a
Solomon's seal, root of S. taketh away bruise, 493a
Solution, attack problems when slight prospect of s., 506a
just but why not experiment, 499a
keep confused until right answer forces s., 529a
one of drugs which carries another in s., 491a
recognition of problem first step in s., 505a
wisdom selecting problems whose s. important, 499a
Solutions, A.M.A. presents no s., 154b
Solve, adequacy of methods to s. conflicts, 470b
Solving, get problems out of system by s., 506b
Somatic, psychic and s. stamina, 610b
splits psychiatrists into psychodynamic and s., 467a
Somebody, life happening to me or s. else, 267b
Something in us can be without us, 285a
Son, cadavers are books your s. will learn, 135b
Charles undresses me, 347a
from father run ill habitudes upon s., 211a
had s. for cradle before husband for bed, 235b
like father like s., 213a
loved sow better than s., 20a
mother's s. none of his, 448b
Queen of Scotlandis is leichter of s., 569b
woman esteems husband adores s., 661a
Song, did Man who wrote S. of Songs write this, 541b
nor in thy marble vault sound my s., 652b
Songs I made for thee, 79b
obsessed with sex and romance in s., 540b
Sonnets, banish dismay write s. gay, 417a
Sons, gallant s. spring from gallant, 210a
give elbow-room to s., 92b
good wombs borne bad s., 210b
grandsons not s. of nature, 315a
healthy s. with healthy daughters pair, 211a

Tempest, from lightning and t., 82b
    hear aloof human t. beat, 342b
    silenced by magic wand, 596a
Temple, art of healing unroofed t., 296b
    work upon t. of God, 593b
Temples, aching t. throb with furious beat, 544b
    conceal by locks on t., 25a
    hospitals t. of medicine, 221a
    rub him about t., 534a
Temporal, before operation arrange t. affairs, 350b
Temporary, action credited to t. insanity, 245a
    crowd device for t. insanity, 470a
Temptation to imagine self a god, 384a
    to toy with press, 63a
Temptations, sick man flee before t. of St. Anthony, 324a
    which men of our profession withstand, 380a
Ten days after woman had company of man, 63b
    dollar bill useful, 177a
    fashioned in t. months, 64a
    lunar months elapsed reap fruit of womb, 448a
    makes man live t. times t., 489a
    ran he on t. winters more, 279a
Tenacity in research admirable, 504b
Tenant, blind and deaf t. in body, 201b
    not go out unprepared, 546b
Tenants, aching teeth ill t., 606a
Tench physician of fishes, 363b
Tendencies, children betray t., 56a
Tender, Leah was t. eyed, 170a
    made nice by plenty t. by indulgence, 660a
Tendons like shrouds, 14b
Tenesmus pain in extremity of urethra, 646b
Tenets of teacher like seed, 134a
    same at last, 67b
Tension, conditions due to t., 49a
    nervous and intellectual system to utmost t., 581b
    relaxation of intellectual t., 663b
Term, difficult transcends useful scientific t., 673a
    foreseeing pernicious uses to which t. put, 610b
    newly created, 610b
    that bolster my thesis, 612a
Terminology, Greek derivatives in scientific t., 610b
    jargon of scientific t., 611a
Terminus, years are stations death t., 271b
Terms, nothing detracts as unfamiliar t., 608b
    producing stupendous while talk in simple t., 611b
    such vague t., 610a
Terrestrial magnetism, 108a
Terrible, human being and t. thing happening, 288a
    medical man sees t. sights, 410a
    nothing more t. than ignorance in action, 234b
Territory, brain is unknown t., 46a

Terror, but for t. where valour, 89b
    my chief cause of t., 453a
    nor conceive such t. in death, 269a
    of death worse than these, 319b
    positive t. in dying, 85b
    so spake grisly t., 90b
Terrors, death in due time shorn of t., 86a
    disarm death of t., 159a
    of disease always with us, 478a
Tertian, burning quotidian t., 283a
Test, cannot t. faith in crucible, 172a
    every t. but critical one done, 99a
    habit with him t. of truth, 145b
    not select good by t., 322b
    repeating laboratory t., 98b
Test tube, answer cry with more than t., 367a
    made sceptics of us, 248a
    seeking reputation at t., 600b
Testaments, laying in wait after t., 294a
Tested, apprentice not permitted advancement until t., 576b
Testimony, pain taken upon t. of patient, 355a
Testing discern fine gold, 497b
    for safety and efficacy of products, 481b
    much t. no guesswork, 527b
    more t. than tolerate with safety, 350a
    natural selection tried by t. of science, 161b
Testy, old men t., 347a
    practice of medicine often t. business, 444a
Tetchy and wayward thy infancy, 55b
Tetter barked about my smooth body, 438b
    fee simple of t., 111b
Textbook, not read chapter in t. myself, 603a
Textbooks become antiquated quickly, 613a
    many facts not in t., 139b
    mistake to believe t. correct, 613a
Thais has black teeth, 604a
Thankless, have t. child, 55b
Thannhauser, Siegfried J., 611b
Theater, nobody care whether you at t., 412b
Theatrical, at end Beaconsfield a little t., 259a
Theatricals, life no better than private t., 265a
Thee, it tolls for t., 78a
Theft, not held responsible for t., 245a
    rational yet commit t., 245a
Theologian begins with soul, 387a
Theologians for personal survival, 384a
Theological, followed calling of t. teacher, 459a
Theology charlatanerie of mind, 615b
    makes sinners, 372b
    new and true not greater in medicine than t., 273b

Theoretical, human nature t. construction, 471a
    physicians perform function, 377b
Theories, accept too readily t., 614a
    applied in face of observation, 277b
    bewitching delusions of t., 136a
    caution in construction of t., 231b
    conceive or accept t., 170b, 614b
    discoveries which correct older t., 309b
    excessive faith in t., 500b
    founded on uncertain data, 450b
    higher intellect for observation than t., 334b
    in terms of notions suggested by fragment, 565b
    keep down luxuriance of t., 135a
    lowest value on visionary t., 231a
    making t. keep window open, 614b
    medical t. more peculiar than facts, 614a
    not dangerous to God or capital, 530b
    outlaw t. from other schools, 466b
    physiologists should have little confidence in t., 613b
    product of Weltanschauung, 614b
    professors prefer own t. to truth, 529b
    treat own t. as dogmas t. of predecessors as myths, 615a
    under sway of rationalized beliefs, 232b
    whose confirmation we seek, 500b
Theorist, empiricist and t. called each other quack, 455a
    we are not t., 450a
Theorizers, America land of doers rather than t., 592a
Theorizing, in t. argue on either side, 615a
    physicians may show as empirics, 615b
Theory, all surgery is t., 593b
    animal that fits in with t., 424a
    anxious for you to believe his t., 549a
    bases of legitimate t., 136b
    causal in t. rule in practice, 561b
    concerned with t. of medical knowledge, 301b
    Darwinian t. support to spiritual nature, 161a
    declares proof of something he requires for t., 549a
    discovery not included in t., 108a
    don't confuse hypothesis and t., 232b, 614b
    establishment of t. purpose of science, 232b, 614b
    even if wrong can bring advance, 507a
    evolution t. abate vehemence, 160b

Tobacco, neither lust after tawney weede t., 621a
none made better than t., 622b
not for body, 488b
oily soot found in t. takers, 620b
outlandish weed, 624a
refuse to take t. accounted peevish, 620b
sometimes medical, 622a
sublime t., 622b
there's nothing like t., 621b
this night leave off t., 622a
three sorts of t. in pocket, 621a
weak dilution, 347b
what pleasure in taking t., 621a
Tobacco's, sound of great t. praise, 621b
Tobago, old man of T., 105a
Toby, send surgeon to Sir T., 585a
Today, he wasn't there again t., 466a
man comes t. gone tomorrow, 286a
never gets enough, 327a
not scorn yesterday because better t., 464a
practically where we are t., 291a
short skirts t. reveal malnutrition, 325a
work t. be happy tomorrow, 384b
Today's facts tomorrow's fallacies, 153a, 171a
Toe, awakened by pain in great t., 189b
explode in volcano in great t., 197b
feel gout hold t. to colchicum, 195b
gout begins in joint of great t., 192b
gout had taken him in t., 196a
pain and redness of t., 198a
pangs arthritic that infest t., 194a
plays rogue with great t., 188b
Toenail, corrects ingrowing t., 177b
Toes grow livid, 81a
joined t. useless, 144b
unplagu'd with corns, 69a
Toga, president of A.M.A. with t., 154a
Toil, earned by exhausting t., 205a
little such men know t., 668a
of ev'ry day supplied, 423a
old age hath honor and t., 343a
perspiration flow only after t., 598b
sleep after t. port after stormie seas, 552b
sleep preparest for t. again, 551b
strung the nerves, 165a
Toilet, take children hurriedly to t., 658a
Toils, few that court retirement aware of t., 512a
light of benevolence around t., 410b
use results without sharing t., 380b
with pain eat with pleasure, 133a

Toilsome, research though t. easy, 235b, 503a
Token of covenant, 59a
Tolls, for whom the bell t., 78a
to him for whom passing bell t., 655b
Tomarters, eat t. daily, 196a
Tomb, for all one t., 405b
from wombe so to t., 284b
have engraven on my t., 258b
old as Pharaoh in t., 179b
rendered less rugged pathway to t., 298b
Tombs abandoned ruins weeping willows, 644b
and worms and tumbling to decay, 348a
Tombstone, compensation gilded t., 444b
Tomorrow, be sure to want guinea t., 176b
eat and drink for t. die, 93b
I shall have read it, 603a
man comes today gone t., 286a
not bother about t., 331a
overeat to feed t., 327a
work today be happy t., 384b
Tomorrow's, today's facts t. fallacies, 153a, 171a
Tomorrows, medicine deals with t., 458b
Tongs, pulses felt with t., 240b
Tongue bitten in agony, 534b
can do most good and evil, 62b
cancers of t. and mouth, 47b
coated t., 181b
every morning look at t., 207a
examining t. of patient, 94b
eye t. sword, 243a
feels harsher, 438a
gain nothing with t. only with works, 363a
given man one t. two ears, 208a
have toothache cut off t., 639a
in surgery t. last and least, 587a
jointed t. beneath rows of teeth, 308a
morphine had loosened my t., 350b
muscle pull not push except t., 314b
never have occasion for t. of one, 456a
our trumpeter, 15a
pen of ready writer, 673b
speak when powers hardly actuate t., 376a
stories from that smoothe t., 432b
symptoms body's mother t., 599b
teach t. to say I do not know, 655b
that bade Romans mark him, 180a
to parch'd mouth t. cleaves, 544b
turning to aching tooth, 606a
wets his parch'd t., 120b
what t. unfold so great wonder, 169a
who unpractised overcultivates t., 399a
Tongues, essential identity of t., 124b
if descend gift of t., 644a
those practice with brains those with t., 381b

Tonic, astringent t. of critical writing, 671a
Tonics, invigorating force of moral t., 603a
visit combines best of t., 365b
Tonsillectomy, owed economic security to t., 624b
Tonsils got into game, 637b
Tool, picks up beautiful new t., 248a
Tools, books and lectures t., 138a
carpenters handle carpenters' t., 666b
doctrines and techniques t., 424b
extensions of limbs, 37b
ill jesting with joiner's t., 534b
Tooth, aching t. better out, 605b
every t. more valuable than diamond, 604a
he looks like t.-drawer, 605a
hollow t. will rage, 69a, 605b
lost one t. walk a little lame, 340b
more deadly than mad dog's t., 483b
one t. with many fangs, 605b
rather have bellies opened than t. pulled, 605a
reason of golden t., 277b
sharper than serpent's t., 55b
sorrow's t. doth never rankle more, 563a
thinking selves in presence of angels when t. out, 546b
tongue turning to aching t., 606a
troubled with raging t., 605b
two years ere could get a t., 604a
Toothache, for t. brimstone and gunpowder with butter, 605b
have t. cut off tongue, 639a
he that sleeps feels not t., 605a
I have t. draw it, 605a
man with t. thinks everyone happy whose teeth sound, 606a
method of relieving t. appendectomy, 637b
music helps not t., 606a
never philosopher endure t. patiently, 605a
speak of evil use t. as example, 606a
Toothaches, no further than curing t., 615a
Toothbrushing, see if t. has effect, 251b
Toothpicks, diseases in gummes bred by t., 604a
Top, scientists on tap not on t., 530b
sleep like a t., 553a
uncovered at t. cracked at foundation, 296b
Tophi in skin, 198a
Topic forbidden to well-bred mortals their distempers, 544a
Topics, king of t. operations, 350b
Topography, science t. of ignorance, 518a
Torment but not destroy, 190a
life to him but t., 159a
of unknown have joy of discovery, 108a
whenever departed from regimen, 249a

Watch, body w. designed to go
given time, 631b
neighbors take nightly w. over
sick, 218b
some must w. some must sleep,
552b
thence to a w., 242b
Watchful, guides Knowledge Experience W. Sincere, 444a
Watchfulness, sleep and w. immoderate constitute disease, 551b
Watching, benefit of sleep and effects of w., 553a
pain of w. with unsatiable man,
607b
that's with w., 199b
Watchmaker cannot open it, 631b
Water, anyone intentionally pollutes w., 655a
bathing feet in cold w. every
morning, 204b
best disinfectant, 19b
better methods than throwing
child into w., 509a
bleeding and drinking warm w.
grand principles, 629b
blood thicker than w., 34b
carry his w. to wise woman,
647b
cast w. of my land, 647a
causes w. to smell bad, 311a
city that does not possess w.
supply, 226b
clean teeth with arquebusade
w., 604b
cold adown warm esophagus,
654b
composed of over 90 per cent
w., 514a
danger inherent in fresh w.
home, 147a
differs as wine and w., 652a
doth deject appetite, 654a
drank prussic acid without w.,
581a
drink no longer w., 11b
drink tea or wine and w., 494b
drinks tumbler of London w.,
655a
drunk sundered in three, 306b
everywhere thirst burns throat,
618a
expect poison from standing w.,
655a
fast and drink w., 362b
fault that w. mend, 598b
fear of w. Greeks call hydrophobia, 483a
feel as if cold w. over them,
189b
feet often used to cold w., 488a
filthy w. not washed, 655a
fire with w. we defeat, 75b
first w. cure the Flood, 225a
foremost medicine, 655a
got w. on knee, 310a
great irritations to make w.,
646b
greatest necessity of soldier w.,
654b
healthy w. but party have diseases, 647a
I am poured out like w., 128a
in June take cold w., 188a
intemperate w. devotees, 197b
invention of soda w., 332b
is free, 163a
letters large through glass filled
with w., 548a

Water, looking at eclipse reflected
in w., 169a
make your mouth w., 23a
makes w. urine congeal'd ice,
647a
man sick of fever bathed in
cold w., 626b
mineral w. reputed capable of
giving fistula, 192b
most salutary beverage, 654b
must not drink cold w., 487a
natural beverage for thirsty w.,
654a
nausea overcome by sipping w.,
173b
neither makes sick, 655a
never miss w. till well dry, 655a
no disease vegetable diet and
pure w. not mitigated, 649a
not drink w. during meals,
101a
not imbibe w. excessively, 101a
one of physicians used drops of
colored w., 428a
one whose name writ in w., 149a
pipes for w. kill everybody except animalcules, 240b
posthaste through sick body,
647b
praised be for sister w., 654a
promotes not infirmities, 59b
put salt in w. shower hour
longer, 496b
reckon what w. worth, 628b
relation infectious agents bear
to w., 451a
remedies of Myddfai w. honey
labour, 497a
render pure w. and food, 451a
resolver of spasms, 654b
rural cleanliness in w. supply,
474a
see your face in her w., 647b
stagnant w. loses purity, 234a
submitted to be half-drowned
in w., 634a
tabetic has power of holding
w., 31a, 236a
take out w. with twopenny pail,
317b
Tantalus seeks w., 618a
thickest stock body's w., 306b
thirst and dread of w. removed
at same time, 618a
throw patient unawares into w.
tank, 483a
till taught by pain know not
what w. worth, 618a
too be saved, 163b
trusteth not single witnesse of
w., 647b
try soap and w., 20a
w. every where, 654b
wagon is place for me, 10a
wash with hot lukewarm tepid
cold w., 226a
what says doctor to my w., 647a
wine and w. against heate of
liver, 275b
Water holes, prose dried up w. of
alkali plains, 672b
Waterloo, loses more by remedies
than W. cost, 396a
Waters, ascent through brackish
w., 163a
at Aix long enough to prove inefficacy of w., 224b
Bath where plans to visit mineral w., 249a

Waters, bathing and drinking w.,
190b, 513b
everyone that thirsteth come to
w., 618b
from Tantalus' lips w. shrink,
120b
men fill selves with w., 110b
office to draw healing w., 380b
peak of life where w. divide,
309a
Watershed, drains large w. of intellect, 330a
Waterworks, physics of circulation
physics of w., 59a
Watson fixed point in changing
age, 419a
work antidote to sorrow W.,
664a
Wax, deafness due to w., 76b
heart like w., 128a
Way, every day in every w. better,
473a
learn more from w. patient tells
story, 97a
of all flesh, 92a
that w. madness lies, 243b
there is no other w., 152b
Wayside, health like happiness
found by w., 206b
Wayward, tetchy and w. thy infancy, 55b
Weak, commit w. condition to raw
morning, 240b
drive w. from marriage hive,
211a
influence of strong upon w.,
444a
legged not in love with Rome,
59b
lunacy refuge of w. nature
against distress, 246a
medical student too w. to labour on farm, 575a
men addicted to drugs, 125b
more w. than child, 25b
old age w., 346a
one of kin has w. pia mater,
244a
only w. can teach, 601b
prevail over strong, 162a
science kill strong keep alive w.,
518a
those w. in mind and will,
535b
thou whose own feet w., 188a
together with most w. hams,
345a
Weakened and wasted to skin and
bone, 654a
spasm may carry off w. body,
345a
Weakens, too much polishing w.
work, 666b
Weaker, promote not infirmities
of w. parts, 59b
Weakest, harm comes to strong
from w., 545b
Weakmindedness, congenital w.,
158b
Weakness, departure from truth
concession to w., 641a
empiric's gains from man's w.,
480a
greater and lasting w., 192b
hurried away from w., 346b
necessary w. of mind, 501a
nor woo means of w., 342a
physician sees w. of our nature,
388b

Well, pity w. person felt for sick, 249b

plenty w. no pray, 239b

say you are w., 206b

set hopes when ill dogs when w., 381b

skilful doctor treats w., 449b

suffer die or get w., 630b

those w. get sick, 360a

to w. baths granted seldom, 372b

treasures in cold deep w., 618b

water supply such as w., 226b

we fail the w., 414a

what may have been w. no longer w., 93a

whatever help patient get w. I in favor of, 635a

within hour will be w., 199b

Well-being regarded as suspect, 116b

Well-read, physician who is w., 398b

Wellspring, difficulties from w. of human condition, 320a

Well-to-do, printing in w. instrument of ignorance, 273a

Well-trained, protection for w. physicians, 299a

Weltanschauung, theories product of W., 614b

Wen, homeopathy like old w., 71b

Wench, brought in beautiful w., 305b

dreaming embracing w. discharged stone, 646a

Wept, mother groan'd father w., 54b

West, impressions that W. obsessed with sex, 540b

people of W. energetic, 201a, 624b

treatment with poison medicines from W., 625a

West Indian, elephantiasis W., 420a

West Side, well known among W. doctors, 407b

Wet, crowd together upon w. gravel, 474a

feet often exposed to w., 488a

mouth w. feet dry, 227a

person not injured getting w., 61a

Wet nurse, intemperance doctor's w., 248b

Wheel, here pivot there w. giving way, 346b

invention of w. more revolutionary than television, 465a

man w. in machine of civilisation, 93a

Wheels of life stood still, 279a

Wheeze, wit began to w., 393b

Wheezes, all that w. not asthma, 13a

with w. and sneezes, 472a

Wheezles, wondered if w. turn into measles, 241a

Whiff of anesthesiologists, 613a

Whim, remedy subject to w., 494b

Whims, surrendering life of sick to w., 634a

Whine less breathe more, 228b

Whips and scorns of time, 580a

Whirlpool, life like w., 267b

Whiskey, beer common instead of w., 8a

Whiskey, gulp of w. at bedtime, 61b

polishes the copper, 9a

soda water whereby w. outdoes champagne, 332b

stupid substitutes for divine Mind, 495b

what butter or w. won't cure, 12b

Whisper, so old that young reach to w. in ear, 416b

Whispering, human w. in steam pipes, 287b

spare me w. room, 84b

White, austere man in w. coat, 251a

black gets w. woman with child, 185b

bull and cow milk-w., 185b

Indian nor more impotent than w., 539a

kidneys large and w., 253b

Laecania has w. teeth, 604a

physician wear w. garments, 398b

Whitehead, conceptual disorder recommended by W., 528b

Whole, half doctor near better than w. far away, 390a

half knowledge dreads w. knowledge, 255a

knows human body as w., 588b

man as part of w., 284b

physician consider more than w. man, 361a

they that w. need not physician, 547a

unless w. is well, 39a

Wholesome, mother's milk only w. food, 289a

Whooping cough, children coughing after cured of w., 496a

Whore, be w. still, 651a

Whoreson cold, 61a

lethargy, 61a

Why, religion deals with w., 491b, 522b

who has *w*. to live bear any *how*, 265b

Wicked, influence of righteous upon w., 444a

would unseen be w., 169b

Wickedness, debasement of arts and sciences to w., 523a

eleven hours sleep, 556a

Wide, nor so w. as church door, 665b

Widow, water neither makes wife w., 655a

Widower, rare that w. not cured, 48a

Widows, made as many w. as Troy, 418a

Wield, know more than able to w., 254b

Wife, anatomical poem on doctor's w., 658b

any evil not evil w., 547a

being doctor's w. occupational hazard, 658a

better without w. than tobacco, 624a

buried head like dutiful w., 658b

clergyman of Stratford killed by w., 495b

deaf husband blind w. happy, 288b

Wife, done better for w. in other calling, 382a

expects doctor's w. set good example, 657b

gives ten dollars a month, 133b

got his w. with child, 447b

help w. could give you, 657a

I am in need of w. think you suit, 656b

in sorrow or sickness w. blessing, 656b

index of character health of w., 658a

joining of bodies without which not have w., 538a

leaving w. and children provided for, 419a

like man and w., 41a

loved no lean, 105a

maid pleased w. and I, 239a

married immediately after w. died, 288b

medicine w. literature mistress, 458b

never like this, 324b

not even in thought seek another's w., 325a

of physician different, 657b

peptic ulcer through which escape w., 646a

physician's w. better diagnostician, 658a

plagued with w., 41a

reduce w. to corrupt breath, 621a

say what thinks about another doctor to w., 658a

wanted to suckle children, 289b

water neither makes w. widow, 655a

Wife's illness strange charm, 645a

liver infected as her life, 275b

mother not think of parting, 311b

opportunity to cure fatigue, 657b

Wig, with long w. cover hair, 397a

Wild goose never laid tame egg, 213a

she was w. sweet witty, 149a

something really w. in universe, 265a

Wilderness, promised land on other side of w., 331b

sleep lay upon the w., 555b

Wildest dreams preludes of truth, 119a

Will, age without a w., 129b

bid sick man make w., 655b

call physician call judge to make w., 397b

courage is w. power, 333b

doctor's error w. of God, 153a

effort to form the life rule the w., 517a

faultless patience unyielding w., 423a

highest vertebrate can say I w., 287b

less master of mind, 41a

madman has no free w., 247a

muscles which obey w., 318b

never directed w. to purpose empty of meaning, 225b

subconscious self lacks w., 469b

those weak in mind and w., 535b

Wonderful, nothing more w. than faith, 172a

Wonders, found man that can do w., 479a

Wood as an hare, 242b
blind man works on w. as surgeon ignorant of anatomy, 584b
have block of w. and saw, 487b
hear scratch of pin at end of w., 570b
resolved on taking the w., 650a
toothpicks made of false w., 604a

Woodland, welcome thee to w. cave, 342b

Wooers, like Penelope's w., 376a

Woof and warp of affairs of men, 302a

Wool obstructs more than cotton, 608a

Woolen clothing keeps skin healthy, 551a

Word, death but little w., 257b
discovery necessitated new w., 611a
encountering new w. two or three times within week, 506a
every w. gaping wound, 665b
ill urg'd to one so ill, 655b
let w. die with thee, 156a
never use long w. where short answer, 609b
newly born w. offers no self-defense, 610b
passed into everyday use, 609a
rightly imposed is landmark, 609b
run pen through every other w., 669a
said master w. of medicine work, 302b
so beautiful must mean something, 612a
Syme never wastes w., 426a
unable to find w. they want, 572b
work of inventor of w., 610b
written w. has part to play, 672a

Words, artists finding mysterious meanings of w., 608b
as long as anacondas, 609b
by poultices not w. pain is ended, 353b
covered with w. *Hic jacet*, 77b
devoid of meaning, 610a
disciplines stake claims on w., 612b
draw lifeblood from my heart, 34a
effect of deeds more than w., 68b
facts nature's w., 609b
from outside source, 76b
getting use of smaller w. first, 572b
give sorrow w., 563a
giving myself out in w., 459a
have no more meaning than tides, 546a
ideas fail invent w., 611a
ill choice of w. obstructs understanding, 608b
in favour of home-made w., 611a
language of medicine sesquipedalian w., 609b
list of w. they want deleted, 671b

Words, man of few w. learns by practice, 399a
man of science uses few hard w., 610a
multitude of w. consume air, 610a
not cumber self with w., 14a
one of most beautiful w. "enthusiasm," 490b
pain by w. eased and diminished, 353b
physicians resort to friendly w., 363a
pleasant w. as honeycomb, 52a
pseudo prestige of difficult w., 673a
quack's w. heard, 478b
received with more attention, 163b
remembered not so much for w., 173a
reveal figure of man in w., 13b
say extraordinary things using ordinary w., 611b
say sweet w., 331b
scrawling cramp w. for slipslop, 449a
should be true signs of facts, 609b
symbols of notions, 276b
thinks by hard w. proves understands hard things, 610a
with long w. doctor like any other, 407a

Work appear in more elegant edition, 149a
benefit if men stopped w. at sixty, 348a
best antidote to sorrow, 664a
by diastole as well as systole, 333b
change of w. equivalent to rest, 511b
consume smoke with w., 63a
cure of all maladies, 663a
day affer day w. all de sam', 412a
devotes self to w., 1a
do day's w. well, 331a
do your w. quick as can, 193a
doctor makes w. for another, 397b
doctors undertake doctor's w., 666b
ease him over hurdles, 577a
effort directed to end, 664a
essential factor of health, 664a
expands to fill time available, 66b
feel love of God in w., 401b
for those who not take it, 635a
great w. to die, 257b
happy in w. three things needed, 663a
hard w. give rest to body peace to mind, 511a
healing fittest emblem of His w., 200b
historic setting of man's w., 215a
if notice of w. when I am gone, 259b
if this doesn't w. we'll try something else, 353a
impressing w. upon memory of nature, 172b
in honest w. ultimate good, 411b
jealous lest other know of w., 454a

Work, kidneys do energetic w., 253a
law of peace w. and health, 330b
life's w. all done, 270b
master-word is W., 663b
more brains to do w. passably, 185a
more than fair day's w., 133a
much w. into narrow compass, 205a
nature does more than half the w., 445a
never hide w. of others under your name, 63a
not care if w. useful to society, 531b
not enough to have begun good w., 327b
not w. kills but worry, 665a
not worry about w. after hours, 531b
nursing hard w. for hands, 322a
of first rate importance, 215a
of noble note yet be done, 343a
of world done between twenty-five and forty, 291a
oppressed by anthills of w., 663b
originator gets credit even if not do w., 233a
own and others' estimation of one's w., 331b
physical defects penalties of w., 424a
play rest in proportion, 488b
poor cured by w., 75b
posterity find worthy w., 461b
prevent disease relieve suffering heal sick our w., 409a
protest at finish of this w., 666b
provided not obliged to w. until better, 545b
pupil who applies self to w., 573a
real w. of doctor, 368b
remembered not so much for w., 173a
said master word of medicine w., 302b
see w. pass into other hands, 502b
shun studies in which w. dies with worker, 497b
still strong beneath steady hand, 89b
stop active w. at sixty, 512b
taking pains means w., 664a
thinking men worry do world's w., 665a
three piles of w., 664a
today be happy tomorrow, 384b
too much polishing weakens w., 666b
too much w. excessive, 657b
useful w. become standard, 68b
value of system in w., 331a
w. w. till eyes heavy and dim, 663a
waiting for practice learn to w., 409b
wanted to w. without having to talk, 459a
which excites opposition, 68b
wife must love your w., 657b
with her w. and be undisturbed, 656b